THE COVID-19 PANDEMIC

A Multidisciplinary Review of Diagnosis, Prevention, and Treatment

THE COVID-19 PANDEMIC

A Multidisciplinary Review of Diagnosis, Prevention, and Treatment

Edited by

Hanadi Talal Ahmedah, PhD

Muhammad Riaz, PhD

Sagheer Ahmed, PhD

Marius Alexandru Moga, PhD

AAP | APPLE ACADEMIC PRESS

First edition published 2023

Apple Academic Press Inc.
1265 Goldenrod Circle, NE,
Palm Bay, FL 32905 USA

4164 Lakeshore Road, Burlington,
ON, L7L 1A4 Canada

CRC Press
6000 Broken Sound Parkway NW,
Suite 300, Boca Raton, FL 33487-2742 USA

2 Park Square, Milton Park,
Abingdon, Oxon, OX14 4RN UK

Library and Archives Canada Cataloguing in Publication

Title: The COVID-19 pandemic : a multidisciplinary review of diagnosis, prevention, and treatment / edited by Hanadi Talal Ahmedah, PhD, Muhammad Riaz, PhD, Sagheer Ahmed, PhD, Marius Alexandru Moga, PhD.
Names: Ahmedah, Hanadi Talal editor. | Riaz, Muhammad (Professor of pharmacy), editor. | Ahmed, Sagheer, editor. | Moga, Marius Alexandru, editor.
Description: First edition. | Includes bibliographical references and index.
Identifiers: Canadiana (print) 2022014074X | Canadiana (ebook) 20220140812 | ISBN 9781774910504 (hardcover) | ISBN 9781774910511 (softcover) | ISBN 9781003283607 (ebook)
Subjects: LCSH: COVID-19 (Disease) | LCSH: COVID-19 (Disease)—Diagnosis. | LCSH: COVID-19 (Disease)—Prevention. | LCSH: COVID-19 (Disease)—Treatment.
Classification: LCC RA644.C67 C68 2022 | DDC 614.5/92414—dc23

Library of Congress Cataloging-in-Publication Data

Names: Ahmedah, Hanadi Talal, editor. | Riaz, Muhammad (Professor of pharmacy) editor. | Aḥmad, Ṣagheer, editor. | Moga, Marius Alexandru, editor.
Title: The COVID-19 pandemic : a multidisciplinary review of diagnosis, prevention, and treatment / edited by Hanadi Talal Ahmedah, Muhammad Riaz, Sagheer Ahmed, Marius Alexandru Moga.
Description: First edition. | Palm Bay, FL : Apple Academic Press, 2022. | Includes bibliographical references and index. | Summary: "The timely volume is a comprehensive review of the evolution, diagnosis, prevention, control, and treatment strategies (both modern as well as complementary and alternative modes) being used against COVID-19. With chapters written by experts in diverse medical fields from around the world, the volume presents authentic and easily understood information on this novel and often deadly virus. The book is organized in sections that cover pathology, epidemiology and diagnosis; prevention strategies; and treatment. The book first covers the morphology, pathogenesis, genome organization and replication of coronavirus (COVID-19) and then goes on to address epidemiology and pathogenesis, the psychological effects, and detection assays and techniques. Chapters on prevention strategies discuss social distancing and quarantine, face masks and hand sanitizers, lockdown strategies, and vaccines. The authors also cover diverse treatment strategies, including using medicinal plants, natural products, and traditional Chinese medicines as well as nanomedicines. A chapter on recent therapeutic developments is also included. The COVID-19 Pandemic: A Multidisciplinary Review of Diagnosis, Prevention, and Treatment is designed for students, teachers and researchers in medical sciences and the allied health professions such as pharmacy, nursing, alternative and complementary medicine. Science journalists writers, and health policymakers will find the volume to be a source of valuable information also"-- Provided by publisher.
Identifiers: LCCN 2022000100 (print) | LCCN 2022000101 (ebook) | ISBN 9781774910504 (hbk) | ISBN 9781774910511 (pbk) | ISBN 9781003283607 (ebk)
Subjects: MESH: COVID-19 | Pandemics
Classification: LCC RA644.C67 (print) | LCC RA644.C67 (ebook) | NLM WC 506 | DDC 616.2/414--dc23/eng/20220110
LC record available at https://lccn.loc.gov/2022000100
LC ebook record available at https://lccn.loc.gov/2022000101

ISBN: 978-1-77491-050-4 (hbk)
ISBN: 978-1-77491-051-1 (pbk)
ISBN: 978-1-00328-360-7 (ebk)

About the Editors

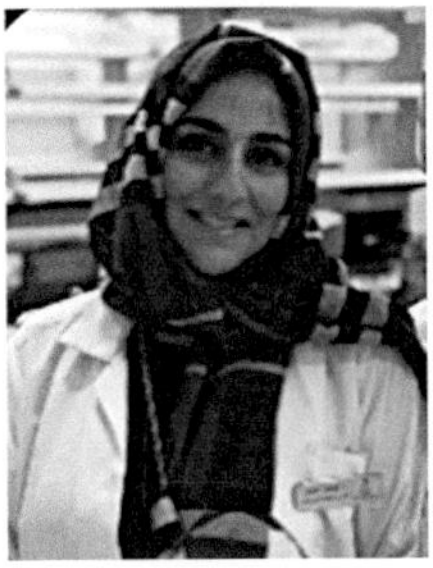

Hanadi Talal Ahmedah, PhD
Assistant Professor, Department of Medical Laboratory Technology, Faculty of Applied Medical Sciences, King Abdulaziz University, Rabigh, Saudi Arabia

Hanadi Talal Ahmedah, PhD, is a lab technologist, researcher, and writer as well as an Assistant Professor in the Department of Medical Laboratory Technology, Faculty of Applied Medical Sciences, King Abdulaziz University, Rabigh, Saudi Arabia. Dr. Ahmedah has published one book with Springer and many articles in journals indexed in the ISI Web of Science. She graduated from King Abdulaziz University (KAU) with a BS in Medical Laboratory Technology and earned an MSc in Pathological Science at Sheffield Hallam University, Sheffield, United Kingdom. She completed her PhD at the Institute of Cancer Therapeutics, University of Bradford, United Kingdom.

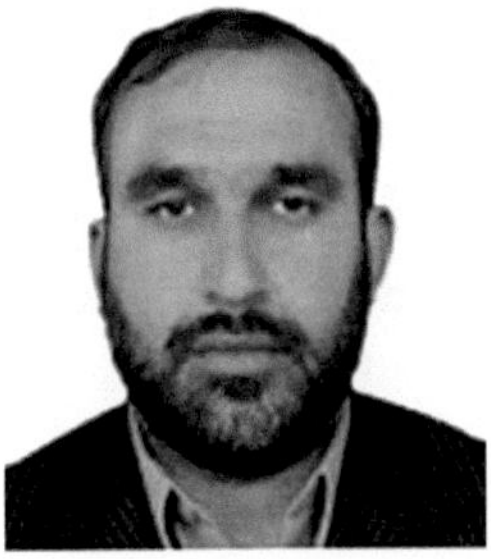

Muhammad Riaz, PhD
Assistant Professor of Pharmacy, Shaheed Benazir Bhutto University Sheringal, Pakistan

Muhammad Riaz, PhD, is an Assistant Professor of Pharmacy, Shaheed Benazir Bhutto University Sheringal, Pakistan. He has authored or co-authored over 30 peer-reviewed publications in renowned journals at the national and international level and two books: *Anthocyanins and Human Health: Biomolecular and Therapeutic Aspects* (2016) and *Carotenoids: Structure and Function in the Human Body* (2021) for Springer. He received his PhD in Pharmacognosy from the University of Karachi, Pakistan, followed by a postdoctoral fellowship in Prof. Dou Deqiang Lab, Liaoning University of Traditional Chinese Medicine, China. During his PhD, Dr. Riaz worked in Prof. Michael Heinrich Labs, UCL School of Pharmacy, London, under the six-month International Research Support Initiative Program of the Higher Education Commission of Pakistan.

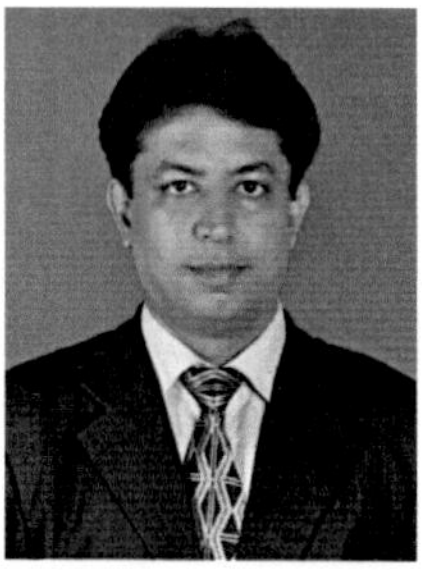

Sagheer Ahmed, PhD
Professor of Pharmacology,
Shifa College of Pharmaceutical Sciences,
Shifa Tameer-e-Millat University, Islamabad

Sagheer Ahmed, PhD, is a Professor of Pharmacology at Shifa College of Pharmaceutical Sciences, Shifa Tameer-e-Millat University, Islamabad. His areas of research interest include pharmacogenetics, cardiovascular, neuropharmacology, and COVID-19. He has contributed to nine patents and over 50 research publications. Dr. Ahmed loves teaching both undergraduate and graduate students and has experience in various problem-based learning approaches, especially the Harvard style and Maastricht style. He has over 20 years of teaching, research, and administrative experience to motivate his students to prepare them for the post-COVID-19 world and take on significant challenges in life.

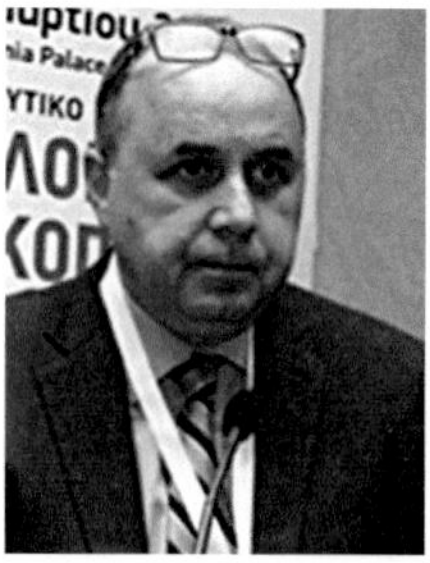

Marius Alexandru Moga, PhD
Professor of Obstetrics and Gynecology,
Faculty of Medicine of Transilvania University of Brasov, Hungary

Marius Alexandru Moga, MD, PhD, born in Brasov, Romania, graduated in 1989 from the Faculty of General Medicine from Cluj-Napoca, Romania, and he became a Specialist (Registrar) in Obstetrics and Gynecology in 1994. As a Senior Doctor/Consultant in Ob-Gyn (1999), he worked at the same Clinical Hospital of Ob-Gyn, I.A.Sbarcea, of Brasov, Romania, where he was nominated in 2007 to run the 4th Clinical Department of Ob-Gyn (32 beds). He obtained certificates of specialization issued by the Ministry of Health in Romania and proved special competency in some ob-gyn subfields, such as ultrasound in obstetrics and gynecology, onco-gynecology, maternal-fetal medicine, colposcopy and cito-diagnosis, laparoscopic surgery, family planning, contraception, and health management. In 2005 he became Associate Professor in the Faculty of Medicine of Brasov, and in 2014 he reached the full professor position at the same Faculty of Medicine. He is currently Professor of Obstetrics and Gynecology at the Faculty of Medicine of Transilvania University of Brasov, Romania, where he was formerly the Dean of the Faculty of Medicine for three terms. Habilitated in 2017, he has eight PhD students under his supervision, with two PhD graduates. He has a Hirsch citation score of 13 and 60 ISI papers with IF (Web of Science-Clarivate Analytics). He has published over 230 medical papers in IDB journals. and he has presented more than 300 papers at national and international conferences. He is also the author or co-author of 11 medical books and 21 book chapters in national and international publications. He has handled many research and educational projects and was the principal investigator of 14 clinical studies as well. He was nominated in 2010 as an International Expert in Environmental Medicine. Dr. Moga founded a master academic Programme in Traditional Chinese Medicine at the Faculty of Medicine of Brasov, Romania.

Contents

Contributors

Roheena Abdullah
Assistant Professor, Department of Biotechnology, Lahore College for Women University, Lahore, Pakistan, E-mail: roheena_abdullah@yahoo.com

Ahmad Adnan
Department of Chemistry, GC University, Lahore–54000, Pakistan

Adeel Ahmad
Department of Agronomy, University of Agriculture Faisalabad–38000, Pakistan, E-mail: adeelahmad772@gmail.com

Asma Ahmad
PhD Scholar, Department of Botany, Lahore College for Women University, Lahore, Pakistan

Izaz Ahmad
Department of Chemistry, GC University, Lahore–54000, Pakistan

Rizwan Ahmad
Assistant Professor, Natural Products and Alternative Medicines, College of Clinical Pharmacy, Imam Abdulrahman Bin Faisal University, Dammam, Kingdom of Saudi Arabia

Sagheer Ahmed
Professor, Shifa College of Pharmaceutical Sciences, Shifa Tameer-e-Millat University, Islamabad, Pakistan, E-mail: sagheer.scps@stmu.edu.pk

Hanadi Talal Ahmedah
Department of Medical Laboratory Technology, Faculty of Applied Medical Sciences, King Abdulaziz University, Rabigh, Saudi Arabia

Iqra Akhtar
PhD Scholar, Department of Botany, Lahore College for Women University, Lahore, Pakistan

Ahmed Akrem
Assistant Professor, Institute of Pure and Applied Biology, Bahauddin Zakariya University, Multan, Pakistan

Naila Ali
Assistant Professor, Institute of Molecular Biology and Biotechnology, The University of Lahore, Lahore, Pakistan

Sumera Anwar
Assistant Professor, Institute of Molecular Biology and Biotechnology, The University of Lahore, Lahore, Pakistan

Muhammad Arfan
Assistant Professor, Department of Botany, Division of Science and Technology, University of Education Lahore, Punjab, Pakistan

M. Yasin Ashraf
Professor, Institute of Molecular Biology and Biotechnology, The University of Lahore, Lahore, Pakistan

Mehvish Azam
MPhil Scholar, Institute of Molecular Biology and Biotechnology, The University of Lahore, Lahore, Pakistan

Naheed Bano
Faculty of Veterinary and Animal Sciences, MNS-University of Agriculture, Multan, Pakistan, E-mail: naheed.bano@mnsuam.edu.pk

Fatima Batool
Department of Botany, Division of Science and Technology, University of Education, Lahore, Punjab, Pakistan

Ayoub Rashid Ch.
Associate Professor, Materials Chemistry Laboratory, Department of Chemistry, GC University Lahore, Lahore–54000, Pakistan

Dou Deqiang
Professor, College of Pharmacy, Liaoning University of Traditional Chinese Medicine, Dalian Campus, China

Muhammad Faheem
Lecturer, Department of Pharmacy, University of Swabi Anbar, Pakistan

Bahzad Ahmad Farhan
Department of Biochemistry, Government College University, Faisalabad, Pakistan

Misbah Hameed
Assistant Professor, Institute of Pharmacy, Lahore College for Women University, Lahore, Pakistan, E-mail: misbahmajid1@gmail.com

Muhammad Hussaan
Department of Botany, Government College University Faisalabad–38000, Pakistan, E-mail: mhussaan7866@gmail.com

Sajjad Hussain
Assistant Professor, School of Chemistry, Faculty of Basic Sciences and Mathematics, Minhaj University, Lahore, Pakistan

Tehreema Iftikhar
Professor, Department of Botany, Government College University Lahore, Pakistan

Mehwish Iqtedar
Department of Biotechnology, Lahore College for Women University, Lahore, Pakistan

Hawa ZE Jaafar
Department of Crop Science, Faculty of Agriculture, University Putra Malaysia, Seri Kembangan–43400, Malaysia

Sumera Javad
Assistant Professor, Department of Botany, Lahore College for Women University, Lahore, Pakistan, E-mail: zif_4@yahoo.com

Sadia Javed
Associate Professor, Department of Biochemistry, Government College University, Faisalabad, Pakistan, E-mail: drsadiajaved@yahoo.com

Afshan Kaleem
Department of Biotechnology, Lahore College for Women University, Lahore, Pakistan

Humaira Kausar
Department of Chemistry, Lahore College for Women University, Lahore–54000, Pakistan

Binish Khaliq
Assistant Professor, Institute of Molecular Biology and Biotechnology, The University of Lahore, Lahore, Pakistan, E-mail: beenish.khaliq@imbb.uol.edu.pk

Majid Khan
PharmD, Department of Pharmacy, Shaheed Benazir Bhutto University, Sheringal, Pakistan

Sidrah Tariq Khan
Research Assistant, Shifa College of Pharmaceutical Sciences, Shifa Tameer-e-Millat University, Islamabad, Pakistan

Zahid Khan
Department of Pharmacognosy, Faculty of Pharmacy, Federal Urdu University, Karachi, Pakistan

Hammad Majeed
Assistant Professor, Knowledge Unit of Science, University of Management and Technology, Iqbal Campus, Sialkot, Pakistan; Department of Biotechnology, Lahore College for Women University, Lahore, Pakistan

Arif Malik
Professor, Institute of Molecular Biology and Biotechnology, The University of Lahore, Lahore, Pakistan

Farkhanda Manzoor
Professor and Chairperson, Department of Zoology, Lahore College for Women University, Lahore, Pakistan

Marius Moga
Professor, Faculty of Medicine, Transilvania University of Brasov, Brasov–500036, Romania

Sahar Mumtaz
Department of Botany, Division of Science and Technology, University of Education, Lahore–54770, Punjab, Pakistan

Zunaira Naeem
Materials Chemistry Laboratory, Department of Chemistry, GC University Lahore, Lahore–54000, Pakistan

Hina Qaiser
Lecturer, Department of Biology, Lahore Garrison University DHA Phase-VI Sector C, Lahore, Pakistan

Najmur Rahman
Assistant Professor, Department of Pharmacy, Shaheed Benazir Bhutto University, Sheringal, Pakistan

Nagina Rehman
Department of Zoology, Government College University Faisalabad, Pakistan

Muhammad Riaz
Assistant Professor, Department of Pharmacy, Shaheed Benazir Bhutto University, Sheringal, Pakistan, E-mail: pharmariaz@gmail.com

Saffora Riaz
Assistant Professor, Department of Zoology, Lahore College for Women University, Lahore, Pakistan, E-mail: riazsaffora@gmail.com

Maham Saeed
Department of Chemistry, GC University, Lahore–54000, Pakistan

Maria Shabbir
Department of Biochemistry, Government College University, Faisalabad, Pakistan

Javed Hussain Shah
Department of Chemistry, GC University, Lahore–54000, Pakistan

Shahzad Sharif
Assistant Professor, Materials Chemistry Laboratory, Department of Chemistry, GC University Lahore, Lahore–54000, Pakistan, E-mail: msharif@gcu.edu.pk

Arifa Tahir
Environmental Science Department, Lahore College for Women University, Lahore–54000, Pakistan

Areeba Tahseen
Department of Biochemistry, Government College University, Faisalabad, Pakistan

Amina Tariq
Assistant Professor, Department of Botany, Lahore College for Women University, Lahore, Pakistan

Ayesha Toor
Department of Biotechnology, Lahore College for Women University, Lahore, Pakistan

Samina Yaqoob
School of Business and Economics, University of Management and Technology, Lahore, Pakistan

Mahnoor Zahid
Department of Chemistry, GC University, Lahore–54000, Pakistan

M. Zia-Ul-Haq
Office of Research, Innovation and Commercialization, Lahore College for Women University, Lahore–54000, Pakistan

Saima Zulfiqar
Materials Chemistry Laboratory, Department of Chemistry, GC University Lahore, Lahore–54000, Pakistan

Abbreviations

AA pathway	arachidonic acid pathway
AAK1	AP2-associated protein kinase 1
ABM	agent-based models
AC	after Christ
ACE	acetylcholinesterase
ACE	angiotensin-converting enzyme
ACE 2 receptor	angiotensin-converting enzymes-2 receptor
Acetyl CO-A	acetyl coenzyme A
ADE	antibody-dependent enhancement
ADR	adverse drug reaction
AEFI	adverse events following immunization
AFM	advanced multi-frequency
Ag	silver
AIDS	acquired immunodeficiency syndrome
AIV	avian influenza virus
AKI	acute kidney injury
AKT/PBK	serine/threonine kinase/protein kinase B
ALI	acute liver infection
ALP	alkaline phosphate
ALT	alanine transaminase
AM- AFM	amplitude modulation atomic force microscopy
Ang	angiotensinogen
ANP	atrial natriuretic peptide
APC	antigen-presenting cell
APN	aminopeptidase N
ARB	angiotensin-receptor blockers
ARDS	acute respiratory distress or syndrome
ASD	acute stress disorder
AST	aspartate aminotransferase
AT1R	angiotensin receptor 1
B cells	B lymphocytes
BALF	bronchoalveolar lavage fluid
BC	before Christ
BCG	Bacille-Calmette-Guerin

BCL 2	B-cell lymphoma 2
BLA	biological license application
BMI	body mass index
CASP	caspase protein
CD	cluster of differentiation
CDC	Center for Disease Control
CDD	cytokine discharge disorder
CEPI	coalition for epidemic preparedness innovations
CFR	case fatality rate
CIOMS	Council of International Organization of Medical Sciences
CK	creatine kinase
CLpro	chymotrypsin-like cysteine protease
CNS	central nervous system
COVID	coronavirus disease
COVID-19	coronavirus disease 2019
CoVn-2019	novel coronavirus 2019
CoVs	coronaviruses
COX	cyclooxygenase
CP	convalescent plasma
CPE	cytopathic effect
CPR	cardiopulmonary resuscitation
CQDs	carbon quantum dots
CRP	C-reactive protein
CRS	cytokine discharge disorder
CT	computed tomography
CXCL8	C-X-C motif chemokine ligand 8
CYP	cytochromes P450 enzymes
DBIL	direct bilirubin
DC	dendritic cell
DMV	double-membrane vesicle
DNA	deoxyribonucleic acid
DS	degree of substitution
E protein	envelope protein
E	envelop
EBOV	Ebola virus
EC_{50}	half-maximal effective concentration
ECA-CoV	epithelial carcinoembryonic antigen coronavirus
ECD	extracellular domain
ECOTOX	ecotoxicology database

EGFR	epidermal growth factor receptor
ELISA	enzyme-linked immunosorbant assay
EMA	European Medicines Agency
ET	endothelin
EUA	emergency use authorization
EV	Eudra vigilance
EV71	enterovirus 71
FDA	Food and Drug Administration
FDA-USA	Food and Drug Administration of USA
FETs	field-effect transistors
FFP	filtering facepiece
Flt-1	vascular endothelial growth factor receptor 1 precursor
FM-AFM	frequency modulation atomic force microscopy
FNW	fluorescent protein nanowire
FRET	fluorescence resonance energy transfer
fRhK-4	fetal rhesus kidney-4 cells
G7	group of seven intergovernmental organization
GDP	gross domestic product
GHE	global health emergency
GI	gastrointestinal
GIT	gastrointestinal tract
GM-CSF	granulocyte macrophage colony-stimulating factor
GTP	guanosine 5'-triphosphate
GVAP	global vaccination action plan
H1F1	histone H1
H1N1	hemagglutinin type 1 and neuraminidase type 1
H2N2	hemagglutinin type 2 and neuraminidase type 2
H3N2	hemagglutinin type 3 and neuraminidase type 2
H5N1	hemagglutinin type 5 and neuraminidase type 1
hACE2	human angiotensin-converting enzyme
HBsAg	surface antigen of HBV
HBV	hepatitis B virus
HCoV	human coronavirus
HCoV-OC43	human coronavirus OC43
HCPs	health care professionals
HCQ	hydroxychloroquine
HCV	hepatitis C virus
HCW	healthcare worker
HE	haemagglutinin-esterase

HIF-1	hypoxia-inducible factor 1
HIV	human immunodeficiency virus
HMGB1	high mobility group box 1 protein
HRCT	high-resolution computed tomography
HSP90AA1	heat shock protein 90 alpha family class A member 1
HSV	herpes simplex virus
IC_{50}	half-maximal inhibitory concentration
ICTV	international committee on taxonomy of viruses
ICTV-CSG	International Committee on Taxonomy of Viruses -Coronaviridae Study Group
ICU	intensive care unit
IEM	immune electron microscopy
iEPO	epoprostenol
IES-R	impact of event scale - revised
IFFIm	finance facility for immunization
IFN	interferon
IFNAR	interferon-α/β receptor
IFN-α	interferon-alpha
IFN-β	interferon beta
IFN-γ	interferon-gamma
Ig	immunoglobulin (A, G, M)
IgG	immunoglobulin G
IL	interleukins (1, 1α/β, 6, 10, 12, 17)
IL-2	interleukin-2
IL-6	interleukin-6
IL-6R	interleukin-6 receptor
IME	immunodeficiency effects
IMV	intrusive mechanical ventilation
INF	interferon
iNO	nitric oxide
IP-10	inducible protein 10
IP-10/CXCL-10	interferon gamma-induced protein 10/C-X-C motif chemokine ligand 10
ISG	interferon-stimulated genes
IV	intravenous
IWVV	inactivated whole virus vaccine
JAK1	Janus kinases 1
JUN	Jun proto-oncogene, activator protein-1 transcription factor subunit

JV virus	John Cunningham virus (human polyomavirus 2)
KDR	kinase insert domain receptor
KOW	octanol to water coefficient
LAV	live attenuated vaccine
LCM	lymphocytic choriomeningitis mammarenavirus
LDH	lactate dehydrogenase
LLC-MK2	cell lines rhesus monkey kidney epithelial cells
LNPs	lipid nanoparticles
LOD	limit of diagnosis
M	membrane
MAC	membrane attack complex
MAPK	mitogen-activated protein kinase
MCP-1	monocyte chemoattractant protein 1
MCP-1/CCL2	monocyte chemoattractant protein 1/chemokine ligand 2
MCP3	monocyte-chemotactic protein 3
MDD	major depressive disorder
MERS	middle east respiratory syndrome
MERS-CoV	middle east respiratory syndrome coronavirus
MHC	histocompatibility complex
MHLW	Ministry of Health, Labor, and Welfare
MIP 1 α	macrophage inflammatory protein 1-α
ML336	antiviral drug
MLV	murine leukemia virus
MMA	methylmalonic acidemia
MMA-SPM	methylmethacrylate-sulfopropylmethacrylate
MNP	methyl-nitrophenol
MNV	murine norovirus
MPEG	methoxy poly(ethylene glycol)
Mpro	main protease
MR	molecular replacement
MRC-5	medical research council cell strain 5
mRNA	messenger ribonucleic acid
MTase	methyltransferase
MW	molecular weight
N protein	nucleocapsid protein
N7-Mtase	N7-methyltransferase
NAB	nucleic acid-binding domain
NCOA2	nuclear receptor coactivator 2
nCoV	novel coronavirus

NEIWPCC	New England Interstate Water Pollution Control Commission
NF-kB	nuclear factor kappa B
NGS	metagenomic next-generation sequencing
NHC	National Health Commission
NIAID	National Institute of Allergy and Infectious Diseases
NIH	National Institute of Health
NIV	nonintrusive ventilation
NK	natural killer cells
NLRs	nucleotide-binding oligomerization domain (NOD) like receptors
NMR	nuclear magnetic resonance
NOS	nitric oxide synthase
NPs	nanoparticles
NPV	net present value
NRA	National Regulatory Authorities
NRSs	N-protein RNA substrates
NRVV	non-replicated viral vaccine
NSAIDs	nonsteroidal anti-inflammatory drugs
NSP	non-structural protein
NTD	N-terminal domain
ORF	open reading frame
P13K-Akt	phosphatidylinositol-3kinase/total protein kinase
P2	pass level 2
PAMP	pathogen-associated molecular patterns
PBMCs	peripheral blood mononuclear cells
PCR	polymerase chain reaction
PCT	pro-calcitonin
PD-1	programmed cell death 1
PD-ACE 2	protease domain of ACE 2
PEDV	porcine epidemic diarrhea virus
PEG	polyethylene glycol
PEG-PLGA	polyethylene glycol-polylactic acid-co-glycolic acid
PEO-PCL	polyethylene oxide-polycaprolactone
PG 12	plasma prostacyclin 12
PG	propylene glycol
PGH_2	prostaglandin H_2
PHEIC	public health emergency of international concern
PLA	polylactic acid

PLGA	polylactic acid-co-glycolic acid
PLP	pyridoxal phosphate
PLpro	papain-like proteinase
PLR	platelet-to-lymphocyte ratio
PMA	phorbol myristate acetate
PMIS	paediatric multi-system inflammatory syndrome
PMMA	poly(methyl methacrylate)
PMN	poly-morpho nuclear
PO	per oral
PP1A	protein phosphatase 1
PPE	personal protective equipment
PRR	pathogen recognition receptors
PTGS	prostaglandin-endoperoxide synthase
PTS	post-traumatic stress
PTSD	post-traumatic stress disorder
QDs	quantum dots
QTc	corrected QT
RAAS	renin angiotensin aldosterone system
RBD	receptor binding domain
RBD-S	RBD of spike
RBP	receptor binding proteins
RdRp	RNA dependent RNA polymerases
RDS	acute state with respiratory distress
RECs	research ethics committees
RELA	REL proto-oncogene, NF-kB subunit
rGO-hpG	graphene oxide-hyper branched glycerol
rhACE2	recombinant human angiotensin-converting enzyme 2
RNA	ribonucleic acid
ROS	reactive oxygen species
RRT	renal replacement therapy
RSV	respiratory syncytial virus
RT	reverse transcriptase
RTC	replication transcription complexes
RTP	replication transcription protein
RVV	replicated viral vaccine
S protein	spike protein
SAGE	scientific advisory group of expert
SAMs	self-assembled monolayers
SARS	severe acute respiratory syndrome

SARS-CoV	severe acute respiratory syndrome coronavirus
SEIR	susceptible exposed infected recovery
SEM	scanning electron microscopy
sgRNA	subgenomic ribonucleic acid
SHLH	secondary hemophagocytic lymph histiocytosis
SIFAP	stroke in young Fabry patients
SIR	susceptible infective recovered type models
SOPs	standard operating procedure
SP	spike protein
SPM	specialized pro-resolving mediators
SPR	surface plasmon resonance
STAT 1	signal transducer and activator of transcription 1
STP	standard temperature and pressure
SUD	SARS unique domain
T cells	T lymphocytes
TCM	traditional Chinese medicine
TGF-β1	transforming growth factor-beta 1
Th	helper T-cells (1 and 2)
Th-1 cells	helper T-cells-1
TibV	trained immunity-based vaccine
TIBV	trained immunity-based vaccines
TLR	toll-like receptors
TM	trans-membrane
TMDC	transition metal dichalcogenides
TMPRSS	transmembrane protein serine 2
TNF	tumor necrosis factor
TNF-α	tumor necrosis factor-alpha
TXA 2	thromoxane A 2
Tyk2	tyrosine kinase 2
Ub	ubiquicin
UNAIDS	United Nations Program on HIV/AIDS
USEPA	United States Environmental Protection Agency
UTRs	untranslated regions
UV	ultraviolet
v/v	volume by volume
VAERS	vaccine adverse event reporting system
VANs	vancomycin resistance genes
VDR	vitamin D receptor
VEGF	vascular endothelial growth factor

VLP	virus-like particle
VOC	variant of concern
VSD	vaccine safety data
VVnr	viral vector (non-replicating)
VVr	viral vector (replicating)
w/w	weight by weight
WBC	white blood cells
WHO	World Health Organization
WRAIR	Walter Reed Army Institute of Research
ZIKV	Zika virus
α-SMA	alpha-smooth muscle actin

Preface

Coronavirus has changed the world's focus as it has changed the economy and health of the world community. Researchers, health care providers, administrators, and policymakers are trying their best to manage the pandemic at their levels. The WHO, UNICEF, European Union, the International Pharmaceutical Federation, and others provide guidelines and provide financial support in the pandemic. Researchers, writers, and publishers play their role in giving timely guidelines to all people to manage the situation to minimize the loss systematically.

Feeling the need for comprehensive coverage of the COVID-19 in an organized way to all healthcare professionals and the general public, we have given a thorough overview of the current situation in this volume. This book is themed with key objectives to provide a state-of-the-art and scientific review of COVID-19 pathogenesis, epidemiology, diagnosis, preventive measures, and different modes of treatment. Various experts wrote on these topics in their respective fields from around the world. The book consists of 14 chapters subcategorized into three parts.

Part I (Pathology, Epidemiology, and Diagnosis) is further divided into four chapters. Chapters 1 and 2 provide detailed information about the COVID historical emergence, morphology, pathology, epidemiology, and symptoms of the infected humans. Chapter 3 is about the psychological effects of the pandemic that have badly affected the everyday life of most of the global population. In Chapter 4, the authors try to educate the readers about the diagnostic tools operated in laboratories through molecular assays, computed tomography (CT), biochemical tests, and biomarkers.

Part II is about the possible prevention strategies; it consists of four chapters. In Chapter 5, the social distancing strategy of COVID prevention is elaborated in-depth. In Chapters 6 and 7, the use of facemasks, nature of materials, sanitizers, and the lockdown strategies in controlling the pandemic are fully described. Chapter 8 is on the importance of vaccines in combating the pandemic, the various stages, types, and firms supporting the vaccine preparation programs and the available vaccines till March 18, 2021.

Part III is covers the various treatment strategies currently being used to manage different disease conditions. This part has six chapters. Chapter 9 describes possible medicinal plants that might be useful as antiviral sources of future anti-COVID drugs. In Chapter 10, the thousands-of-years-old system of traditional Chinese medicines (TCM) and its quick-acting treatment formulas to manage the COVID-19 are summarized. Chapters 11 and 12 encompass the historical aspects and role of natural products in treating diseases and the role of nanotechnology-based strategies to combat the pandemic. In Chapter 13, the recent developments in therapies and techniques, especially Western medicine, are elaborated. Types of symptomatic and supportive remedies for COVID-19 are explained. And Chapter 14 gives "An Overview of COVID-19 Treatment."

We hope that researchers in the medical and allied health professions will find this book valuable and exciting. We hope this book will also attract the attention of researchers in several fields of biology. Finally, this book is written in an easy-to-understand style keeping in mind the general public, so we hope that the layman will be interested in this book, as it presents existing literature in simple language.

We want to thank each of the authors for their contributions and dedicated efforts to provide prepared chapters according to the instructions of the AAP.

The editors believe that this book is of benefit and will be a reference source to anyone researching the COVID-19 diagnosis, prevention, and treatment options. We tried to include existing pertinent literature in the book; however, we might have missed some essential papers due to the massive literature on this topic. Our apologies to the authors whose articles we could not include.

We are obligated to the staff at Apple Academic Press for their support in assembling this work and their efforts in keeping this book on schedule.

Finally, we have a message for every reader of this book. These collaborative book projects of hundreds of thousands of words may always contain some errors or gaps. Therefore, instructive comments or even criticism are always welcome.

—Hanadi Talal Ahmedah, PhD
Muhammad Riaz, PhD
Sagheer Ahmed, PhD
Marius Alexandru Moga, PhD

PART I

Pathology, Epidemiology, and Diagnosis

CHAPTER 1

Morphology, Pathogenesis, Genome Organization, and Replication of Coronavirus (COVID-19)

SADIA JAVED,[1] BAHZAD AHMAD FARHAN,[1] MARIA SHABBIR,[1] AREEBA TAHSEEN,[1] HANADI TALAL AHMEDAH,[2] and MARIUS MOGA[3]

[1]*Department of Biochemistry, Government College University, Faisalabad, Pakistan, E-mail: drsadiajaved@yahoo.com (S. Javed)*

[2]*Department of Medical Laboratory Technology, Faculty of Applied Medical Sciences, King Abdulaziz University, Rabigh, Saudi Arabia*

[3]*Faculty of Medicine, Transilvania University of Brasov, Brasov–500036, Romania*

ABSTRACT

Coronaviruses (COVID-19), the family of Coronaviridae, is a universally contagious and pathogenic viral infection which is known to contaminate humans and cause severe respiratory diseases. COVID-19 recently appears, and the World Health Organization (WHO) proclaimed it is a pandemic disease. A new family of Coronavirus named the novel CoV was recognized in Wuhan, the city of China, in December 2019, resulting in a redoubtable eruption in many of China's cities and expanding worldwide. On February 11, 2020, the viral pandemic disease was named the COVID-19 by WHO. Genomic research reveals that the COVID-19 virus is bat originating from the Wuhan Seafood market, China, and has been transmitted to people via unknown intermediate hosts. The COVID-19 viral genome is +ssRNA (~30 kb) ORFs from 6 to 11 having 50 and 30 untranslated regions (UTRs) are included in the genome. COVID-19 has a composition same as SARS-CoV. Spike protein, membrane protein, viral envelope surface protein is incorporated into a host membrane lipid bilayer that encapsulates viral RNA viral helical nucleocapsids. Inhaling or contact with infected droplets is the transmission of the disease and the 2–14 days of incubation time. Symptoms for COVID-19 disease include high fever, weakness, and cough are usually initiated by non-specific syndromes. Special biochemical techniques are used for the diagnosis of the virus in respiratory secretions; Standard laboratory results include low WBC levels and abnormal CRP levels. The computed tomography (CT) chest scan is normally irregular, even though there are no signs or symptoms of sickness. Since the therapy is mostly successful, it is also necessary to decide how antiviral agents work. Home quarantine of suspected and minor illness cases is one way of preventing, and the implementation of strict hospital infection prevention measures, including touch and droplet precautions. The vaccine against COVID-19 has been developed in around 90 institutions worldwide, and it is considered to be an effective prophylactic strategy for control and prevention. Sadly, the WHO on world health scientific advancement to combat the new Coronavirus is addressed.

1.1 INTRODUCTION

For human beings and vertebrates, coronaviruses (CoVs) are major pathogens and can cause the degenerative infectious effects on the respiratory system, nervous system, hepatic, and digestive system of various vertebrates like humans, birds, bats, and other wild animals. The epidemic SARS in 2002/2003 and MERS in 2012 demonstrated the potential for newly developed CoVs to propagate from wild animals to human beings and then transferred exponentially from human to human. Since December 2019, a mystery pneumonia epidemic in Wuhan has drawn immense interest around the globe. The Chinese government and researchers have taken rapid steps to monitor the epidemic and carry out etiological studies. At least five different laboratories in China have detected the mystery pneumonia infectious virus as a novel coronavirus through DNA (deoxyribonucleic acid) sequencing and etiological tests (nCoV). World Health Organization (WHO) on January 12, 2020 designated the infectious virus as the 2019-nCoV (novel coronavirus 2019) [1]. The MERS-CoV, SARS-CoV, and SARS-CoV-2 are all members of the Corona family Coronaviridae, with SARS-CoV-2 having the genomic sequence structure that is identical to SARS-CoV. COVID-19 disease is the diagnosed viral strain that is infected by the exposure of SARS-CoV-2 [1].

SARS CoV-2 was spread all over the world. SARS CoV-2 virus was bat-borne and transferred to human beings through an unidentified middle hosts in the Wuhan the city of China. Since December 2019, the Coronavirus

(SARS-CoV-2) has been circulating globally [2]. The COVID-19 (SARS-CoV-2) is spreading internationally since December 2019, with hundreds of thousands of deaths, millions of virus-infected (COVID-19), and millions more [3]. Corona is a corona spike on the virus' outer surface; it was sometimes referred to as a coronavirus [4]. Coronavirus (CoV) is a +ssRNA genome sequence, that is around 26–32 kb in genome size, the largest known RNA virus genome. Coronavirus infection mostly affects humans in the upper respiratory and gastrointestinal tract (GIT) and ranges from moderate, self-limiting conditions such as the common cold to severe symptoms of bronchitis and renal pneumonia [5]. Bronchoalveolar secretion and nasal swabs were obtained to identify the novel coronavirus from 9 infected patients that came from the market of Wuhan seafood after their preliminary outburst. Special pathogen-free cells from human airways (HAE) were used to capture the virus. Inoculation was done in the human alveoli cells via the apical surfaces. For RT-PCR experiments, HAE cells were tracked and supernatants obtained [6]. However, in nasopharyngeal and or pharyngeal samples were collected with symptoms of COVID-19 disease. The COVID-19 viral structure was detected by analyzing the SARS-CoV coronavirus morphology was discovered by electron microscopy of infected cells after 3 days of infection, with viral sizes varying from 70 to 90 nm, most often in vesicles [6]. However, conventionally been known that the intermediate source of transmission to humans is not understood. No antiviral medications or vaccines that have been clinically approved for COVID-19 use are eligible. Nevertheless, COVID-19 has been studied for therapeutic therapy in clinical experiments with few broad-spectrum antivirals [4].

1.2 COVID-19 HISTORY AND ORIGIN

RNA viruses containing single-stranded genome sequence that are enveloped present in infected persons, but also a huge diversity of species, are CoVs. On January 30, 2020, the WHO Emergency Committee raises up an international health threat, citing an increasing alert rate in China and other countries. Tyrell and Bynoe, who cultivated the virus in common cold patients in 1966, were the first to identify CoVs family [7]. The very first incident occurred in China the province of Guangdong, in 2002–2003, when a new genus Coronaviridae circulating in bats was transmitted from bats to human beings by the intermediate host for viral infection of palm civet cats. This viral infection is estimated to affect 8,422 persons, mainly in Hong Kong and China, contributing to 916 deaths before it was discovered (11% mortality rate) [8]. In

Saudi Arabia, bat-borne respiratory syndrome (MERS-CoV) with dromedary camels has become the intermediary host almost 10 years later those results in 858 deaths in 2494 people (34% fatality rate; Figure 1.1) [9, 10].

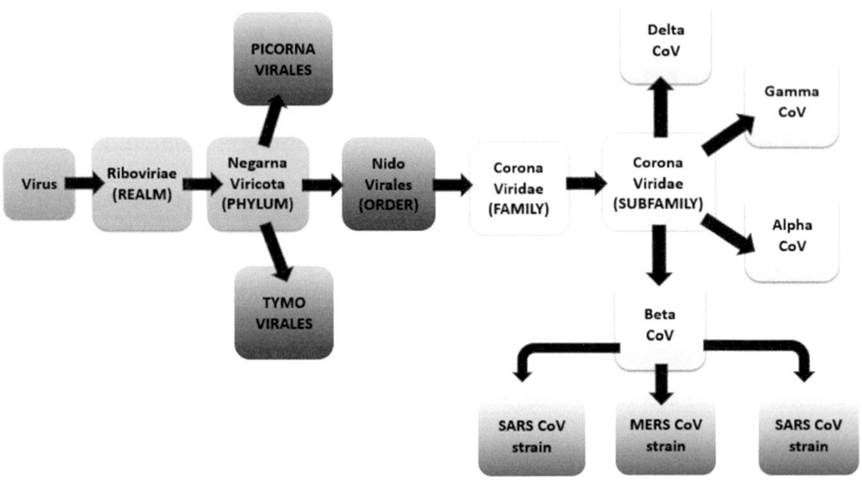

FIGURE 1.1 Classification of coronavirus.

As a result, on the 26th of December 2019, six days after onset of the infection, a 41 years old person was reported to Wuhan Central Hospital. He has no diagnosis of tuberculosis, hepatitis or diabetes and had been recorded for one week for pneumonia, chest infection, unproductive cough, pain, and exhaustion. The Wuhan CDCP performed an epidemiological study. The infected persons worked in a neighboring indoor marine store, which sold live marine wildlife (such as badgers, hedgehogs, birds, rabbits) as well as dead animals and shellfish and fish. No bats were there saleable, though, and while he may have contacted wild animals, the patient did not mention exposure to live poultry [11]. Between December 31, 2019 and January 3, 2020, public government in China reported 44 unspecified infected persons with causative pneumonia with the WHO. During this process of identification, no cause was found. WHO then received more information on the outbreak in Wuhan City in conjunction with one of the marine markets on 11 and 12 January 2020 by the China's National Health Commission (NHC) on 7 January the Chinese extracted a new form of Coronaviridae and identified it in order to establish unique diagnostic kits for other countries. On January 12, 2020, China declared the genomic sequence of a novel coronavirus [12].

Thailand's Ministry of Health announced the very first confirmed case from laboratory (nCoV-2019) transmitted case from Wuhan origin, Hubei Province, China, on January 13, 2020. The MHLW (Ministry of Health, Labor, and welfare) of Japan identified a novel coronavirus patient (COVID-19) from the similar origin on 15 January, 2020. The first novel coronavirus outbreak in Korea, similar in Wuhan, China, was verified by the National IHR Focal Point (NFP) for Korea on January 20, 2020 [13, 14].

1.3 SYMPTOMS

COVID-19 incubation, on the other hand, is predicted to last 14 days, with a mean interval from indication of symptoms of 4–5 days. In one study, 97.5% of patients were diagnosed with the symptoms of COVID-19 illnesses within 11.5 days of respiratory distress disorder, according to the CDCP. COVID-19 signs normally occur between 2–14 days of infection, with normal duration of 5.2 days [15]. Pneumonia, now known as COVID-19 disease, is a common symptom of a contaminated patient, as shown by a computed tomography (CT) examination or chest X-ray [16]. Early on, infected person showed signs of severe respiratory disease, with certain developing chronic obstructive pulmonary failure and other potential complications. The first three infected persons identified by the China's novel SARS-CoV-2 discovering and testing team had severe illness, and 2 out of the 3 infected persons with relevant clinical profiling had a distinct fever condition [17]. At the beginning of COVID-19 disease, typical signs include fever, dry cough, muscle weakness, and disease, as well as other symptoms such as headache, lymphopenia, and dyspnea. However, 1 to 2 days before infection, some individuals can develop diarrhea or nausea [18, 19]. Patients may report problems with breathability 5 days after the onset of infection and ARDS on day 8 of infection. Abdominal pain and pneumonia will occur if the patient's condition worsens; most physiological deficiencies depend on your immune state and health history [20].

As a result, the interval between diagnosis and death varies from 6 to 40 days, with an average range of 14 days [21]. The length is determined by a number of factors, including age and health, and is lower for infection above the age of 70 who have comorbidities [21]. The type of the disease differs from the symptoms. Cough, fever, and difficulty breathing are more frequent than people with milder illnesses (non-hospitable patients) among persons who are diagnosed with COVID-19. There are common symptoms of fever and respiratory infection in aged persons and infected persons with the exposure to COVID-19 [22]. Tiredness, nausea, and myalgia are one of the most usual recorded signs in non-hospitalized patients, and stiff neck and nasal inflammation, or nasal congestion (rhinorrhea), are therefore common. Gastrointestinal (GI) discomfort such as fever, vomit, or diarrhea may appear prior to the onset of an initial illness and lower respiratory problems. COVID-19 has also been linked to a lack of scent (anosmia) or flavor (ageusia) even before the appearance of respiratory problems, particularly in young females and intermediate-aged infected patients who do not require hospitalization [23, 24]. However, certain signs of COVID-19 are characteristic of other respiratory and viral diseases; COVID-19 anosmia appears to be more severe [23]. The common signs of COVID-19 disease in children differ by age difference and are generally slower in adulthood, according to several studies [24, 25].

1.3.1 ASYMPTOMATIC AND PRE-SYMPTOMATIC INFECTION

COVID-19 disease infections have been identified in asymptomatic (non-symptomatic) and symptomatic (symptomatic) patients in several studies (pre-symptomatic) [25]. Until RT-PCR or other laboratory tests are not confirmed, asymptomatic infections can not usually be identified, and symptomatic cases cannot be detected until medical treatment is obtained [26]. Because of the right-hand side of the equation, the sensitivity of RT-PCR is decreased. It should be remembered that the asymptomatic ratio measurement is not influenced by it. However, the drawback of this study is that the samples were based on the Wuhan exile from Japan, which indicated that there was little consideration of age dependence and other aspects of heterogeneity. Although, this prediction shows that maybe less than half of COVID-19 affected people are asymptomatic, due to the restricted sample size. Significantly, this ratio is lower than the influenza ratio of 56–80% [26]. Patients with asymptomatic COVID-19 are those that have good outcomes in viral nucleic acidified or antibodies tests but have not display traditional signs (e.g., fever, dry cough, fatigue). Just 889 cases were identified in a survey of the initial 72,314 cases of COVID-19 disease in China, with the percentage of asymptomatic cases being 1%. As far as the infectiousness in disorder without any symptoms and pre-symptomatic cases is concerned, it is necessary to notice that the existence of +ssRNA sequence of virus (i.e., +ve results of the virus genome sequence test) does not generally mean the existence of an active virus that can be spread [27].

An investigation showed that up to 13% of the RT-PCR checked in children were symptomless cases of SARS-CoV 2 infection [25]. Patients may experience chest-imaging abnormalities after the symptoms begin [28, 29].

1.3.2 ASYMPTOMATIC AND PRE-SYMPTOMATIC TRANSMISSION

Asymptomatic patients are described as the persons that test positive of RT-PCR but do not have any symptoms that show COVID-19. Whereas certain people may go through the whole cycle of exposure and never have signs, there might be others that immediately show indication in certain days or a week later. Persons who eventually undergo symptoms are identified as pre-symptomatic [30].

However, increased viral infections of epidemiological research have reported COVID-19 exposure throughout pre-symptomatic incubation [28, 31].

In virological studies using RT-PCR, low-cycle tests showing significant numbers of viral RNA genome sequence and viability of virus from asymptomatic to pre-symptomatic COVID-19 infections have been published [32–34]. On the Diamond Princess Cruise ship, the primary vast-level testing for asymptomatic COVID disease was conducted, with an asymptomatic 17.9% of all vessel cases predicted [35].

A tendency of asymptomatic COVID-19 exposure was determined in many research, that includes a UCSF study, that 53% of people with positive tested positive did not have any signs when they had the test [30]. Since then, in several trials, symptomless COVID-19 infection has been identified.

Consequently, including a UCSF report, 53% of individuals whose tests are positive at the time of checkup had no signs.

The connection between asymptomatic exposure and pre-symptomatic exposure of virus events and their distribution is not quite well understood. The RT-PCR test will diagnose whether the virus can be identified, but this will not tell us whether or not someone is infected [36]. Virulence in cell culture is used to determine whether or not a patient has been infected to a viral strain. In the lack of virus sample data, RT-PCR data such as viral load or cyclical thresholds (Ct) parameters were used as a guideline for spread possibility. The Ct is the total number of cycles needed to pass a certain limit in an RT-PCR signal [30]. This variable is not proportional to the number of targeted viral genome sequences or viral sample loaded, particularly when virus levels are low, as indicated by higher Ct measurement. The virus was not successfully eliminated unless Ct was smaller than 24 among 90 infected persons with COVID-19 infection, according to Bullard and colleagues

[38]. The connection among COVID-19 virus RNA elimination and the mode of transmission remains unknown. The percentage of symptomless or pre-symptomatic exposure of COVID-19 infection is not apparent when compared to symptomatic infection [39].

1.4 MODE OF TRANSMISSION

Corona viral genome is positive sense non-segmented RNA and have more similarity with SARS-CoV. The genome of the virus is determined to be 96.2% similar to the SARS CoV sequence of RaTG13. It is considered that Bat is the natural host for All types of CoVs, and it is assumed that it could traveled to humans and cause infection in humans through an unknown intermediate host like SARS CoV-2 [40]. This virulence is then transferred from human to human through coughing or sneezing that produce droplets or aerosol formation in the air and can be entered to other person by inhaling, as these viruses primarily cause respiratory infection in the throat and lungs. In the respiratory cells, their present receptor site on their cell allows the virus to enter the cell and cause the infection in these lungs' cells [41]. Therefore, there are many modes of transmission of corona viral infections like by touching the exposed sites and then touching eye, mouth, and nose with contaminated bare hands, air droplets by coughing and sneezing and inhaling aerosols contaminated with virus, pregnant mother to child and eating viral exposed animal host to human and cause mild respiratory illness to serious illness and disturbance in breathing and even cause the death at this serious condition (Figure 1.2) [42]. There are variety of mode of transmission of this viral infection and because of respiratory illness it is very easy to transmit though air in the critical pandemic condition it is crucial to take much hard steps for government to take. For the prevention of this pandemic condition, it is necessary to use N95 masks and surgical masks to get rid of SARS CoV-2 [42].

There are three modes of transmission of COVID-19 disease including:

- Mouth droplets;
- Touch; and
- Aerosols during sneezing.

SARS CoV-2 spread was happening through touch transmission of droplet transmission and droplet transmission of aerosol spread that occurs when respiratory aerosols are produced when diseased individual coughs or sneezes and a nearby person inhales them. Transmission of contact happens when a human contact viral contaminated substance and then touches with contaminated hands his mouth or eyes. When the Coronavirus containing the virus, blend is inhaled into the air, aerosol transmission happens and again inhaled [43].

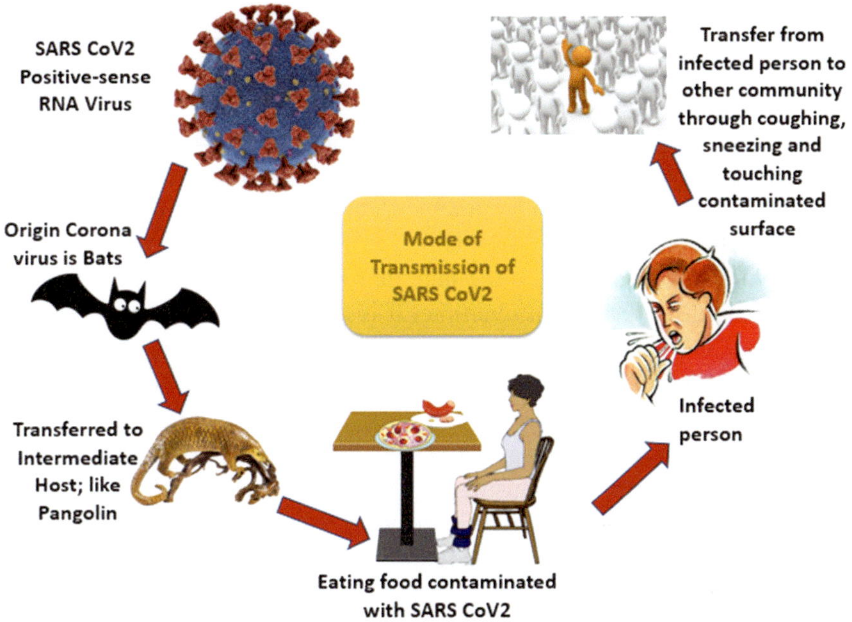

FIGURE 1.2 The life cycle and mode of transmission of COVID-19 by using animal intermediate host to the human being.

COVID-19 is stable on the surface for up to 24 hours, stainless steel, and plastics for two to three days, and aerosols like rain, wet mud, air pollution and smoke for up to three hours [44]. It is also possible to get sick by touching a polluted substance or by air. The incubation time is the duration between initial symptoms and infection for the COVID-19 disease calculation [42]. The time of incubation ranges from 2 to 14 days, although it is normally believed that it is about 5 days. There is further discussion on the latent time between contamination and infection. It is now considered that before displaying symptoms, persons may be contagious and therefore dormant. When a tourist is ill in one country and registered as sick in another area, a significant case happens [6]. Local dissemination happens if the traveler infects others or if a cluster of cases is found and the distribution is readily traced when neighborhood transmission occurs where Ro can be used to quantify no clear cause of infection infectivity [45]. R_0 is the reproduction number, the figure of cases a viral exposed person can cause on average during their infections [46]. Therefore, if R_0 is equal to 2, then an infected human will infect an average of two other individuals when they are contagious, the basic reproduction number reflects the overall capacity of a virus to infect individuals. In essence, what would happen if an infected person joined a population without previous immunity? The effective reproduction number represents a population's present susceptibility depending on whether individuals possess immunity or previous exposure [47].

Over the duration of an epidemic, the Effective Reproduction Number does not decline. Notice that, Basic, and Effective reproduction number depends on environmental conditions, demographics, and infectiousness of the pathogen [48]. The aim of public health initiatives is to minimize Ro to less than one as this will cause illness as the seasonal flu has and would not range from 0.9 to 2.1 as the disease dies out overtime. It is estimates from more recent data that R_0 for COVID-19 ranging from 2.7 to 4.2. There has been a much higher possibility for COVID-19 to spread than for influenza [49]. For example, flu is R_0 = 1.5 and COVID-19 R_0 is = 3 after 3 periods of infection 11 people had influenza and 40 individuals have been affected by COVID-19. Although subsequently 10 periods of transmission, 171 people became ill with influenza and almost 88,000 people become infected by COVID-19 virus [49].

While coughing, sneezing, and talking with friend there is the great risks of transferring SARS CoV-2 from infected person to healthy person [47]. Small droplets or aerosols are produced in the air and remain still for a long time because of low weight and if contaminated droplets are inhaled by the other person from mouth or nasal cavity, there are the high risks of infecting the person with serious condition of SARS CoV-2 that cause the difficulty in breathing and even cause the death of the patient. These aerosols when landed on certain surface then there remain the virus for a long period of time (Figure 1.3) [43].

1.5 VIROLOGY

Scientists have rapidly recognized the pathogen after the COVID-19 outbreak in January 2020, which has been confirm as a new viral strain of Coronaviridae, that was discovered as category β coronavirus and was first called WHO 2019-nCoV [51]. Since 70% of the SARS-CoV genetic sequences are similar, it was later named SARS-CoV-2 [52]. CoVs, with their genome structure, are the most common viruses of all RNA viruses [53]. The pathogenic function of COVID-19 looks to be unclear and is believed to be closely related to viral species [15]. Structural biology, however, discloses how viruses enter cells. The only receptor for COVID-19 is determined to be the ACE-2 [54]. In rare cases, CoVs are enveloped with 26 to 32 kb (CoV; Nidovirales, Coronaviridae family, Coronavirinae, and Torovirinae subfamily, Torovirus genus) large, more-beached RNA genomes [55]. One of the most common pathogenic viruses that chiefly affect the respirational mechanism of human is the Coronavirus. (MERS)-CoV and extreme SARS-CoV's are past coronavirus outbreaks (CoVs) that have significantly posed a danger to individuals [56]. Genotypically and serologically, CoVs are broken down into four subfamilies: α, β and ϒ CoV. Such viruses may contribute to pulmonary, hepatic, enteric, and neurological illnesses [57].

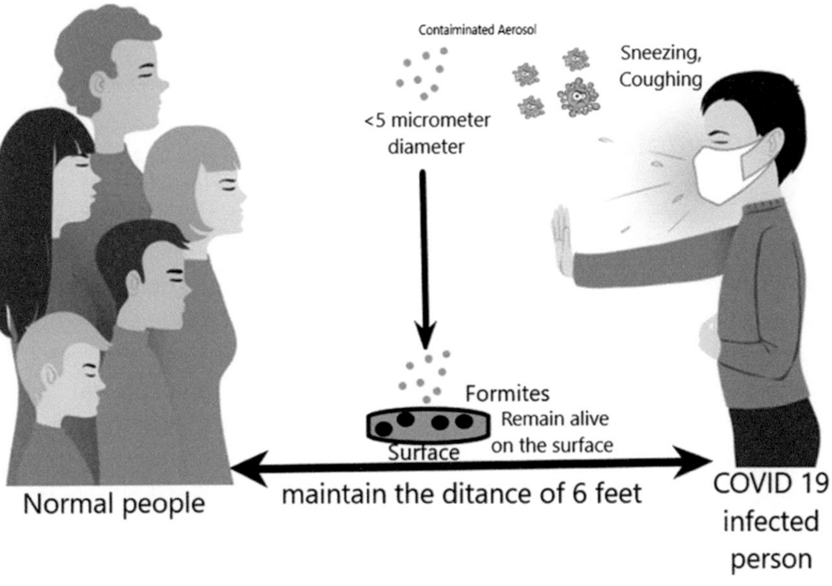

FIGURE 1.3 This diagram represents that how SARS-CoV-2 transmits from the infected host to the susceptible host through aerosols droplet and touching the surface contaminated with COVID-19 fomites. To prevent your family, maintain the social distancing.

Source: Adapted from https://www.bizimkose.com/06/13/hofstedenin-guc-mesafesi-ve-belirsizlikten-kacinma-kavramlari-uzerinden-covid-19-salgini-analizi/

Mammalian pathogenic viruses (Alpha-and Beta-coronavirus), above all, bird viruses (Gamma-coronavirus). CoV sets 1, 2, and 3 are also mentioned to as α, β and ϒ CoVs [58]. There are four subtypes of human CoV's that effect blood flow and severe respiratory diseases, that include 229E and NL63 human alpha CoVs and OC43 and HKU11 human beta CoVs [59]. An additional human beta coronavirus that spread briefly in the human population during 2002 and 2003 was SARS-CoV, resulting in a SARS outbreak with a 10% case fatality risk [60, 61]. Coronavirus that belongs to the pandemic caused by MERS-CoV originated from the β coronaviridae and it was first identified in 2012. MERS coronavirus nay effect serious diseases in human beings and infect multiple host species [62]. The typical cases of pneumonia, due to new coronavirus COVID-19, was first determined and confirmed in the last month of 2019 the city of China, Wuhan, has turned into a worldwide disease outbreak. COVID-19 virus is a mutated pathogenic strain of the β coronaviridae family that has similarities in their genome sequences to the SARS, MERS, and other bat originated CoVs [63]. As compared with SARS and MERS pandemic, the novel mutated strain is more pathogenic and have much more spread speed as compared with other CoV's as declared by the WHO [63].

1.6 MORPHOLOGY

After the clear examination and analysis of Coronavirus by cryo-electron tomography and microscopic studies, it is determined that COVID-19 are spherical and diameter with 125 nm [64, 65] CoV's are all zoonotic pathogens that cause pathogenic effects in the animals, and it is assumed that all CoV's are originated from animals specially COVID-19 derived from bats [2]. It is decided that samples from Nasopharyngeal and Oropharyngeal samples of SARS COVID inoculate with Vero cells for the clear examination of the morphology of COVID-19 virus. Inoculated Vero cells were then fixed by using 2.5% Glutaraldehyde and 2% of Formaldehyde for the classification of SARS COVID 2 and microbial examination off virion. It is observed that after three days of infection of it is determined that a large peplums was examined it is Crown like structure and the name of Corona was originated from "Crown" or "halo" shape [2]. This was found that size of particles of virus ranging from 70–90 nm And most commonly found in Intracellular organelles [2]. It is determined that Coronavirus Contains a single positive sense-RNA strand that is similar to host messenger RNA, Which is about 26 to 30 kb [13, 66]. The RNA of COVID-19 has single-stranded RNA with positive charge having 4 major types of structural proteins that are envelope-protein (E), Transmembrane protein (M), Nucleocapsid protein (N), and Spike protein (S) [67]. Figure 1.4 shows the sequence of these structural proteins in COVID-19 genome is directive as S, E, M, and N. Protein

Specialized for the assembly of budding of viruses And morphogenesis, while S protein are fusion virus protein that comprised of two subunits S1 And S2 [14]. S proteins are made up of receptor binding sites that bind to the human ACE-2 receptor [6].

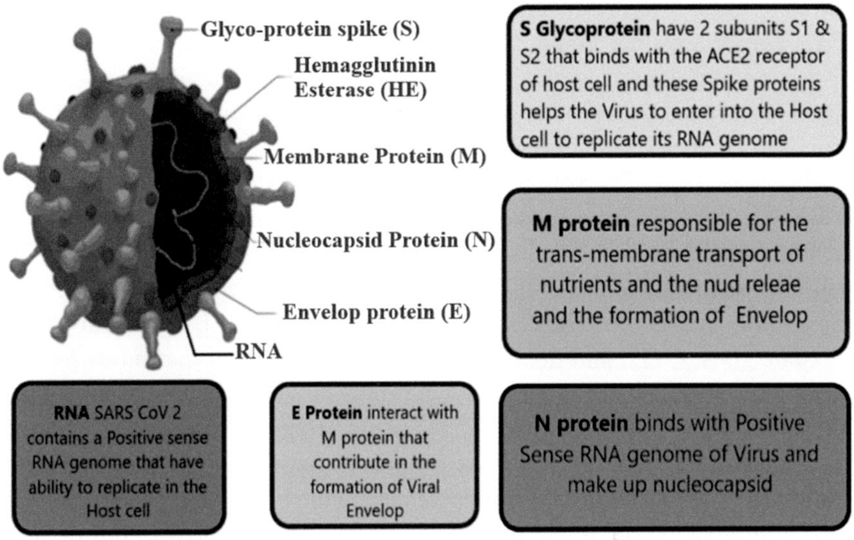

FIGURE 1.4 Structural representation of (COVID-19) is made of virus surface proteins, i.e., glycoprotein spikes (S). The COVID-19 viral membrane glycoprotein (M) and envelope (E) are enclosed in a lipid bilayer originating from the host membrane, encapsulating helical nucleocapsids of viral RNA.

1.6.1 N PROTEIN

SARS is a pandemic disease that emerge in the early 21 century in 2002 in the middle-east and has the death rate of 8% and is because of a new SARS-associated coronavirus (SARS-CoV) [68, 69]. The viral packing of viral positive-sense RNA is the main process in the organization of SARS-CoV and other types of CoVs. When Coronavirus is exposed to a Host cell Viral spike protein bind with specialized receptors on the host cells and fuse with the host cell to insert Viral genome and Nucleocapsid protein and these viral RNA and N-protein work together that interfere with the cellular machinery of the Host cell [70]. It is determined that COVID-19 Viral RNA and N-protein binds with the cellular DNA *in vitro* and block functionality of DNA for its own cell and modify cellular DNA to work for viral genome. This interaction of RNA and N-protein have the role in pathogenesis of virus [71].

The COVID-19 N-protein attached to the viral +ssRNA that makes a structured helical capsid that allows the virus to function properly. COVID-19 and N-protein are made up of two structural domains that are linked by these parts, according to previous nuclear magnetic resonance (NMR) work [72]. These two structural regions share order-disorder characteristics and inferred secondary structure with all Coronavirus N-proteins [73]. The N-terminal Domain (NTD, residues 45–181) of the SARS-CoV N-protein functions as a prospective RNA-binding site, while the C-terminal site (CTD, residues 248–365) functions as a dimerization site, according to structure determination [74].

There is the on N-protein that allow to form Nucleocapsid protein that it binds to the positive-sense RNA of Coronavirus [14]. N-protein have an important part in the transcriptional function and pathogenesis of Viral +ssRNA sequence and the expression of N-protein enhance the process of replication and recover the cDNA clones effectively [75]. It contains of two separate sites, CTD, and the NTD and the, both regions that binds positive sense RNAs *in vitro*. Perfect RNA binding has been proposed to contain assistance from both domains [76, 77] the N protein is also strongly bonded by phosphorylation [78], and it is proposed that this phosphorylation will cause some types of deformation that enhance the non-viral versus viral RNA attraction to bind each other. In a Beads of-string change in the confirmation, Nucleocapsid-protein bound to the viral positive-sense RNA. There are two groups of N-protein RNA substrates (NRSs): the genomic packing signal and the N-protein RNA substrates (NRSs) [79, 80]. The viral RNA packing signal is significantly connected to the other type of domain or C-terminal RNA binding domain [81]. nsp3 also attached with N-protein [77, 82]. This is the main constituent of the complex of replicase enzyme, and the Myoprotein interactions directly help to attach the RNA viral genomic sequence to the reverse transcriptase, and the condensed viral genomic sequence into particulates shown in Figure 1.6 [83].

1.6.2 S GLYCOPROTEIN

Spike protein, also called S-protein, is basically composed of two subunits S1 and S2. S-glycoprotein is composed of RBP. These binding proteins bind with the ACE-2 receptors in the surface of human cells. ACE-2 when exposed with the receptor-binding protein in S1 and S2 subunits of S-glycoprotein then this complex of ACE-2 and receptor binding protein evolve in the lysis of cell membrane of human cell and insertion of viral genome into the human cell where viral genome use the components of cellular-machinery for the replication of viral single-stranded positive-sense RNA and providing toxin for degeneration or infection of cell [84].

The size of S-protein in 180–200 kDa. The length of SARS CoV-2 is 1273 amino acid residues length which consists of 1–13 residues of N-terminus with a single peptide. The polypeptide for S1 subunit from 14–686 aa residues and for S2 subunit, it is from 687–1273 aa residues. Spike protein consists of transmembrane TM domain and extracellular domain (ECD). TM anchor on the viral envelop and there also consists of Short intracellular C domain segment [85]. Extracellular S-protein domain having receptor binding proteins (RBP) that binds with the ACE-2 receptor site of host cell by some conformational changing in the S-protein and allow viral strain to attach the ACE-2 receptors of Host-cell. Spike protein is coated with poly-saccharide molecules that prevent the spike protein form immune response of host immune system (Figure 1.5) [86].

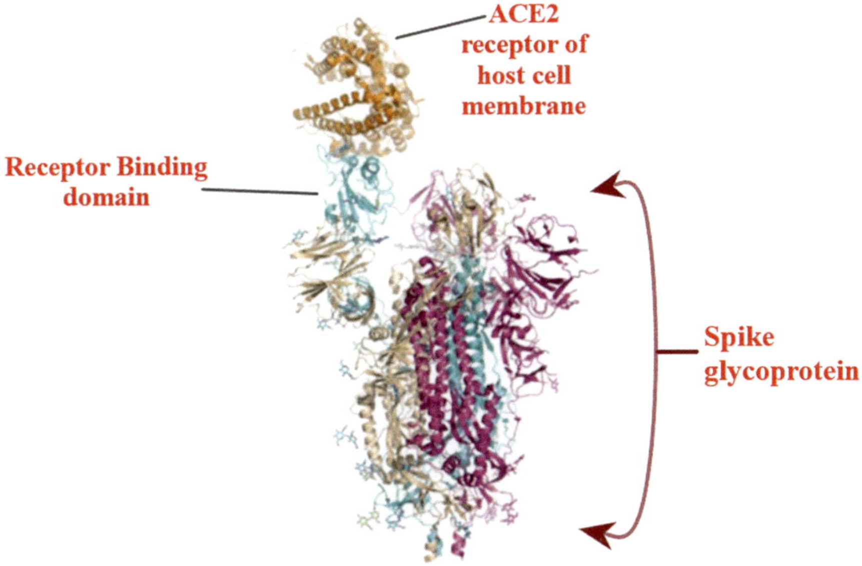

FIGURE 1.5 Spike glycoprotein which projects from the membrane of mature virions having receptor binding domain.

Source: Adapted from https://www.rcsb.org/structure/7cwm

It is very important to know about the structure and functions of all proteins of Coronavirus because it will help to develop better vaccines, screening kits, and cures to fight COVID-19 and so every single Coronavirus is coded with these spike proteins [6]. These spike proteins help to involved in how this virus is affecting host cells and so one of these spike proteins have something that looks like spike-like structures and each one of these spike proteins is composed of three domains the outermost domain is transferred to as the receptor-binding domain (RBD) [87]. RBD has to job sticking to some receptor site referred to as the ACE-2 receptor on host cells that it is about to impact as well as getting cleaved off in order to activate underlying domains inside of the spike protein and one of the spike proteins is going to essentially anchor itself onto the ACE-2 receptor on the host cell and an additional spike protein on this Coronavirus is going to actually do the work of fusing the membrane of the Coronavirus into the host membrane [84]. Some types of cleaving enzyme released and cleave off the cell membrane of the host cell and genomic material of COVID-19 is inserted in a Host cell that taking control over the cellular machinery of the Host cell to replicate the Viral genome in multiple copies and causing the toxic effects on the host cells and producing disease [19].

1.6.3 M PROTEIN

The shape of viral is defined due to the membrane protein. Some virus is spherical, rod, tadpole, and hexagonal crystalline type structure. Basically, these variant structures are due to the arrangement of membrane (M) and envelop (E) protein proteins. Membrane-protein is most abundantly present protein in Coronavirus. It defines the shape and assembly of Viral genome, it interacts with the proteins of viral structures. It also binds with the nucleocapsids that directly attached with the positive-sense RNA of SARS CoV 2 viral genome [88]. Membrane protein gives the virus a definite shape and protection in *in-vitro* environments. This membrane protein interacts with the other envelop protein and give them perfect arrangements to these proteins. Membrane protein also interact in the assembly of structural protein of virus and specialized assembly to the viral genome [75]. The virion is a less molecular weight (MW) protein of almost 25–30 kDa MW, having 3 transmembrane (TM) domains [89]. The glycosylated short N terminal outer domain has more larger C terminal endo-domain that are spreading 6–8 almost nm into the viral crystal-molecule [90]. Although, implanted into the endoplasmic reticulum membrane transnationally, the most of Membrane proteins do not consists signal sequence. The Membrane protein is originating as a di-molecular form in the virion and take two variant forms that promote both membrane twisting and bind to nucleocapsids that directly binds with the viral genome. Recent researches determined that in certainty, the COVID-19 M-proteins was assumed to be tangled in host interactions that apart from its importance in viral structures arrangements [91]. The glycosylated O (group I and III) or N (group II) can also be made. Glycosylation is not important for mobility or pathogenesis but is important that perform a greater part in the interaction between the virus and host in the glycosylated form of the M-protein [75].

1.6.4 E PROTEIN

In less amounts in the virion, the E protein with MW of (~8–12 kDa) can be present. The proteins of coronavirus E have variant structures but have a general architecture [92] Although the E-protein membrane structure analysis is not conclusive, most evidence suggests that it is primarily a membrane structural protein. The E-protein has N-terminal exo-domain and the ion channel functionality of the C-terminal endo-domain. Unlike, other types of structural proteins, the Envelop protein recombinant viruses are not more dangerous and more lethal, but they are basically on the virus from [93] Coronavirus E is a membrane protein that integrates. E proteins plays an important function in viral organization along with the M-protein. E protein binds virus-like particles when expressed by itself or in combination with M [75].

1.7 GENOME ORGANIZATION

COVID-19 viral morphology defines the club-shaped projection that is similar to the solar-corona and Crown-shaped virus. On the viral surface, just because of the presence of most abundant S (spike) proteins this virus shows crown-like shape [67]. Coronavirus contains approximately 26–32 kb of non-segmented +ssRNA which shows similarity with the host's mRNA and it is considered the largest known viral genome. In the genome of SARS-COVID-2, with 5 prime end 265 and 3 prime end 358 nucleotides there are two flanking untranslated regions (UTRs) [6]. Corona viral genome have open reading frame (ORF) with variable numbers (6–11). The 2/3 parts of this viral genome consisting of two open reading frames (ORFs) ORF1a and ORF1b, which are used to translate the 2 Polyproteins PP1a and

PP1ab and many other proteins including 16 structural and non-structural are also expressed in this viral genome. Glycosylated S proteins, M protein, N protein and E protein, these are four basic structuralizing proteins which are encoded by the viral genome [40]. In viral genome, there are 14 ORFs and TRSs are used to regulate these frames [11]. The two basic transcriptional units of ORF1a and ORF1ab are used to translate two key proteins. Therefore, main polyprotein pp1ab combine with non-structural protein and form complex replica mechanism. This activate enzymes which is an unusual phenomenon in the positive-sense RNA families of virus [94]. COVID-19 contains 38% of GC nucleotides and comprised of 30,000 nucleotides there are unknown function of non-essential proteins many of the protein encoded by viral genome are still undetected [75, 96]. Their comprised 5' cap and 3' prime poly-A tail end and similar to mRNA of Host and transcribed by a host ribosome to translate viral polyprotein immediately [75]. Furthermore, there are organized UTRs present in the viral genome, which are crucial for viral RNA transcription and translation 5' (UTRs) also present seven stem-loops and 3' end contains pseudo-knot and stem-loop and these structures plus important role in transcriptional regulator regime shown in Figure 1.6 [97].

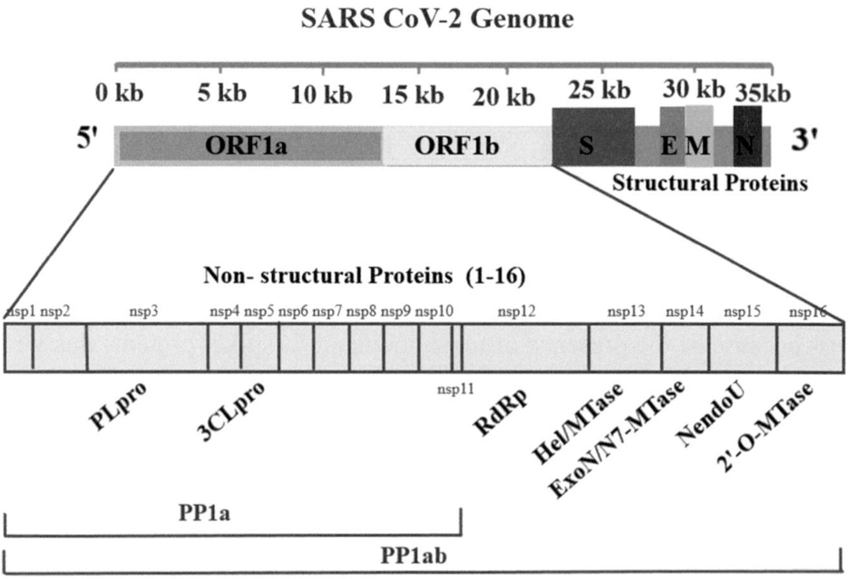

FIGURE 1.6 COVID-19 polycistronic genome sequence containing non-structural proteins and (having 1–16 nsp) and structural proteins (S, E, M, and N).

1.8 REPLICATION

However, COVID-19 virus is composed of S-protein and many structural proteins including N-protein and M-proteins like RNA polymerase, helicase, 3-chymotrypsin-like protease, glycoprotein, and other required protein papain-like protease [4]. By following the joining and translation of the viral replication complex, viral RNA is synthesized [98]. As with the binding of envelop spike glycoproteins to ACE-2 receptors, SARS-COVID-2 life cycle begins and either directly from the host cells or from endocytic membrane, fusion of membrane takes place. After attachment to the cell membrane, the transported viral genomic sequence in the cytoplasm causes the conversion of non-coated RNA into the two polyproteins. Consequently, Polyproteins are reduced to 16 nsps by the protease encoded by ORF1a, which can also form a complex RNA replica-transcriptase complex [98, 100].

The development of negative RNA, used as a full-length (+) RNA genome template, is regulated by this complex. Sub-genomic RNAs in transcription are produced by transcription and decoded by sub-genomic (+) mRNA into different structural proteins. From the transcription, transcripts are produced. A nucleocapsid constitutes the freshly formed structural protein and viral genomic RNA. Viral particles are then emitted from the infected cells to the ER-Golgi C (ERGIC) intermediate compartment [101].

Therefore, after the entrance of SARS-COVID-2 into the body, the next step is viral replication. In order to bind to their mobile receptors, CoVs use homotrimer spike glycoprotein (including S1 in each spike monomer and S2 in each subunit) on the envelope. In the event of cell entry, such a bond triggers a subsequent cascade that leads to cell-viral membrane fusion [101]. In Coronavirus, there are six ORF regions that act as models by which sub-genomic mRNA structures the protein, spike, nucleocapsid, and diaphragm-proteins. The polypeptides derived from pp1a and pp1ab are generated by ORFs [102].

A virus normally requires a series of primary interactions to reach the host cell. First of all, with the help of cellular receptors, it binds with the target host cell, second one is the combination of shell with a cell membrane; and then leaving the genetic material within the cell (Figure 1.7). However, it depends heavily on receptor binding specificity, efficiency of endocytosis and proteolytic activation that which mechanism is used for viral genomic transmission of nucleic acids into host cells [41]. The SARS-CoV is triggered with TMPRSS2 proteolytically *in vitro* and *in vivo*. Therefore, we tried VeroE6/TMPRSS2 cells that constitutively express TMPRSS2, to separate COVID-19. The expression frequency of TMPRSS2 of messenger RNA is around 10 times higher in VeroE6/TMPRSS2 cells than in human cell lines like lungs cells and other cell linings [103]. A functional, *in vitro* and *in vivo*, COVID-19 viral receptor is the ACE-2 angiotensin-converting enzymes. Entry into host cells and subsequent replication of viruses are important (Figure 1.7) [5, 104].

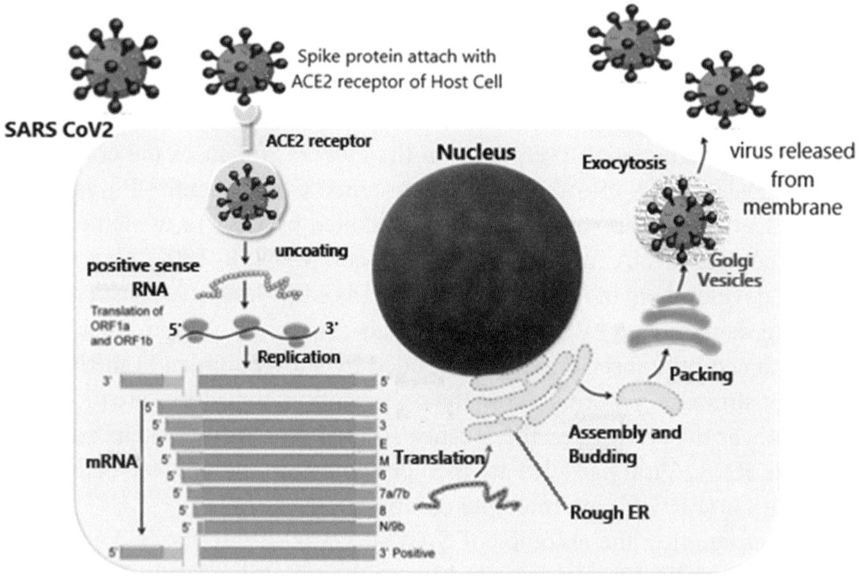

FIGURE 1.7 The replication of COVID-19 in the host body. The binding of the spike protein to the binding receptors (ACE-2) initiates the life cycle, accompanied by conformation shifts in the S protein, further facilitating the integration of host cell membrane and viral envelope.

Source: Reprinted and modified with permission from Ref. [5]. © 2020 Springer Nature.

An important component of transmission over species is cell entry, specifically for beta coronavirus. The S protein sits are known as the RBD in beta CoVs that can stimulate the association with binding receptor of the host cell linings. However, upon binding to the membrane receptor, protease binds the spike protein and produces the spike binding peptide that allows viruses to reach. The host-recognized receptors of beta coronavirus have included COVID-19 enzyme 2 (ACE-2) that transforms angiotensin [105]. In the average adult human lung, ACE-2 is predominantly expressed as a viral reservoir in alveolar epithelial type II cells [106]. To facilitate the binding of virus spike protein and host cell membrane binding receptors, the particles of coronavirus spike protein (S) react to cellular receptor. For the conversion of huge overlapping ORF1a/b into the host cell, the +ssRNA genome is then transferred into the cytoplasm. The RNA-dependent viral polymerase enzyme subsequently produces the number of sub-genomic messenger RNAs by recreating the viral genome. These include protein nucleocapsid N and E glycoprotein encoding RNAs, M protein, S-protein unknown function, and 8 proteins. In ER-Golgi system, the proteins in the envelope are recycled and transferred to a budding compartment in which the M-protein is bound to helical N-protein and the envelope and spike-proteins. After that, by the process of exocytosis, the transgenic virions are expelled out from infected cells [107]. This causes the growth of enormous multi-nucleated cells that can multiply without virus-specific antibodies inside an infected organism [98].

1.9 PATHOGENESIS

COVID-19 tends to be spread mainly during the winter season in temperate-climate nations. COVID-19 infections mainly involve human upper breath and GIT, ranging from minor, egregious diseases like common cold, to more extreme causes along with bronchitis and renal pneumonia [5]. However, in the person who are exposed with COVID-19 disease have an increased number of leukocytes, prominent respiratory infection results and the highest level of inflammatory cytokinesis in plasma had verified the indications at five days of fever such as coarse coughing noises from lungs with high fever with body temperature of 39°C have shown after the analysis of one of the COVID-19 patients [108]. To improvise the detection of COVID-19 virus, the pathogens of SARS-COVID and MERS-COVID can also be used in related processes to provide a great deal of information about SARS-COVID-2 because there is a little information about pathogenicity of COVID-19 [109].

Therefore, in order to different disease aspects, there are three classifications of COVID-19 can be done. In Asymptomatic disease, reaction of upper airways and airways (next days) and hypoxia, ground glass penetration and development into ARDS [110]. The virus spreads and tends to move across the breathing tract through the respiratory airways, and as a result, an involuntary, larger immune response is stimulated. However, it is estimated that nasal swab and sputum may be included in the initial's markers of innate immune response against the virus. Currently, COVID-19 is scientifically manifested [111]. Unfortunately, approximately 20% of affected people, those with very severe conditions, can experience stage 3 diseases and pulmonary infiltration. Initial fatality rates are about 2%, although this varies significantly with age [112]. The virus joins the network for lung gas exchange and infects alveolar type II cells [113]. As in the case of SARS, the pathogenesis of COVID-19 involves immune-mediated inflammation. The development of COVID-19 was correlated with a continuous decrease of lymphocyte numbers and a significant rise of neutrophils [114].

However, in the clinical findings of COVID-19, three forms of individual reaction to COVID-19 occur. The first form involves individuals who respond ineffectively to an infection and that are unable to control the virus. This results in an exhilarating inflammatory reaction in some individuals. Consequently, virus replication occurs. The second form consists of people who, following infection with immune responses, are asymptomatic or minimally symptomatic and controls the virus successfully without causing undue host damage to disrupt homeostasis. In the third form, those individuals include that either initially respond to damage to COVID-19 tissue or are increasingly inflamed in the lungs by unregulated viral replication [115].

In the samples of liver biopsy, moderate microvascular steatosis and minor lobular and portal activity were identified that may be produced by COVID virus or the medicines that were used for treatment [116]. In COVID-19 affected death cases, in both lungs, large mucous secretions were found as compare to the SARS and MERS [117].

1.9.1 FACTORS INFLUENCING THE VIRAL PATHOGENICITY

Conjunction lies between CVD and neurological conditions and also in diabetes. Many other aberrations have been identified, involving cellular immune deficiencies, myocardial injuries, liver, and renal injuries, and secondary bacterial infections [118]. Lymphopenia and chronic soreness were reported in most of the severe illness and death cases. After the outbreak of COVID in 2003, in the patients of acute respiratory syndrome, such findings are very normal [117]. Previously, multiple types of S protein-based vaccines and antivirals have been studied. A full-size Spike protein, viral vector, DNA, recombinant Spike, and RBDs protein may be vaccines' components seen on the S protein [84]. Some recombinant compounds have only a slight COVID-19 infection effect, like ribavirin IFN [119]. To bind with the RBDs of COVID-19 virus is more closely associated to ACE-2 [120]. On the other hand, ACE-2 is the attachment site for COVID-19. On the basis of this information, Gurwitz introduced the use of accessible antagonists, such as angiotensin receptor 1 (AT1R), to suppress COVID-19 diseases [121].

The research is currently focused on detecting and developing strong, selective monoclonal antibodies to COVID-19 and introducing remdesivir as a new analog nuclear antibody drug that was applied as an Ebola virus (EBOV) treatment [117, 122]. Therefore, in the aspect to increase the binding with human infection receptors, its degree of mutation has to be considered. It is important to see how COVID-20 mutates in an attempt to comprehend the rate of transmission of the virus to humans. Any improvement in the COVID-19 sequences which might enable interaction between individuals might also increase its pathogenicity [123]. COVID-19 is predicted to become less infectious by transmission from human-to-human due to RNA virus genetic bottlenecks that frequently exist during respiratory transmissions [124, 125].

1.9.1.1 IMMUNE DYSFUNCTION

Defects of the immune system contribute to heightened susceptibility to infection, autoimmune conditions, asthma, and often even cancer (such as chronic rheumatism). The most prevalent causes include poor health factors and malnutrition worldwide. Secondary hemophagocytic lymph histiocytosis (SHLH), typically attributed to adult virus infection, is a disease under which so many stimulated immune cells (macrophages and lymphocytes) are generated by the body [126]. The modification of the activity of the antigen-presenting cell (APC) and the disrupted migration of the dendritic cell (DC) leading to lower T cell priming are also potential causes to decrease the T cells number [127]. CD4 + and CD8+ T cells decreased in numbers are known to be associated with SARS-COVID-2 mortality in terms of adaptive immunity [17].

1.9.1.2 CYTOKINE STORM

In all of the sickest people with COVID-19, their blood is full of high amounts of immune system proteins called cytokines. In autoimmune disorders such as juvenile arthritis, storms with cytokines are known to occur. Cytokines are the proteins that take part in chemical signaling for a pathogenic invasion-resistant reaction. The production of a variety of cytokines gives the ability of the host body to remove the illness as a reaction to an infectious pathogen such as a virus. Various classes of cytokines are chemokines, IFNs, and interleukins [117]. The main cause of severe coronavirus infection may be the cytokine storm, which reinforces the related severity of SARS-CoV and COVID-19 [126, 128].

They primarily start with increase viral replication and may lead to significant epithelial and endothelial cell deaths, as a result of acute lung injury [57].

1.9.1.3 RDS (ACUTE STATE WITH RESPIRATORY DISTRESS)

ARDS is a deadly respiratory state which restricts the absorption and delivery of adequate oxygen into the lungs, leading to some breathing difficulties and acute lung injury [129]. Male, obese, smokers, and those with essential co-morbidities (such as elevated blood pressure, coronary disorders, asthma, chronic lung disease) above 60 years, the high-risk patients that require hospitalization for severe ARS-CoV-2 [130]. In severe conditions of human corona viral infections, patients suffer from extreme respiratory failure that involves artificial ventilation, and histopathological observations help Acute State Respiratory Distress (ARDS) [131]. Over 40 genes associated with ARDS development or results, including ACE-2 interleukin 10 (IL-10), tumor necrosis factor (TNF) and vascular endothelial growth factor (VEGF), have been identified [132]. There has also been evidence that the adverse effects of ARDS are linked with elevated plasma levels of interleukin-6 and interleukin-8 [57].

1.10 PHASE OF THE IMMUNE RESPONSE IN HUMAN BODY AGAINST COVID-19

We are protected by the immune system against infections and disease. This creates an antibody for pathogen-killing. The whole body is made up of cells from the immune system that protects against disease. In maintaining pathogenesis and well-being, it plays a key role [133, 134]. The major players in the immune response are WBCs, that can move throughout the body's circulating. In order to determine invading bacteria, and the body transfers blood and lymph channels to activate the lymphatic function. Antigens are processed, operated on, and used to control them in the lymph nodes and spleen cells [134, 135].

COVID-19 viral infection supported by the adaptive and innate immune response of COVID viral pathogens. A rapid and well-coordinated immune response can inflict damaging of tissue at the region of viral infection and at systemic speeds, too strong an inflammatory inborn response, or deregulated adaptive immune protection [112, 135]. Significant pro-inflammatory host reactions are predicted to induce immunological pathology in COVID-19 infected patients, results in instant progression of ARDS and acute liver infection (ALI) [110, 136]. The vast release of cytokines and chemokines, clearly mirrors a generally unregulated deregulation of host immune response. Therefore, in view of the main role the immune response plays in COVID infection, a complete knowledge of the function of the immune system and the immune escape mechanisms of COVID-19 will provide us with insights into the therapeutic handling of serious cases and the avoidance of changes between mild and extreme phases. Potential analysis on the structural effect of the uncontrolled immune system on the GIT, neuroendocrine, renal, and cardiovascular processes are also relevant throughout the present research, however the current review may not support it [137].

1.10.1 IMMUNE RESPONSE FOR SARS-COVID-2

In normal course of 1–2 weeks, a multiphase process is the development of immunity to the wretched by natural infection. With a non-specific innate response, the body responds to a viral infection that can slow the propagation of the virus by macrophages, neutrophils, and DCs, and can also resist symptoms [20]. In the immune system of COVID-19 patients, significant changes have been observed, both inborn and adaptive, in some research. In fact, lymphocytopenia is common, and the difference in total neutrophils is closely linked to the seriousness of the illness and death [24, 135]. In patients of COVID-19, a significant reduction in the number of cells flowing in the blood like CD8 + cells, CD4 + cells, NK cells and B-cells, [24]. The response of the immune system of the host cell is based on the intrusion and pathogenicity of SARS-COVID-2. The viral spike glycoprotein (S protein) protects the ACE-2 of its receptor on the cell membrane of human cell linings [116, 138].

An electron microscopy of the COVID-19 of Spike protein structure and its binding affinity for ACE-2 indicated that the COVID-19 S protein structure was very similar to that of SARS, although with slight variations. COVID-19 Spike protein is 10–20 times higher than SARS CoV spike protein and can thus be quickly moved with COVID-19 protein affinity from human to human [86]. Natural immunity response represents the initial defense line in response to viral insertion. Coronavirus infection in vertebrates activated intermembrane binding receptors, which are pathogenic to molecular structures [16]. Cytotoxic T cells were activated that can terminate viral-infected body cells and the target virus-specific antigens, anti-organ-generating B-cells, also have a major function in viral elimination. A variety of cytokines that cause inflammation, includes interleukin-6 and TNF, have been documented to be slightly lower and higher in COVID-19 patients and, in particular, in patients with extreme pneumonia [21, 110, 136, 139].

Conversely, mass development of inflammatory cytokines and damages to the host cells may also be caused by a powerful and sustained immune response. To eradicate the invading virus, the immune response of the virus is important [138, 140]. As overproduction caused by aberrant immune activation, cytokines are referred to as cytokine tempests. In fact, late-stage cytokine storms of coronavirus diseases (COVID), have been the significant reason of development and eventual death [141] [142]. Huang and colleagues have observed elevated plasma levels of both Th1 (e.g., IL-1β) and Th2 (e.g., IL-10) cytokines [139].

As in the situation of MERS-CoV and SARS-CoV, no particular antiviral agent against COVID-19 infection is currently available with scientifically proven efficacy [100]. Various animal models were also used to explain SARS-CoV replication and they reported extreme signs of infection. On the other hand, owing to DDP4 receptor non-compatibility in mice, no pathogenesis was observed in the condition of MERS-CoV [143]. SARS-CoV animal models should be used for testing COVID-19 virulence factors since COVID-19 is 80% identical to SARS-CoV. It is believed that COVID-19 entry into host cells is identical to SARS-CoV, likely through ACE-2 cell receptors [139]. As per separate studies of genomic structure and COVID-19 pathogenesis molecular pathways, [144]. There are several targets that may be used as therapeutic agents in various ways to prevent replication of the virus or to create an antibody that could be successful against COVID-19 [145, 146]. Many types of therapeutic strategies like antiviral drugs, immunotherapeutic techniques and vaccination methods that are under consideration are mentioned in the table 1.1.

1.10.2 ACE-2/TMPRSS2 RECEPTOR INHIBITION

At first, a virus binds to a host cell using specific receptors. As the result of previous research on SARS-CoV, it is revealed that the presence of macrophages and epithelial cells in the lungs are the basic targets for this viral attack. Many of these cells have ACE-2, which is used for attachment and entry by SARS-CoV [155]. Another immune response kinetics research has reported that cell spike (S) and hemagglutinin (H) are the associated proteins COVID-19 virus that are used to attach with the cells of the host by the

TABLE 1.1 The Therapeutic Strategies, Procedure Used and Mode of Action of Drugs That are Under Consideration

Strategy of Therapy	Methods	Mode of Action	Under Trial Drugs	References
Receptor inhibition	• Inhibition of ACE-2 receptor • Inhibition of TMPRSS2 receptor	Inhibitor that resembles the structure of ACE-2 receptors interfere the spike protein and or binds on the other side of Spike proteins and inhibit the original functioning.	Baricitinib, ruxolitinib, natural hesperidin, nafamostat mesylate, camostat mesylate and other antiviral drugs	[87, 112, 139]
Immunotherapy	• IL-6 inhibitors • Complement system • NK cell therapy • mTOR inhibitors	In this type of therapy drugs that boost up the immune system or drugs that suppress the immune system of the body, are used	C3a, C5a inhibitors, CYNK-001, tocilizumab, rapamycin	[15, 147]
Vaccination	• DNA vaccines • RNA vaccines • Recombinant protein vaccines • Killed/inactivated vaccines • Live attenuated vaccines • Viral vector-based vaccines	An acquired immunity is provided by injecting the live or attenuated vaccines that produce antibodies in the body that fight against the virion	Currently, more than 115 vaccines are developing for example: mRNA-1273 (RNA vaccine by Moderna Inc.), INO-4800 (DNA vaccine by Inovio Pharmaceuticals Inc.), ChAdOx1nCov-19 (killed/inactivated vaccine by Oxford University, AstraZeneca Plc.), Ad5-nCov (live attenuated vaccine by CanSino Biologics Inc.) and NVX-CoV2373 (recombinant protein vaccine by Novavax Inc and by Clover biopharmaceuticals).	[148–150]

TABLE 1.1 *(Continued)*

Strategy of Therapy	Methods	Mode of Action	Under Trial Drugs	References
Antiviral drugs	• Antiviral drugs specifically designed for COVID-19 • Antiviral drugs already used for other viral infections (such as HIV, hepatitis, influenza, etc.), are now under clinical research against novel coronavirus	–	Lopinavir/ritonavir, IFN-α, arbidol, favipiravir, and darunavir, etc., (all these drugs are already approved for other viral infections but now are under clinical trial against COVID-19). Remdesivir, chloroquine, and ivermectin are recently US FDA accepted drugs for COVID-19 infection.	[151]
Other therapies	• Plasma therapy • Medicinal plants • Protease inhibitors • Monoclonal antibody	–	Inhibit viral replication or to boost body immune response	[152–154]

virus. On the surface of the virus, the presence of S and H proteins play an important role to bind with the ACE-2 and sialic acid receptors of host cells, respectively [156]. However, as compared to the SARS-COVID the increase in pathogenicity of SARS-COVID-2 is considered because of the occurrence of Furin-like cleavage region on the S protein [116]. The entrance of the host cell and SARS-COVID-2 spike protein synthesis along with furin pre-cleavage is also involved in TMPRSS2 [87].

It was hypothesized that to prevent SARS-COVID-2 infection, one way is the use of various molecules and antibiotics to saturate or block the ACE-2 receptors or TMPRSS2, thus restricting the Coronavirus from binding to the membrane receptors of the host cell and thereby preventing the replication cycle [135]. However, except camostat mesylate, which proves effective against the entrance of virus into lung cells, no other therapeutic agent has yet been directly checked for TMPRSS2 inhibition in the case of COVID-19 [87].

1.10.3 ANTIVIRAL DRUGS

Instead of destroying them as antimicrobials do, antiviral drugs are intended to recognize the viral proteins to stop virus replication. They appear to reduce the number of viruses to a certain stage by restricting the replication cycle, where they are unable to cause pathogenesis and allow the body immune system to neutralize the viral infection [151].

Hundreds of clinical trials to perform and assess post-infection treatments for COVID-19 infections have been licensed by the WHO International Clinical Trials Registry Platform [157]. Although several antiviral medications are now being used for other treatment therapies [158]. These medications have already been evaluated and used against HIV, malarial bugs, hepatitis C virus (HCV), influenza viruses, etc. Any of the antiviral drugs studied *in vitro* as COVID-19 infection inhibitors are: IFN-alpha, which was historically used to treat hepatitis infection, which can be used to prevent the replication of SARS-COVID-2 [151]. This drug can also theoretically inhibit SARS-CoV2 replication.

Ivermectin, an antiparasitic drug, was also recently approved by the FDA to avoid Coronavirus infection following the effective inhibition of *in vitro* COVID-19 viral replication [159]. The most important component of the human body's innate defense mechanism, which act as a connection between adaptive and innate immunity, is the complement system, which is made up of more than 35 proteins and regulators. Following the establishment of its function in inflammation and a possible therapeutic impact against some diseases, research on the complement system is advancing quickly [149].

The respiratory distress COVID-19 infection, the C3 component of complement activation was found to further exacerbate the disease. Since SARS-COVID is closely linked to SARS-COVID-2, it can be assumed that COVID-19 may likely have the same function. SARS-CoV animal models have also demonstrated that mice deficient in C3 have shown minimal respiratory dysfunction. Therefore, against SARS-COVID 2, C3 inhibition may be used as an efficacious treatment [160].

1.10.4 VACCINATION STRATEGIES

Vaccination is one of the most active methods of stopping a disease. By triggering acquired immunity, the vaccine allows the body's immune system to recognize and combat infectious diseases. A vaccination that aims to reduce the severity, shedding, and dissemination of the virus must be made to manage coronavirus outbreak [148].

COVID-19 vaccination methods, like recombinant protein vaccines, killed/inactivated vaccines, RNA vaccines, DNA vaccines, live attenuated vaccines, and vaccines centered on viral vectors, are diverse. The target is S protein in all these vaccines, except for the live-attenuated and killed vaccine for which the entire virion is targeted. They have many drawbacks, together with their benefits [149]. These methods have also been determined by trail animal-based research against Coronaviridae infections, and they are all in the first stage of clinical trials. It could take many months to several years to produce a final vaccine after these trials. The S protein is considered an optimal treatment for the SARS-COVID and MERS-COVID vaccines [150].

1.10.5 PLASMA THERAPY

Another treatment technique used against COVID-19 patients is plasma therapy, much as coronavirus infections in this method, plasma was pumped into affected persons from, treated patients [152]. Previously, in patients of COVID-19 positive results are shown, more thorough studies are needed to explore if this procedure is worth applying, taking into account complications associated with other plasma proteins [153].

In his study, Contini proposed two protease inhibitors for the cure of novel coronavirus pandemic, commonly used against HIV infection. Another hopeful therapeutic treatment of infections caused by COVID-19 is the recombinant human monoclonal antibody. In the treatment of SARS-COVID-2, certain monoclonal antibodies previously used against SARS-COVID can be used as an alternative method for treating infection [154].

1.11 EPIDEMIOLOGY

In the short term, the geographic spread of the causative agent and worldwide dispersal have become a significant health concern [154]. According to the Wuhan Municipal Health Commission, 27 pneumonia patients were associated with the South China seafood industry, that was announced on December 31, 2019, the earliest finding of COVID-19 [21]. Conversely, after China's New Year, there is dramatic development in the infected patients. COVID-19 had exposed more than 200 countries on 16 May 2020, and the confirmed number of individuals infected by virus was 4,425,485 worldwide [161].

A major part of epidemiological research is the SARS-COVID-2 mode of propagation. However, It's really clear that COVID-19's human-human transmission occurs predominantly through respiratory droplet molecules [162]. Even though it is unclear if the eyes will transmit COVID-19 [163]. It must be noticed that some researchers have indicated that some infected persons with COVID pandemic have substantial digestive symptom reports and that COVID-19 genomic sequence has been detected in samples of fecal or swabs of anal of infected patients, suggesting the existence of oral-fecal connexins [21, 164]. B y contact trace, four patients (22%) were detected, while 3 (17%) were detected by boundary scanning. The patients traveled to Wuhan, China, 14 days before the disease emerged. Around 16 (89%) of the 18 respondents were Chinese citizens, while 2 (11%) were Singaporeans [34].

To date, 86.6% of infected patients are almost 31 and 79 years of age, 1% below one year, 1% below 10–19 years of age, and 3% above 1980 years of age have been registered in China's most important case sequence. For men, the number of patients is 51%, while the number of females is 49% and 4% are medical staff [99]. In the United States, 31% of all COVID-19 casualties are elderly (over 65 years of age), 45% are injured, 53% are ICU patients (over 65 years of age) and 80% are deceased [95]. A total patient of 1,285,257 COVID-19 infected present in almost 170 countries at about 5.4% (70,344/1,285,257) by 6 April 2020. Much of these were patients between the ages of 60 and 80, in these age classes, the highest number of fatalities (20.3%) [119]. Younger children (0–9 years of age) had relatively fewer reported cases. Luckily, although the male-to-female ratio varies when it relies on multiple demographic categories, in the most affected cases; COVID-19 pneumonia was moderate. Actually, this pathogen has become highly contagious; there have not been mild or even extreme deaths [50].

Basic reproductive numbers and death rates are important in terms of epidemiology. A broad index for forecasting the development of an outbreak is known to be Common reproductive numbers (R0). In order to predict the disease pattern, the main approach to estimating R0 is to construct an accurate statistical model using data from infected individuals, such as serial time and latent duration. On the basis of broad epidemiologic findings of 425 confirmed patients, the baseline reproductive number of COVID-19 was 2.2, and each patient was able to infect 2.2 other individuals [29]. The estimated mortality risk is about 2% for patients seeking care so far, but this is true will not be verified for some time [37]. However, the mortality ratio for COVID-19 still continues to rise just because of the enormous number of COVID-19 patients. Epidemic zone statistics also indicate that the highest mortality rate for people between the ages of 30–59 years and year after year has raised the incidence of symptomatic infection for people of all ages [27].

1.12 CONCLUSION

In the past 50 years, a vast range of human and animal host diseases have been produced in various CoVs. The fact that these viruses are able to mutate, or infect other organisms and cells that will possibly continue to develop and cause human as well as veterinary outbreaks. CoVs are an interesting community of viruses that include natural pathogenesis models, remarkable molecular transcription and recombination processes and pathogens that are emerging. Structural analysis of the cells infected by viruses revealed about SARS-COVID 2 and this virus is about 70 to 90 nanometer in size. SARS-COVID is predominantly transmitted by the inhalation and direct or indirect communication with the respiratory system, while for infection, the estimated incubation time is about 5.2 days. Older age and concurrent disease are the mutual factors behind COVID-19 infection death rate. No specific COVID-19 treatment is currently available. Since the virus was so close to its relatives, attempts were made to supply COVID-19 drugs and vaccines. Nevertheless, it is important to recognize the particular molecular features of the infection.

KEYWORDS

- **coronavirus (COVID-19)**
- **genome organization**
- **morphology**
- **pathogenesis**
- **replication**
- **vaccination**

REFERENCES

1. Hamer, O. W., et al., (2020). CT morphology of COVID-19: Case report and review of literature. In: *RöFo-Fortschritte Auf Dem Gebiet Der Röntgenstrahlen Und Der Bildgebenden Verfahren*. © Georg Thieme Verlag KG.
2. Alanagreh, L. A., Alzoughool, F., & Atoum, M., (2020). The human coronavirus disease COVID-19: Its origin, characteristics, and insights into potential drugs and its mechanisms. *Pathogens, 9*(5), 331.
3. Rose-Redwood, R., et al., (2020). Geographies of the COVID-19 pandemic. *Dialogues in Human Geography.*
4. Shereen, M. A., et al., (2020). COVID-19 infection: Origin, transmission, and characteristics of human coronaviruses. *Journal of Advanced Research.*
5. Su, S., et al., (2016). Epidemiology, genetic recombination, and pathogenesis of coronaviruses. *Trends in Microbiology, 24*(6), 490–502.
6. Kumar, S., et al., (2020). Morphology, genome organization, replication, and pathogenesis of severe acute respiratory syndrome coronavirus 2 (SARS-CoV-2). In: *Coronavirus Disease 2019 (COVID-19)* (pp. 23–31). Springer.
7. Velavan, T. P., & Meyer, C. G., (2020). The COVID-19 epidemic. *Tropical Medicine & International Health, 25*(3), 278.
8. Chan-Yeung, M., & Xu, R., (2003). SARS: Epidemiology. *Respirology,* (Suppl 8), S9–14.
9. Singhal, T., (2020). A review of coronavirus disease-2019 (COVID-19). *The Indian Journal of Pediatrics*, 1–6.
10. Memish, Z. A., et al., (2020). Middle east respiratory syndrome. *The Lancet.*
11. Fan, W., et al., (2020). In: Holmes, E. C., & Yong-Zhen, Z., (eds.), a new coronavirus associated with human respiratory disease in China. *Nature, 579*(7798), 265–269.
12. Lu, R. Z., & Yang, B. W., (2020). Genomic characterization and epidemiology of 2019 novel Coronavirus: Implications for virus origins and receptor binding. *Lancet, 395*, 565–574.
13. Park, W. B., et al., (2019). Virus isolation from the first patient with SARS-CoV-2 in Korea. *Journal of Korean Medical Science, 35*(7).
14. Hasöksüz, M., Kiliç, S., & Saraç, F., (2020). Coronaviruses and SARS-CoV-2. *Turkish Journal of Medical Sciences, 50*(SI-1), 549–556.

15. Risitano, A. M., et al., (2020). Complement as a target in COVID-19? *Nature Reviews Immunology, 20*(6), 343, 344.
16. Zhong, N., et al., (2003). Epidemiology and cause of severe acute respiratory syndrome (SARS) in Guangdong, people's Republic of China, in February, 2003. *The Lancet, 362*(9393), 1353–1358.
17. Zheng, J., (2020). SARS-CoV-2: An emerging coronavirus that causes a global threat. *International Journal of Biological Sciences, 16*(10), 1678.
18. Carlos, W. G., et al., (2020). Novel Wuhan (2019-nCoV) Coronavirus. *American Journal of Respiratory and Critical Care Medicine, 201*(4), P7.
19. Wang, W., Tang, J., & Wei, F., (2020). Updated understanding of the outbreak of 2019 novel coronavirus (2019-nCoV) in Wuhan, China. *Journal of Medical Virology, 92*(4), 441–447.
20. Organization, W. H., (2020). *Modes of Transmission of Virus Causing COVID-19: Implications for IPC Precaution Recommendations: Scientific Brief.* World Health Organization.
21. Wang, W., et al., (2020). Detection of SARS-CoV-2 in different types of clinical specimens. *JAMA, 323*(18), 1843–1844.
22. Guan, W. J., et al., (2020). Clinical characteristics of coronavirus disease 2019 in China. *New England Journal of Medicine, 382*(18), 1708–1720.
23. Giacomelli, A., et al., (2020). Self-reported olfactory and taste disorders in patients with severe acute respiratory Coronavirus 2 infection: A cross-sectional study. *Clinical Infectious Diseases*.
24. Xu, J., et al., (2020). Use of angiotensin-converting enzyme inhibitors and angiotensin II receptor blockers in context of COVID-19 outbreak: A retrospective analysis. *Frontiers of Medicine, 14*(5), 601–612.
25. Hua, C. Z., et al., (2020). Epidemiological features and viral shedding in children with SARS-CoV-2 infection. *Journal of Medical Virology.*
26. Nishiura, H., et al., (2020). Estimation of the asymptomatic ratio of novel coronavirus infections (COVID-19). *International Journal of Infectious Diseases, 94*, 154.
27. Wu, J. T., et al., (2020). Estimating clinical severity of COVID-19 from the transmission dynamics in Wuhan, China. *Nature Medicine, 26*(4), 506–510.
28. Pan, X., et al., (2020). Asymptomatic cases in a family cluster with SARS-CoV-2 infection. *The Lancet Infectious Diseases, 20*(4), 410–411.
29. Bai, Y., et al., (2020). Presumed asymptomatic carrier transmission of COVID-19. *JAMA, 323*(14), 1406–1407.
30. Savvides, C., & Siegel, R., (2020). *Asymptomatic and Presymptomatic Transmission of SARS-CoV-2: A Systematic Review.* Department of Biomedical Informatics, Stanford University, Stanford, California, USA 2. Department of Microbiology and Immunology, Stanford University, Stanford, California, USA.
31. Qian, G., et al., (2020). COVID-19 transmission within a family cluster by presymptomatic carriers in China. *Clinical Infectious Diseases*.
32. Kimball, A., et al., (2020). Asymptomatic and presymptomatic SARS-CoV-2 infections in residents of a long-term care skilled nursing facility—King County, Washington. *Morbidity and Mortality Weekly Report, 69*(13), 377.
33. Tong, Z. D., et al., (2020). Potential presymptomatic transmission of SARS-CoV-2, Zhejiang province, China, 2020. *Emerging Infectious Diseases, 26*(5), 1052.
34. Young, B. E., et al., (2020). Epidemiologic features and clinical course of patients infected with SARS-CoV-2 in Singapore. *JAMA, 323*(15), 1488–1494.

35. Mizumoto, K., et al., (2020). Estimating the asymptomatic proportion of coronavirus disease 2019 (COVID-19) cases on board the diamond princess cruise ship, Yokohama, Japan. *Euro Surveillance, 25*(10), 2000180.
36. Min, C. O. W., (2020). *Position Statement from the National Centre for Infectious Diseases and the Chapter of Infectious Disease Physicians, Academy of Medicine, Singapore: Period of Infectivity to Inform Strategies for De-isolation for COVID-19 Patients*, 109–112.
37. Lipsitch, M., Swerdlow, D. L., & Finelli, L., (2020). Defining the epidemiology of Covid-19—studies needed. *New England Journal of Medicine, 382*(13), 1194–1196.
38. Bullard, J., et al., (2020). Predicting infectious SARS-CoV-2 from diagnostic samples. *Clinical Infectious Diseases.*
39. Liu, Y., et al., (2020). Viral dynamics in mild and severe cases of COVID-19. *The Lancet Infectious Diseases.*
40. Guo, Y. R., et al., (2020). The origin, transmission and clinical therapies on coronavirus disease 2019 (COVID-19) outbreak-an update on the status. *Military Medical Research, 7*(1), 1–10.
41. Khan, S., Liu, J., & Xue, M., (2020). Transmission of SARS-CoV-2 required developments in research and associated public health concerns. *Frontiers in Medicine, 7*, 310.
42. Organization, W. H. (*2020*). *Transmission of SARS-CoV-2: Implications for Infection Prevention Precautions: Scientific Brief.* World Health Organization.
43. Morawska, L., & Cao, J., (2020). Airborne transmission of SARS-CoV-2: The world should face the reality. *Environment International, 139*, 105730.
44. Edwards, D. A., et al., (2004). Inhaling to mitigate exhaled bioaerosols. *Proceedings of the National Academy of Sciences, 101*(50), 17383–17388.
45. Van, D. N., Lloyd-Smith, J. O., et al., (2020). Aerosol and surface stability of SARS-CoV-2 as compared with SARS-CoV-1. *New England Journal of Medicine.*
46. Pfaender, S., et al., (2020). LY6E impairs coronavirus fusion and confers immune control of viral disease. *Nature Microbiology, 5*(11), 1330–1339.
47. Meselson, M., (2020). Droplets and aerosols in the transmission of SARS-CoV-2. *New England Journal of Medicine.*
48. You, C., et al., (2020). Estimation of the time-varying reproduction number of COVID-19 outbreak in China. *International Journal of Hygiene and Environmental Health, 228*, 113555.
49. Del, R. C., & Malani, P. N., (2020). COVID-19—new insights on a rapidly changing epidemic. *JAMA, 323*(14), 1339–1340.
50. Tu, Y. F., et al., (2020). A review of SARS-CoV-2 and the ongoing clinical trials. *International Journal of Molecular Sciences, 21*(7), 2657.
51. Zhu, N., Zhang, D., & Wang, W., (2020). China novel coronavirus investigating and research team. A novel coronavirus from patients with pneumonia in China 2019. *N. Engl. J. Med.*
52. Gorbalenya, A., et al., (2020). *Coronaviridae* study group of the international committee on taxonomy of viruses. The species severe acute respiratory syndrome-related Coronavirus: Classifying 2019-nCoV and naming it SARS-CoV-2. *Nature Microbiology*, 3, 4.
53. Zhu, N., et al., (2020). A novel coronavirus from patients with pneumonia in China, 2019. *New England Journal of Medicine.*
54. Zhou, P., et al., (2020). A pneumonia outbreak associated with a new coronavirus of probable bat origin. In: Zhang W., Si, H., Zhu, Y., Li, B., Huan, G. C., Chen, H. D., Chen, J., et al., (eds.), *Nature* (Vol. 579, pp. 270–273).

55. Becker, M. M., et al., (2008). Synthetic recombinant bat SARS-like Coronavirus is infectious in cultured cells and in mice. *Proceedings of the National Academy of Sciences, 105*(50), 19944–19949.
56. Hamid, S., Mir, M. Y., & Rohela, G. K., (2020). Noval coronavirus disease (COVID-19): A pandemic (Epidemiology, Pathogenesis and potential therapeutics). *New Microbes and New Infections*, 100679.
57. Jin, Y., et al., (2020). Virology, epidemiology, pathogenesis, and control of COVID-19. *Viruses, 12*(4), 372.
58. Cavanagh, D., (1997). *Nidovirales*: A new order comprising *Coronaviridae* and *Arteriviridae*. *Archives of Virology, 142*(3), 629–633.
59. Isaacs, D., et al., (1983). Epidemiology of coronavirus respiratory infections. *Archives of Disease in Childhood, 58*(7), 500–503.
60. Eickmann, M., et al., (2003). *Phylogeny of the SARS coronavirus. Science, 302*(5650), 1504–1506.
61. Drexler, J. F., et al., (2010). Genomic characterization of severe acute respiratory syndrome-related Coronavirus in European bats and classification of coronaviruses based on partial RNA-dependent RNA polymerase gene sequences. *Journal of Virology, 84*(21), 11336–11349.
62. Zhang, Z., Shen, L., & Gu, X., (2016). Evolutionary dynamics of MERS-CoV: Potential recombination, positive selection and transmission. *Scientific Reports, 6*(1), 1–10.
63. Gao, Y., et al., (2020). Structure of the RNA-dependent RNA polymerase from COVID-19 virus. *Science, 368*(6492), 779–782.
64. Bárcena, M., et al., (2009). Cryo-electron tomography of mouse hepatitis virus: Insights into the structure of the corona virion. *Proceedings of the National Academy of Sciences, 106*(2), 582–587.
65. Neuman, B. W., et al., (2006). Supramolecular architecture of severe acute respiratory syndrome coronavirus revealed by electron cryomicroscopy. *Journal of Virology, 80*(16), 7918–7928.
66. Walls, A. C., et al., (2020). Structure, function, and antigenicity of the SARS-CoV-2 spike glycoprotein. *Cell.*
67. Bergmann, C. C., & Silverman, R. H., (2020). COVID-19: Coronavirus replication, pathogenesis, and therapeutic strategies. *Cleveland Clinic Journal of Medicine.*
68. Kuiken, T., et al., (2003). *Newly Discovered Coronavirus as the Primary Cause of Severe Acute Respiratory Syndrome, 362*(9380), 263–270.
69. Drosten, C., et al., (2003). *Identification of a Novel Coronavirus in Patients with Severe Acute Respiratory Syndrome, 348*(20), 1967–1976.
70. Ng, M., et al., (2003). *Early Events of SARS Coronavirus Infection in Vero Cells, 71*(3), 323–331.
71. Tang, T. K., et al., (2005). *Biochemical and Immunological Studies of Nucleocapsid Proteins of Severe Acute Respiratory Syndrome and 229E Human Coronaviruses, 5*(4), 925–937.
72. Chang, C. K., et al., (2006). *Modular Organization of SARS Coronavirus Nucleocapsid Protein, 13*(1), 59–72.
73. Chang, C. K., et al., (2005). *The Dimer Interface of the SARS Coronavirus Nucleocapsid Protein Adapts a Porcine Respiratory and Reproductive Syndrome Virus-Like Structure, 579*(25), 5663–5668.

74. Yu, I. M., et al., (2006). Crystal structure of the SARS coronavirus nucleocapsid protein dimerization domain reveals evolutionary linkage between corona-and *Arteriviridae*. *Journal of Biological Chemistry, 281*(25), 17134–17139.
75. Weiss, S. R., (2005). Coronavirus pathogenesis and the emerging pathogen severe acute respiratory syndrome coronavirus. In: Navas-Martin, (ed.), *Microbiol. Mol. Biol. Rev.* (Vol. 69, No. 4, pp. 635–664).
76. Chang, C. K., et al., (2006). Modular organization of SARS coronavirus nucleocapsid protein. *Journal of Biomedical Science, 13*(1), 59–72.
77. Hurst, K. R., Koetzner, C. A., & Masters, P. S., (2009). Identification of in vivo-interacting domains of the murine coronavirus nucleocapsid protein. *Journal of Virology, 83*(14), 7221–7234.
78. Stohlman, S. A., & Lai, M., (1979). Phosphoproteins of murine hepatitis viruses. *Journal of Virology, 32*(2), 672–675.
79. Stohlman, S., et al., (1988). Specific interaction between coronavirus leader RNA and nucleocapsid protein. *Journal of Virology, 62*(11), 4288–4295.
80. Molenkamp, R., & Spaan, W. J., (1997). Identification of a specific interaction between the coronavirus mouse hepatitis virus A59 nucleocapsid protein and packaging signal. *Virology, 239*(1), 78–86.
81. Kuo, L., & Masters, P. S., (2013). Functional analysis of the murine coronavirus genomic RNA packaging signal. *Journal of Virology, 87*(9), 5182–5192.
82. Hurst, K. R., Koetzner, C. A., & Masters, P. S., (2013). Characterization of a critical interaction between the coronavirus nucleocapsid protein and nonstructural protein 3 of the viral replicase-transcriptase complex. *Journal of Virology, 87*(16), 9159–9172.
83. Klausegger, A., et al., (1999). Identification of a coronavirus hemagglutinin-esterase with a substrate specificity different from those of influenza C virus and bovine Coronavirus. *Journal of Virology, 73*(5), 3737–3743.
84. Du, L., et al., (2009). The spike protein of SARS-CoV—a target for vaccine and therapeutic development. *Nature Reviews Microbiology, 7*(3), 226–236.
85. Bosch, B. J., et al., (2003). The coronavirus spike protein is a class I virus fusion protein: Structural and functional characterization of the fusion core complex. *Journal of Virology, 77*(16), 8801–8811.
86. Watanabe, Y., et al., (2020). Site-specific glycan analysis of the SARS-CoV-2 spike. *Science, 369*(6501), 330–333.
87. Hoffmann, M., et al., ((2020)). SARS-CoV-2 cell entry depends on ACE2 and TMPRSS2 and is blocked by a clinically proven protease inhibitor. *Cell, 181*(2), 271–280. e8.
88. Alsaadi, E. A., & Jones, I. M., (2019). Membrane binding proteins of coronaviruses. *Future Virology, 14*(4), 275.
89. Armstrong, J., et al., (1984). Sequence and topology of a model intracellular membrane protein, E1 glycoprotein, from a coronavirus. *Nature, 308*(5961), 751, 752.
90. Nal, B., et al., (2005). Differential maturation and subcellular localization of severe acute respiratory syndrome coronavirus surface proteins S, M and E. *Journal of General Virology, 86*(5), 1423–1434.
91. Timani, K. A., et al., (2004). Cloning, sequencing, expression, and purification of SARS-associated coronavirus nucleocapsid protein for serodiagnosis of SARS. *Journal of Clinical Virology, 30*(4), 309–312.
92. Godet, M., et al., (1992). TGEV coronavirus ORF4 encodes a membrane protein that is incorporated into virions. *Virology, 188*(2), 666–675.

93. DeDiego, M. L., et al., (2007). A severe acute respiratory syndrome coronavirus that lacks the E gene is attenuated in vitro and in vivo. *Journal of Virology, 81*(4), 1701–1713.
94. Romano, M., et al., (2020). A structural view of SARS-CoV-2 RNA replication machinery: RNA synthesis, proofreading and final capping. *Cells, 9*(5), 1267.
95. Team, C., (2020). Severe outcomes among patients with coronavirus disease 2019 (COVID-19)-United States. *MMWR Morb. Mortal. Wkly Rep., 69*(12), 343–346.
96. Naqvi, A. A. T., et al., (2020). Insights into SARS-CoV-2 genome, structure, evolution, pathogenesis and therapies: Structural genomics approach. *Biochimica et Biophysica Acta (BBA)-Molecular Basis of Disease*, 165878.
97. Sola, I., et al., (2015). Continuous and discontinuous RNA synthesis in coronaviruses. *Annual Review of Virology, 2*, 265–288.
98. Fehr, A. R., & Perlman, S., (2015). Coronaviruses: An overview of their replication and pathogenesis. In: *Coronaviruses*, (pp. 1–23). Springer.
99. Zhang, Y., (2020). Analysis of epidemiological characteristics of new coronavirus pneumonia. *Chin. J. Epidemiol, 41*(2), 1–7.
100. De Wit, E., et al., (2016). SARS and MERS: Recent insights into emerging coronaviruses. *Nature Reviews Microbiology, 14*(8), 523.
101. Lan, J., et al., (2020). Structure of the SARS-CoV-2 spike receptor-binding domain bound to the ACE2 receptor. *Nature, 581*(7807), 215–220.
102. Dong, N., et al., (2020). *Genomic and Protein Structure Modeling Analysis Depicts the Origin and Infectivity of 2019-nCoV: A New Coronavirus which Caused a Pneumonia Outbreak in Wuhan, China.* BioRxiv.
103. Matsuyama, S., et al., (2020). Enhanced isolation of SARS-CoV-2 by TMPRSS2-expressing cells. *Proceedings of the National Academy of Sciences, 117*(13), 7001–7003.
104. Zhang, H., et al., (2020). Angiotensin-converting enzyme 2 (ACE2) as a SARS-CoV-2 receptor: Molecular mechanisms and potential therapeutic target. *Intensive Care Medicine, 46*(4), 586–590.
105. Letko, M., Marzi, A., & Munster, V., (2020). Functional assessment of cell entry and receptor usage for SARS-CoV-2 and other lineage B beta coronaviruses. *Nature Microbiology,* 5(4), 562–569.
106. Monteil, V., et al., (2020). Inhibition of SARS-CoV-2 infections in engineered human tissues using clinical-grade soluble human ACE2. *Cell.*
107. Hofmann, H., & Pöhlmann, S., (2004). Cellular entry of the SARS coronavirus. *Trends in Microbiology, 12*(10), 466–472.
108. Rothan, H. A., & Byrareddy, S. N., (2020). The epidemiology and pathogenesis of coronavirus disease (COVID-19) outbreak. *Journal of Autoimmunity*, 102433.
109. Li, X., et al., (2020). Molecular immune pathogenesis and diagnosis of COVID-19. *Journal of Pharmaceutical Analysis.*
110. Mason, R. J., (2020). Pathogenesis of COVID-19 from a cell biology perspective. *Eur. Respiratory Soc.*
111. Tang, N. L. S., et al., (2005). Early enhanced expression of interferon-inducible protein-10 (CXCL-10) and other chemokines predicts adverse outcome in severe acute respiratory syndrome. *Clinical Chemistry, 51*(12), 2333–2340.
112. Wu, Z., & McGoogan, J. M., (2020). Characteristics of and important lessons from the coronavirus disease 2019 (COVID-19) outbreak in China: Summary of a report of 72 314 cases from the Chinese Center for Disease Control and Prevention. *JAMA, 323*(13), 1239–1242.

113. Mossel, E. C., et al., (2008). SARS-CoV replicates in primary human alveolar type II cell cultures but not in type I-like cells. *Virology, 372*(1), 127–135.
114. Cao, W., & Li, T., (2020). COVID-19: Towards understanding of pathogenesis. *Cell Research, 30*(5), 367–369.
115. Pirofski, L. A., & Casadevall, A., (2020). Pathogenesis of COVID-19 from the perspective of the damage-response framework. *Mbio, 11*(4).
116. Yang, X., et al., (2020). Clinical course and outcomes of critically ill patients with SARS-CoV-2 pneumonia in Wuhan, China: A single-centered, retrospective, observational study. *The Lancet Respiratory Medicine.*
117. Liu, T., et al., (2020). *Transmission Dynamics of 2019 Novel Coronavirus (2019-nCoV)*, 187–190.
118. Chen, Y., Liu, Q., & Guo, D., (2020). Emerging coronaviruses: Genome structure, replication, and pathogenesis. *Journal of Medical Virology, 92*(4), 418–423.
119. Chen, N., et al., (2020). Epidemiological and clinical characteristics of 99 cases of 2019 novel coronavirus pneumonia in Wuhan, China: A descriptive study. *The Lancet, 395*(10223), 507–513.
120. Prabakaran, S., et al., (2004). Mitochondrial dysfunction in schizophrenia: Evidence for compromised brain metabolism and oxidative stress. *Molecular Psychiatry, 9*(7), 684–697.
121. Gurwitz, D., (2020). Angiotensin receptor blockers as tentative SARS-CoV-2 therapeutics. *Drug Development Research, 81*(5), 537–540.
122. Sheahan, T. P., et al., (2017). Broad-spectrum antiviral GS-5734 inhibits both epidemic and zoonotic coronaviruses. *Science Translational Medicine,* 9(396).
123. Hou, Y. J., et al., (2020) SARS-CoV-2 reverse genetics reveals a variable infection gradient in the respiratory tract. *Cell, 182*(2), 429–446. e14.
124. Cascella, M., et al., (2020). *Features, Evaluation and Treatment Coronavirus (COVID-19)*. Statpearls [internet].
125. Mousavizadeh, L., & Ghasemi, S., (2020). Genotype and phenotype of COVID-19: Their roles in pathogenesis. *Journal of Microbiology, Immunology, and Infection.*
126. Liang, W., et al., (2020). Cancer patients in SARS-CoV-2 infection: A nationwide analysis in China. *The Lancet Oncology, 21*(3), 335–337.
127. Iwata-Yoshikawa, N., et al., (2019). TMPRSS2 contributes to virus spread and immunopathology in the airways of murine models after coronavirus infection. *Journal of Virology, 93*(6).
128. Pedersen, S. F., & Ho, Y. C., (2020). SARS-CoV-2: A storm is raging. *The Journal of Clinical Investigation, 130*(5).
129. Thompson, B. T., Chambers, R. C., & Liu, K. D., (2017). Acute respiratory distress syndrome. *New England Journal of Medicine, 377*(6), 562–572.
130. Lipworth, B., et al., (2020). Weathering the cytokine storm in susceptible patients with severe SARS-CoV-2 infection. *The Journal of Allergy and Clinical Immunology: In Practice, 8*(6), 1798–1801.
131. Ng, O. W., et al., (2016). Memory T cell responses targeting the SARS coronavirus persist up to 11 years post-infection. *Vaccine, 34*(17), 2008–2014.
132. Mikkelsen, M. E., et al., (2013). The epidemiology of acute respiratory distress syndrome in patients presenting to the emergency department with severe sepsis. *Shock (Augusta, Ga.), 40*(5), 375.
133. Yazdanpanah, F., Hamblin, M. R., & Rezaei, N., (2020). The immune system and COVID-19: Friend or foe? *Life Sciences*, 117900.

134. Chowdhury, R., et al., (2020). Dynamic interventions to control COVID-19 pandemic: A multivariate prediction modelling study comparing 16 worldwide countries. *European Journal of Epidemiology, 35*(5), 389–399.
135. Paces, J., et al., (2020). COVID-19 and the immune system. *Physiological Research, 69*(3).
136. Hung, H. C., et al., (2020). Discovery of M protease inhibitors encoded by SARS-CoV-*2. Antimicrobial Agents and Chemotherapy, 64*(9).
137. Catanzaro, M., et al., (2020). Immune response in COVID-19: Addressing a pharmacological challenge by targeting pathways triggered by SARS-CoV-2. *Signal Transduction and Targeted Therapy, 5*(1), 1–10.
138. Hu, Z., et al., (2020). Clinical characteristics of 24 asymptomatic infections with COVID-19 screened among close contacts in Nanjing, China. *Science China Life Sciences, 63*(5), 706–711.
139. Wan, Y., et al., (2020). Receptor recognition by the novel Coronavirus from Wuhan: An analysis based on decade-long structural studies of SARS coronavirus. *Journal of Virology, 94*(7).
140. Shahrajabian, M. H., et al., (2020). Chinese herbal medicine for SARS and SARS-CoV-2 treatment and prevention, encouraging using herbal medicine for COVID-19 outbreak. *Acta Agriculturae Scandinavica, Section B—Soil & Plant Science, 70*(5), 437–443.
141. Mahallawi, W. H., et al., (2018). MERS-CoV infection in humans is associated with a pro-inflammatory Th1 and Th17 cytokine profile. *Cytokine, 104*, 8–13.
142. Lee, N., et al., (2004). Effects of early corticosteroid treatment on plasma SARS-associated Coronavirus RNA concentrations in adult patients. *Journal of Clinical Virology, 31*(4), 304–309.
143. Cockrell, A. S., et al., (2014). Mouse dipeptidyl peptidase 4 is not a functional receptor for Middle East respiratory syndrome coronavirus infection. *Journal of Virology, 88*(9), 5195–5199.
144. Lu, R., et al., (2020). Genomic characterization and epidemiology of 2019 novel Coronavirus: Implications for virus origins and receptor binding. *The Lancet, 395*(10224), 565–574.
145. Zia-Ul-Haq, M., et al., (2021). *Alternative Medicine Interventions for COVID-19* (Vol. XII, p. 284). Springer, Cham: Springer Nature Switzerland AG.
146. Zia-Ul-Haq, M., Dewanjee, S., & Riaz, M., (2021). *Carotenoids: Structure and Function in the Human Body* (Vol. XVI, p. 859) Springer Nature Switzerland AG: Springer International Publishing.
147. Celularity, I., (2020). *Celularity Announces FDA Clearance of IND Application for CYNK-001 in Coronavirus, First in Cellular Therapy*, 85, 86.
148. Graham, R. L., Donaldson, E. F., & Baric, R. S., (2013). A decade after SARS: Strategies for controlling emerging coronaviruses. *Nature Reviews Microbiology, 11*(12), 836–848.
149. Qu, H., Ricklin, D., & Lambris, J. D., (2009). Recent developments in low molecular weight complement inhibitors. *Molecular Immunology, 47*(2, 3), 185–195.
150. Nascimento, I., & Leite, L., (2012). Recombinant vaccines and the development of new vaccine strategies. *Brazilian Journal of Medical and Biological Research, 45*(12), 1102–1111.
151. Welliver, R., et al., (2001). Effectiveness of oseltamivir in preventing influenza in household contacts: A randomized controlled trial. *JAMA, 285*(6), 748–754.
152. Mair-Jenkins, J., et al., (2015). The effectiveness of convalescent plasma and hyperimmune immunoglobulin for the treatment of severe acute respiratory infections of viral etiology: A systematic review and exploratory meta-analysis. *The Journal of Infectious Diseases, 211*(1), 80–90.

153. Koenig, K. L., (2015). Identify-isolate-inform: A modified tool for initial detection and management of middle east respiratory syndrome patients in the emergency department. *Western Journal of Emergency Medicine, 16*(5), 619.
154. Zhang, L., & Liu, Y., (2020*)*. Potential interventions for novel Coronavirus in China: A systematic review. *Journal of Medical Virology, 92*(5), 479–490.
155. Hamming, I., et al., (2004). Tissue distribution of ACE2 protein, the functional receptor for SARS coronavirus. A first step in understanding SARS pathogenesis. *The Journal of Pathology: A Journal of the Pathological Society of Great Britain and Ireland, 203*(2), 631–637.
156. Jia, H. P., et al., (2005). ACE2 receptor expression and severe acute respiratory syndrome coronavirus infection depend on the differentiation of human airway epithelia. *Journal of Virology, 79*(23), 14614–14621.
157. Cattani, M., (2020). Global coalition to accelerate COVID-19 clinical research in resource-limited settings. *Lancet, 395*(10233), P1322–P1325.
158. Harrison, E. A., & Wu, J. W., (2020). Vaccine confidence in the time of COVID-19. *European Journal of Epidemiology, 35*(4), 325–330.
159. Caly, L., et al., (2020). The FDA-approved drug ivermectin inhibits the replication of SARS-CoV-2 in vitro. *Antiviral Research, 178*, 104787.
160. Wraith, D. C., (2017). The future of immunotherapy: A 20-year perspective. *Frontiers in Immunology, 8*, 1668.
161. Fan, J., et al., (2020). Epidemiology of coronavirus disease in Gansu province, China. *Emerging Infectious Diseases, 26*(6), 1257–1265.
162. Chan, J. F. W., et al., (2020). A familial cluster of pneumonia associated with the 2019 novel coronavirus indicating person-to-person transmission: A study of a family cluster. *The Lancet, 395*(10223), 514–523.
163. Wu, P., et al., (2020) Characteristics of ocular findings of patients with Coronavirus disease 2019 (COVID-19) in Hubei Province, China [published online ahead of print March 31, 2020]. *JAMA Ophthalmol.*
164. Yeo, C., Kaushal, S., & Yeo, D., (2020). Enteric involvement of coronaviruses: Is faecal-oral transmission of SARS-CoV-2 possible? *The Lancet Gastroenterology & Hepatology, 5*(4), 335–337.

CHAPTER 2

Epidemiology and Pathogenesis of COVID-19

SIDRAH TARIQ KHAN and SAGHEER AHMED

Shifa College of Pharmaceutical Sciences, Shifa Tameer-e-Millat University, Islamabad, Pakistan, E-mail: sagheer.scps@stmu.edu.pk (S. Ahmed)

ABSTRACT

As soon as the first case of COVID-19 was reported in China in December 2019, it spread throughout the entire country within a matter of a few weeks and soon after to other countries like Italy, the United States, and Germany. This high pace of its spread is attributed to its mode of transmission, which is through respiratory droplets of an infected individual from where the virus spreads person to person, either directly by being in contact or through contaminated surfaces/fomites. Moreover, intra-country traveling has also been a major role player in the spread of this virus. Everyone can be infected by the virus, but some people show more symptoms than others, especially the elderly, males, and people with certain blood groups and co-morbid conditions. The virus enters the human body and primarily infects lung cells, where it binds through its S protein to a host cellular receptor known as the ACE-2 or angiotensin-converting enzyme-2. The genome of the virus was sequenced quickly after its isolation and millions of complete and partial genome sequences are now available. Although a number of vaccines have been developed recently, there is not enough evidence if it will completely cure the disease. The research community is working hard, utilizing the biochemical, pathophysiological, and genomic information to develop safe and effective drugs and vaccines in order to overcome this deadly pandemic.

2.1 INTRODUCTION

The entire world's focus since 2020 has been on the novel coronavirus. In order to eradicate this pandemic, scientists all over the world have put all their effort into developing vaccines effective against this virus. But before going into vaccines and drugs, it is crucial to understand what the virus is, where it comes from and how it transmits. Initially, when the virus spread, a number of individuals exhibiting symptoms closely related to those seen in pneumonia patients, in the city of Wuhan, China. Due to recent advances in the fields of science and technology, sequencing results were quickly obtained showing that the symptoms were caused by a new strain of coronavirus and in much less time, scientists had sequenced the virus's entire genome to decipher its structural and functional components after which, owing to its similarities with the 2002–2003 SARS coronavirus. The international committee on taxonomy of viruses (ICTV) officially gave the virus it is now known name; SARS-CoV-2.

To ascertain the origins of the virus, contact tracing was carried out, after which the Center of Disease Control found that the virus may have originated from a wholesale seafood market in Huanan, Wuhan, where a variety of wild animals were also sold. Fortunately, studies from previous coronavirus outbreaks such as the SARS outbreak in 2002–2003 and the MERS 2012 has given us some insight as to how the virus spreads and what kind of symptoms the viruses from this family can cause. Generally, coronaviruses (CoVs) attack the respiratory airways of the host causing symptoms resembling those of pneumonia and lymphopenia, i.e., shortness of breath, coughing, fever, fatigue, and muscle pain and because the virus grows in the respiratory tract of the host, it transmits through the respiratory droplets of the infected person. These droplets can be acquired by a healthy person either by being in direct contact with the infected person, i.e., within a 1-meter distance or indirectly through contaminated fomites. Clinical trials for vaccines have been fast tracked and are being given top priority in 2020. Management of disease includes prevention through face masks and social distancing, early detection through PCR and antibody tests and antiviral therapy. However, at the moment, doctors are mostly aiming to reduce disease severity via symptom control.

2.2 EPIDEMIOLOGY

In December 2019, a considerable number of individuals in a city inside Hubei, China, presented with a viral infection of unknown etiology and their symptoms resembled that of a severe pneumonia infection. The origin of this novel infection was traced back to a seafood market (Huanan seafood market), that sold all manners of wild animals. All the early patients presenting with the infection visited this market within a period of the past 2–14 days. Upon isolation and identification, it was found that the pathogen infecting these people was a novel strain of a virus belonging to a family of viruses called the CoVs that typically cause respiratory illnesses in their hosts. The virus possesses much resemblance to the previous viruses; middle east respiratory syndrome virus (MERS-CoV) and severe acute respiratory syndrome virus (SARS-CoV) which fall under the same family of viruses. SARS-CoV-2 is a beta-coronavirus of the family Coronaviridae (order Nidovirales) and the viruses from this family typically cause respiratory infections in humans and mammals. Using Bayesian statistical tools, it was found that the virus was introduced into humans approximately on the day of 13th December 2019 (CI 95%), and by day 7, the viral population had doubled (CI 95%). On January 12th 2020, the WHO named the virus 2019-nCoV (n for novel) and later, on 11th February 2020, the ICTV officially named this novel coronavirus 'SARS-CoV-2.' Much like the SARS virus from 2002, SARS-COV-2 too is a zoonotic virus and is thought to have been originated from bats (that are frequently sold at the Huanan Seafood market). However, the evidence on that is not entirely conclusive.

The first fatality due to COVID-19 in China transpired on the 11th of January 2020. After Wuhan, the virus quickly spread to other countries such as Thailand (first case outside China reported (January 13th), Italy, UK, Spain, Iran, France, and USA. On January 23rd, travel restrictions were imposed on citizens of Wuhan where entry and exit from the city were banned [1], but reports of confirmed COVID-19 cases had already started flowing in from other parts of the country and later, similar restrictions were imposed worldwide. However, these restrictions alone did not help, and most governments were unable to control it completely. The WHO on 30th January 202 declared these events as a Public Health Emergency of International Concern (PHEIC) and a little later, a global health emergency (GHE) on 11th March 2020, which is when the world had become witness to the catastrophic effects of SARS-CoV-2. By April 23rd, 2020, the virus had reached 2,649,680 confirmed and 1,743,688 active cases, respectively, and the overall fatalities were estimated to be 184,643 people.

Initial data from the city of Wuhan suggested that 73% of the infected individuals were male, and 32% had some sort of co-morbid disease such as mainly diabetes and hypertension. The median age of all patients was found to be over 50 years, showing that males of ages around 50 and above with underlying co-morbidities were amongst the most vulnerable group of people [2]. This was evident from another report involving 425 confirmed COVID-19 cases with the average age of 59 years and of which 56% were of the male gender. Average period of incubation of the virus is estimated to be 5.2 days (CI= 95%, 4.1 to 7.0), with the 95th percentile of the distribution at 12.5 days. Every 7.4 days, the pandemic doubled in magnitude in the earlier stages [3].

The most important mode of transmission is through respiratory droplets of an infected individual from where the virus spreads person to person, either directly by being in contact or through contaminated surfaces/fomites. After entering host cells, the virus incubates for a period of 2–14 days, during which times it migrates to the lower respiratory tract and causes serious lung damage. Symptoms include fever, myalgia, fatigue, cough, dyspnea, headaches, and diarrhea, etc. The virus causes different symptoms in different people with different genders, genetics, and different health conditions [2]. At first, it was believed that the virus only causes disease in adults, i.e., adults were more susceptible to severe illness, however recent studies have shown us that the virus affects individuals from all age groups. However, due to several unconfirmed reasons, different individuals react differently to the virus and on April 26th, 2020, reports started originated from the UK of a serious inflammatory syndrome now called Pediatric Multi-System Inflammatory Syndrome (PMIS) which was shown to be closely related to the pediatric Kawasaki Disease, in its symptoms which included fever, hypotension, multiple organ involvement and high levels of severe inflammation. Most of these individuals were also infected with SARS-CoV-2, however not all patients showed respiratory symptoms [4].

The United States as of now has been most severely hit by the pandemic with 31 million cases and over 572,000 fatalities [5] and as of April 8th, 2021 with over 133 million cases confirmed to have COVID-19 and over 2.9 million deaths have been confirmed [6].

2.3 CONTRIBUTIONS OF TRAVEL

COVID-19 is a virus capable of spreading at an exponential rate due to being aerosol and because the virus incubates for 2–14 days before it really starts showing symptoms. Early detection can only be possible if tests are performed on every single individual. But since the virus was a mystery in December 2019, nobody had predicted what devastating effects the virus will have in the near future and how quickly it would spread. It is no doubt that travel restrictions would have had a greater impact had they been imposed early on, but something like this is not possible to achieve before there is evidence of local transmission within the country. The local transmission of the virus was only established between January 1st and January 8th 2020 in China and it was on the 8th of January 2020 when the cause of this mysterious pneumonia like disease was credited to a novel coronavirus and still its mode of transmission was not yet established. Soon after discovering SARS-CoV-2, Thailand reported the first case of COVID-19 infection on January 13th, making it the first infection to have been reported away from China. On 15th January 2020, another case emerged from Japan, and on the 20th January, another one from Korea and all cases had been imported from Wuhan, China. USA reported its first infection on 20th January 2020 from Washington, a man in his mid-30s who had just visited the city of Wuhan recently.

When reports from across the world started emerging, the Chinese authorities, on January 23rd 2020 placed Wuhan under strict quarantine and shortly after on the 31st of January the United States government imposed a ban on any US national returning from China to enter the US. On February 19th cases started emerging in Iran, and on the 21st, the Italy devastation began, followed by Spain on 3rd March 2020. When the cases in Italy began to spike, the government imposed a lockdown across the entire country on 8th March 2020, soon after which COVID-19 was declared a GHE, after which on March 11th US government banned travel from 26 European countries to the US. By April 2nd, 2020, COVID-19 had affected 1 million people across the globe and the death toll was at 100,000. On April 24th, 2020, the virus reached Brazil, in May 2020, COVID-19 had spread across all 7 continents, and by September 2020, there were over 1 million deaths across the globe [7]. This trajectory of COVID-19 transmission from country to country could not have been foreseen in early December, 2019. By the time we knew more about the virus, about its relatively facile mode of transmission, Wuhan residents had already traveled to other cities and also the world, and only little could have been done to contain it (Figure 2.1).

2.4 TRANSMISSION

The reason why COVID-19 became a pandemic was due to its mode of transmission. We know through evidence that this virus spreads between individuals via direct or indirect contact with respiratory droplets of an infected patient. These respiratory droplets generally range from 5–10 μm and can traverse up to a 1-meter distance and recent studies have also shown that viable infected droplets may also remain suspended in air for up to a period of 3 hours. Droplets are let out when an infected person speaks, coughs or even sneezes at anyone standing within a 1-meter distance. The respiratory droplets can also fall onto surfaces such as stainless steel, cloth, and plastic, etc., and anyone who touches contaminated surfaces is at a very high risk of getting infected, especially if they touch their mucous membranes such as the nose, mouth, and eyes afterwards.

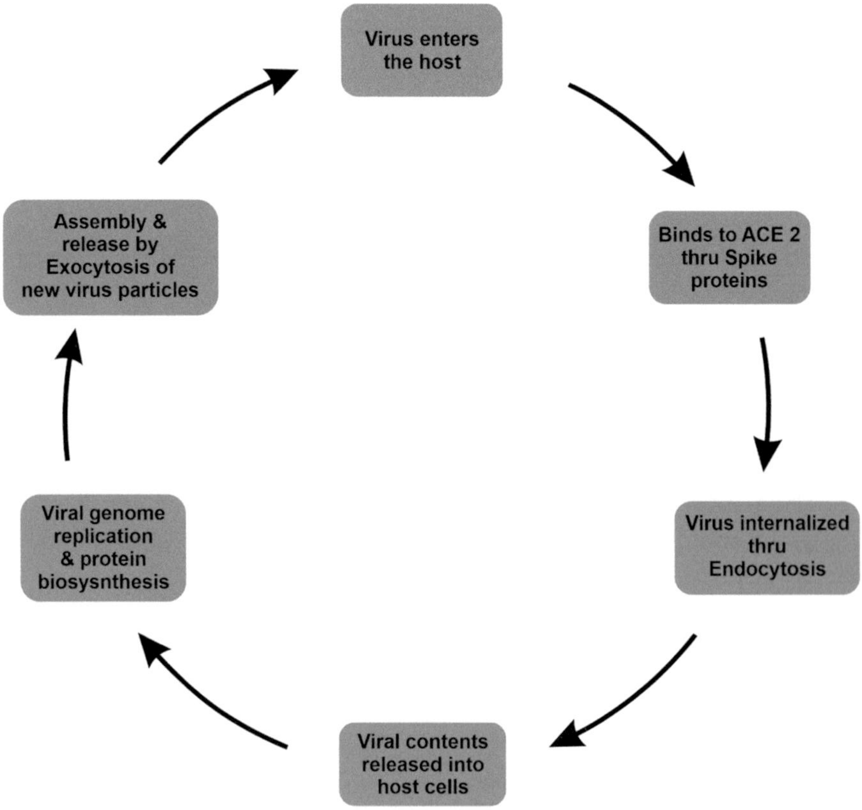

FIGURE 2.1 Flow diagram showing viral entry and important host interactions.

Airborne transmission occurs when the contaminants are present inside a droplet that is < 5 μm in size, and these droplets are capable of traversing distances greater than 1 meter and remain floating in air for certain time spans. Transmission of SARS-CoV-2 through air possibly occurs during certain aerosol-generating medical procedures such as manual ventilation, endotracheal intubation, bronchoscopy, tracheotomy, and CPR (cardiopulmonary resuscitation). Studies have also been carried out to test the possible airborne transmission of COVID-19 via normal speech, but these investigations have not been validated. Other studies suggest that the respiratory particle emission during normal speech varies from person to person, i.e., a high amplitude of vocalization generally results in higher particle emission. However, the relativeness of these findings to COVID-19 requires further research. Moreover, the possibility of aerosol transmission mostly arises during prolonged exposure in closed gatherings such as gyms, indoor areas without proper ventilation and restaurants, etc. In these areas, transmission through respiratory droplets and contaminated surfaces also becomes possible, resulting in a large number of people getting infected by the virus [8].

Although stool samples of some patients have shown to contain viable viral agents, the WHO has not considered the fecal-oral route as an important factor in transmission. Moreover, there have been no reports suggestive of sexual transmission, However, there have been some reports where serum samples of newborn infants have shown levels of IgM antibodies against SARS-CoV-2 because of which fetal transmission has not been completely ruled out but requires further evidence. There have also been reports suggesting asymptomatic transmission of COVID-19 is possible, and patients who have recovered from the disease may still be able to transmit the virus to other people while being symptom free themselves.

2.5 SIGNS AND SYMPTOMS

Signs and symptoms of coronavirus do not manifest immediately but after an incubation period of anywhere between 2–14 days, during which time the infected person is asymptomatic, i.e., a person can get infected and still be unaware of it during the incubation period. Common symptoms that are shown in most, if not all, patients are as follows: high temperature (fever), continuous cough, mostly dry, fatigue, loss of smell, shortness of breath, sore throat. Other symptoms that have been observed are myalgia, chills, flu, headache, chest pain, conjunctivitis, and severe diarrhea.

Still, these symptoms of COVID-19 are not conclusive. Newer studies are revealing more symptoms and newer risk factors. However, certain symptoms are more alarming and require emergency medical attention, these include: confusion, troubled breathing, pain in the chest, loss of focus, hypersomnia, and bluish lips/nails [9].

2.6 PATHOGENESIS

The CoVs are enveloped and positively charged single-stranded RNA based viruses of zoonotic origins. The viruses are much larger in size and range from about 26–32 kb. They are also frequently the reason behind a number of respiratory diseases, much like those seen in the 2002–2003 SARS and the 2012 MERS outbreaks. In fact, according to sequencing results, SARS-CoV-2 does belong to the same subgroup of CoVs that also contains the 2002–2003 SARS virus and several other bat CoVs, although it is much more similar to the SARS virus and is only distantly similar to the MERS virus, its closest resemblance is to 2 bat CoVs. Moreover, sequencing results have also suggested bats and pangolins as the primary source of the virus from where it was spread to humans, but it is unclear whether it originated in the bats or if they were only an intermediate host. As for most CoVs, studies have shown lungs to be the main tropism of this virus as well, i.e., SARS-CoV-2 targets the host respiratory cells, particularly the alveolar epithelial type 2 cells, alveolar macrophages and the vascular endothelial cells that also serve as an entry gateway for SARS-CoV-2 due to the high expression of the ACE-2 receptors in these cells. Moreover, it is important to note that, as with many other mammalian species, human beings also have an abundance of ACE-2 receptors in the intestinal tract, which could be the reason behind diarrhea experienced by many COVID-19 patients.

The four structural proteins that make up the CoVs are the Spike Proteins (S1 and S2), nucleocapsid proteins, membrane proteins and envelop proteins. These viruses use the S1 spike proteins to attach themselves to the host cellular receptor ACE-2 and the S2 spike protein to fuse themselves to cellular membranes in order to penetrate inside the host cells. The spike proteins on this virus are of particular importance. These proteins give the virus its unique crown shape and range in size from 9–12 nm. The S1 spike protein has further been divided into A, B, and C domains. The SARS-Cov-2 virus mainly utilizes the S1 B domain to gain entry into the host cell. Apart from the structural proteins, 2/3rd of the total open reading frames (ORFs) comprises of the non-structural proteins (replicase complex, nsp 1–16) responsible for replication and transcription, and the remaining consists of accessory proteins. These together comprise the functional proteins of the SARS-CoV-2 virus (Figure 2.2).

SARS-CoV-2 has shown certain alterations in S1 spike protein RBD which along with the existence of a unique polybasic furin cleavage site (present at the fusion site of both spike protein subunits) and O-linked glycans, which reflect in its much higher binding affinity towards the ACE-2

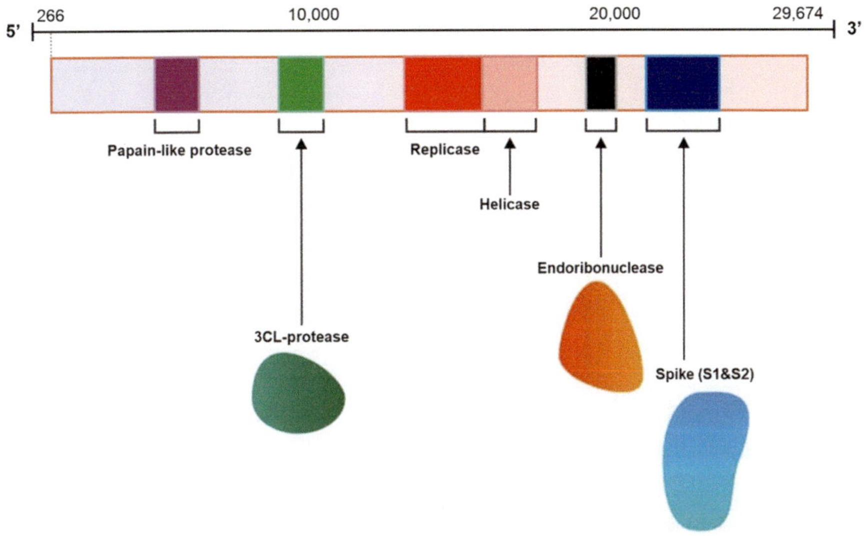

FIGURE 2.2 SARS-COV-2 genomic organization.

receptor in the human lung epithelial cells than its predecessors, giving it a much smoother entry into the host cell and a much greater ability to infect the upper respiratory tract in human beings. The binding between the S1 proteins and the ACE-2 receptor is mediated by Vander Waal forces and the entire process of entry into the host cell occurs in two steps; the initial priming is mediated via the transmembrane protease serine 2 (TMPRSS2) and cathepsin L also present in the lung epithelial cells and is involved in the cleavage of the enzyme ACE-2 followed by cleavage within S2 protein that leads conformational changes in the spike protein resulting in its activation which results in fusion with the host alveolar epithelial type 2 cell membrane via the S2 subunit of the spike protein. The virus then enters inside the host cell by the process of endocytosis. After gaining entry inside the host cells, nucleocapsid releases its cellular contents inside the host cells and initiates cellular replication; the viral open reading frames types a and b, are converted to replicate proteins which in turn with the help of protease enzymes are spliced into non-structural proteins, nsp12 which is formed via this mechanism from open reading frame type a and is also responsible for the formation of RNA dependent RNA polymerases. The replicase proteins formed during this process are also responsible for repositioning of the host cell's endoplasmic reticulum converting it into vesicles with double membranes that later aid in the replication process. Once that process is complete, the cell membrane of the host is ruptured to release viral content into the extracellular spaces to infect other cells.

2.7 COMMON HOST RESPONSES

Studying host responses when it comes to viruses becomes especially important when trying to find effective treatments. In order to control the pandemic, it is crucial to understand how human beings react to this virus. We now know that SARS-CoV-2 causes a more severe disease in the elderly than those of young age and in people with pre-existing co-morbidities such as cardiac diseases, respiratory diseases, diabetes, HIV infections and those receiving immune-suppressant therapy. We also know that the once the virus gains entry into the host cells, it carries out incubation for somewhere between 2 days to 2 weeks, replicating in the upper respiratory tract, before it causes symptomatic infection. Once it travels to the lower parts of the respiratory tract, it triggers a highly profound immune response that leads to a 'cytokine storm in patients who then start exhibiting more severe symptoms such as Acute Respiratory Distress Syndrome (ARDS), pulmonary edema and most severely multiorgan dysfunction and, death. However, the most commonly occurring symptoms in these patients are; dry cough, high fever and extreme myalgia and fatigue. Some patients have also exhibited chest pain, diarrhea, sore throat, nausea, headaches, chills, ageusia, and anosmia.

The mechanism of host response is as follows: Once the virus gains entry into the human body, the first thing the body does is: recognize the invader. Our immune cells have evolved to use certain receptors that are equipped to recognize pathogens. These are known as the pathogen recognition receptors (PRR). Toll-like receptors (TLR) belong to this class and perform the function of identifying pathogen associated molecular patterns (PAMP) on the virus and promote the relevant immune response, in this case, production of interferons. Studies on previous CoVs have shown us that the B-cell antibody response during a coronavirus infection occurs much earlier for the smaller (but more immunogenic) N-protein than the S-protein where the response is seen after 4–8 days of symptom onset. This could be due to the absence of glycosylation sites on the N-protein making it an easier target for neutralization.

The humoral immunity response, i.e., production of immunoglobulins IgG and IgM, in the case of this virus has much similarity to the immune responses in other CoVs. At different time intervals, patients show different levels of immunoglobulins where IgG levels are detected 14 days after symptoms onset and also persist the longest, whereas IgA and IgM levels rise after 5 days of symptom onset and the latter shows a decreasing pattern after a period of 3 months. Moreover, severe morbidity and mortality has been attributed to a strong IgG response in patients as compared to weaker responders for IgG, where high viral clearance was observed [10]. A study was carried out on COVID-19 patients to observe the different levels of antibodies produced after infection. Results showed a presence of Anti-N IgG along with anti-S-RBD IgM in 15 out of the total 16 patients, 14 patients showed presence of anti-N IgM, whereas all 16 patients had anti-S-RBD IgG present [11].

Other cells released in the event of a viral infection include inflammatory cytokines; TNF-α, IL-6, 2, and 10, IFN-α/-γ, Granulocyte-macrophage colony-stimulating factor (GM-CSF), monocyte chemotactic protein 3 (MCP3), macrophage inflammatory protein 1-α (MIP 1 α), which have shown enhanced levels after infection with a coronavirus leading to the migration of inflammatory cells in the lungs resulting in ARDS which has a high mortality rate especially in critical patients. Along with cytokines, increased levels of chemokines such as CCL2/MCP1, interferon gamma-induced protein *10* (IP-10), CXCL1 as well as CXCL5 have also been observed. One study carried out a transcriptomic analysis on infected peripheral blood mononuclear cells (PBMCs) and infected cells from the patient's bronchoalveolar lavage fluid (BALF) to ascertain host responses. The results showed an upregulation of inflammatory cytokines such as CCL2, CXCL2, CCL8, CXCL1, IL33, CCL3L1 in the BALF and CXCL10, TNFSF10, TIMP1, C5, IL18, AREG, NRG1, IL10 in the PBMCs which led to a cytokine storm in patients causing severe inflammation in the lungs. Moreover, further analysis also revealed activated apoptotic and P53 signaling pathways that could be the reason behind the lymphopenia seen in many severely ill COVID-19 patients [12].

2.8 DIFFERENTIAL HOST RESPONSES

We know that different people react differently to SARS-CoV-2, the elderly (age > 65 years) are generally more susceptible to severe disease, and children and younger people mostly experience milder symptoms. However, to say that only the aged population is at risk would be false. The underlying reason for this variability in disease response could be anything from genetics to underlying diseases, making it extremely important to study host and viral genetics. A large amount of research is being carried out to pinpoint genetic factors that are playing a pivotal role in COVID-19 related disease susceptibility, severity, and treatment responses.

2.8.1 MALE SUSCEPTIBILITY

Differences in biological sex are known to be an important factor when it comes to disease susceptibility, immune responses, and clinical outcomes, etc., which could be due to their underlying differences in the sex-determining chromosomes, in reproductive organs or in their distinct sex-related hormones such as estrogen and testosterone. With COVID-19, it is becoming increasingly important to study the effects of gender differences on disease outcomes as there had been numerous reports placing males at a heightened risk of severe morbidity and mortality, which is consistent with what we have seen in other coronavirus outbreaks (SARS, MERS).

A study was carried out on 41 confirmed COVID-19 patients in Wuhan, China, shortly after the outbreak had begun. Out of the 41 cases, 30 (73%) patients were identified as males [2]. Moreover, case by case deaths occurring due to COVID-19 were analyzed across 38 countries and reports showed that, in the case of women, the case fatality rate (CFR) was 1.7 times lower than that of men ($P<0.0001$) female CFR 4.4 (95% CI 3.4–5.5)); (male CFR 7.3 (95% CI 5.4–9.2)) [13]. These findings are consistent with other reports on gender-associated disease severity. The prevalence of male gender-associated fatality in COVID-19 is also coherent with findings from the previous SARS and MERS outbreaks.

These differences could be due to the different genetics or due to the lifestyles/underlying co-morbidities. Studies carried out on mice models to determine the fatality rates between males and females attributed the high fatality rate in men to the steroid hormones (testosterone, etc.), which along with other epigenetic and chromosomal differences in males and females can result in a contrasting immune response to COVID-19. Further studies are also being carried out to determine whether the sex-specific gene regulation of ACE-2 enzyme and the transmembrane serine protease 2 (regulated by androgen receptor signaling) are important contributors to the higher mortality rate in men [14]. As to the reason why women are spared from such serious illness, it could be due to the extra X chromosome that provides protection and is also a significant role-player in the development of both types of immunity [15].

2.8.2 ABO BLOOD GROUP

There had also been an increase in reports of association of the ABO blood type with disease susceptibility and severity. Several studies had been carried out to investigate these findings, but the results showed conflicting patterns. A meta-analysis on 4 studies comprising of a total of 139 128 participants against 135 940 controls showed prevalence of type A blood group across infected patients at 36.22%, 29.67% for type O, 24.99% for type B and 9.29% for AB. The frequency of the blood types associated with death in COVID-19 patients was 40% for type A, 29% for type O, 23% for type B and 8% for type AB suggesting that people with type A blood groups are at a partial risk of contracting COVID-19 whereas those with type O blood groups had a protective advantage. The statistical results for the association of type B and type AB blood types with COVID-19 infections were concluded to be insignificant [16]. Moreover, the CFRs for type A blood group patients were also significantly higher (OR 1·482; P = 0·008), than those with type O blood group, connecting type O to a much lower risk of death than the other blood types (OR 0·660; P =0·014). Although these findings are not conclusive, there are previous reports for diseases such as malaria that have shown an association between infectivity, severity of disease and the blood group systems [17]. However, findings such as these require further evidence.

2.8.3 DIFFERENTIAL RESPONSE IN CHILDREN

In the beginning of the pandemic, it was believed that children less <18 years of age were spared from severe symptoms and were generally less vulnerable to the SARS-CoV-2 virus. A study carried out on 500 COVID-19 patients found that only 1% of the cases were of age <19 years [18], supporting the notion that children are spared from the disease. Another survey carried out in the US found that out of the 149,082 confirmed COVID-19 cases in the united states at the time (June 2020), only 1.7% (2,572) were children under 18 years of age. Of these 2,572 cases, 73% experienced symptoms such as fever, cough, and shortness of breath. Only 5.7% of all the patients had to be hospitalized, and 3 deaths were reported in children [19]. Although these numbers are much lower than those for adults and children do experience symptoms much less severe than adults, they are in fact at equal risk of contracting COVID-19.

Scientists have been working to find the pathophysiological differences in children and adults that lead to the reduced severity of infection in children. One study suggested that this could be the result of differences in levels of the mediators, i.e., ACE 2 and the transmembrane serine protease 2, that are required by the virus to enter host respiratory cells. There have been several studies suggesting that the expression of these mediators actually increases with age (which tells us why adults are most vulnerable), meaning children generally show significantly lower concentration of these mediators in their bodies, causing hindrance in viral entry into the respiratory epithelium, ultimately 'sparing' the children from severe lung disease [20].

Most of the severe symptoms in COVID-19 such as ARDS occur as a result of the overactivity of our own immune systems. Infiltration of pro-inflammatory cells in the lung tissue leads to a large amount of lung damage. In children, especially in neonates, the immune system is not yet completely developed and is considered to be evolving or 'immature' at that stage which could be the reason why children are relatively less likely to fall victim to the immune-mediated phase 2 of the disease. Moreover, it has also been reported that the number of T-cells (CD4+ and CD8+) in the immune system were generally much lower in adults while children have shown a relative abundance of these cells which even in the absence of a fully developed innate immune system can help in tackling the infection. Moreover, children also have much lower levels of neutrophils, pro-inflammatory cytokines, and a higher level of immunomodulatory cells, protecting them from severe infection [20]. Children are generally more resilient when it comes to diseases and their lungs are better capable of recovering and healing than adults.

Although children are spared from severe lung disease, they are not entirely spared from other effects of the virus. There had been reports where children had started developing late-onset symptoms in response to the virus, now called Pediatric multisystem inflammatory syndrome (PMIS). This syndrome is a result of post-infection spike in the immune system of children and shares much resemblance to Kawasaki disease with symptoms such as fever, inflammatory shock, rashes, conjunctivitis arterial damage (We now know that SARS-CoV-2 can destroy endothelial cells in adults causing inflammation and excess clotting, leading to cardiac complications) [21]. The CDC has reported 570 PMIS patients who also tested positive for COVID-19, of whom 2/3 had no underlying condition and obesity was the most common underlying condition in the rest [22]. Based on these findings, we know that children exhibit a much different reaction to the SARS-CoV-2 Infection. In addition, it would be incorrect to suggest that children are spared from disease. Children are in fact as much a victim of COVID-19 as any adult and should follow the same precautions as older adults.

2.8.4 RESPONSE IN THE ELDERLY

As we age, our body's defense systems start to lose their power, our cells lose their healing properties, and as a result, we fall victim to countless diseases/ co-morbidities which predispose us to infections such as COVID-19. We know that people with elder age (>65 years) are a particularly vulnerable group when it comes SARS-CoV-2 infection susceptibility, and not only that, they are also at the highest risk of becoming critically ill and mortality, mainly because of their already deteriorating health conditions.

2.9 RISK FACTORS FOR SEVERE INFECTION

COVID-19 is a disease that spares no one, it can affect any person of any age and can produce symptoms that could range from none to mild to severe. Although we know that there are certain pre-requisites that can predispose people to severe illness, scientists are still trying to find further evidence as to why patients are exhibiting such a wide range of symptoms. Some factors that bring people under the high-risk radar for severe infection are as follows:

- Age above 65 years;
- Male gender;
- Underlying co-morbidities such as diabetes type-2, hypertension, asthma, certain blood and bone marrow cancers and other cardiovascular and respiratory diseases;
- High levels of C-reactive protein (CRP) and lactate dehydrogenase;
- Immunosuppressant therapy.

Moreover, there have also been reports where people with hematological diseases were developing severe illness in response to COVID-19. This is thought to be a result of a dysfunctional immune system (a result of their hematological illness) and the immunosuppressants they receive for treatment [23]. There is also some indication that a higher body-mass index (BMI) or obesity can also be a major risk factor for severe disease. As we know, obesity does in fact, exposes people to a high risk of heart diseases and usually have a higher expression level of ACE-2 enzyme, all of which coupled with SARS-CoV-2 can have devastating outcomes, [24]. Moreover, higher levels of certain proteins and enzymes in the body can also indicate disease progression and severity, these include:

- High WBC count;
- High aspartate aminotransferase (AST), and alanine transaminase (ALT);
- High C-reactive protein (CRP);
- High pro-calcitonin (PCT);
- High creatine kinase (CK);
- High lactate dehydrogenase (LDH);
- High D-dimers.

Other clinical symptoms such as shortness of breath, difficulty breathing, and high-grade fever are also associated with disease progression [15]. Moreover, vitamin-D has been known to possess some immune-modulatory properties which include reducing the overexpression of pro-inflammatory cytokines. Deficiency of vitamin D has also been associated with conditions such as hypertension and diabetes, and some recent studies are suggesting that vitamin D deficiency can be another risk factor for severe ARDS through an indirect mechanism, which involves not being unable to suppress the cytokine storm in lungs of COVID-19 patients. However, these studies do not support the use of vitamin D supplementation for managing critically ill patients [25, 26].

2.10 POTENTIAL TREATMENT OPTIONS

As of March 2021, there have been no completely effective treatments developed for the treatment of COVID-19. Certain drugs and therapies have provided some benefit in managing symptoms of the disease; however, not many have been successful in alleviating the root cause. The following paragraphs enlist a few therapies that have been used or possess the potential to treat COVID-19:

2.10.1 IMMUNO-MODULATORS

The reason why patients get severely ill in COVID-19 is due to their body's initiation of a strong immune response to the virus, which results in a 'cytokine storm' for which the use of immunomodulatory drugs may prove beneficial but only as adjuncts together with other therapies. Monoclonal antibodies such as Bevacizumab, Sarilumab, Ezulizumab, and Tocilizuab are being used for the treating COVID-19. Our most important defense against the coronavirus is the interferon response that inhibit replication of the coronavirus. Drugs such as INF-α and INF type-1 have shown very promising results against COVID-19 and multiple trials are underway to test their efficacy in the treatment of COVID-19.

Bevacizumab, an anti-VEGF drug has the ability to attenuate pulmonary edema in critically ill patients. The anti-rheumatoid IL-6 receptor-specific antibodies Sarilumab and Tocilizumab have shown to be very effective in controlling cytokine storm in critically ill COVID-19 patients, however their use in such instances requires further study. Currently, corticosteroids such as dexamethasone are being used in severely ill patients and has been shown to reduce fatalities caused by severe COVID-19 by at least $1/3^{rd}$. However, these drugs have not shown any significant benefit in treating non-critical patients.

2.10.2 VIRAL ENTRY BLOCKERS

Drugs that have the ability to block the interaction between viral proteins and human Ace-2 receptors may result in a reduction in viral load in infected patients and prove to be beneficial in treating the disease. Japan has approved the use of the antiviral drug Camostat mesylate, which is responsible for inhibiting serine protease enzymes such as TMPRSS2, which results in a reduction in viral entry into the host cell and also prevent the patient from reaching severe disease. Unfortunately, at present there is not enough clinical data to support the use of this drug in COVID-19 patients. In patients with milder disease, Umifenovir has been shown to be much more effective than ritonavir. However, the drug has not shown much promise when it comes to treating more severe COVID-19 cases. Previously, antimalarial drugs Chloroquine and hydroxychloroquine (HCQ) were being used to treat COVID-19 due to their ability to block viral entry via multiple mechanisms such as raising the endosomal PH making it more acidic and inhibition of receptor glycosylation thereby interfering with membrane fusion. However, due to their debilitating adverse effects, especially those related to the cardiovascular systems, the FDA has now unauthorized the use of these drugs in emergency cases.

2.10.3 REPLICATION INHIBITORS

Drugs that inhibit the replication and spread of viruses include favilavir, ribavirin, lopinavir, remdesivir, and ritonavir, etc. The influenza drug favilavir has been shown to speed up viral clearance from the body where the drug showed improvement in patients with severe disease by 40–60% and in patients with mild disease by approximately 73–87%. Unfortunately, these results are concluded from small scale studies and, therefore, need further validation. Remdesivir, on the other hand has shown promising activity against COVID-19 in both *in vivo* and *in vitro* studies. The drug has shown a reduction in the total time for recovery and also in the need for O_2 support in severely ill patients and has been granted emergency use approval from the FDA in such cases.

2.10.4 CONVALESCENT PLASMA (CP)

IgG therapy in the form of convalescent plasma (CP) from recovered patients has been also been used for treating COVID-19 and has been approved by the FDA for emergency use. There are, however, many downsides with this treatment, such as transfusion reactions and antibody mediated exacerbation of infection. Moreover, these antibodies cannot be produced at a mass scale the way monoclonal antibodies can.

2.11 NEW VIRAL VARIANTS

Up until now, four different variants of COVID-19 have been identified, which reflects the fact that; being an RNA virus, SARS-CoV-2 has a very high capability of undergoing genetic mutations, and there has been some speculation that the rate of fatalities caused by COVID-19 may differ across different geographical regions. There are 13 different sites on the virus's genome that have a very high probability of undergoing mutations with the site 28144 in the Open Reading Frame 8 having the highest probability of mutation (30.5%). The RNA dependent RNA polymerases (RdRp) are a major element in the virus's replication process, this virus has a higher expression of the non-structural protein 12, reflecting a well-established mechanism of infection. Other non-structural proteins such as 7, 8, and 14 have also been associated with proofreading and correction of any errors during the addition of nucleotides in the replication process and thereby increase the integrity of RNA synthesis. These polymerases have been viewed as major targets for the development of antiviral drugs such as Remdesivir and Ribavirin, etc.

Soon after becoming a GHE, the first variant of this virus; D614G, was identified in February 2020 in China, although this variant did not cause more severe disease, it did prove to be more virulent and had a much higher rate of transmission and later became the more dominant virus than its predecessor. A little later, in August 2020, the Danish authorities identified a novel variant of SARS-CoV-2 that had not been seen previously and was named the 'cluster 5' variant. This strain did not have a higher rate of transmission. However, it did turn down the post-infection/vaccination neutralization in people. Fortunately, the variant does not seem to have spread across the country and was only seen in a dozen patients in September 2020.

In December 2020, 2 new strains; N501Y and 501Y.V2 of SARS-CoV-2 emerged in the UK and South Africa, respectively. Although similar, the two strains are phylogenetically very different. The UK variant was then introduced as the variant of concern (VOC) and by late December, was being detected at a much higher rate throughout the Kingdom and has now been identified in 31 countries across the globe. The South Africa strain has been seen in four different countries up until now. Moreover, much like the D614G strain, these two strains have not been associated with critical disease, however, their transmissibility is much higher than their predecessors. The UK strain was found to be approximately 70% more contagious than the previous virus and after the identification of the strain, the UK was seeing 50,000 new cases every day with 1,000 fatalities. As of April 2021, the UK has been reporting a reduction in cases across the country. However, cases across other countries are on the rise, which includes Pakistan, for which reason all incoming flights from Pakistan to UK have been banned effective 08-April-2021. The Danish, South African and UK strains, although have a very high rate of transmission, these variants are not immune against the vaccines that are being developed. Companies such as Pfizer, Moderna, and AstraZeneca are now claiming that their vaccines will be effective against the new strains that have been identified up until now.

2.12 CONCLUSION

SARS-COV-2 has many similarities to SARS-COV and MERS. It is likely that bats are an important host for the virus. The infection is spreading through the inhalation of respiratory droplets. The symptoms of the disease vary but mostly include a flu-like condition. After entering the body, the virus usually targets the lungs where its spike proteins interact with the human ACE2 receptors to help the virus enter the host cells. The severity of the disease is different in different sections of the population and different populations across the world, more generally, the elderly and male are more susceptible to the disease, as are patients with co-morbid conditions. The virus has a much higher probability of undergoing genetic mutations with an increase in transmissibility, for which reason the most immediate task is to develop small molecule inhibitors and vaccines for the effective control of this pandemic which has already infected more than 133 million people. SARS-CoV-2 is a virus that will live amongst us for many years to come. Our only defense against this virus at this time will be to aim towards vaccinating each and every individual in order to dampen the extent of damage that this virus has caused to our society, economy, and the world as a whole.

KEYWORDS

- **COVID-19**
- **COVID-19 epidemiology**
- **COVID-19 treatments**
- **monocyte-chemotactic protein 3**
- **pediatric multisystem inflammatory syndrome**
- **pro-calcitonin**
- **SARS-CoV-2**

REFERENCES

1. Chinazzi, M., Davis, J. T., Ajelli, M., et al., (2020). The effect of travel restrictions on the spread of the 2019 novel coronavirus (COVID-19) outbreak. *Science, 368*, 395–400.
2. Huang, C., Wang, Y., Li, X., et al., (2020). Clinical features of patients infected with 2019 novel coronavirus in Wuhan, China. *The Lancet, 395*, 497–506.
3. Li, Q., Guan, X., Wu, P., et al., (2020). Early transmission dynamics in Wuhan, China, of novel coronavirus-infected pneumonia. *The New England Journal of Medicine, 382*, 1199–1207.
4. (2020). *HAN Archive-00432|Health Alert Network (HAN)*. https://emergency.cdc.gov/han/2020/han00432.asp (accessed on 5 August 2021).
5. *United States of America: WHO Coronavirus Disease (COVID-19) Dashboard*. https://covid19.who.int (accessed on 5 August 2021).
6. *WHO Coronavirus Disease (COVID-19) Dashboard.* https://covid19.who.int (accessed on 5 August 2021).
7. Mosher, S. N., & Aylin, W. D., (2020). *A Comprehensive Timeline of the Coronavirus Pandemic at 9 Months, from China's First Case to the Present*. In business insider.

https://www.businessinsider.com/coronavirus-pandemic-timeline-history-major-events-2020-3 (accessed on 5 August 2021).
8. *Transmission of SARS-CoV-2: Implications for Infection Prevention Precautions*. https://www.who.int/news-room/commentaries/detail/transmission-of-sars-cov-2-implications-for-infection-prevention-precautions (accessed on 5 August 2021).
9. CDC, (2020). *Coronavirus Disease 2019 (COVID-19) – Symptoms*. In: Centers for Disease Control and Prevention. https://www.cdc.gov/coronavirus/2019-ncov/symptoms-testing/symptoms.html (accessed on 5 August 2021).
10. Shah, V. K., Firmal, P., Alam, A., Ganguly, D., & Chattopadhyay, S., (2020). Overview of immune response during SARS-CoV-2 infection: Lessons from the past. *Front. Immunol*. https://doi.org/10.3389/fimmu.2020.01949.
11. *Temporal Profiles of Viral Load in Posterior Oropharyngeal Saliva Samples and Serum Antibody Responses During Infection by SARS-CoV-2: An Observational Cohort Study*. PubMed. https://pubmed.ncbi.nlm.nih.gov/32213337/ (accessed on 5 August 2021).
12. Full Article. *Transcriptomic Characteristics of Bronchoalveolar Lavage Fluid and Peripheral Blood Mononuclear Cells in COVID-19 Patients*. https://www.tandfonline.com/doi/full/10.1080/22221751.2020.1747363 (accessed on 5 August 2021).
13. Jin, J. M., Bai, P., He, W., Wu, F., Liu, X. F., Han, D. M., Liu, S., & Yang, J. K., (2020). Gender Differences in patients with COVID-19: Focus on severity and mortality. *Front. Public Health*. https://doi.org/10.3389/fpubh.2020.00152.
14. Scully, E. P., Haverfield, J., Ursin, R. L., Tannenbaum, C., & Klein, S. L., (2020). Considering how biological sex impacts immune responses and COVID-19 outcomes. *Nature Reviews Immunology, 20*, 442–447.
15. Xu, L., Mao, Y., & Chen, G., (2020). Risk factors for 2019 novel coronavirus disease (COVID-19) patients progressing to critical illness: A systematic review and meta-analysis. *Aging, 12*, 12410–12421. Albany NY.
16. *Relationship Between Blood Group and Risk of Infection and Death in COVID-19: A Live Meta-Analysis*. https://www.ncbi.nlm.nih.gov/pmc/articles/PMC7418722/ (accessed on 5 August 2021).
17. Zaidi, F., Zaidi, A. R., Abdullah, S. M., & Zaidi, S., (2020). COVID-19 and the ABO blood group connection. *Transfusion and Apheresis Science*, 102838.
18. Rachael R., (2020). *Not All Children are Spared from Coronavirus*. In: livescience.com. https://www.livescience.com/coronavirus-children-serious-illness.html (accessed on 5 August 2021).
19. CDCMMWR, (2020). Coronavirus Disease 2019 in Children-United States. *MMWR Morb. Mortal. Wkly. Rep*. https://doi.org/10.15585/mmwr.mm6914e4.
20. Lingappan, K., Karmouty-Quintana, H., Davies, J., Akkanti, B., & Harting, M. T., (2020). Understanding the age divide in COVID-19: Why are children overwhelmingly spared? *American Journal of Physiology-Lung Cellular and Molecular Physiology, 319*, L39–L44.
21. Zhang, S., (2020). *Why the Coronavirus Hits Kids and Adults So Differently*. In: The Atlantic. https://www.theatlantic.com/science/archive/2020/05/covid-19-kids/611728/ (accessed on 5 August 2021).
22. Godfred-Cato, S., (2020). COVID-19–associated multisystem inflammatory syndrome in children-United States. *MMWR Morb. Mortal. Wkly. Rep*. https://doi.org/10.15585/mmwr.mm6932e2.

23. Fox, T. A., Troy-Barnes, E., & Kirkwood, A. A., et al., (2020). Clinical outcomes and risk factors for severe COVID-19 in patients with hematological disorders receiving chemo- or immunotherapy. *British Journal of Hematology*. https://doi.org/10.1111/bjh.17027.
24. Ryan, D. H., Ravussin, E., & Heymsfield, S., (2020). COVID 19 and the patient with obesity-the editors speak out. *Obesity (Silver Spring)*. https://doi.org/10.1002/oby.22808.
25. Panarese, A., & Shahini, E., (2020). Letter: Covid-19, and vitamin D. *Aliment. Pharmacol. Ther., 51*, 993–995.
26. Rhodes, J. M., Subramanian, S., Laird, E., Griffin, G., & Kenny, R. A., (2021). Perspective: Vitamin D deficiency and COVID-19 severity - plausibly linked by latitude, ethnicity, impacts on cytokines, ACE2 and thrombosis. *Journal of Internal Medicine*. https://doi.org/10.1111/joim.13149.
27. Tony, K., (2021). New variant of SARS-CoV-2 in UK causes surge of COVID-19. *Lancet Respir Med., 9*(2), e20, e21. 10.1016/S2213-2600(21)00005-9.

CHAPTER 3

Psychological Effects of COVID-19

BINISH KHALIQ,[1] MEHVISH AZAM,[1] AHMED AKREM,[2]
M. YASIN ASHRAF,[1] SUMERA ANWAR,[1] ARIF MALIK,[1]
SAMINA YAQOOB,[3] and HAWA ZE JAAFAR[4]

[1]*Institute of Molecular Biology and Biotechnology,
The University of Lahore, Lahore, Pakistan,
E-mail: beenish.khaliq@imbb.uol.edu.pk (B. Khaliq)*

[2]*Institute of Pure and Applied Biology, Bahauddin Zakariya University,
Multan, Pakistan*

[3]*School of Business and Economics, University of Management and
Technology, Lahore, Pakistan*

[4]*Department of Crop Science, Faculty of Agriculture,
University Putra Malaysia, Seri Kembangan–43400, Malaysia*

ABSTRACT

COVID-19 is worldwide, and due to this, the whole world is fear and disorder in the people. Due to COVID-19 rate of anxiety and stress in the people had become increase worldwide. Coronavirus disease worldwide spread in 198 countries since February, 2020. This worldwide disease has health-related effect and caused the change in the psychological behavior. The world has been trying on testing, sort out the cure, and inhibiting the transmission, and people are going to numerous psychological issues in the lifestyles and fear of the disease. In addition, a lack of researches on this pandemic and due this worldwide disease causes the fear, depression, and anxiety symptoms in the people. During the COVID-19 anxiety, fear, and depressive symptoms were remained common in the people. Due to COVID-19 diseases, the mental health issues were common, and frontline healthcare workers (HCWs) overlook the higher risk of this pandemics and also have a negative effect on the mental health of HCWs. Due to the COVID-19 disease the medical care workers faced a lot of pressure and over workload.

3.1 PSYCHOLOGICAL IMPACT OF COVID-19

Epidemic coronavirus disease (COVID-19) commonly a severe acute respiratory syndrome (SARS) that have been started in Wuhan, a city of China [1]. During the pandemic (COVID-19) social activities became restricted to all over the world due to quarantine situation. Human activities were also banned. During the quarantine time period, most of the people were badly affected by COVID-19. This pandemic disease caused a number of mental illnesses, i.e., depression, anxiety, emotional disruption, nervousness, restlessness, insecurity, distress, and changes in mood. Emotional collapse, trauma, and annoyance were rapidly appeared due to loss of sleep-in human. A report showed that 9.6% population have great chance to get infection of swine flu (influenza A H1N1) and 32.9% moderately affected [2]. During SARS, Ebola, and MERS pandemic situation, serious mental health issues were appeared in humans [3]. A significant relationship in between the anxiety and avoiding behavior was observed during the MERS outbreak in Jeddah (Saudi Arabia) [4]. Around 53.8% of citizens of China were moderately shown psychological disorders, 16.5% affected by depressive disorders, 28.8% and 8.1% showed anxiety problem and great levels of stress, respectively, during COVID-19. There was no decrease in anxiety and depression about four weeks of COVID-19 [5, 6].

The lifestyle of people has significantly changed almost all over the world within few days during COVID-19 lockdown. The population has been experienced unpredictable and speedily changing situation. People were restricted to stay at home. Family dynamics was extraordinarily affected due to restricted traveling condition. Social and leisure activities also have been reduced during lockdown. Owing to COVID-19, the working situation was badly affected, most of the people were lost their jobs temporary and most of them lost permanently, and many people worked from their homes. Health system of Spanish, USA, and Italy was overwhelmed because hospitals have been faced a lot of difficulties due to lack of space (especially in emergency and in ICU) and shortage of health equipment. This condition has spread extraordinary fear about this pandemic among people. In fact, by seeing this situation, health crises have been compared with 'the end of the world' [7]. Mostly researchers relate COVID-19 to its experimental characteristics [8], chances of survival [9], genomic characteristics of virus and remedy therapeutic possibilities [10].

Considerably very few logical struggles have been found to analyze the psychological influence of coronavirus infection. Additionally, scarce literature relates psychological concerns of international health crises to the Chinese population during outbreak in China. According to Xiang et al. [1], persons confirmed to COVID-19 or with similar symptoms spread anxiety and fear about this infection and some signs, i.e., fever, and difficulty in breathing caused psychological disorders and depression. Furthermore, the volatility of the existing crisis, and the wrong information spreading from it creates the entire situation more tense [11]. Extreme actions were taken by Governments to cope with the spreading of psychological problems by restricting the people quarantine to stop the spreading of the virus. These psychological troubles to manage with the present-day situation are worse with the risky processes taken by the Governments of different countries to stop the spreading of virus specifically by staying people in home. According to a review reported in Ref. [12], people faced serious psychological effects, i.e., anger, fear, and frustration due to being stay at home. The quarantine condition may impact negative and long-lasting effects. During outbreak in China, people experienced loneliness, anger, and boredom. However, being restricted, psychological problems (stress, depression, and anxiety) have been increasing among people [13].

In such a harsh environment, many writers admit to take care of human's mental health is necessary [3, 13–15] and further research is required to completely understand the damaging psychological consequences of pandemic and needed to lessen the psychological effects in all over the world [1]. The frequency of depression was 21.3% that is in between the current literature (16 to 28%) [16], research conducted in Pakistan showed (45%), Spain (34.1%) [12, 13], in Iran (15%) and in India (13.97%) [17, 18]. Increased anxiety condition being infected to COVID-19 was found to be a major factor of chronic disorders among students. A research related the chronic disorders with the rise in IES-R, anxiety, and depression. Someone having a friend infected to COVID-19 increasing the cause of IES-R.

The scores of anxieties to affected with PSS, IES-R, and COVID-19 got from pre-clinic students were found to be considerably greater than clinic students. As in such pandemic, a standard procedure (lockdown) and by retaining social distance in public place was imposed to decrease the spreading of disease [19]. The public agree to undertakes such preventive measures but unfortunately, health care professionals (HCPs) are left to exposed with many issues because of this situation. Firstly, HCPs face gradually extensive work hours with limited medical resources and uncertain arrangement because of the increasing rate of pandemic cases [20]. Secondly, they faced physical irritation even breathing complications while having personal protective equipment (PPE) that is essential to stay away from virus [21].

Another huge problem faced to HCPs is because of little knowledge about this new viral disease, and there was no recognized or evidence-based protocols for their treatment. Many HCPs were unable to perform their duties [4], and there is effective fear of autoinoculation and great risk of spreading this pandemic disease to their friends and family [1, 22]. Due to this fear, HCPs were bound to quarantine from their family members, daily routine was also disturbed, even social support was also reduced to keep everybody safe from them [19]. A significant Pakistani citizen was depressed with stress and anxiety. Approximately 89% HCPs were scared about their families and 80% HCPs be afraid of getting COVID-19 themselves. This data can be related to HCPs that looked after the patients of COVID-19 in Wuhan, 50.4% was depressed, 44.6% suffered in anxiety, 34% had insomnia. However, a significant percentage of people was depressed (634 [50.4%]) and (560 [44.6%]), (427 [34.0%]), (899 [71.5%]) showed symptoms of fear, depression, insomnia, and distress, respectively [23].

In 2003, around 18–57% of HCPs was suffered with emotional disorders and psychiatric symptoms for the period of outbreak of (SARS) [24]. In 2015, HCPs was suffered with dysphoria and stress when another disorder middle east respiratory syndrome (MERS) was emerged that also affected by coronavirus [7]. Many other research reports revealed that during the pandemic and epidemic mental health illness for healthcare professionals would have long lasting effects. Even after a while of such events, fear, posttraumatic stress disorder (PTSD), stress, and hopelessness were noted in many cases [25, 26].

High levels of anxiety, stress, and depression in Pakistan have been increasing due to improper supervision of patients, shortness of masses awareness, reduced submission with preventive measures. Additional to this, the most important effect is the mental health persistence of healthcare workers (HCWs). Various research reported that a significant number of HCPs have been facing extraordinary level of trauma, anxiety, PTSD, and depression even after a long time of an epidemic. Moreover, the HCPs also suffered to stigma that was directly involved for the treatment of extremely infectious disease such as the COVID-19 while, at the other end of the spectrum, this pandemic has led to HCPs being given the ‘superhero’ status. As this enhanced the importance and gratification toward their jobs, it also put extra pressure on workers having no margin of mistake. Due to extraordinary effort toward worldwide pandemic, the status of 'superhero' being secured by media, encouraging the basics for appreciation and emotional support. The psychological effects of COVID-19 may lead from panic or collective hysteria to universal feelings of desperation and hopelessness that results to negative effects especially suicidal attempt.

The most important and great perception of social support is related with reduced probability of psychological disorders and psychiatric distress. On the other hand, according to the latest survey in South Korea [27], about 72% of respondents said that they might get someone's support in case of quarantine due to COVID-19 and about 28% reported that they would not have social funding and support. Social support plays an important role towards general population during this COVID situation, social support should be provided to infected persons, medical professionals, and quarantined persons according to reliable and scientifically evidence. Relevantly, a significant number of mental health associated policies are mandatory in pandemic areas to facilitate lifestyle and rewind activities are necessary after invalidating lockdown.

3.2 BEHAVIORAL IMPACT OF COVID-19

In the period of COVID-19 associated fear (COVID-19 personal experience, illness or other significant persons, ingestion of psychiatric medicines, revealing a psychiatric distress), to analyze behavioral responses including safety and checking behaviors, in addition to evaluate compliance concerns with public health strategies and motivation of social responsibility [28]. The relationship between behavior and psychological effects was observed during MERS, SARS, and Ebola. Similarly, outbreak of COVID-19 causes major psychological disorders (anxiety, depression, and fear) along with behavioral practices (avoidance behavior and application of non-pharmacological precautionary measures. However, by discussing appropriate solution may change the situation effectively. Approximately 74.5% were limited to their physical contact with other people avoiding their healthcare facilities, 84.5% canceled their family trips, social gathering, and business meetings or traveling, 87% frequently washed their hands. However, few participants avoided going on prayer places, 56.8% has hand sanitizer in their pockets, 44.3% wore mask. Meanwhile, 35% of people avoided to watch, listen, or read the current news about pandemic as it increases the anxiety and depression level.

As the most research reports revolve about clinical manifestation, treatment of disease, pathophysiology effects, and diagnosis of disease, the mental health issues of outbreak often ignored and no research data was given for psychological effects and behavioral fluctuations in the affected population [29, 30]. Moreover, regular collection and analysis of data in controlling an outbreak situation include people beliefs, attitude, public perception, and practices concerns the overwhelming situation. Seeing the current situation, major mental health illness is caused due to heavy toll-paying by most of the people. Special consideration released by WHO should be adopted during this situation. Out of them, the most important is to stay connected with beloved relations by using digital media, avoid to watch or listen the news regularly, supporting, and cheering each other, along with take care of own by taking proper diet, sleeping well, and exercising regularly. In this research, our goal is to highlight the psycho behavioral changes related to psychological disorders among the population in Karachi, Pakistan, after the lockdown of COVID-19. Furthermore, it is significantly reported that up to now, no research focusing on psychological and behavioral effects of pandemic was conducted in the region.

During a survey, about 62.5% of respondents stated that they are anxious because of the fast-spreading of coronavirus, that is a very disturbing situation. According to the survey report, approximately 28.8% of people claimed to be affected by severe anxiety disorders during the initial period of COVID-19 in China [5]. In a limited month of pandemic, it is suggested to control the increasing level of anxiety and mental health in the population. Interestingly, about two-thirds of our people were frightened to leave their house, while 83.3% felt anxious. This situation points out that, being possessive for their family members play an important role to increase the fear in the time of crises. From the start of the lockdown in Wuhan to current situation, 88.8% of respondents feared to visiting crowded areas. This is happening due to the relationship between anxiety and avoidance behavior (traveling and visiting to public place) has been established [4].

At the initial time period of lockdown in China due to COVID-19 internet was the only source to provide general information about public health [5]. However, it is a frightening situation that 82.8% of the population was panic due to social media. It was also found that 71% of people expressed anxiety over the control measures of current infection, thus this study indicated that high level of anxiety lead to dis satisfaction and mistrust in preventive measures taken by government [31]. A study reported on SARS in 2003 revealed that few people avoid visiting hospitals [32]. This finding is opposite to our survey report according to that higher number of people (74.5%) avoided to health care facilities [33].

It was revealed that higher than 80% of our people were restricted for their physical contact and 84.5% canceled their planes. This awareness may cause the positive changes among people. As preventive measures are highlighted to control the spreading of disease from the very beginning of this pandemic. However, everyone should have kept in mind that sudden change in life activities and social interaction may lead to trigger anxiety. According to this survey, it is clearly indicated that certain preventive measures are closely associated to epidemic transmission and virus transmission [34].

As males are the main source of income in Pakistan, they were certainly more worried to leave their home and even in case of leaving the house they were feel more anxious, that negates the survey report in Saudi Arabia [35]. In addition to this, our research also highlighted that apart from males, graduates, and individuals above than 35 years that are the main labor forced agents in Pakistan also suffered with anxiety due to COVID-19 lockdown. The shutdown of global economy is the major factor of increasing fear and anxiety [36]. In this research, there are various methods to stabilize the outbreak in an effective way. Firstly, there is a need to stop the spreading of wrong information through social media and portal from where individuals obtain news from reliable government source. Secondly, there is a need for government to plan their activities stronger and be responsible for accurate and update news to both health care workers and the general public in order to lighten their fear and anxiety level and develop their trust in government to make sure future cooperation. Undergraduate medical students should be trained enough that they provide psychotherapy counseling due to the increased rate of contact transmission cases, medical help provided from medical volunteers play a crucial role in this situation [26].

While one third of our people continued to go prayer places (36.5%), it is request for consideration of spiritual leaders to clear the mistaken believes of people to clarify them that visiting in these places would be one of the main factors for spreading of disease during an outbreak. Meanwhile they are providing by alternate means to continue their religious events. In order to elude the vast business loss, participants should train to work from their homes in every field where possible and as young participants are more interested in smartphone uses, they should be engaged with online classes that may help the country to save from long-lasting losses [37]. In the last, it has been found that increasing level of anxiety may lead to additional diseases, so few preventive measures should be adapted by individuals to decrease their anxiety and fear. Avoiding too much coverage of news could be helpful to decrease the stress. Similarly, sustaining a healthy routine not only boost the immunity but also help to refresh the mood. However, conversation with friends and family members is another method to improve emotional support and retain person to feel more comfortable and relax [38].

3.3 INITIAL PSYCHOLOGICAL IMPACT OF COVID-19 AND ITS CORRELATES IN COMMUNITY

Around the world, primary psychological influence was travel during lock-down of COVID-19. As with the spreading of disease, anxieties regarding economy, business, job, and health increased day to day. The results of pandemic effect on mental health may help the public to plan mental health interventions for needy persons [39]. World Health Organization (WHO) advised continually to adopt essential precautions to switch of the negative effects of spreading of coronavirus on psychological health and comfort [40]. The research conducted in China by Wang et al. showed that from 1210 respondents about 53.8% suffered to psychological disorders from outbreak [5]. In the past, national, and international individuals faced a wide range of psychosocial effects during the outbreak due to the Ebola virus (EBOV). People are probability concerning the virus fall in sickness, hopelessness, stigma, helplessness, and even death [41].

People faced mental health distress, i.e., anxiety, fear, and insomnia mainly after the declaration of the outbreak. Governments provided helpline numbers for guidance and counseling with the collaboration of different national and international institutes [40]. First aid psychological counseling act as quintessential in the period of an epidemic. It helps people to lessen their psychological fear and support to coping policies to deal effectively with situation [42]. Although, the outbreak of COVID-19 imposed by WHO and other health authorities creating stress all over the country [43], much similar to its effects on worldwide counterparts [44]. Continuous caring of mental and psychological comforts should be in highest priority in different regions during the lockdown [45].

3.4 ALEXITHYMIA

In addition to psychological disorders, people faced cognitive and emotional disorders during COVID-19 outbreak. People with alexithymia have ordinarily high levels of depression, apprehension problems and psychosomatic problems as compared to non-alexithymic during COVID-19 situation [46]. It was noted that a high level of depression is due to the alexithymia, that was reliable to previous research on alexithymia and depressing feelings [47]. Alexithymia is an emotional disorder and appearance of scarcity disorder that is described by condensed capability to recognize and expressing the emotions [48]. People affected in alexithymia feel difficult to avail social support [49] and may develop harsh interpersonal lifestyle [50], also fail to identify their emotions or to respond to other's emotions [51].

Limited societal support has been linked with despair [52], and it is reported that individuals facing anxiety disorders usually involve in sensitive inhibition policies and have been facing complications in personally recognizing and expressing their emotions [53]. It was also reported that PTSD is a major cause for the connection between depressive symptoms and alexithymia in-home quarantined individuals. It was also studied that alexithymia had a solid influence on ESTD, that was constant with former reports in which it was reported that alexithymia paid significant role towards hyperarousal PTSD features [54]. Unexpectedly, it was also reported that PTSD had strong relation with depression in self-quarantined university students [55]. However, the current survey confirmed that both PTSD and alexithymia play crucial role in the expansion and spreading of despair in severe stage resulting in distress. However, it is expected that alexithymia may change as a part of surviving mechanism [55] to lessen the fear and anxiety depressions related to COVID-19. Stepwise regression analysis was conducted to identify major factors of alexithymia that caused depression and PSTD independently (Figure 3.1).

Alexithymia as a negotiator between depression, anxiety, and exposure, as shown in Figure 3.1. Hébert et al. [56] reported the similar results that alexithymia is an intercessor PTSD, depression, earthquake trauma and interpersonal trauma [56, 57]. These results showed that exposures are a very important factor because it led to more and acute alexithymia [58]. During COVID-19 disease a lot of public health reverse was observed, people, and students self-quarantined and tried to change by denying, distancing, and suppressing their own needs [59]. The fighting mechanism between the fear of COVID-19 pandemic and control of emotion provided the survival of fitness. However, it was observed that the alexithymia may arise as part of fighting mechanism to prevent the anxiety and worry linked with this COVID-19 pandemic [60]. Due to the compatible analysis, alexithymia existed in the people trying to fight overcome the stressor [61] However it can be ceased that emotional disturbance caused by the traumatic factors in the people.

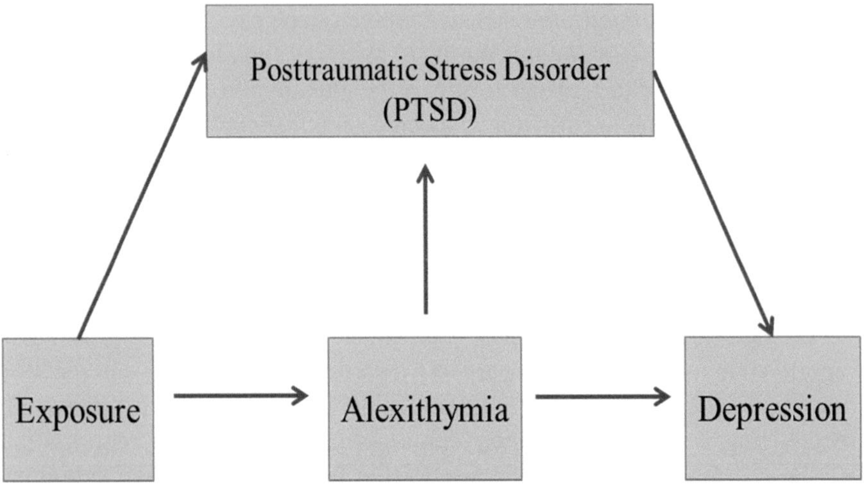

FIGURE 3.1 Relationship between the posttraumatic stress disorder (PTSD), exposure, alexithymia, and depression.

Secondly, the risk factor for depression was increased by alexithymia, which was described in the earlier study that association exist between alexithymia and anxiety, depressive feelings, and fear [47]. Due to the alexithymia is a lack of emotion, anxiety, and deficiency of expression [48]. Due to the fear of COVID-19, people developed the alexithymia and became to live isolate and cut off the social life, may adapt the truculent lifestyles [55]. Less social activities were linked with anxiety and depression [52], it has been observed that those people with mental stress, alexithymia, and under depression typically hide their emotions and have faced the difficulties to identify their emotions and feeling [53].

In the study it was observed that posttraumatic stress disorder (PTSD) was indirectly associated between alexithymia and depression features in quarantined people. It was observed that posttraumatic stress disorder was directly influenced under the alexithymia because it was seen that alexithymia significantly increased the anesthetic and hyperarousal posttraumatic stress disorder symptoms [54]. It was seen that posttraumatic stress disorder (PTSD) has been found to show the depression in the self-quarantined people [55, 63]. However, it was seen that both alexithymia and PSTD took a part to develop and creation of depression in the severe condition of a trauma.

The possibility risk of quarantine disorders may also be due to the existence of alexithymic characters that can reduce psychological possibilities in some individuals [46, 64, 65]. Alexithymia literally means 'no words for mood' was primarily identified to describe mental and affective conditions in patients suffering from psychosomatic diseases. Alexithmic person show considerably greater level of depression, psychological disorders, and anxiety than non alexithymic persons. In short, alexithymia caused major depressive disorder (MDD) showed a significant association between alexithymia, MDD and increasing threat of suicidal behavior.

3.5 DEPRESSION, ANXIETY, AND STRESS SCALES

COVID-19 is most challenging and disturbing public health disaster since the influenza pandemic in 1918. From 14th May 2020, higher than 4.2 million individuals being infected and 292,046 individuals died internationally according to WHO 2020. It has carried to discomfort and sorrow to all nations. It is certainly true that this disease caused high level of fear, disturbance, and anxiety in individuals of all ages. Concern to anxiety and fear, around 34% [GAD-7: moderate anxiety (19.8%) and severe anxiety (13.7%)] and 45% [PHQ-9: moderate (21%), moderately severe (13.6%) and severe depression (10.4%)] individuals had scored $\geq$ 10 on both above-mentioned methods, respectively. Contrasting to our result [66] stated that Chinese students suffering 21.3% (mild), 2.7% (moderate) and 0.9% (severe) anxiety. Considerably higher percentage of students suffering in anxiety and depression may be responsible for circumstances that 21.8% of our research issues related to someone (fellows, neighbors, family members, relatives, and colleagues) that have been detecting COVID-19 that was less than 1% in previous report [11].

Research that evaluates the emotional effects of SARS and MERS, COVID-19 lockdown also found considerable influence of these infections on intellectual psychological health of students [67, 68]. Upon examining that effect of anxiety or depression on lifestyle, 48% somewhat and 6.5% felt extreme troubles in responsibility of work, take carefulness about work at home or receiving alongside with others. It is necessary of the time that educational organizations needed work with the collaboration of government to encourage methods advised by WHO [111] in order to maintain the psychological health of pupils during COVID-19 outbreak. Any other epidemic lockdown would cause damaging effects on people and society. A report on public psychological situation during COVID-19 lockdown showed that SAS record was 36.92% and 6.33% suffered in anxiety. Studies recommended that public health crises may cause severe psychological impacts on college students that may be expressed as fear, worry, and anxiety, among others [69].

There was no national data about anxiety level for college students of China, but we related our results with SAS scores of Chinese university students for the period of SARS and H1N1 and assuming that university students faced a higher level of anxiety during outbreak of COVID-19 than SARS and H1N1. Further, it is indicated that 24.9% of medical students were suffered with anxiety due to COVID-19 lockdown. As comparing to our report, medical students faced anxiety greater than general university students during COVID-19.

It was noted that approximately 66.99% of individuals faced different stages of challenges and 15.43% were detected with different levels of anxiety. There were 20.3% students that felt weakness got exhausted easily. The majority of the Chinese individual were recommended to quarantine in their homes for almost about a month to avoid the spreading of coronavirus, and our students had lost their temper and also not having proper exercise and social activities. Social media and news also major factor of causing complex mental issues, i.e., anxiety, upset, depression, stress, anger, and frustration, etc., according to response from psychological advising telephone helpline set up around China, anxiety was the major feature of callers. Research have confirmed that people that was experienced with public health emergency they are still facing higher level of stress diseases even after the incidence is over and they have been recovered [70].

Significant sex alterations were reported, and female students exhibited more anxiety than male students. This is confirmed with former reports that females were extraordinary suffered with anxiety [71], such as frequency of anxiety and depression in Pakistan is about 34% (range 29 to 66% in females and 10 to 33% in males) [72]. But significant difference was not observed among science and arts students. However, students of grade two had complex anxiety level than grade three and grade one students had lower anxiety than grade two and three. This is due to the fact that students of grade two and three had extra academic burdens.

Throughout the COVID-19, it was point out that the frequency of anxiety was 27.1%, this conclusion is sustained with a survey report completed in China (24.9%) and review of current literature (16–28%), [16, 66] but greater than Iran (20%), Spain (21.3%) and India (12.63%), [13–15] and lower than a study completed in Jordan (69.5%), Turkey (69.9%), Pakistan (34%) and France (60.2%), [73–76]. The fraction of stress was 32.5%. This result is sustained with a survey done in Spain (28.14%), [76] but greater than Indian (15.57%), [3] and lower than a survey completed in Jordan (69.5%) and France (61.6%), [3, 51]. The reason for the difference is due to change in strict isolation, extraordinary prevalence level, effect of outbreak, dissimilarity in learning level and sessions of study. For the duration of the COVID-19 pandemic showed that sex is considerably linked with anxiety. Female students of university faced 2.1 times greater risk of having anxiety comparing to men. This outcome is supported by a survey completed in India [16].

This was happened because females being usually exposed to economic deprivation, mental disorder, traditional aspects and because of hormonal instabilities [77]. Students that quarantined in their home showed 3.6 times greater threat of developing anxious disorders comparing to those students that did not quarantined in their homes. This is all due to the fact of quarantine that social isolation and great variations in regular life is the main source of medical despair due to coronavirus [78].

There are some other factors that cause anxiety. Students that did not live with their family members exhibited a 3.3 times greater possibility of having depressive disorders as compared to students that are living with their family members. Previous research showed that higher levels of emotional and anxiety risk factors in adults are because of the death of parents in their childhood, parent's psychological disorders or mental illness, and not living with their parents [66]. It was studied that students belongs to family whose income is less than 2500 ETB, they had 2.8 times greater risk factors to suffered in anxiety and fear as compared to counterparts, that might increase the psychological and economic stress. This is supported by a survey completed among student colleges in China [66]. Students whose relatives being suspected to COVID-19 have greater risk factors of developing anxiety, that might be associated with high contagiousness infection of coronavirus pneumonia [79]. Furthermore, this research also represented major issues that rise the stress disorders related to COVID-19 among university students. The students that suffered from depressive and anxious disorders showed 2.3 and 2.8 more risk of having stress as compared to students that did not suffer from depression and anxiety. This is due to the distribution of fake news about health, societal issues, and financial pressure of COVID-19. This result is link with the current status of COVID-19 and psychological health outcomes [80].

Students with weak social support faced a 2.8 times greater threat of having stress and depression as compared to counterparts. Shortage of social funding also increase the burden to financial crises, health, and social issues. Data also indicated that isolation or weak social support cause higher level of stress and depression [81]. Furthermore, the students that used constituent faced 3.4 times greater risk of having stress as compared to students who did not use constituent. People that use substances are supposed to be marginalized and stigmatized groups having poor immunity responses and susceptibility to stress [78]. This result is supported with a survey completed in Dessie and Ethiopia and substance that was used considerably linked with psychological disorders of students [82].

Social boycott related to lockdown and restriction measures cause the feeling of uncertainty about future, fear of new infection and unknown infectious agents brings abnormal and high level of anxiety [83]. Anxiety is directly linked to sensorial scarcity and universal loneliness may lead to insomnia in starting but in future depression and posttraumatic disorders occurred. Furthermore, anxiety is closely related to fatigue and poor performance in HCWs, although boredom and being alone are directly interrelated to frustration, anger, and distresses linked to quarantine limits [84]. Moreover, additional awful effects related to general anxiety in a pandemic time period may include to lower social support, parting from loved ones, uncertainty, boredom, and loss of freedom [27].

Distress, social isolation, boredom, and frustration are directly linked to limitation, abnormally lack of social and physical contact with others and loss of habitual activities [85–90]. As reported by Jeong et al. [91] obstruction and general loneliness seem to develop by the cut down from daily activities, disturbance of social requirements, not participating in social network activities. Unluckily, in this situation, hopelessness, together with other individual activities such as the practice of childhood cruelty as well as life-threatening sensory processing's may considerably and independently expect suicidal attempts [92, 93], but even the intolerable rage related to the burden of quarantine may cause negative outcomes. The final effect of quarantine is persistent isolation and boredom, that have intense effects on individual both physically and mentally. Pervasive loneliness might be linked with increased level of depression and suicidal behavior. Unfortunately, the loneliness is gradually increased by anxiety, collective hysteria, and panic. Thinking abilities and decision making are primarily reduced by anxiety and hyperarousal and later by restricting mental state of loneliness. Generally, it is acknowledged that long time periods of social boycott or quarantine for specific infections may have harmful effects on mental health.

3.6 THE MENTAL HEALTH BURDEN OF THE EMERGING CORONAVIRUS DISEASE

COVID-19 pandemic caused severe mental health problems, including psychological effects among the common individuals and patients with previous psychiatric disorders due to declines and exacerbations after it has followed. Early report in China described some attitudes of the initial mental disorders that have arisen during the time period of COVID-19 [13]. Patients suffering in mental disorders had a great chance of being infected with COVID-19. A number of patients with mental illness may hinder identification and visit to a hospital and therefore not receive satisfactory mental health care. Special attention towards children suffered from autism spectrum disease were who found it hard to change their routines. Children were suffered greatly with behavioral and emotional disorders during lock-down [94].

Alexithymia was an intermediary between contact and mental health supported results found that alexithymia act as intermediated between interpersonal shock and depression [56], PTSD, and earthquake trauma [57]. The most vital lane in this report was high coverages that going to a stark alexithymia [58]. The quarantined students were most likely to attempted by suppressing their thoughts, denying, and distancing from their emotions during COVID-19 outbreak [59]. These surviving strategies, while valuable in expressively insecure environments, could affect in reduced awareness of emotions when laboring over time, probably increase the cases of alexithymia [95]. Hence, it is possible that alexithymia may progress as a part of a dealing mechanism [60] avoid to spreading the fear of anxiety and depressive disorders related to coronavirus. Regular analyzes about alexithymia was observed in people who trying to survive with the feelings related to tremendous stressor [61, 96]. As a result, in accordance with earlier findings [97, 98], it might be reported that shocking events may be the major reason of emotional disorders that persons seek to handle by retreating from detecting and recounting their feelings. So, recognizing the highly experienced students and low experienced students is essential while pursuing to improve preventive methods and interferences against COVID-19 related alexithymia indications.

3.7 THE PSYCHOLOGICAL EFFECTS OF COVID-19 ON FRONTLINE HEALTHCARE WORKERS (HCWS)

The psychological facts of frontline employees are complicated and partly understood during an epidemic of COVID-19. Unavoidable fear, anxiety, and stress about a poorly recognized contagious infection outbreaks like COVID-19, may be profound between the higher threat groups, such as HCPs and other frontline employees, including policemen, bankers, and armed forces, etc. Being exposed to quarantined during COVID-19 cases in hospitals, the death or disorder of a relative or friend from COVID-19 and sensitive self-perception of hazard by the lethality of the virus can all damagingly influence the mental safety of health workers [94, 99, 100]. Medical specialists from severely COVID-infected countries like China experienced enormous performance stress, as well as higher unfavorable psychological outcomes due to unexpected surge of overwork, insufficient protection from infection, frustration from disappointment to give ideal patient care and quarantine [22, 23]. Numerous varieties of psychologically stressful happenings associated with "vicarious traumatization" in the nursing staff have been reported during the time period spreading and controlling of the COVID-19 pandemic in China [22].

In the developing countries where the health care mechanism is already overloaded, rushes of COVID-19 cases are likely to enhance acute anxiety, stress, and irritation in nurses and doctors. This might be due to the inadequate hospital supply of necessary health hygiene equipment's [101] and significant limited supply of personal protective equipment (PPE) in HCPs that are at the peak of transmission [102]. Li et al. in their general study amongst HCPs employed in fever clinics or dealing with COVID-19 patients, showed that half of the individuals recognized the smallest mild depression and one third identified insomnia while 14% of doctors and 16% of nurses having moderate and severe depressive indication during the outbreak of COVID-19. The investigators pointed out that being female and employed in the frontline were direct and self-determining risk factors for emerging abnormal stress indications [18]. Addressing the psychological features, like fear and anxiety of unfavorably illness of COVID-19 patients, appears furthermore problematic disorders in most of the hospitals and their employees have scarce proper training on appropriate infection control events [103].

Along with behavioral issues and mental health interferences during and after infectious disease [1]. It is extremely difficult for health workers to deal with panic stricken, dismayed, uncooperative, and stigmatized patient of COVID-19 as previously practiced by medical teams in China [19], and this might produce laziness among clinicians. Providing medical precaution in the time of over-all epidemic causes depressive and surges anxiety to a large scale [104] according to a report about 70% acknowledged that becoming ill was utmost disturbing. HCWs was faced with high infection threats and dying, ethical problems in determining which is the most suitable for ICU and extreme work-loads. The whole knowledge might be traumatizing and increase the threat of psychological health problems among individuals that are evenly at the peak of the risk, in order to HCWs were at greater chances of suicide than the common individuals [105].

It is possible that emotional adverse effects of COVID-19 on HCWs are changeable through diverse situations by number of surveys representing as high threat of attaining a distress or anxious disorders. The possibility of the mental health of HCWs are possible to be aspects and advance research is required to explain the fundamental procedures that can actually be diminished by means of suitable methods. Assemblage of correct information is immediately wanted, specifically for susceptible individuals bare of pandemic. Mediations to ease the sickness and harshness of emotional disorders in HCWs in the initial phase that may possibly stop adverse short term as well as long term effects.

It is essential to remind that expert's appreciation and beliefs may absolutely emphasize to great effort, but the importance of this factor is reduced when they are used in a disciplinary manner that categorizes HCWs. The importance on their self-discipline however giving the needed and life-saving facilities becomes expanded in the middle of an epidemic and regularly HCWs are described as heroes. In short, this might be turned to carry out positive expectations from them, by establishing individual strength and spirit both passionately and professionally. Though, this situation also lessens their talent to identify susceptibilities or stressful practices, comparable in some traits to army workers. This could accidentally raiseraise their psychological health problems and stigmatizing views, consequently avoid them for looking of emotional help [106]. As HCWs must be able to direct their feelings freely and even share their both positive and negative experiences when the people of the whole world reveal them as unknown masked agents and called them as heroes. Through admitting the positive extents of any overall health disorder, it is appropriate to recognize features that may provide greater spirit in HCWs either employed as entities or in groups.

HCWs during the SARS outcome, 82% stated emotion respected by their manager and 77% by their society. HCWs reported that they were more enthusiastic about serving other people. Experts and moral ethics were acknowledged as major persuade energetic HCWs to complete their responsibilities for the duration of the MERS outcome [107]. Therefore, it is essential and persistent to learning scientifically the flexibility factors that may stimulate the psychological health of HCWs at the practiced workplace, psychological, and social planes.

A range of emotional methods were reported to describe the psychological health experiments during former infections, through controlling of stress level, workplace, and education supports to increase the recovery and comfort. Strategies can be enhanced to local perspectives, flexible surroundings and be ascended or descended depends on the requirements of HCWs overtime. PFA might be responsible for support to fighters during a severe emergency event, as it lessens the early pain of the distressing event by improving adaptive operational and managing in the aspect of unexpected trauma [108]. On the other hand, this is basically not sufficient in surviving to the outbreak of corona. The most basic awareness must also be reflected to control the recognized emotional health difficulties in an efficient, practical manner. Moreover, even in the rescue period of an infection, there is a strong requirement for regular and long duration care to stimulate and defend the mental health of HCWs.

During COVID-19 the psychological health issue of frontline healthcare employees may increase the value in the mid of east and Africa of pre-existing literature in Asian countries [24, 109]. The emotional reaction of healthcare employees to the outbreak of contagious infection is complicated and may be associated with diverse issues. Causes of depression and anxiety in healthcare employees enhance the emotional state of vulnerability, loss of control and anxieties about someone's condition and chances of being contamination of coworkers, spreading of virus among others, well-being of family members especially children and old aged people. Further work associated issues to study are insecurity of employment, economic fears, shortage of taking rest, experience to severe happenings such as death and being quarantined for extensive-time period. Furthermore, Expected lack of goods and an enhancing influx of doubted and real cases of coronavirus may increase the burdens and distresses of medical employees [110, 111].

In addition to all this, high level of transmission and doubts about the method of transmission of coronavirus enhance the fear of this group. It is universally reported that droplet transmission is a key method. On the other hand, it was supposed that coronavirus also found on surfaces of doors, mobile phones and toilets, etc. So, medical employees are more attentive regarding their activities and keep on harmless (not to touch their skin after get in touch with patients or their caretakers) that may also increase their depression and fear levels [112]. It is usually observed that forefront employees feel anxiety greatly during the whole time period because there is no existing treatment and a certain protective vaccine. However, there is no any adequate confirmation that those who stay alive during infection have established resistance against the virus [113]. Furthermore, there is no compromise on the organization of ill people and restricted amounts of Intensive Care beds that medical employees are conscious and recognize the grieve of the condition.

Unluckily, the broadcasting sources influence has not been supportive, particularly social news in this situation. Scattering of wrong evidence and distribution of unverified news about the records of infections played a significant role in enhancing the anxieties, even among specialists. At times, message from Governments was so strong and threatening for need of people to take the right direction, that also prompted anxiety in different classes as well as medical employees. The significant feature necessary to be emphasized is the part of public broadcasting and skill in such matter. WHO has recognized the pandemic of 'COVID-19 lockdown and reaction have been complemented by an immense "infodemic" the large quantity evidence-some correct and some incorrect that marks it difficult for society to discover reliable foundations and consistent guidance' [114]. Reports point to social media involvement for the period of pandemics may be linked to mental health problems at greater risk. A current Chinese report revealed that a greater frequency of psychological health issues generally anxiety and depression was certainly connected with regularly social broadcasting coverage for the period of the COVID-19 lockdown, that was already stated before in a report showed that social media contact may certainly correlated with making risk perceptions during the MERS lockdown in South Korea [115]. Furthermore, many medical employees used social news to share their own skills, objections about deficiency of defensive tools and tributes of their missing colleagues and family members.

3.8 PSYCHOLOGICAL EFFECT OF COVID-19 ON MEDICAL WORKERS

It has also been reported that medical health workers faced extraordinary level of anxiety, posttraumatic stress (PTS), despair, and emotional stress for the period of infection and even after COVID-9 lockdown. Acute stress disorder (ASD) has related symptoms to post traumatic stress disorder (PTSD), is identified 3 to 30 days post-trauma, and is a noble forecaster of PTSD [116]. The extent of spreading of COVID-19 outbreak and the trauma experienced by the health care employees, adversarial emotional effects are likely to happen in them, specifically the individuals on the forward-facing line. Until now, slight is identified about the emotional control of corona-virus infection on health care employees in the rigorously affected countries. Opposing to emotional and psychological results in health care employees are usually suffered in a diversity of issues for the period of lockdown of contagious disease through great level of humanity, as well as indefinite isolation time period, insufficient therapeutic materials, stigma, discrimination, and worries of contamination, etc. [3, 117].

For the time being, the care from others and to hold plans that they accepted during the incident had been stated to be linked with their emotional issues by the time of pandemic of contagious disease [118]. The results of COVID-19 exposed a dominance of PTS issues in Chinese health care employees for the period of lockdown of coronavirus. Almost half of the individuals infected with PTS meeting medical cut-off of PTSD and 97.9% had at least one PTSD symptom, that was far complex than in other residents in the same study (34.0 and 94.0% respectively in university students). The ratio was also out of the range of 10–27% and medical PTSD analysis reported in the Ebola epidemic during 2014–2016 among general people [117] and in SARS outbreak in health care employees in 2003 [119]. By Comparing to PTS symptoms, the (13.6%) chances of despair were indicated by DASS-21 were lesser, but still considerably greater than the all-age incidence rate of 3.2% in Chinese individuals in latest eras [120]. For the moment, through the outbreak of cities or even countries due to the COVID lockdown, the medical employees turn out to be clearly the great risk in population to transfer the virus to those who have close relations with them, and surprisingly, were below the condition of being defamed or by escaped from others. In our study, EFA generated 3 extents from the 8 recognized warning items, namely stigmatization or separation, worries of being infected and apparent greater threat of their profession. These are vastly disturbed problems by medical employees during the COVID-19 lockdown and in other alike infection, and were showed to be linked to contrary emotional effects in this study, especially PTSD symptoms.

The most basic challenges encountered to control this widespread infection is the extreme scarcity of PPEs [121]. An extremely infective disorder trials previously cooperated with health organizations with subsequent lacks in supplies and PPEs. However, for the period of the Ebola outbreak, several countries cope with PPE shortages [122, 123]. During the infection, approving the emergency medical materials is relatable to national general health emergency response systems [120]. Consequently, it is appropriate to found an emergency reserve health materials package to make sure the delivery of materials based on type, quality, needs, and amount.

Pandemics employ significant psychological influences on HCWs, importance the need for suitable emotional support, interferences, and team support dealings. Specific psychological interventions related to COVID-19 for medical staff in China comprised psychological mediation care teams, spiritual advising, online platforms for medical assistance, availability of helpline, establishing the shift systems in hospitals, encouragements, providing sufficient breaks and time offs, given a plate form to take some rest and sleep, free time events such as yoga, musing, exercise, and motivational settings [22, 102]. Caring for the mental health of HCWs, by adopting suitable methods is a vital instrument in national emergency general health response to struggle during the lockdown. If appropriate dealings are adapted, the disease will finally diminish, in another case, a new flow of individuals distress from psychological sickness will arise [6, 124].

During the COVID-19, women, and young adults was shown the great psychological impact. These results do not show that this disease has shown the greater impact one gander specific [125]. However, most the industries influenced through this pandemic disease and mostly the women affected with this pandemic [126]. In addition to, usually the women mostly take care of her child and limited measures such as increase their burden at home, such as schools and childcare facilities closures [62].

3.9 CONCLUSION

COVID-19 has a significant opposing impact on psychological in the form of behavior impact, alexithymia, depression, anxiety. COVID-19 showed the significant negative effects on frontline healthcare and medical care workers all over the world population.

KEYWORDS

- **alexithymia**
- **anxiety**
- **behavioral impact**
- **COVID-19**
- **healthcare workers**
- **psychological impact**

REFERENCES

1. Xiang, Y. T., et al., (2020). Timely mental health care for the 2019 novel coronavirus outbreak is urgently needed. *The Lancet Psychiatry, 7*(3), 228, 229.
2. Rubin, G. J., Potts, H., & Michie, S., (2010). The impact of communications about swine flu (influenza A H1N1v) on public responses to the outbreak: Results from 36 national telephone surveys in the UK. *Health Technology Assessment, 14*(34), 183–266.

3. Brooks, S. K., et al., (2020). The psychological impact of quarantine and how to reduce it: Rapid review of the evidence. *The Lancet.*
4. Al Najjar, N., et al., (2016). Psychobehavioral responses to the 2014 middle east respiratory syndrome-novel coronavirus [MERS CoV] among adults in two shopping malls in Jeddah, western Saudi Arabia. *EMHJ-Eastern Mediterranean Health Journal, 22*(11), 817–823.
5. Wang, C., et al., (2020). Immediate psychological responses and associated factors during the initial stage of the 2019 coronavirus disease (COVID-19) epidemic among the general population in China. *International Journal of Environmental Research and Public Health, 17*(5), 1729.
6. Zia-Ul-Haq, M., et al., (2021). *Alternative Medicine Interventions for COVID-19* (Vol. XII, p. 284). Springer, Cham: Springer Nature Switzerland AG.
7. Lima, C. K. T., et al., (2020). The emotional impact of Coronavirus 2019-nCoV (new Coronavirus disease). *Psychiatry Research*, 112915.
8. Xu, Z., et al., (2020). Pathological findings of COVID-19 associated with acute respiratory distress syndrome. *The Lancet Respiratory Medicine, 8*(4), 420–422.
9. Ruan, S., (2020). Likelihood of survival of coronavirus disease 2019. *The Lancet Infectious Diseases, 20*(6), 630, 631.
10. Al-Tawfiq, J. A., Al-Homoud, A. H., & Memish, Z. A., (2020). Remdesivir as a possible therapeutic option for the COVID-19. *Travel Medicine and Infectious Disease.*
11. Bao, Y., et al., (2020). 2019-nCoV epidemic: Address mental health care to empower society. *The Lancet, 395*(10224), e37, e38.
12. Brooks, A. S., & Smith, C. C., (1987). Ishango Revisited: New age determinations and cultural interpretations. *African Archaeological Review, 5*(1), 65–78.
13. Duan, L., & Zhu, G., (2020). Psychological interventions for people affected by the COVID-19 epidemic. *The Lancet Psychiatry, 7*(4), 300–302.
14. De Medeiros, C. P. M., et al., (2020). The psychiatric impact of the novel coronavirus outbreak. *Psychiatry Research, 286*, 112902.
15. Zandifar, A., & Badrfam, R., (2020). Iranian mental health during the COVID-19 epidemic. *Asian Journal of Psychiatry, 51.*
16. Rajkumar, R. P., (2020). COVID-19 and mental health: A review of the existing literature. *Asian Journal of Psychiatry*, 102066.
17. Shahriarirad, R., et al., (2020). *The Mental Impact of COVID-19 Outbreak: A Population-Based Survey in Iran*, 1–21. Springer Nature.
18. Rehman, U., et al., (2020). Depression, anxiety and stress among Indians in times of Covid-19 lockdown. *Community Mental Health Journal*, 1–7.
19. Wilder-Smith, A., & Freedman, D. O., (2020*). Isolation, quarantine, social distancing and community containment: Pivotal role for old-style public health measures in the novel coronavirus (2019-nCoV) outbreak. Journal of Travel Medicine, 27*(2), taaa020.
20. Shigemura, J., et al., (2020). Public responses to the novel 2019 coronavirus (2019-nCoV) in Japan: Mental health consequences and target populations. *Psychiatry and Clinical Neurosciences, 74*(4), 281.
21. Huang, J. Z., et al., (2020). Mental health survey of 230 medical staff in a tertiary infectious disease hospital for COVID-19. *Zhonghua Lao dong wei sheng zhi ye bing za zhi= Zhonghua laodong weisheng zhiyebing zazhi= Chinese Journal of Industrial Hygiene and Occupational Diseases, 3*8, E001–E001.
22. Kang, L., et al., (2020). The mental health of medical workers in Wuhan, China dealing with the 2019 novel coronavirus. *The Lancet Psychiatry, 7*(3), e14.

23. Lai, J., et al., (2020). Factors associated with mental health outcomes among health care workers exposed to coronavirus disease 2019. *JAMA Network Open, 3*(3), e203976–e203976.
24. Lee, S. M., et al., (2018). Psychological impact of the 2015 MERS outbreak on hospital workers and quarantined hemodialysis patients. *Comprehensive Psychiatry, 87*, 123–127.
25. Li, Z., et al., (2020). Vicarious traumatization in the general public, members, and non-members of medical teams aiding in COVID-19 control. *Brain, Behavior, and Immunity*.
26. Ornell, F., et al., (2020). "Pandemic fear" and COVID-19: Mental health burden and strategies. *Brazilian Journal of Psychiatry, 42*(3), 232–235.
27. Lee, M., & You, M., (2020). Psychological and behavioral responses in South Korea during the early stages of coronavirus disease 2019 (COVID-19). *International Journal of Environmental Research and Public Health, 17*(9), 2977.
28. Parlapani, E., et al., (2020). Psychological and behavioral responses to the COVID-19 pandemic in Greece. *Frontiers in Psychiatry, 11*, 821.
29. Chan, J. F. W., et al., (2020). A familial cluster of pneumonia associated with the 2019 novel coronavirus indicating person-to-person transmission: A study of a family cluster. *The Lancet, 395*(10223), 514–523.
30. Tang, X., et al., (2020). On the origin and continuing evolution of SARS-CoV-2. *National Science Review*.
31. Balkhi, F., et al., (2020). Psychological and behavioral response to the coronavirus (COVID-19) pandemic. *Cureus, 12*(5).
32. Lau, J., et al., (2003). Monitoring community responses to the SARS epidemic in Hong Kong: From day 10 to day 62. *Journal of Epidemiology & Community Health, 57*(11), 864–870.
33. Rosen, A. B., Tsai, J. S., & Downs, S. M., (2003). Variations in risk attitude across race, gender, and education. *Medical Decision Making, 23*(6), 511–517.
34. Jin, Z., et al., (2020). *Psychological Responses to the Coronavirus Disease (COVID-19) outbreak, 14,* 1. China.
35. Bukhari, E. E., et al., (2016). Middle East respiratory syndrome coronavirus (MERS-CoV) outbreak perceptions of risk and stress evaluation in nurses. *The Journal of Infection in Developing Countries, 10*(08), 845–850.
36. Onyeaka, H. K., Zahid, S., & Patel, R. S., (2020). The unaddressed behavioral health aspect during the coronavirus pandemic. *Cureus, 12*(3).
37. Do, T. T. T., et al., (2018). Receptiveness and preferences of health-related smartphone applications among Vietnamese youth and young adults. *BMC Public Health, 18*(1), 764.
38. Shah, K., et al., (2020). Focus on mental health during the coronavirus (COVID-19) pandemic: Applying learnings from the past outbreaks. *Cureus, 12*(3).
39. Banerjee, D., (2020). The COVID-19 outbreak: Crucial role the psychiatrists can play. *Asian Journal of Psychiatry, 50*, 102014.
40. Yao, H., Chen, J. H., & Xu, Y. F., (2020). Rethinking online mental health services in China during the COVID-19 epidemic. *Asian Journal of Psychiatry, 50*, 102015.
41. Hall, R. C., Hall, R. C., & Chapman, M. J., (2008). The 1995 Kikwit Ebola outbreak: Lessons hospitals and physicians can apply to future viral epidemics. *General Hospital Psychiatry, 30*(5), 446–452.
42. Patel, A., & Jernigan, D. B., (2020). Initial public health response and interim clinical guidance for the 2019 novel coronavirus outbreak—United States. *Morbidity and Mortality Weekly Report, 69*(5), 140.

43. Chaturvedi, S. K., (2020). Covid-19, coronavirus and mental health rehabilitation at times of crisis. *Journal of Psychosocial Rehabilitation and Mental Health*, 1–2.
44. Holmes, E. A., et al., (2020). Multidisciplinary research priorities for the COVID-19 pandemic: A call for action for mental health science. *The Lancet Psychiatry.*
45. Dong, L., & Bouey, J., (2020). *Early Release-Public Mental Health Crisis During COVID-19 Pandemic, 26*(7), 1616. China.
46. De Berardis, D., et al., (2020). Alexithymia, resilience, somatic sensations and their relationships with suicide ideation in drug naïve patients with first-episode major depression: An exploratory study in the "real world" everyday clinical practice. *Early Intervention in Psychiatry, 14*(3), 336–342.
47. Lankes, F., et al., (2020). The effect of alexithymia and depressive feelings on pain perception in somatoform pain disorder. *Journal of Psychosomatic Research*, 110101.
48. McCaslin, S. E., et al., (2006). Alexithymia and PTSD symptoms in urban police officers: Cross-sectional and prospective findings. *Journal of Traumatic Stress: Official Publication of The International Society for Traumatic Stress Studies, 19*(3), 361–373.
49. Wells, R., Rehman, U. S., & Sutherland, S., (2016). Alexithymia and social support in romantic relationships. *Personality and Individual Differences, 90*, 371–376.
50. Grynberg, D., et al., (2010). Alexithymia in the interpersonal domain: A general deficit of empathy? *Personality and Individual Differences, 49*(8), 845–850.
51. Kojima, M., et al., (2003). Alexithymia, depression and social support among Japanese workers. *Psychotherapy and Psychosomatics, 72*(6), 307–314.
52. Stice, E., Ragan, J., & Randall, P., (2004). Prospective relations between social support and depression: Differential direction of effects for parent and peer support? *Journal of Abnormal Psychology, 113*(1), 155.
53. Hwa, S. S., et al., (2012). A comparative study on alexithymia in depressive, somatoform, anxiety, and psychotic disorders among Koreans. *Psychiatry Investigation, 9*(4), 325.
54. Declercq, F., Vanheule, S., & Deheegher, J., (2010). Alexithymia and posttraumatic stress: Subscales and symptom clusters. *Journal of Clinical Psychology, 66*(10), 1076–1089.
55. Ginzburg, K., Ein-Dor, T., & Solomon, Z., (2010). Comorbidity of posttraumatic stress disorder, anxiety and depression: A 20-year longitudinal study of war veterans. *Journal of Affective Disorders, 123*(1–3), 249–257.
56. Hébert, M., et al., (2018). Alexithymia as a mediator of the relationship between child sexual abuse and psychological distress in adolescence: A short-term longitudinal study. *Psychiatry Research, 260*, 468–472.
57. Tang, W., Xu, D., & Xu, J., (2020). The mediating role of alexithymia between earthquake exposure and psychopathology among adolescents 8.5 years after the Wenchuan earthquake. *Personality and Individual Differences, 159,* 109881.
58. Eichhorn, S., et al., (2014). Traumatic experiences, alexithymia, and posttraumatic symptomatology: A cross-sectional population-based study in Germany. *European Journal of Psychotraumatology, 5*(1), 23870.
59. Spaccarelli, S., (1994). Stress, appraisal, and coping in child sexual abuse: A theoretical and empirical review. *Psychological Bulletin, 116*(2), 340.
60. Parker, J. D., Taylor, G. J., & Bagby, R. M., (1998). Alexithymia: Relationship with ego defense and coping styles. *Comprehensive Psychiatry, 39*(2), 91–98.
61. Karukivi, M., et al., (2010). Alexithymia is associated with anxiety among adolescents. *Journal of Affective Disorders, 125*(1–3), 383–387.

62. Mantovani, A., Dalbeni, A., & Beatrice, G., (2020). Coronavirus disease 2019 (COVID-19): We don't leave women alone. *International Journal of Public Health, 65*(3), 235, 236.
63. Tang, W., et al., (2017). Mental health problems among children and adolescents experiencing two major earthquakes in remote mountainous regions: A longitudinal study. *Comprehensive Psychiatry, 72*, 66–73.
64. De Berardis, D., et al., (2020). Alexithymia, suicide ideation, affective temperaments and homocysteine levels in drug naïve patients with posttraumatic stress disorder: An exploratory study in the everyday 'real world' clinical practice. *International Journal of Psychiatry in Clinical Practice, 24*(1), 83–87.
65. De Berardis, D., et al., (2017). Alexithymia and suicide risk in psychiatric disorders: A mini-review. *Frontiers in Psychiatry, 8*, 148.
66. Cao, W., et al., (2020). The psychological impact of the COVID-19 epidemic on college students in China. *Psychiatry Research*, 112934.
67. Wong, T. W., Gao, Y., & Tam, W. W. S., (2007). Anxiety among university students during the SARS epidemic in Hong Kong. *Stress and Health: Journal of the International Society for the Investigation of Stress, 23*(1), 31–35.
68. Al-Rabiaah, A., et al., (2020). Middle east respiratory syndrome-corona virus (MERS-CoV) associated stress among medical students at a university teaching hospital in Saudi Arabia. *Journal of Infection and Public Health.*
69. Mei, S., et al., (2011). Psychological investigation of university students in a university in Jilin Province. *Medicine and Society, 24*(05), 84–86.
70. Cheng, S. K., et al., (2004). Psychological distress and negative appraisals in survivors of severe acute respiratory syndrome (SARS). *Psychological Medicine, 34*(7), 1187.
71. Azad, N., et al., (2017). Anxiety and depression in medical students of a private medical college. *Journal of Ayub Medical College Abbottabad, 29*(1), 123–127.
72. Mirza, I., & Jenkins, R., (2004). Risk factors, prevalence, risk factors, prevalence, and treatment of anxiety and depressive disorders in and treatment of anxiety and depressive disorders in Pakistan: Systematic review. Pakistan: Systematic review. *BMJ, 328*, 794.
73. Salman, M., et al., (2020). *Psychological Impact of COVID-19 on Pakistani University Students and How They are Coping.* MedRxiv.
74. Al-Tammemi, A., Akour, A., & Alfalah, L., (2020). *Is it Just About Physical Health? An Internet-Based Cross-Sectional Study Exploring the Psychological Impacts of COVID-19 Pandemic on University Students in Jordan Using Kessler Psychological Distress Scale.*
75. Husky, M. M., Kovess-Masfety, V., & Swendsen, J. D., (2020). Stress and anxiety among university students in France during Covid-19 mandatory confinement. *Comprehensive Psychiatry, 102*, 152191.
76. Özdede, M., & Sahin, S., (2020). Views and anxiety levels of Turkish dental students during the COVID-19 pandemic. *Journal of Stomatology, 73*(3), 123–128.
77. Albert, P. R., (2015). Why is depression more prevalent in women? *Journal of Psychiatry & Neuroscience: JPN, 40*(4), 219.
78. Aylie, N. S., Mekonen, M. A., & Mekuria, R. M., (2020). The psychological impacts of COVID-19 pandemic among university students in Bench-Sheko Zone, South-west Ethiopia: A community-based cross-sectional study. *Psychology Research and Behavior Management, 13*, 813.
79. Read, M. C., (2020). EID: High contagiousness and rapid spread of severe acute respiratory syndrome coronavirus 2. *Emerg. Infect. Dis, 26.*

80. Vindegaard, N., & Benros, M. E., (2020). COVID-19 pandemic and mental health consequences: Systematic review of the current evidence. *Brain, Behavior, and Immunity*.
81. Wang, J., et al., (2018). Associations between loneliness and perceived social support and outcomes of mental health problems: A systematic review. *BMC Psychiatry, 18*(1), 156.
82. Tesfaye, K. R., Bayray, K. A., & Ahmed, K. Y., (2020). Prevalence of mental distress and associated factors among Samara university students, Northeast Ethiopia. *Depression Research and Treatment*.
83. Khan, S., et al., (2020). Impact of coronavirus outbreak on psychological health. *Journal of Global Health, 10*(1).
84. Torales, J., et al., (2020). The outbreak of COVID-19 coronavirus and its impact on global mental health. *International Journal of Social Psychiatry*, 0020764020915212.
85. Reynolds, D. L., et al., (2008). Understanding, compliance and psychological impact of the SARS quarantine experience. *Epidemiology & Infection, 136*(7), 997–1007.
86. Hawryluck, L., et al., (2004). SARS control and psychological effects of quarantine, Toronto, Canada. *Emerging Infectious Diseases, 10*(7), 1206.
87. DiGiovanni, C., et al., (2004). Factors influencing compliance with quarantine in Toronto during the 2003 SARS outbreak. *Biosecurity and Bioterrorism: Biodefense Strategy, Practice, and Science, 2*(4), 265–272.
88. Cava, M. A., et al., (2005). The experience of quarantine for individuals affected by SARS in Toronto. *Public Health Nursing, 22*(5), 398–406.
89. Desclaux, A., et al., (2017). Accepted monitoring or endured quarantine? Ebola contacts' perceptions in Senegal. *Social Science & Medicine, 178*, 38–45.
90. Braunack-Mayer, A., et al., (2013). Understanding the school community's response to school closures during the H1N1 2009 influenza pandemic. *BMC Public Health, 13*(1), 344.
91. Jeong, H., et al., (2016). Mental health status of people isolated due to Middle East Respiratory Syndrome. *Epidemiology and Health, 38*.
92. Pompili, M., et al., (2014). The associations among childhood maltreatment, "male depression" and suicide risk in psychiatric patients. *Psychiatry Research, 220*(1, 2), 571–578.
93. Engel-Yeger, B., et al., (2016). Extreme sensory processing patterns and their relation with clinical conditions among individuals with major affective disorders. *Psychiatry Research, 236*, 112–118.
94. Narzisi, A., (2020). *Handle the Autism Spectrum Condition During Coronavirus (COVID-19) Stay at Home Period: Ten Tips for Helping Parents and Caregivers of Young Children*. Multidisciplinary Digital Publishing Institute.
95. Canning, E. H., Canning, R. D., & Boyce, W. T., (1992). Depressive symptoms and adaptive style in children with cancer. Journal *of the American Academy of Child & Adolescent Psychiatry, 31*(6), 1120–1124.
96. Devine, H., Stewart, S. H., & Watt, M. C., (1999). Relations between anxiety sensitivity and dimensions of alexithymia in a young adult sample. *Journal of Psychosomatic Research, 47*(2), 145–158.
97. Craparo, G., et al., (2014). Posttraumatic stress symptoms, dissociation, and alexithymia in an Italian sample of flood victims. *Neuropsychiatric Disease and Treatment, 10*, 2281.
98. Güleç, M. Y., et al., (2013). Effects of childhood trauma on somatization in major depressive disorder: The role of alexithymia. *Journal of Affective Disorders, 146*(1), 137–141.

99. Liu, X., et al., (2012). Depression after exposure to stressful events: Lessons learned from the severe acute respiratory syndrome epidemic. *Comprehensive Psychiatry, 53*(1), 15–23.
100. Greenberg, N., et al., (2020). Managing mental health challenges faced by healthcare workers during covid-19 pandemic. *BMJ, 368*.
101. Biswas, P., & Chatterjee, S., (2014). Hand hygiene compliance among doctors in a tertiary care hospital of India. *The Indian Journal of Pediatrics, 81*(9), 967–968.
102. Chen, Q., et al., (2020). Mental health care for medical staff in China during the COVID-19 outbreak. *The Lancet Psychiatry, 7*(4), e15–e16.
103. Chan-Yeung, M., (2004). Severe acute respiratory syndrome (SARS) and healthcare workers. *International Journal of Occupational and Environmental Health, 10*(4), 421–427.
104. Tam, C. W., et al., (2004). Severe acute respiratory syndrome (SARS) in Hong Kong in 2003: Stress and psychological impact among frontline healthcare workers. *Psychological Medicine, 34*(7), 1197.
105. Dutheil, F., et al., (2019). Suicide among physicians and healthcare workers: A systematic review and meta-analysis. *PloS One, 14*(12), e0226361.
106. Jones, N., Whybrow, D., & Coetzee, R., (2018). UK military doctors; stigma, mental health and help-seeking: A comparative cohort study. *BMJ Military Health, 164*(4), 259–266.
107. Khalid, I., et al., (2016). Healthcare workers emotions, perceived stressors and coping strategies during a MERS-CoV outbreak. *Clinical Medicine & Research, 14*(1), 7–14.
108. Pekevski, J., (2013). First responders and psychological first aid. *Journal of Emergency Management, 11*(1), 39–48. *Weston, Mass.*
109. Zhang, C., et al., (2020). Survey of insomnia and related social psychological factors among medical staff involved in the 2019 novel coronavirus disease outbreak. *Frontiers in Psychiatry, 11*, 306.
110. Spitzer, R. L., et al., (1999). Validation and utility of a self-report version of PRIME-MD: The PHQ primary care study. *JAMA, 282*(18), 1737–1744.
111. World Health Organization, (2020). *"Immunity Passports" in the Context of COVID-19: Scientific Brief.*
112. Hassany, M., et al., (2020). Estimation of COVID-19 burden in Egypt. *The Lancet Infectious Diseases.*
113. Organization, W. H., (2020). *Novel Coronavirus (2019-nCoV): Situation Report, 13.*
114. Zhang, W. R., et al., (2020). Mental health and psychosocial problems of medical health workers during the COVID-19 epidemic in China. *Psychotherapy and Psychosomatics, 89*(4), 242–250.
115. Chua, S. E., et al., (2004). Psychological effects of the SARS outbreak in Hong Kong on high-risk health care workers. *The Canadian Journal of Psychiatry, 49*(6), 391–393.
116. Bryant, R. A., (2010). Acute stress disorder as a predictor of posttraumatic stress disorder: A systematic review. *The Journal of Clinical Psychiatry, 72*(2), 233–239.
117. Jalloh, M. F., et al., (2018). Impact of Ebola experiences and risk perceptions on mental health in Sierra Leone. *BMJ Global Health, 3*(2), e000471.
118. Raven, J., Wurie, H., & Witter, S., (2018). Health workers' experiences of coping with the Ebola epidemic in Sierra Leone's health system: A qualitative study. *BMC Health Services Research, 18*(1), 251.
119. Wu, P., et al., (2009). The psychological impact of the SARS epidemic on hospital employees in China: Exposure, risk perception, and altruistic acceptance of risk. *The Canadian Journal of Psychiatry, 54*(5), 302–311.

120. Ren, X., et al., (2020) Burden of depression in China, 1990–2017: Findings from the global burden of disease study 2017. *Journal of Affective Disorders*.
121. Wang, X., Zhang, X., & He, J., (2020). Challenges to the system of reserve medical supplies for public health emergencies: Reflections on the outbreak of the severe acute respiratory syndrome coronavirus 2 (SARS-CoV-2) epidemic in China. *Bioscience Trends, 14*(1), 3–8.
122. Shaukat, N., Ali, D. M., & Razzak, J., (2020). Physical and mental health impacts of COVID-19 on healthcare workers: A scoping review. *International Journal of Emergency Medicine, 13*(1), 1–8.
123. Selvaraj, S. A., et al., (2018). Infection rates and risk factors for infection among health workers during Ebola and Marburg virus outbreaks: A systematic review. *The Journal of Infectious Diseases, 218*(suppl_5), S679–S689.
124. Zia-Ul-Haq, M., Dewanjee, S., & Riaz, M., (2021). *Carotenoids: Structure and Function in the Human Body* (Vol. XVI, p. 859). Springer Nature Switzerland AG: Springer International Publishing.
125. Wenham, C., Smith, J., & Morgan, R., (2020). COVID-19: The gendered impacts of the outbreak. *The Lancet, 395*(10227), 846–848.
126. Rodríguez-Rey, R., Garrido-Hernansaiz, H., & Collado, S., (2020). Psychological impact and associated factors during the initial stage of the coronavirus (COVID-19) pandemic among the general population in Spain. *Frontiers in Psychology, 11*, 1540.

CHAPTER 4

Detection Assays and Techniques Against COVID-19

SHAHZAD SHARIF,[1] MAHAM SAEED,[1] JAVED HUSSAIN SHAH,[1] SAJJAD HUSSAIN,[2] AHMAD ADNAN,[1] HANADI TALAL AHMEDAH,[3] and MUHAMMAD RIAZ[4]

[1]*Department of Chemistry, GC University, Lahore–54000, Pakistan, E-mail: mssharif@gcu.edu.pk (S. Sharif)*

[2]*School of Chemistry, Faculty of Basic Sciences and Mathematics, Minhaj University, Lahore, Pakistan*

[3]*Department of Medical Laboratory Technology, Faculty of Applied Medical Sciences, King Abdulaziz University, Rabigh, Saudi Arabia*

[4]*Department of Pharmacy, Shaheed Benazir Bhutto University, Sheringal, Pakistan*

ABSTRACT

A viral disease, COVID-19, is an emerging health threat to the public and has caused large-scale deaths throughout the world. Since its outbreak, scientists are working on sequencing its genome, understanding its targets, mechanism, and way of transfer from animal to humans. It is necessary to detect and prevent the disease outbreak at a large scale near to an early stage. This virus is visually characterized via electron microscopy, x-ray diffraction, and atomic force microscopy as well as can be detected in the laboratory through molecular assays, computed tomography (CT), biochemical tests, biomarkers such as an inflammatory biomarker, cardiac biomarkers, hepatic biomarkers, renal biomarkers, serological assays including enzyme-linked immunosorbent assay (ELIZA), lateral flow immunoassay, neutralization assay, luminescent immunoassay, rapid antigen assay, contact tracing, and potentially small molecule biomarkers in blood. In this chapter, we have summarized the possible methods for the detection and characterization of this new virus. Developing plug-and-play diagnostics to manage the COVID-19 outbreak may be helpful for prevention of ahead epidemics.

4.1 INTRODUCTION

By going through history, it has been observed that the world has faced five major deadly widespread viruses the most recent is COVID-19, while previously reported are Ebola, Severe acute respiratory syndrome (SARS), The middle east respiratory syndrome (MERS) and Swine flu occurred in previous 15 years. The world community has to face the severity of both deadly pandemics, i.e., MERS, and COVID-19 but the latter is more active in severity and infection nowadays [1]. China was the first country where an eruption of COVID-19 was appeared in December 2019 [2]. Many patients were admitted to the hospital with symptoms of temperature, difficulty in respiration, hawk (cough) with many others [3]. In contrast to images of healthy lungs, scanning of virus-infected individuals through computed tomography (CT) showed variations in lungs, i.e., effusive, tributary, and compact [4]. These results guide to early detection of pneumonia. To suggest the unfamiliar reasons for pneumonia, evaluation of nucleic acid with multiplex real-time polymerase chain reaction (PCR) can be done.

Human interaction with each other is happened to be the major cause of SARS-CoV-2 spread. The occurrence of 1st communication is done between bats and unfamiliar host cells [2]. Analysis has been done that infection of 3 new people will occur due to 1 SARS-CoV2 patient (Ratio is 1 to 3.28) [5]. Some patients show symptoms, while others do not show any, mostly observed symptoms are fever, cough, and fatigue. COVID-19 patients' main symptoms are common with symptoms of influenza. Direct contact and droplet spread have become the major reasons for transmission [6].

Globally, SARS-CoV-2 directing to COVID-19 prevalent has affected world community, till now, there are confirmed cases of almost 20,730,456, and deaths of almost 751,154, as of August 15, 2020, reported by World Health Organization (WHO). Partially and completely lockdown and social distancing have modified and disturbed the working life of billions of people worldwide in many cities. Resultantly, winding up of business and almost every hindrance on trade and tours the world economy has to face a big decrease. The present situation focuses on making certain the worldwide attainability of fast, cheap, and accessible diagnosis tools to decrease the severity involved in the SARS-CoV2 virus and immunity. It is also a need of time to give the best support and opportunities to universities, companies, and laboratories all over the world to produce test kits on an urgent basis. On the basis of positive test results, fear is that the affected virus patients are supposed to be more as compared to present today [7]. Unexpressed proliferation/transmission of COVID-19 can be finished by applying fast, easy, and accurate testing.

SARS-CoV2 also called Severe Acute Respiratory Syndrome Corona-virus-2 has become the main source of this infectious pandemic [8]. SARS-CoV-2 recently joins the family of *Corona* and the genus *Betacoronavirus* as compared to MERS-CoV and SARS-CoV. Having their *CORONA*-like resemblance, these viruses are named so. Corona has been derived from the Latin word known as *CROWN*. Coronavirus-induced Acute Respiratory Distress Syndrome (ARDS) is almost similar to Cytokine Storm Syndrome, causing fluid extravasation and a leap of pulmonary inflammation resulting in breathing collapse. Breathing hindrance, cardiac issues or ARDS may be the main causes. Secondary bacterial infection causes sepsis followed by death due to COVID-19 (Figure 4.1) [9].

4.2 PECULIAR PROPERTIES OF COVID-19 PANDEMIC

It cannot be confirmed accurately the symptoms of COVID-19 patients as these are nonspecific for early and perfect detection. According to Guan et al. research, fever is the main symptom, as in China, almost 44% of 1099 COVID-19 infected persons caught temperature by admitting in hospitals while 89% of patients got temperature during hospitalizing [10]. Researchers also concluded the infected persons had Shortness of breath (19%), sputum production (34%), fatigue (38%), and cough (68%) were the symptoms of patients. Most symptoms can be correlated with other breathing viruses. For screening and diagnosing of COVID-19 CT scans and Nucleic acid, testing has been used.

Many clinical expressions from mild to life-threatening conditions have been observed due to COVID-19. To differentiate COVID-19 patients from other diseases, the main key is to have an accurate and fast diagnosis. This will help accurate quarantining of COVID-19 positive while separating negative patients. Physicians having early and accurate diagnosis would be able to offer developed treatment as compared to patients who are at a lower risk.

Food and Drug Administration of USA (FDA-USA) have authorized vaccination and therapeutics of COVID-19 infected persons, while they work on vaccination and therapeutics is under process [11–13]. First case is identification, second includes isolation and third is related to identification of patients that may have in contact with infected patients, i.e., contact pacing, play a vital role in countering COVID-19 patients. Quick, accurate, and reliable diagnosis can help to save lives from this pandemic disease. It is believed that adopting precautions and timely diagnosis can help to save humanity. The immunity level of individuals can be increased by following WHO health guidelines of COVID-19. Early diagnosis, timely treatment, and increasing immunity are remarkable to face this infectious disease.

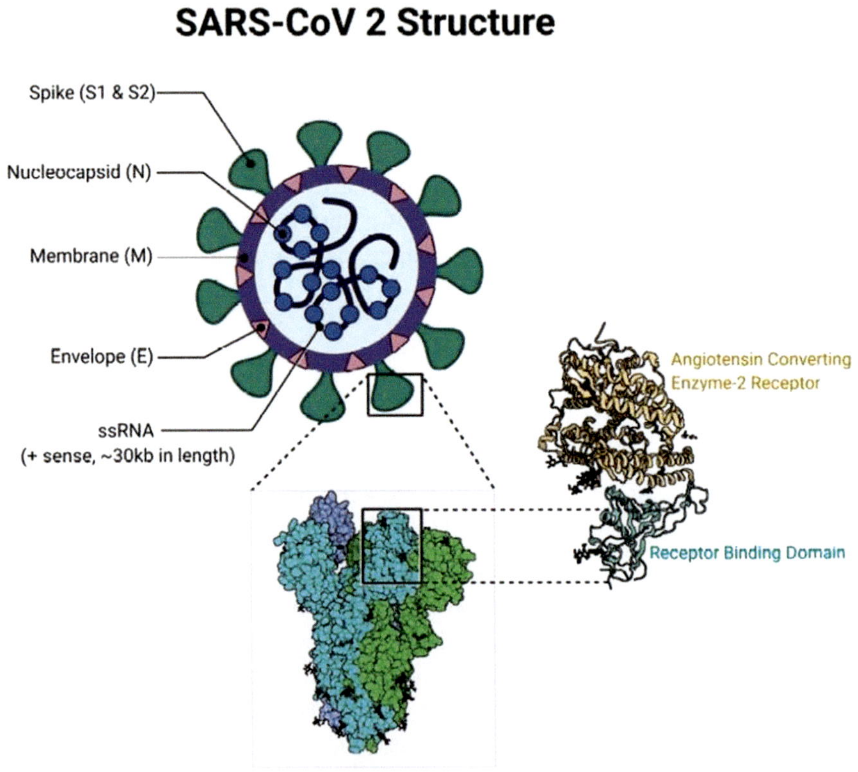

FIGURE 4.1 Structure and surface proteins of SARS-CoV-2.

Source: Reprinted with permission from Ref. [134]. © Copyright © 2021, StatPearls Publishing LLC. Figure contributed by Rohan Bir Singh, MD; Made with Biorender.com http://creativecommons.org/licenses/by/4.0/.

4.3 DEVELOPMENTAL STRATEGIES FOR ANALYSIS

For the COVID-19 virus, there must be specific criteria and developmental strategies for its accurate and best analysis. For the management of

COVID-19, we have to focus on accurate and early diagnosis, best treatment and adopting precautions. In the present situation, it is necessary to use testing kits and biochemical tests in a laboratory that are simple and accurate ways of detecting this infection at an early stage. To boost up the ongoing innovation of testing, we can develop methods for the analysis of COVID-19 diagnosis and applied strategies depending on methods that are conventional and novel including CRISPR. These strategies also include published information from the CAS research conclusions and MEDLINE for the development and improvement of diagnosis and testing kits on the COVID-19 pandemic.

Bio-chemical sensors with the developmental strategy of analysis have excitation to detect quickly, perfectly, and before the time current with scientific opportunities and challenges. The remarkable technologies and instruments in connection with COVID-19 can be analyzed to be best utilized for widespread strains. Commonly, diagnosis of viruses can be categorized into three major types:

- Diagnosis of antibody;
- Direct detection of disease; and
- Diagnosis of DNA-RNA viral.

Further analyzing strategies are elaborated as the techniques involved in characterization or structure elucidation like EM, XRD, and AFM that exhibit a full range of techniques that can be strongly employed to detect drug discovery, analysis, and ultimate results for ensuring public health and welfare. The use of advanced technology for scientific development, for example, the improvement of Corona detection bio-sensors, there should be a strong contribution in shaping a new era utilizing the best technical tools for future utilizations. Hence, differences must be highlighted with similarities among the different viral RNA infections and the COVID-19 disease. This will serve the understanding between the present technology and that which will sensitize and characterize the SARS-CoV2 virus [14].

4.4 COMMERCIALLY AVAILABLE METHODS FOR THE DETECTION OF COVID-19

The commercially available tests for COVID-19 have been categorized into:

- Polymerase chain reaction (PCR) techniques or nucleic acid hybridized relevant techniques are used for the study of molecular assays to detect RNA viral of SARS-CoV-2;

- Serological and immunological assays, in which antibodies, and antigenic proteins are detected in the samples collected from the infected individuals.

The former helps to find the infection at an acute phase; while the latter antibodies developed against the virus, these antibodies could be donated to other individuals. These both drive towards contact tracing as well as monitoring the immune status for both individuals and groups over time [15].

At present diagnosis of Corona-19 is originally composed of the collaboration of two or more than two techniques that contain CT scans, chest X-ray and RTPCR, with the identification of biomarkers in blood. These approved tests of biomarker with diagnosis of high concentration of C-reactive protein (CRP), low value of interleukin 6 and interleukin 10, low lymphocyte counts and low procalcitonin. Detection assay and techniques against COVID-19 are described as in subsections.

4.4.1 MOLECULAR ASSAYS FOR DETECTION OF COVID-19

Around 8 million cases of COVID-19 and 430,000 casualties are reported globally. The major infectious factor for this pandemic is found to be Severe Acute Respiratory Syndrome Coronavirus-2 called (SARS-CoV-2) [2, 8, 16, 17]. Recent addition to the Betacoronavirus genus and Coronaviridae family, SARS-CoV-2 linked the already existed MERS-CoV and SARS-CoV. These viruses are categorized because of their *corona*-like (crown) appearance and also having their ability to cause ARDS (Acute Respiratory Distress Syndrome). The presence of Coronavirus compels the ARDS through syndrome cytokine storm which enhances fluid extravasations and pulmonary inflammation at the end cause lungs failure [9, 18, 19].

By the study shows that SARS-CoV-2 contains RNA, which is a single-stranded (ssRNA) virus enveloped by capsid in the bilayer of lipids and the viral genome encodes proteins of viruses. Coronavirus genome is the biggest having 26 kb–32 kb. An infectious SARS-CoV-2 virus constitute structural proteins of 4 kinds; 1) envelop (E), 2) nucleocapsid (N), 3) spike proteins (S); and, 4) membrane (M) along with 29,903 nucleotides (nt) [20, 21]. N proteins and RNA genome join in a helical way just like rosary beads, and this resultant structure is enveloped by a bilayer of lipids as well as proteins of E, S, and M.

SARS-CoV-2 contagion infects a person when spike proteins interact with Angiotensin-converting enzyme 2 (ACE2) receptors onto the layers of the host cells [22, 23]. Inside the host body, the multiplication genome of RNA of SARS-CoV-2 leads to development of four structural type proteins as well as 25 non-structural proteins [15, 24]. SARS-CoV-2 viruses are produced when genome RNA assembles with structural proteins.

Molecular detection of COVID-19 is fundamentally based upon the recognition of RNA of SARS-CoV-2 [25–27]. Identification of viral proteins is helpful as well, even though it is not implemented in the diagnosis of COVID-19 yet. Seroconversion takes place within about 13 days for IgG as well as IgM [28]. Many test kits are being used to detect IgG and IgM antibodies in the blood. The challenges and potentials of antibody testing captured worldwide attention [29, 30]. However, a molecular assay of COVID-19 faces various challenges.

For instance, due to changing molecular structure and very low viral concentrations in samples, there are many challenges from collecting samples, treatment, and handling to limit detection and analytical specificity. Serological testing is a challenge when there is a response of antibodies against SARS-CoV-2, affecting the trustworthiness of diagnosis arising questions on clinical sensitivity (percentage of ill persons) and ratio of healthy individuals.

➢ **Step 1: Detection of Viral RNA:** During the initial outburst, SARS-Cov-2 presence was used to investigate the NGS (Metagenomic next-generation sequencing) have been utilized for detection of SARS-CoV-2 virus, leading towards COVID-19 infection [31]. Complete RNA molecule was removed from a broncho lavage specimen fluid. This RNA had been changed into DNA through reverse transcription and was followed by amplification of DNA through PCR. The Amplified DNA is sequenced by forming new templates. Various fluorometers were used to detect four different nucleotides; this helps to determine the exact sequence of DNA by tracing the fluorescence produced during polymerase elongation. Short length reads (150 bp) were joined and arranged with databases. SARS-Cov-2 was obtained by analyzing the longest overlapping regions of DNA. These DNA regions were sequenced in a highly concentrated sample. First-ever SARS-CoV-2 genomic sequence was passed on, January 7, 2020, by Wu et al. Since then, a large number of SARS-CoV-2 has been analyzed. Global initiative on sharing all influenza data plays a vital role to identify affected people. More than 460,000 people were identified by this center till 15 June 2020 [32].

RT (Reverse Transcriptase) PCR technique was used for diagnosis of peculiar arrangements of the SARS-CoV-2 genome [33], during the start of the COVID-19 pandemic. Due to expensiveness and much time taking conditions, RT-PCR is preferred to detect the infections caused by COVID-19. Even though RT-PCR is a recognized technique, but there are still challenges in the overall procedure from an initial collection of samples and treatment to gradual amplification and diagnosis.

- **Step 2: Collection of Samples:** Concentrations of SARS-CoV-2 vary in uninvolved samples depending upon the infectious phase. Clinical samples were analyzed through RT-PCR and their results were compared: fibro-bronchoscope brush biopsy, nasal swabs, bronchoalveolar lavage fluid (BALF), sputum, blood [34]. Largest positive results (93%) appeared for BALF, following by sputum (72%), nasal swab (63%), fiber bronchoscope brush biopsy (46%), pharyngeal swabs (32%), stool (29%), blood (1%) and urine (0%). Hence, respiratory samples are usually gathered to diagnose SARS-CoV-2 [35–37]. New researches show that concentrations of SARS-CoV-2 in different acute samples come up to maximum extent in a short time after the onset of symptoms and lower by the time after a week. The symptoms of SARS-CoV-2 and influenza are similar; symptoms of Influenza are severe at the time of onset of symptoms. In comparison, the viral concentrations of MERS-CoV, as well as SARS-CoV, reach maximum, respectively about a period of 10 days and 14 days.

  To use nasal and oral pharyngeal swabs along with endotracheal and nasopharyngeal washes to take a sample of the affected persons, the idea was proposed by WHO [38]. Samples collection from nasopharyngeal swab is relatively simple. Lower respiratory samples constitute endotracheal aspirate, bronchoalveolar lavage and sputum. Sputum generation depends upon repetitive coughs in individuals. Patients, who have asymptomatic or pre-symptomatic conditions of infection, may not produce sputum. A person supposed to collect the samples from the individual infected with SARS-CoV-2 may get encountered with it due to close contact as well as breathing process. Sputum directly from the patients as well as from nasopharyngeal swabs gives rise to coughing or sneezing and generation of aerosols.

  WHO proposed employing polyester or Dacron embedded swabs for collection of samples from the oropharyngeal vs. nasopharyngeal swabs as well as sterilized pots to oropharyngeal and nasopharyngeal,

BALF, endotracheal aspirates, and sputum [39]. The collected samples after proper seal and storage at 2–8°C should be transferred to the laboratory very early for testing.

Oropharyngeal or nasopharyngeal washes, endotracheal aspirate, bronchoalveolar lavage and sputum can be intact for two days; while, serum, oropharyngeal, and nasopharyngeal swabs, and blood for five days [40]. If these are required to be preserved for a longer time, then these must be placed at –70°C. It has been significant to ascertain practice for appropriate preventive measures while sample gathering, reposition, packing with shipping.

➢ **Step 3: Deliverance of RNA Viral:** This virus RNA has been enveloped with nucleocapsid, during determination of SARS-CoV-2, it is necessary to remove top-standard RNA viral in samples. RNA has been denatured by RNases (ribonucleases). RNA removal via inappropriate way leading to degradation or loss of viral RNA is one of the reasons behind poor clinical sensitivity [41]. In addition, the RNA removal procedure is time taking and needs well-trained personnel and laboratory instruments.

Fundamentally, RNA is removed with the help of organic solvents. One of them is phenol-guanidine isothiocyanate (GTTC) that has the potential to quickly degrade nuclease-like enzymes and stabilize RNA. However, this process of RNA removal needs much time, critical conditions as well as corrosive GITC reagent. The removed RNA is being contaminated by natural salts and organic liquids. These contaminants include positive ions which may restrict PCR that is downstream. RNA purification employing spin columns and magnetic particles evaporate contaminants and organic solvents. RNA purification tools and kits are successfully developed by using strategies that have been proposed by CDC [36, 37, 42, 43]. However, the enhancing requirement for RNA removal kits forces manufacturers and suppliers globally that restricts the capability of COVID-19 diagnosis quickly.

4.4.2 COMPUTED TOMOGRAPHY (CT)

The term CT is generally recognized as CT scan which is a detection technique used for confirming inaccurate hits obtained from RT-PCR of SARS-CoV2 virus. This may either be used as a single detection tool or in combination with other techniques. In CT, examination of the chest via X-rays with various directions has been done to get three-dimensional pictures having different contrasts. Afterwards, the obtained images are analyzed by field specialists or radiologists to detect any abnormality to ascertain the infection of SARS-CoV2. COVID-19 infection is confirmed from CT scans by ground-glass opacification of areas of sub-pleural regions; As a result, both lobes of the chest cavity affected depends upon the infection severity [44]. Moreover, data collected from COVID-19 affected people showed solidification of fluids in the lungs. In addition, CT scan images also helped in serving as the most suitable tool for COVID-19 so far. For instance, at the start of the infection, the CT images look like a normal chest. The opacity of images increases with the spread of infection; for example, ground-glass opacity has been observed in patients after 4th day of onset, it is confirmed by random patterns obtained in scan [41].

To diagnose COVID-19 in the early time, a CT scan is a suitable technique. There is similarity between symptoms of COVID-19 and common respiratory infections and pneumonia so, it is difficult for the radiologist and other doctors to identify this disease. The main idea of using a CT scan to detect this virus comes from literature which indicates that the specific detection of this tool is about 25% because it shows resemblance with pneumonia and respiratory infections. For operation and analysis, a CT scan is used. It is a highly advanced and expensive technique. That is why this technique is used along with RT-PCR for COVID-19 virus detection.

4.4.3 BIOCHEMICAL TESTS

The importance of clinical laboratories during this pandemic surpasses early diagnosis and epidemiological monitoring. Regular hematological, biochemical, and immune-chemical laboratory testing is necessary to analyze the severity of the disease, selection of proper therapeutic choices and following treatment response. As the numbers of ascertained COVID-19 patients are continuously increasing worldwide, laboratory malfunctions linked with the increased severity of disease are increasingly transparent.

4.4.3.1 BIOMARKERS

There is a list of various biomarkers linked to COVID-19 disease and can be used as diagnostic tools in the laboratories.

4.4.3.1.1 Inflammatory Biomarkers

Different inflammatory biomarkers are involved in serious COVID-19, indicating an immune-chemical profile related to the said cytokine storm. Shortly, pro-inflammation cytokinesis and necrosis factor increased in the persons having a severe infection and are greatly linked with casualty [44–47]. It is necessary to consider that pro-inflammatory Cytokinesis not only acted as environment pollution indicators but also a major cause to spread COVID-19. Even though cytokine calculation is not usual in clinical lab practices, complementary biochemical markers for inflammation are all applied in serious cases of COVID-19 and may be found useful in analyzing the seriousness of disease [19, 48, 49]. The increased concentration of pro-calcitonin is appeared in serious COVID-19, with the indication of bacterial co-or supra infection in individuals who are severely ill [50]. Besides biochemical markers of inflammation, hematological results indicate that elevation in neutrophil-to-lymphocyte ratio, lymphopenia as well as platelet-to-lymphocyte ratio (PLR) were found to have warning potential. Enhancement of D-diameter coagulation factor was reported continuously and linked with a huge risk of multiple thromboembolic reactions development in COVID-19 victims and severing disease, involving in different processes [51–55].

Generally, this data ascertained that serious cases of COVID-19 were assessed by a huge pro-inflammatory reaction or increased cytokine level that was analyzed to promote MOF n serious cases. In short, biochemical analyzes of COVID-19 cases involve timely identification of renal, hepatic, and cardiac injury by common testing in labs and analyzing the inflammatory response.

4.4.3.1.2 Cardiac Biomarkers

When clinical data was collected it indicated clear cardio-vascular malfunction in serious COVID-19 cases [48, 56, 57]. Early reports in China discovered that almost 12% of reported cases and ICU cases of about 31% were diagnosed with a serious myocardial injury which is indicated by a high concentration of cardiac troponin I [50]. Cases with increased cardiac troponin levels needed to be admitted to ICU and exhibited enhanced hospital casualty [58–63]. In one of the cases of this virus, the detailed study indicates that 27.8% of affected patient had a myocardial injury, that is ultimately responsible for cardiac and asthma diseases [64]. These data confirmed that analyzing cardiac biomarkers like natriuretic peptides and cardiac troponin throughout the disease would be necessary for adequate assessment of risk initialization in the patients. An official statement has been published by the American college of cardiology on the function of cardiovascular biomarkers analysis in COVID-19 cases. They published that on clinical grounds if the diagnosis of myocardial infarction is analyzed, clinicians are suggested to measure troponin level [65].

This medicinal suggestion was to stop unauthentic diagnosis of COVID-19 cases and reduced down-stream processes and consultations involving angiography and bedside echocardiography [66]. However, a lot of people rules out this stance, forcing that cardiac troponin must not be only taken as a secondary test for diagnosis of myocardial infarction, instead of as a helpful diagnostic indicator for both non-ischemic and ischemic reasons of cardiac malfunction that could be very useful in patients' trial as well as appropriate treatment selection [67].

Supposed mechanisms for cardio-vascular severities of COVID-19 involve direct myocardial injury, exacerbation of coronary artery disease, viral myocarditis, and cytokine-driven myocardial damage. Nowadays, not a single of these recommended mechanisms are explained as the major participant of the cardio-vascular severities found in serious COVID-19 cases. More clinical research would be necessary to indicate the major factor of Heart disorders for proper treatment and guidelines for laboratory investigation [15, 25, 32, 33, 68, 69].

4.4.3.1.3 Hepatic Biomarkers

Lately, evidence suggested that in serious COVID-19 cases, liver dysfunction has also been traced. Researches in some large hospitals also reported a rise in the level of enzymes of hepatic and mixed nature like gamma-glutamyl-transferase-GGT, alanine aminotransferase-ALT and aspartate aminotransferase (AST) [70–77]. New research by Cai et al. completed an anticipated review of laboratory and clinical results from 417 confirmed COVID-19 patients. About 76.3% of reported patients showed an abnormal levels of liver markers, and the remaining 21.5% were found to suffer from liver injury after getting hospitalized. Interesting to note that while alkaline phosphate (ALP) and GGT were both considered enzymes related to cholangiocyte and GGT was only found to be increased in the COVID-19 disease, indicating that the complication was likely drug-related instead of bile duct injury [78]. As it was certain that liver damage was linked with an increased chance of developing serious COVID-19, thus most of the concern relies on diagnostic tests in liver injury to know the reasons for associated complications. Reasonable biochemical mechanisms related to liver damage in COVID-19 involve direct cytotoxicity because of potential viral multiplication in biliary epithelial cells expressing ACE2, drug-induced liver damage, immune-mediated damage because of serious inflammatory reaction following infection and hypoxic hepatitis due to anoxia [79–81].

While the participation of intrinsic hepatic situations, as well as biochemical processes behind liver damage, remained vague, it was, nevertheless, clear that LFTs must be considered commonly to analyze all the hepatic injuries associated in the clinical labs, especially for patients having treatment against viruses.

4.4.3.1.4 Renal Biomarkers

Reported data of SARS pandemic in 2002 to 2003 revealed that 6.7% of cases had severe damage in kidney and the casualty of SARS individual having "acute kidney injury" (AKI) was huge as 91.7% [82]. As there is much relatedness between different causative factors, therefore, the emphasis is on analyzing kidney impairment in the COVID-19 patients. Recently reported data revealed that the chance of spreading AKI is relatively less and different researches showed its fluctuation between 0.5 to 19.1%. Serum creatinine and blood urea nitrogen both are considered common markers of kidney damage [83]. Certainly, the current process for AKI detection is actually based on serious variations in serum creatinine, and the rate of detection is strongly affected by testing through serum creatinine [84, 85]. In advanced research by Cheng and colleagues, individuals with increased basic serum creatinine were at high risk that they could be admitted to the "intensive care unit (ICU)" as well as to give mechanical ventilation [86]. These results recommend that initial diagnosis and treatment of kidney damage involving appropriate hemodynamic support and reducing nephrotoxic medicines can prove important in COVID-19 cases and a greater number of creatinine and related markers of kidney testing must be assured. Urinary albumin, serum, and total protein are considered helpful diagnostic indicators in COVID-19. Just like liver damage, the pathophysiological processes associated with renal impairment in COVID-19 cases are not known and prone to be multi-causative. Active processes involve direct cytopathic impacts on renal tissues, organ cross-talk like cardiomyopathy as well as myocarditis and intrarenal inflammation and damage because of cytokine inflammatory reaction towards infections can cause renal vein blockage, renal hypoperfusion as well as hypotension [87].

4.4.4 SEROLOGICAL AND IMMUNOLOGICAL ASSAYS

While viral RNA detections based on RT-PCR is vastly employed in COVID-19 diagnosis, it cannot be utilized for monitoring of advanced stages in disease and also cannot be employed in broad identification of previous immunity and infections. Serological testing consists of an analysis of plasma or blood serum and is operationally extended to accommodate testing of biological fluids, saliva, and sputum to check the appearance of immunoglobulin G (IgG) and M (IgM). This analysis is significant in vaccine development and epidemiology, giving an idea of short and long duration traces of antibody retaliation, diversity, and abundance. After some days, IgM can be detected, and it also remains for some weeks after infection and then switched to IgG. Hence, IgM can be considered as a sign of present or previous infection. IgG can also be utilized in suggesting the onset of immunity after infection. In last year's, immunological tests selectivity and sensitivity have not only increased but it is also used in the analysis of derived antigens from pathogens and applications of antibiotics. These all tests can be proved very helpful in the epidemics of COVID-19 however, the consequences may be affected through the following situations:

- Due to a halt in the production of antibodies after infection with SARS-CoV-2, the subjects combined with positive results obtained after analysis by "Molecular Genetics" are considered as seronegative.
- The subjects which are seropositive but results after analysis by molecular genetics are negative then there are chances of mild infection.
- Restriction comes in the sensitivity and specificity of the analyzes [88–92].

The third problem is specifically more important due to the lower percentage of incorrect positive result having less specificity that can cause the prediction of excessive misleading antibodies in a population with unwanted effects on a socioeconomic decision and mass confidence [93, 94].

Detection of different viral antigens has a strong influence on the determination of SARS-CoV-2 including nucleocapsid proteins and spike glycoprotein which are S1/S2 subunits binding sites for a receptor. The methods for these tests constitute fundamental enzyme-linked immunosorbent assay (ELISA), neutralization bioassay, specific chemosensors and immunochromatographic lateral flow assay. Each assay has its particular advantages like multiplexing, speed, and automation and disadvantages such as dedicated laboratories, trained personnel, etc. In addition to testing procedures for antibodies, there are fast antigen detection tests where antibodies have been employed for the diagnosis of viral antigens through a blood serum specimen. Currently, the development of high-throughput serological tests falls in major concerns of companies undergoing diagnosis [95].

4.4.4.1 ENZYME-LINKED IMMUNOSORBENT ASSAY (ELISA)

This technique may be recognized as microwell assay that is plate-based particularly to detect as quantification of substances such as proteins, peptides, hormones, and antibodies. These assays may be quantitative, qualitative, and commonly results are obtained from 1 to 5 hours. In the SARS-CoV-2 case, viral proteins are specifically used to cover the plate wells. If the patient samples contain antibodies, they will particularly bind and the complex is utilized for further process. ELISA is fast, capable of automation for increased response and can test various samples collectively but can have varied sensitivity and is appropriate for POC determinations.

4.4.4.2 LATERAL FLOW IMMUNOASSAY

This type has been a qualitative chromatographic analysis which may be portable and small and further utilized. Such techniques has been simply a fast detection test (RTD) because results can be collected within half an hour. Practically, the substrate is loaded with fluid specimen permitting the specimen to flow over a non-mobile band of viral antigen. If the antibodies for anti-COVID are found there, they start accumulating at the band, and in addition to other antibodies (tracer), there is an appearance of color indicating the results. This is an inexpensive technique and does not need any trained person, but it is for qualitative analysis only. When combined with symptomology, the infection can be detected feasibly. Rapid techniques for antigen diagnosis where antibodies against COVID-19 are employed instead of static viral antigen, permit a more accurate analysis for the proceeding infection.

4.4.4.3 NEUTRALIZATION ASSAY

This test is an analysis of an antibody potential to develop resistance for viral infections of prepared cells and the virus undergoing replication process with cytopathic impacts consequently. The serum, whole blood or plasma samples of patients are diluted for this test, and their decreasing concentrations are in the cultures of cells. If the neutralizing antibodies are present, the point at which antibodies resist against the multiplication of virus can be utilized to determine their concentration in the infection causing cell medium. The obtained results from this test are achieved in 3–5 days with advanced methods had lessened time to hours [95, 96]. That kind of detection needs facilities of cell cultures, and in the SARS-CoV case, BSL3, i.e., Biosafety Level-3 laboratories. For the vaccine development and medicinal implications of convalescent plasma (CP), neutralizing antibody detection in a small duration of time is significant instead of the mentioned restrictions.

4.4.4.4 LUMINESCENT IMMUNOASSAY

This type of essay consists of methods that reduce the LOD (Limit of Diagnosis) for the antibodies. In general, it includes fluorescence and chemiluminescence. Cai et al. have developed a method to detect COVID-19 by constructing a magnetic chemiluminescence enzyme immunoassay and Diazyme. Laboratories also confirmed the accessibility of 2 novel serological diagnosis of SARS-CoV-2 which have been completely automated.

4.4.4.5 BIOSENSOR TEST

These are based on detection of a readout signal through particular interactions of biomolecules developed by enzymatic, electrical, optical, and further methods. An analysis that determines light incident interference phenomenon at boundary-line of solid is known as Surface Plasmon Resonance (SPR). A biosensor based on SPR had been invented for SARS testing with the implementation of SCVme, i.e., coronaviral surface antigen upon a substrate of gold [97]. The developed SPR chip displayed a 200 ng/mL limit of detection for anti-SCVme antibodies in 10 minutes.

4.4.4.6 RAPID ANTIGEN TEST

In addition to tests of molecular genetics, some fast antigen tests are also there which permit the detection of the viral antigen [98, 99]. These types of tests involve the viral antigens containment forming a specific specimen for analysis to give a proper mechanism to this type of analysis test primarily entail monoclonal antibodies forming a particular specimen for analysis. These tests do not have limitations for a specific format [100], an enhancement for chemiluminescence based immunoassay for COVID-19 in 2005 [101] and a fluorescence lateral flow assay to diagnose nucleocapsid protein related to SARS-CoV [102].

Detection of SARS-CoV at a higher level can be based upon serological and immunological assay:

Ultimately, where these analysis trials having a heavy capability to pursue the SARS-CoV-2 virus, various techniques have been developing. Infection status, Immune protection status and seroprevalence for the personnel's healthcare can be diagnosed via a combination of serological detection and molecular genetic tests but with a limitation.

The technique is affected by the reason that due to delay in the generation of antibodies, few patients with positive results for the molecular genetic assay are "seropositive." Currently, no strong evidence has been found for a combination of seropositivity and the immune system.

4.4.5 CONTACT TRACING

Contact tracing is a procedure of identifying, analyzing, and managing individuals who have encountered an infectious disease to restrict the further spread of disease. If implemented gradually, contact tracing can break the strings of the prevalence of infection and hence, is an important public health measure for monitoring infectious disease outbursts. Contact tracing for coronavirus disease needs tracing people who might have encountered COVID-19 and monitoring them regularly for 2 weeks (14 days) from the last day of the encounter.

Important elements of the application of contact tracing are public support and community participation; careful strategies and understanding of local contexts, cultures, and communities; professional contact tracers and supervisors; transportation facility to contact tracing units and a database to gather, arrange, and analyze data in a short time. For effective contact tracing, nations must have enough resources to test possible cases on time. When it is not possible, testing and contact tracing planning should focus on particular high-risk arrangements with on risk persons, like care homes, hospitals, or other related spaces [103].

As people can transmit COVID-19 at the pre-symptomatic or asymptomatic stage, these guidelines also signify the importance of isolation to decrease the risk of secondary transmission [104].

4.4.5.1 COMMUNITY ENGAGEMENT

Contact tracing starts with guiding communities about disease, how to save people and surrounding societies and how to reduce transmission. Contact tracing needs people to be convinced to regular monitoring, to agree to report initial signs of COVID-19 actively, and to prepare themselves to isolate for minimum 2 weeks if the symptoms appear. Interaction with communities and their spokespersons can assist in pointing out possible challenges in the path of contact tracing involving language and educational barriers, information, availability of food and medical facility, stigma, and marginalization. Special importance should be put on planning contact tracing for vulnerable groups involving homeless individuals, refugees, minority groups, migrants, and others.

Communication about contact tracing must signify reciprocity, common good and solidarity. By engaging in contact tracing, societies will participate in monitoring the local prevalence of infection, individuals at risk will be saved more preventive measures like staying at homes and lockdowns can be minimized. All societies are prone to have concerns about the confidentiality and privacy of their private medical information. Public health organizations that employ contact tracing for COVID-19 must be ready to communicate how data would be collected, stored, used, and accessed and how to protect people from dangerous disclosure.

It is crucial that contact tracing and related stages like isolation of affected people must not be used punishingly or related to security parameters, migration problems or other issues outside the boundary of public health. Contact tracing facilities must be accessible to every community. WHO proposed on purpose involvement by cases and contacts.

4.4.5.2 EPIDEMIOLOGICAL SCENARIOS

Contact tracing readiness, alertness, and performance will rely on four major transmission scenes:

i. **No Cases:** A well-organized contact tracing team should be selected, trained, and on alert, prepared to approach to first cases.
ii. **Sporadic Cases/Clusters:** Comprehensive contact tracing is crucial to quickly decrease the transmission.
iii. **Clusters:** Contact tracing is necessary for reducing spread within clusters.

iv. **Community Transmission:** Contact tracing can be complicated when the spread is severe but must be done as much as possible, targeting household contacts, high-risk closed settings, healthcare employees, and at-risk individuals, and keeping powerful contact tracing capacity in small clusters regions.

When nations have passed, the surge of spread and confirmed cases were declining, specifically when strict social and public health steps were settled, quick identification of cases and contact tracing were crucial to keep reduced levels of prevalence and quickly trace and break new spread strings.

4.4.5.3 STEPS OF CONTACT TRACING

Contact tracing is necessary to be carried out for every confirmed case and can be required for might be cases without comprehensive testing potential.

Defining Contacts: Contact may be defined as any person having the following encounters to COVID-19 confirmed case from 2 days before 2 weeks after the start of disease (Figure 4.2):

i. Presence at 1 m distance for more than 15 minutes near to COVID-19 case;
ii. With a confirmed case of COVID direct physical contact;
iii. Without using standard (PPE) Personal Protective Equipment giving direct caution to patients of COVID-19.

If ascertained cases do not show any symptoms, i.e., are asymptomatic, contacts must be dealt similarly as asymptomatic cases with an encounter time from 2 days prior the case was confirmed or after 2 weeks.

4.4.5.4 IDENTIFICATION OF CONTACTS

As already explained, contact identification can be conducted in community households, healthcare units and hospitals and areas in close vicinities like dormitories, living spaces, prisons, shelters, etc., public transport, well-defined places like schools, gatherings, private, and public events. Data that is gathered is the distance between the infected and healthy individuals, closed relationship, sharing of living spaces, physical contact, etc. Information and guidance about these scenarios can be provided to the masses through current media, social media applications, telecommunication authorities, influential personals, newspapers, television, information technology sources, etc.

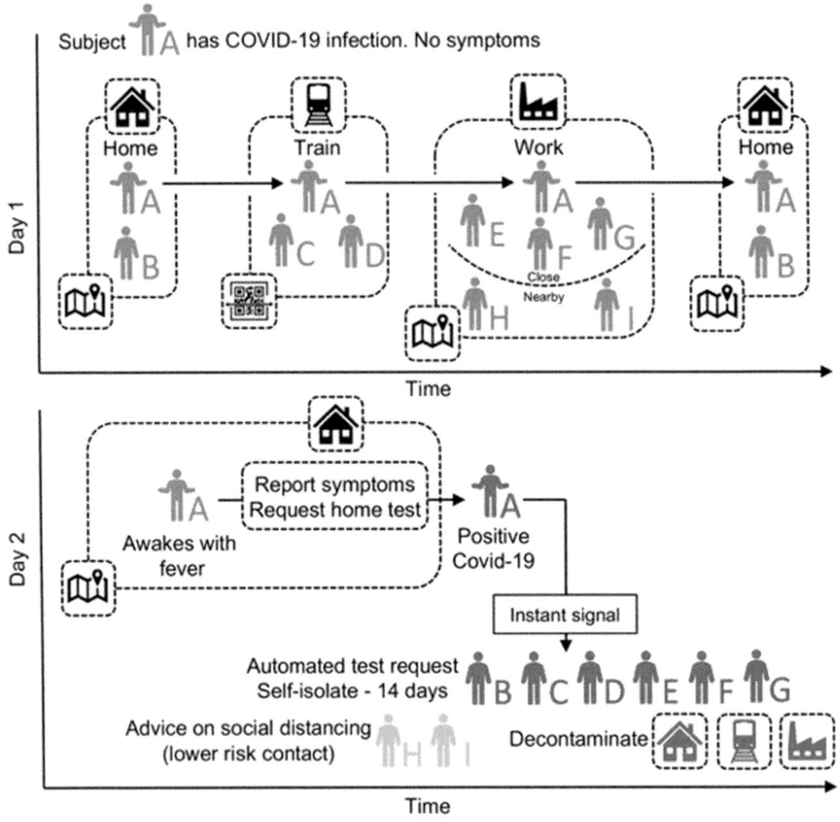

FIGURE 4.2 Application of contact tracing.

Source: Reprinted with permission from Ref. 135.

4.4.5.5 INFORMING CONTACTS

Contact tracing units should prepare a list of individuals who were in the vicinity of COVID-19 confirmed cases. Every individual should be initially contacted over the phone or personally to check if they fulfill the contact definition and so, need monitoring. Every person confirmed as a contact must be given information on the following:

i. The procedure of contact tracing and information on quarantine;
ii. The place where they will be isolated and how to be cared;
iii. What signs to care for during the monitoring time? This involves any signs, particularly fever, chills, cough, nasal congestion, sore throat,

difficulty breathing, running nose, diarrhea, nasal dysfunction, muscle pain, etc.;

iv. What actions to take if contacts become unwell, such as whom to call, how to quarantine and take precautions and what procedures are present for test and treatment;
v. Data saving involving how to use, analyze, and store personal information;
vi. Other particular queries or concerns of contacts.

Information can be given personally or over the phone, and complementary approaches like emails or text messages can be used.

4.4.5.6 MANAGING AND MONITORING CONTACTS REGULARLY

i. **Quarantine:** of individuals is the reduction of actions or the separation of individuals who are not currently infected but might have encountered a disease or an infectious agent, with the sole purpose of analyzing their signs and ascertaining the timely identification of cases. Quarantine must not be confused with isolation which is the parting of diseased or infected individuals from the healthy ones to stop spreading the virus or contamination.
ii. **Daily Monitoring:** This means the regular two-way communication between the contact tracing unit and the contacts they are given to monitor to check any symptom of infection. Daily monitoring options involve:

   Direct monitoring by the contact tracing unit: monitoring possible symptoms and signs over the phone or visiting the contacts personally. Contact tracers should take necessary precautions and social distancing.
iii. **Self-Reporting:** Where contacts monitor their own selves and report every symptom to contact tracers. This process must be carried out regularly, even in the absence of signs (zero reporting).

   The contact tracing team gathers data on symptoms and signs from every contact regularly on a contact tracing form. Electronic tools or gadgets can be used where possible.

   The key data on the contact tracing form include:

   a. **Contact Identification:** Such as full name, contact ID, phone number, address, etc.

b. **Demographic Information:** Involving gender, date of birth, language, marital status, and occupation.
c. **Type of Contact:** Such as a workplace, household, health facility, community, date of the last contact, number, and duration of exposure and factors affecting contact vulnerability should be a follow-up daily already.
d. **Absence of Follow-Up:** Like causes of not reporting routine signs, altered address, etc.
e. **Steps to Take if Symptomatic:** Such as date of onset of signs, contact's location, date of data collection, etc.
f. **Out of Reach Contacts:** In this case, contact tracers can ask friends and relatives or consider other sources to locate contacts. If contact moves to a known area in the same region, contact tracers can check them. If contact moves to another region, contact tracers covering that region must be informed and follow-up. Contacts with symptoms must quarantine and follow developed referral routes for diagnosis and treatment. The monitoring phase ends up after 14 days of an encounter of contact with an infectious person, or if contact shows signs of COVID-19. If contacts are in close vicinity of each other, and one of them develops symptoms, the follow-up duration is reset to 14 days after the last encounter to a new patient.

iv. **Particular Population Groups:** For potentially susceptible health-care personals caring for COVID-19 patients, a complete encounter risk assessment must be implemented to analyze the type of encounter and PPE usage at the exposure time:
   a. An encountered staff member not wearing specific PPE at the exposure time must give up working, take quarantine and self-analyze themselves for 2 weeks following the last encounter.
   b. Staff who were in close distance of COVID-19 cases but were wearing proper PPE at the exposure time may carry on working.
   c. Staff must regularly respond to COVID-19 focal person at a workplace for any disease.
   d. Healthcare workers (HCWs) near of COVID-19 cases outside the boundary of a healthcare unit will abide by the same guidelines and monitoring laws as community contacts.

For other people, contact tracing can be adapted for the regions with restricted human facilities and technological resources involving quite low-income groups or humanitarian viewpoint; it can emphasize considering only severe contacts and regions not having a community-to-community transmission. In areas with restricted facilities, the provision of necessary facilities like clean water and soap must be ascertained to control the spread of infection.

v. **Data Processing and Analysis:**

   a. **Flow of Data:** The information that contact tracers collect about every contact must be included to proper databank involving information of data origin and further details. Database must be upgraded and sequence wise information must be added to it. Detailed analysis and related performance indicators must be arranged regularly and contacted to contact tracer teams and their supervisors. If a contact develops symptoms of the disease, the changes in condition must be linked, using a common indicator, to a contact's database. The proper utilization of routine indicators of contact tracing and private laboratory results are necessary.

   b. **Analysis:** Important monitoring indicators must be arranged regularly and communicated to contact tracing teams.

   c. **Workforce Requirements for Contact Tracing:** Analyzing workforce requirements for contact tracing relies on different factors involving the required number of contacts which need tracing, technological, and physical transportation to reach affected areas, cultural point of views, socio-political point of views, security aspects and contact tracing protocols like regular personal visits versus self-reports. Public health organizations should assess their basic requirements and make a strategy for a properly managed workforce for contact tracing.

   d. **Profile of Contact Tracers:** Contact tracers are selected from their region and must have an adequate literacy level, proficiency in the local language, cultural understanding, and communication skills. Contact tracers must be familiar with and trained on the fundamentals of COVID-19 spread, prevention, control parameters, monitoring of symptoms, signs, and the morals of public health analysis and quarantine. Contact tracers' team must be selected from different settings involving civil society, local government and non-governmental bodies, community volunteers, university students, etc. Medical staff must not be permitted to do contact tracing until situations require. Supervisory staff must be assigned to every contact tracing unit to provide technical and transportation facility, better monitoring and problem-solving. Every contact tracer needs to keep a safe distance while interacting with contacts and probable COVID-19 cases and do interviews outside or well-arranged settings.

e. **Equipment and Transportation:** Contact tracers may need administrative, logistics, and material support like paper or electronic substances for recording data, transport, mobile phones and credits, etc. The contact tracing team must be given proper PPEs.

f. **Information Technology:**
   - **Types of Tools:** Electronic gadgets and information technology are not necessary for contact tracing but may facilitate applications on large scales and make them better. Other devices are present for self-reporting of signs by contacts and related apps that trace individuals' movement to point out possible encounter to and from other individuals.
   - **Data Protection:** The moral values of public health information, data saving and data privacy should be ensured during the whole contact tracing procedure. Particularly:
     - Safeguards should be present to ascertain data protection and privacy according to the legal infrastructure of the nations where systems are applied.
     - Every individual involved in contact tracing should consider the moral principles of personal information handling to ascertain privacy and data management throughout the procedure.
     - How to handle, use, and store data requires to be exchanged to those related to transparent and clear ways. It is necessary for engaging and avoiding misunderstandings that can spoil the credibility of the contact tracing technique.
     - Digital devices used in this regard must be checked before use to ascertain data protection according to national laws.

4.4.6 POTENTIAL SMALL MOLECULE BIOMARKERS IN BLOOD

Recently, a variety of molecular biomarkers has been detected in blood for the detection of COVID-19 patients in the whole world. Although various biomarkers have not been determined as unique as analysis or viral DNA or RNA testing is, their value in blood during testing of the COVID-19 has been found to help.

It is actually due to the various protein-based compounds in blood that automatically act as the disease biomarkers, increase, or decline the concentrations for fighting the infection. That is why many of such biomarkers are in direct link with the severity of the disease. Specifically, concentrations of CREA, serum urea, C (Cys-C), CHE, LDH (lactate dehydrogenase), and serum direct bilirubin (DBIL) were detected as particularly increased as in serious COVID-19 patients as compared to mild COVID-19 patients [105]. Most latterly, the inability to sniff was regarded as a COVID-19 biomarker. The nasal mucous secretions constitute many proteins assisting metabolizing xenobiotics and support epithelial coordination necessary for smelling. Hence, manufacturing biosensors for identifying proteins present in mucous may also prove helpful for the timely SARS-CoV2 detection. But it must be considered that these biomarkers are not exclusive to COVID-19 as loss of smell is also associated with other diseases such as Parkinson's disorder [106]. This surely gives initial information for the development of biosensors to start planning for specifying either one or more than one candidate to construct test kits for exact and accurate COVID-19.

Poly-morpho nuclear leukocytes (PMN) moving in the blood, exhibit increased levels as a defense strategy of the host during infections. PMN constitutes various fragments of knowledge about various etiological factors that stimulate the immune system. These result in stimulation of PMN, and enhanced molecular oxygen utilization leading towards the generation of reactive oxygen species (ROS), a procedure jointly known as respiratory burst. Several biosensors were developed in biomedical history for ROS identification from different viruses, and on the same ground, detection of SARS-CoV2 disease ROS may cause a complementary way for COVID-19 detection [107].

4.4.6.1 BIOSENSORS FOR EARLY DETECTION AND PROGNOSIS OF PANDEMIC VIRAL STRAINS

Biosensors have been the chemical sensing tools having a biologically derived recognition coupled to a transducer, allowing quantitative development of some complicated biochemical parameters. Generally, biosensors comprise a biological element which may be enzymes, nucleic acids, plant proteins, tissue slices, microorganisms, organelles or antibodies and an electrical element that is a transducer. The elements interact with the analyte present in the sample to be tested, and the response may be biological, optical, or thermal, which is converted into an appropriate electrical parameter like voltage or current with the help of the transducer.

These biosensors are becoming highly sophisticated primarily due to the combination of advances in biotechnology and microelectronics. These are greatly valuable tools for measuring a wide range of analytes from organic compounds to bacteria and viruses.

4.4.6.2 CHARACTERISTICS OF BIOSENSORS

Biosensors are highly valuable due to their advanced characteristics which give them an edge over other detection devices:

1. **High Selectivity:** Selectivity is referred to the potential of biosensors to particularly identify the desired substance even in the presence of other similar substances and impurities. Usually, viruses show similar structures due to their required genome and protein capsule covering the genome. In few species, a membrane covers genetic material and the protein coat. The protein coat of viruses is their distinguishing character from bacteria. Specific identification and targeting a few proteins present on the capsule with other proteins through protein-protein attractive links probably help in the selective virus detection. Selectivity can be made better by ascertaining that the single layer of probes targeting the selected sensor surface on the analyte biomarkers is optimally static. Mostly it is a research field and commonly requires selected personnel containing time of 6 months to a year for constructing required-specific probes. Such aspect has been certainly a chokepoint for the rapid promotion of biosensors in the course of pandemics like COVID-19. However, the advances in nanotechnology and the momentum of discoveries and inventions of substances present a good prospect for researchers to construct target-specific probes. While the development of particular probes is certainly challenging, new research has illustrated a transparent covering for the electrodes comprising biological molecules blended with conductive nanomaterials' web [108]. Such transparent coatings are tested to retain 88% of actual detection after a month of disclosure to the sample concluding original patient original plasma for IL-responses.

2. **High Sensitivity:** The characteristics like attraction, spacing, and target probes' specificity in the single layer, sometimes known as bio-recognition elements or self-assembled monolayers (SAMs) measure the fixing of the substances on the sensors' surface. Moreover, the electrical or optical characteristics of the transducer affect the net sensitivity of the biosensor; for example, the number of molecules attached with the sensor before a response can be easily detected from the noise it makes. If the monolayer's specificity is ascertained, then it is probable to determine different small-sized biomarkers of size <150 kDa even at a single molecular stage. For detecting biomarkers related to pandemic strains like COVID-19, the prepared sensor must be able to determine the biomarkers particular for the disease at reduced concentrations, specifically at only one molecule stage and generate a feasible readable response for the desired quantity. For example, a big hurdle is directly detecting viral RNA or DNA in an unprocessed blood sample without requiring signal strengthening through PCR. It would make the basis of studies for quick testing of worldwide viral strains. Some additional devices like microfluidics and nanoparticle-based detection tools may also be used to resolve some of the basic issues constituting on the surface of sensor handling of biological fluid [109].
3. **Rapid Response Time:** To effectively avail diagnostic tool during pandemics, the sensor response is the significant aspect. Theoretically, the majority of transducers in the sensors give an instantaneous response to the applied stimulus taking <1s, for example, on the interaction of biomolecules with the surfaces of sensors. However, sometimes these signals need post-processing with the help of new computing systems and electronics for exact analysis of the measured concentration. For example, identification of background noise and its removal and temperature correction can often cause enhanced sensor response time. Hence, the role and design of signal processing circuits are of great significance in ascertaining rapid response times of the measurement.
4. **Multiplexing:** During the initial levels of the disease when there is less comprehension of the properties of virus strains, it is sometimes the number of usual biomarkers in the blood (like interleukin and CRP as explained for COVID-19) that work as the indication of infection. For the detection of COVID-19, currently, more than two biomarkers are used in combination to ascertain the disease. That

is why a multiplexed system allowing determination of different biomarkers is required for a rapid, early, and exact testing of the infection. The phenomenon by physically separating many parts of the sensor surface multiplexing phenomenon can be acquired where every separated part functions as an individual sensor [110, 111]. Every single part could further be made specifically for one biomarker [112–114]. Measurements can be taken by either a single transducer scanning the individual parts of the sensing surface or by combining more than one transducer fixed to a single sensing area [115].

5. **Multimode Sensing:** For detecting the viral strains, the sensor which gives rapid response must be reliable as well. To enhance the reproducibility in the functioning of the sensor, multiple sensing processes could give cross-confirmation of the obtained signals. The fundamental compromise of using this type of sensing is a rise in computation time of sensor and the size of physical dimensions, leading to an enhanced power utilization, slow response time and cost concerns. However, the better aspect is that mostly these barriers are quickly looked after. Optical and electrochemical techniques on one platform that can feasibly be converted into multimode panels are greatly acquiring an interest in the industry as well as academia [116]. This may be able to fulfill the need for enhanced strength and reliability in the medical sensors through quick authentication of data.
6. **Disposable:** As the pandemic viral species are greatly infectious, like COVID-19 having a higher multiplication number than that of SARS and H1N1, there is a great need for single-use sensors to avoid impurities from sensors. The most reasonable way to construct disposable sensors is the modular approach. In this method, readout modules and electrodes could be individually constructed with disposable electrodes and cost-effectiveness. The available substances for constructing such waste-able electrodes could primarily constitute glass, plastic, metal, paper, or ceramic substances that may be utilized to immobilize bio-probes exclusive for our desired biomolecules. Among these electrodes, paper-based bio-sensing electrodes which gathered concern of the community recently, give the most reasonable disposable characteristics which classify these electrodes as burnable waste after use. In contrast, signal readouts in the form of cell phone app-based readouts will give multiple advantages (like a link with the centralized healthcare unit and periodic collection of data) other than cost-effectiveness.

7. **Longtime Shelf Life and Trouble-Free to Utilize:** The advanced electrodes must be easy to utilize and must have at least one month. It would make clear huge numbers of detection tools can be developed and exported to the medical units as well as to the supermarket racks. The ease of using these testing kits could help people to test them own and make compulsory and informed decisions to quarantine themselves to hamper the transmission of the infection [117].
8. **Cost-Effective:** The major plus point of the inexpensive availability of a biosensor is related to its affordability. Fundamentally, the lesser the cost of a particular biosensor, the more approachable it is. To keep the price low and to make it affordable for all the members of the community in the time of pandemics, a biosensor can be studied in two parts. The first part could be a single-use electrode like a paper-based electrode or a screen-printed electrode easily available at the healthcare section of any supermarket. These electrodes may directly touch through body fluid, for example, saliva for rapid determination of virus. The other part of the sensing device might be a cell phone application, particularly serving the need for a direct readout device. These apps might primarily be made approachable by medical authority units situated in the affected neighborhood.

   Whereas, an individual portable and data collection operations having data collectors for single-use devices might also be constructed, which might be employed at boundary check posts of a nation or in hospitals. Surely, there would be a few bio-sensors that can be approached easily in big markets currently, for sexually transmitted disorders strips of lateral flow glucose meters or pregnancy test kits [117]. It is obvious that if rapid response sensors are developed, they may prove to be very helpful for the self-testing of viral strains. Moreover, this will reduce the burden on the government medical units to determine the infection in huge populations, leading to on-time prevention of the virus spreading.

   At the times of pandemics like COVID-19, there is a large and severe need for sensors to detect the rapidly spreading disease quickly and precisely. Lack of availability of sensors leads to the fewer numbers of testing even in the countries having excellent health infrastructure. It has been published that the number of detections performed for the determination of COVID-19 is less as compared to the total population. In ideal conditions, the number of biosensors should be comparable to the number of individuals living in a given geographical region under monitoring to ascertain that every member living in the society which may transmit infection gets detected during the early stages. Where there is a major technological hurdle to develop sensing devices in great quantities, recent advances in the development like machine molding and 3-D printing may assist in manufacturing large numbers of devices in a much short period [118].

9. **Autonomy and Connectivity to Central Healthcare Systems:** Autonomous systems of biosensors may ascertain a higher link between the readout modules and electrodes. In addition to autonomy, the measurement systems of sensors during pandemics must be capable of joining itself with a basic database of the medical or health care center, which will accumulate actual data from the signals. For example, a cell phone app collecting data from the sensors might be linked with cross-communication medium to:

    i. Provide better therapeutic involvement or ease the severity with paramedical personnel being dispatched;
    ii. Send data to the basic database unit.

Interlinked healthcare services can also troubleshoot and maintain through additional know-how of functioning of the sensors. Moreover, positive cases, location, personal information like gender, age, and contact details can conveniently be added to the basic databases. This process will provide the healthcare policymakers and government with actual data to accurately and rapidly take necessary decisions like locking down specific areas to resist and lessen the quick spread of infection.

Among the 10 major aspects discussed earlier, the most significant focus of recent innovations in biosensing systems must be the specificity and sensitivity of the tests performed for the timely determination of COVID-19 or related pandemic species. It is mandatory to remove the vagueness relating to the diversity of recent assay technology involving pin-point testing of viral RNA by CRISPR biosensors and lateral flow assays. Reusing some instruments like 96-well microliter plate readouts can also actively give many duplicates of bioassays in reduced time. These absorbance readers are very common and almost every laboratory providing routine CBC profile, involving in remote sensing, may use this base for rapid detection. For example, absorbance readouts are utilized in advanced works on rapid COVID-19 detection recommending the resources needed for newly developed procedures are present within various test centers beforehand. The other significant aspect actively leading to a rapid solution needed during pandemics is the soft-biosensors utilization. Like, recent advanced software can be equipped in portable thermometers that are largely employed nowadays for identifying COVID-19 probable patients. Perhaps, the software can be arranged such that the IR signals assessed through the detector give important knowledge, in addition to temperature sensing, on some important biomarkers present on the skin of patients similar to non-invasive biosensing.

4.4.6.3 TYPES OF BIOSENSORS

4.4.6.3.1 Electronic Sensors

Three-electrode potentiometric and ampere metric systems and FETs (field-effect transistors) are the major electronic biosensors greatly used for the detection of pathogens as well as biomolecules. The important advantages of electronic biosensors include low cost, mass manufacturing and miniaturization. Moreover, the ideas of a-modular sensors for parting readouts and electrodes in an android phone can be employed effectively. For example, field-effect transistors are feasibly developed in CMOS plants, on the other hand, a large amount of electrochemical sensing devices are currently approachable on a commercial scale as portable devices in the markets. In previous time, various kinds of electrochemical devices were manufactured for pandemic species. For example, Han et al. manufactured a micro-fluidic electro-chemical bio-sensor to detect and determine of H1N1, H5N1 and H7N9 with further details. Li et al. [119], electrochemical determination of MERs by Layqah et al. [89] determination of SARS by Iskhikawa et al. [120] and a lot of research in which paper-based substrates and disposable screen-printed electrodes were utilized for testing pandemic virus. Most researches absolutely motivated scientists for making novel plans for timely testing of COVID-19. Seo et al. pointed out a field-effect transistor device to detect SARS-CoV2 in various specimens. Required working of biosensor had been checked for detections carried out for processed viral strains, nasal swabs, and antigens as protein specimens from patients of COVID-19. The device which is used for detection can detect SARS-CoV2 proteins that may have a range from 1 mg/mL to 100 mg/mL buffer solvent. This device was mostly utilized for accurate determination of viral species in culture media with a LOD in different samples. It can be explained by how devices may determine viruses' minimum concentrations with no analyte processing. In a recent study, Mahari et al. manufactured the device employing different electrochemical setups. The LOD of this device, eCovSens, was measured around 120 FM in buffer solvents. Although test had been done in a non-clinical specimen, the electrodes remained unaffected for about 4 weeks, indicating that these electrodes might be constructed in large numbers, exported, and then distributed in the society in a comparable period amid pandemics. Seo et al. constructed a special Transistor to test SARS-CoV2 in clinical specimens [121].

4.4.6.3.2 Optical Biosensors

These biosensors fundamentally originated on principles of plasmonics, particularly where transduction principles use optical constituents for example, fiber optics, lasers, waveguides, and photonic crystals have been divided as optical biosensors. Optical biosensors of different types like (SPR) and (LSPR), are present on a commercial scale since the early 1990s, [117]. Whereas, some of the developed plasmonics techniques having developed surface chemistry give accurate selection, rapid response time with sensitivity for detecting the viral strains, but their utilization is significant.

Although, if utilization of such sensors is vague for self-testing by individuals and mass production, these biosensors are better developed recently to be widely used to diagnose virus. At present, Qiu et al. had manufactured biosensor to exact determination of COVID-19. Fundamentally, DNA receptors have been employed for the diagnosis of desired arrangements through SARS-CoV2. Through usage of light and nanoparticles in LSPR, it is reported that LSPR bio-sensor not only exhibited the best level of diagnosis but also responsive to different values which led to better sensitivity towards desired SARS-CoV-2.

It must be considered that through present improvements of joining of microfluidics to LSPR, extra improvements are possible. Hence, LSPR which has very large potential to detect precision in various tests and reduce extra burden through best-trained staff with better equipped lab because of unavailability of means. As described, Wei et al. exhibited the usage of sensors to check virus [117]. The main mechanism that has been developed for this purpose is further applied.

4.4.6.3.3 Microfluidic Biosensors

A technique known as microfluidics is employed to get exact control and a perfect way to handle the microscale fluids. The basic units under operation for transferring through analysis on the microchip are preparation, extraction, reaction, and detection. By employing the micromachining method, small to moderate type routes having fluid, detectors, pumps, valves, checkpoints with various stages are possible for construction to a silicon surface, polymers, metals, and other substances. Till now, microfluidic media have been employed by various techniques analytically involving fluorescence analysis, MS, chemiluminescence, and electrochemical analysis. Platforms of microfluidic might be divided into pressure-driven, capillary, acoustic, centrifugal, and electro-kinetic methods regarding their liquid propulsion laws. During the ancient times, these bio-sensors were manufactured to diagnose different diseases. Such ailments have been commonly detected through bacteria (such as *E. coli*, *S. agal*), pathogens that are foodborne (like listeria, cholera toxin, salmonella), and the viruses (like dengue virus, influenza, hepatitis C). For instance, an extreme horizontal shaped surface wave of acoustic biosensors was manufactured to diagnose anti-gp41 and anti-p24 antibodies of HIV [122].

Main developed biochip is made up of a sensitive part towards bio-folding arrangements as well as miniaturization configuration. These biosensors may identify HIV bio-markers in only 5 minutes utilizing a 6 μL plasma sample, it increases the chances of the next level of quick, point-of-care, and cost-effective detection for restrict HIV virus. Main biosensor was manufactured as well for the detection of RT-PCR result of dengue fever type 2. It proceeds by detection of less than 10 fM within 30 minutes which was 3 times less in magnitude than that gained through probes 32P-labeled and 4 times less in magnitude than that obtained through the staining of ethidium bromide. Amid the COVID-19 pandemic, the initial diagnosis is important for treatment. Even though molecular techniques and culture-based procedures are usually utilized in the clinical identification of diseases, recently introduced microfluidic biosensors are identified to portability, cheapness, high accuracy, fast response, low sample consumption, high reproducibility, high throughput parallel processing and easy application. Hence, microfluidic biosensors can follow the WHO guidelines "ASSURED" (able to afford, Specific, Sensitivity, In use friendly, active, and sturdy, Free Equipment, Easy to deliver to the user) that have excellent potential for SARS-CoV2 identification, in important COVID-19 diagnosis [123]. Although, more energy must be put into improving specificity and sensitivity, reducing manufacturing time, enhancing stability, and lowering detection period to control virus.

4.4.6.3.4 Wastewater Biosensors

WBE, i.e., Wastewater-based epidemiology is being utilized to identify different bio-markers, involving illegal and legal chemicals, markers of population size, pharmaceutical, and personal care products, industrial, and biological chemicals. Human viruses (like enteroviruses, astroviruses, noroviruses, saliviruses, rotaviruses, etc.), these also recognized in wastewater, pointing WBE have high value potential in viral outbreaks, timely detection by properly monitoring the quantity and types of varieties of viruses in wastewaters. In general, WBE may permit data for virus as well as within the boundary of treatment plants lead to the existence of viruses in the watershed. The COVID-19 outburst is because of SARS-CoV2 which has caused the clear-cut danger for humanity. This has been proposed as COVID-19 can be confirmed in patient's fecal specimens, SARS-CoV2 can be identified from countries, e.g., China, US Germany, Korea, and Singapore. The research including 10 confirmed pediatric COVID-19 patients provided clear evidence of SARS-CoV2 [124]. Sewage system of target cities in connection with sewage samples of virus SARS-CoV2 can be determined.

New declaration indicates identification of SARS-CoV2 in wastewaters helps examine the transmission of the virus in human beings as SARS-CoV2 might be expelled in urine or stool. Many attempts were done to test SARS-CoV2 in wastewaters in countries like the US, Australia, Netherlands, France, Sweden, and Spain. The SARS-CoV2 report identification in wastewaters was published by Gertjan Medema et al. [125]. The research studies of Netherlands, through RT-PCR in the wastewater analytes to detect existence of SARSCoV2. None of both genes on February 6 was detected, but detection of gene N1 in six regions. On February 27, it is the first-ever reported case in concurrence in the Netherlands. On the other hand, Massachusetts state of USA showing research that in sewage samples SARS-CoV2 may be detected. This study exhibited that the longitudinal assay of sewage can supplement an idea of the concentration level of SARS-CoV2 with no availability of onsite diagnosis.

Hence, WBE can be relied upon as an initial equipment that warns of the COVID-19 disease check with spread and give a more precise idea than clinical testing, of the extent to which COVID-19 infections can prevail for analysis of RT-PCR have been generally used for the identification of SARS-CoV2 in many research. But RT-PCR has few drawbacks which can lower its applications in the whole world. For instance, expensive equipment, laborious processes, complete facilities, and skilled technicians are required for RT-PCR. By the fast increase of cases that are confirmed of COVID-19 globally, RT-PCR has been proved not to be able to fulfill detecting requirements of various doubtful cases with a short period. Although for some of the reports, PCR is detected as maximum sensitive and specific. Best treatment of sample getting time (4–6 hours) and skilled personnel are not feasible to quick and effective sample monitoring on position. Therefore, it needs a strong transportable and analytical device for verification which quickly detect SARS-COV on a very low level without using high laboratories on sewage collection point the using of WBE planning is beneficial. Recently, we have to introduce the paper-based tool to check WBE. Advancements in signal strengthening techniques have also led to increased sensitivity in paper-based analytical devices for different sensing applications. In addition, biosensors can be used for multiplex diagnosis of infectious diseases. For example, Men et al. [126] expressed a multifunctional fluorescent protein nanowire (FNW) for multiplex identification of p24 and gp120 protein from HIV. The FNW mixed through various green fluorescent proteins can strengthen the signal and increase sensitivity. Moreover, for the diagnosis of infectious diseases in that area where there are no source biosensors can be manufactured into integrated medical tools. For instance, Choi et al. [127] has used a well-developed coordinated paper-based sample-to-response biosensor for testing of nucleic acid. For the first time for nucleic acid extraction, new technology was introduced called glass fiber, which is used for amplification, eye detection as well as android phone quantification.

In POC setting a portable heating tool known as battery-powered was introduced for LAMP amplification. And hence biosensors are used for warning sensing systems to control the system to assist the government to take considerable steps initially to avoid infectious diseases spread. Biosensors have the ability for SARS-CoV2 detection in sewage. It has been known that sewage is a complicated mixture; recently, we have developed a paper-based tool that has exhibited the high value for the identification of pathogens in wastewaters. The obtained results were further cross-checked with an agarose gel image analysis and robust electrophoresis, exhibiting enhanced reliability for waste analysis. The advantages of the biosensor are rapid response, specificity, sensitivity, low cost, friendly usage of tools, and very friendly testing analysis. One of the most important advantages is SARS-CoV2 detection in waste in an early stage so that treatment is possible at early stages. It is because new research shows that it is also found in urine and stools, which then enter sewage treatment plants.

4.5 NANOSCALE VISUALIZATION AND CHARACTERIZATION TOOLS

It can be described that main important techniques that are being utilized for the visualization which are EM, XRD, and AFM through which we can easily study the structure and characterization of the virus and also can monitor their environment and the host-guest relation through which we can also work on drugs against the virus [128].

4.5.1 ELECTRON MICROSCOPY

It is a device that is based on an electronic system due to its short wavelength, and it has 100,000 times more resolution power than a compound microscope. The electronic microscope is used for the study of the structure of the nanoparticle. It has a very high-resolution and detection power. So here it is used to study the detection of viruses and their structure. As every test needs some specification to study the specific pathogen or any microorganism but the electronic microscope does not need such kind of tests. So, we can say that an electron microscope helps us to identify the virus and its structure and also help in designing the medicine or vaccine for the appropriate pathogen [129].

The key methods of electron microscopy are to identify the structures of viruses are: thin sectioning, IEM (immune electron microscopy), negative staining, cryo-electron microscopy (cryo-EM), SEM (Scanning Electron Microscopy) and tomography. The background is stained in negative staining by leaving unchanged original sample so it may be visible easily. So, it compresses the thin layer of a virus which becomes transparent for an Electron microscope. In the past, SARS was classified, using Electron Microscopy techniques, as a coronavirus. EM was utilized in the identification of MERS, and the COVID-19 virus image was taken by TEM.

Presently, cryo-EM is used to elaborate various monoclonal antibodies that target SARS-Cov-2, mainly to the S protein that was present in memory B cells of an infected person of SARS-CoV-2 in 2003. An antibody, known as S309, effectively makes neutral SARS-CoV2 and by using cryo-EM and binding analysis, it was cleared that S-309 was recognized as a glycan comprising epitome that was saved within the sarbecovirus genus in the absence of receptor attached site competing. This involved increased visualization of the trimeric structure in the 10–20 nm spikes of the virus surfaces. These data supported the characterization of the SARS agent and antiviral development planning, and we assume that such procedures can easily be expanded to demonstrate the details of CoV-19.

4.5.2 X-RAY CRYSTALLOGRAPHY

The analysis of single-crystal through X-ray diffraction is an excellent process for achieving the best resolution of virus with visualization of the macromolecular network. In general, structure of virus may be determined through five steps employing X-ray crystallography techniques which include:

- Preparation and purification of virus particles;
- Crystallization and mounting the particle crystal;
- Measurement of diffracted data;
- Calculation of phase through molecular replacement (MR) or isomorphism replacement;
- Interpretation of map and model building.

For purification and preparation of the viruses through the extracellular/tissue culture media, commercial sources have kits for purification. In preparation steps, for keeping the icosahedral geometry of the virus, the way of handling should be perfect. After the purification and crystallization are needed. There are two stages in crystallization: nucleation and growth. In first, the nucleus crystal is assembled on the critical point of molecular aggregation, and then the following growth process is started. For the growth of virus sample crystals, there are four procedures, dialysis, vapor diffusion, batch crystallization and liquid–liquid diffusion [130].

EM and XRD processes are mainly used to collect any particles that present in electron micrographs. Due to this reason, a restriction occurs through data specifying changes with single particles in the form of a huge population. These methods also require an appropriate environment that is away from the physiological situations, because in these situations, viruses usually grow and, in reality, remove the characterization of diverse qualities. This character of virus creates a difficulty in its structural analysis of viruses that have no proper shape for example SARS-Cov-2 as an envelope virus. AFM is another important technique that impacts a significant effect on the virus.

4.5.3 ATOMIC FORCE MICROSCOPY

This microscopy is turned into a quick and appropriate device to visualize and characterize nano-scale pictures of analytes in aqueous and aerial medium. Basically, through AFM analysis, analysis of micro-cantilever has been employed to develop interactions among sample and nano-metric tip situated at the extreme of micro-cantilever. Depending on its function, it reflects a vast level information as working with respect to time involving explanation of atomic, mechanical, chemical, surface, thermal, viscoelastic, and physical characteristics of nanomaterials can be collected. The contact mode has been recognized as initially manufactured mode of microscopy to be explained further. The major challenge for utilizing this mode for picturing soft substances as clinical samples and viruses are forces applied to restrict the irreversible or reversible imaging, damage, and control to the specimen.

There are two basic modes of microscopy:

- AM-AFM (amplitude modulation atomic force microscopy); and
- FM-AFM (frequency modulation atomic force microscopy).

In the first mode, because of the decline in contact time between sample and tip during the further process, the sample damage risk is greatly minimized. Moreover, day by day new techniques are developed through which we can enhance the resolution and get more information from the specimen during the study, due to this diversity and advancement it is called multi-frequency processes, [109] in which cantilever is fixed at various frequencies having various signals which are utilized as parameters for feedback. With the capability to show an image of the particles of a virus, AFM shows the ability to quantify and measure the structural and mechanical characteristics of particles of the virus. Furthermore, AFM may be used to handle and dissect the biological specimen in which viruses are included. To quantify and separate chemical, physical, and viscoelastic characteristics of viruses, common methods are AFM (advanced multi-frequency method) and FD-Based AFM (force-distance curve base).

Main task of AFM based on FD is the large amount and data analysis time. Enhancement of resolution rate of an image and to get more information during the study AFM procedure is used. Different types of multi-frequency-based AFM processes are being recommended, nevertheless, because of its complicated principles, and methods of describing data and theoretical development are under investigation. At start investigations of coronaviruses (CoVs) by using AFM procedures exhibited AFM best function for imaging, visualization, and elaboration of structural aspects of SARS-CoV virus. In general, visualization/characterization tools provide the following information: (i) detect various diverse relation between host and SARS-CoV2 virus; (ii) surface quantification and its characteristics of a cell which is damaged by COVID-19; (iii) Study the entrance mechanism of virus that how it crosses the membrane; (iv) Mechanism of replication inside the host and its properties.

For advanced studies, a nano-scale map direction flow pattern is used to study the pH and its properties in the host. Not long ago, Yang et al.

investigated these processes in research describing interactions of SARS-CoV2 and AFM [131].

4.6 RESEMBLANCES AMONG SARS-COV-2 AND OTHER VIRUSES

COVID-19 pandemic is bitterly transmittable because communication is caused by tiny drops of air and human to a human association. The most general indication of the pandemic is influenza, and hence, its accurate and fast detection is not insignificant. Relative investigation of SARS-CoV2 and other epidemics provides the bulk data to be utilized by researchers to create such quick and implementable processes for human welfare. There are various similar and different characteristics among these viruses. Such properties can be employed for researchers who are working in the regions of biosensors and to characterize or visualize surfaces for its best diagnosis and structural analysis of SARS-CoV2. One of the major resemblances among SARS-CoV2 pandemic with other viruses, especially flu, SARS-CoV, H1NI, and MERS has been elaborated as they all keep RNA as hereditary particles, hence called RNA contagious. Comparison between RNA and DNA viruses, RNA viruses being highly dangerous technically because they affect cells by introducing RNA in the replication and transcription of viral proteins in host cells.

Diagnosis of RNA at an initial stage is also a big challenge. In comparison to all available techniques, nucleic acid-based tests and cell culture are being used as gold standards. DNA viruses have polymerase machinery while RNA has supplementary processes to go back from RNA to DNA formerly of its amplification. Viruses of SARS, COVID-19 and MERS correspond structurally to a homogenous type of “Beta Coronavirus” origin, which being globular, often multi-shapes [132]. Various properties of the above-mentioned viruses including average diameter are “125 nm,” capsid layer “85 nm” and surface diameter of “Spikes” is 20 nm. Early detection of COVID-19 may be done by correlating hereditary properties of SARS-CoV2 with other viruses.

In addition, to manufacture sensors for analysis of drug detection and disease structure, COVID-19 viruses may infect other cells. In short, protein-protein interactions is the major way by which the SARS-CoV2 virus penetrates the cell and glycoprotein points correspond to the cell surface’s angiotensin-converting enzyme 2 (ACE2) [133]. Association of contagious and entry of cell is supported by protease enzyme named TMPRSS2.

4.7 CONCLUSIONS

It has been observed in the last few months that rapid progress is being done for promotion and progression in detecting kits of COVID-19, attempts at a vast level are also being done for the development of accurate, quick, easy, and cheap laboratory tools and methods to be utilized all over the world. This chapter explains the most accurate and efficient tests and techniques to detect the COVID-19 virus. Diagnosis of SARS-CoV2 at the initial stage depends on reverse transcription-PCR but best substitutes are also available like transcription-mediated methodology, CRISPR-based methodologies, and nucleic acid amplification methodology. This chapter describes that to detect COVID-19 pandemic immunological, serological, and molecular genetic tools are also being used. To diagnose RNA strains, RT-PCR is being utilized as the most dominant tool. Other techniques as CRISPR-based technologies, nucleic acid-based are under the process of completion to justify best-recognized tests. Remarkable improvements have been made for effective and valid diagnosis. Some COVID-19 diagnostic kits and tools have been recognized by FDA, EUA but various new techniques and methodologies are under process.

KEYWORDS

- **acute respiratory distress syndrome**
- **assays**
- **biosensor**
- **computed tomography**
- **CRISPER**
- **polymerase chain reaction**
- **RNA**
- **severe acute respiratory syndrome**

REFERENCES

1. Walls, A. C., et al., (2020). Structure, function, and antigenicity of the SARS-CoV-2 spike glycoprotein. *Cell*.

2. Zhou, P., et al., (2020). A pneumonia outbreak associated with a new coronavirus of probable bat origin. *Nature, 579*(7798), 270–273.
3. Wang, J., Zhou, M., & Liu, F., (2020). Reasons for healthcare workers becoming infected with novel coronavirus disease 2019 (COVID-19) in China. *J. Hosp. Infect., 105*(1).
4. Ai, T., et al., (2020). Correlation of chest CT and RT-PCR testing in coronavirus disease 2019 (COVID-19) in China: A report of 1014 cases. *Radiology*, 200642.
5. Mizumoto, K., et al., (2020). Estimating the asymptomatic proportion of coronavirus disease 2019 (COVID-19) cases on board the diamond princess cruise ship, Yokohama, Japan, 2020. *Eurosurveillance, 25*(10), 2000180.
6. Liu, Y., et al., (2020). The reproductive number of COVID-19 is higher compared to SARS coronavirus. *Journal of Travel Medicine.*
7. Bendavid, E., et al., (2020). *COVID-19 Antibody Seroprevalence in Santa Clara County, California.* MedRxiv.
8. Wu, Z., & McGoogan, J. M., (2020). Characteristics of and important lessons from the coronavirus disease 2019 (COVID-19) outbreak in China: Summary of a report of 72 314 cases from the Chinese Center for Disease Control and Prevention. *JAMA, 323*(13), 1239–1242.
9. Zhou, F., et al., (2020). Clinical course and risk factors for mortality of adult inpatients with COVID-19 in Wuhan, China: A retrospective cohort study. *The Lancet.*
10. Alhazzani, W., Du, B., et al., (2020). Surviving sepsis campaign: Guidelines on the management of critically ill adults with coronavirus disease-2019 (COVID-19). *Intensive Care Medicine*, 1–34.
11. Ahmed, R., Oldstone, M. B., & Palese, P., (2007). Protective immunity and susceptibility to infectious diseases: Lessons from the 1918 influenza pandemic. *Nature Immunology, 8*(11), 1188–1193.
12. Zia-Ul-Haq, M., et al., (2021). *Alternative Medicine Interventions for COVID-19* (Vol. XII, p. 284). Springer, Cham: Springer Nature Switzerland AG.
13. Zia-Ul-Haq, M., Dewanjee, S., & Riaz, M., (2021). *Carotenoids: Structure and Function in the Human Body* (Vol. XVI, p. 859). Springer Nature Switzerland AG: Springer International Publishing.
14. Ramanathan, K., et al., (2020). Planning and provision of ECMO services for severe ARDS during the COVID-19 pandemic and other outbreaks of emerging infectious diseases. *The Lancet Respiratory Medicine.*
15. Carter, L. J., et al., (2020). *Assay Techniques and Test Development for COVID-19 Diagnosis.* ACS Publications.
16. Wu, F., et al., (2020). A new coronavirus associated with human respiratory disease in China. *Nature, 579*(7798), 265–269.
17. Zhu, N., et al., (2020). A novel coronavirus from patients with pneumonia in China, 2019. *New England Journal of Medicine.*
18. Wang, D., et al., (2020). Clinical characteristics of 138 hospitalized patients with 2019 novel coronavirus-infected pneumonia in Wuhan, China. *JAMA, 323*(11), 1061–1069.
19. Huang, C., et al., (2020). Clinical features of patients infected with 2019 novel coronavirus in Wuhan, China. The *Lancet, 395*(10223), 497–506.
20. Letko, M., Marzi, A., & Munster, V., (2020). Functional assessment of cell entry and receptor usage for SARS-CoV-2 and other lineage B beta coronaviruses. *Nature Microbiology, 5*(4), 562–569.

21. Hoffmann, M., et al., (2020). SARS-CoV-2 cell entry depends on ACE2 and TMPRSS2 and is blocked by a clinically proven protease inhibitor. *Cell.*
22. Du, L., et al., (2009). The spike protein of SARS-CoV—a target for vaccine and therapeutic development. *Nature Reviews Microbiology, 7*(3), 226–236.
23. Kim, D., et al., (2020). The architecture of SARS-CoV-2 transcriptome. *Cell.*
24. Chavez, S., et al., (2020). Coronavirus Disease (COVID-19): A primer for emergency physicians. *The American Journal of Emergency Medicine.*
25. Udugama, B., et al., (2020). Diagnosing COVID-19: The disease and tools for detection. *ACS Nano, 14*(4), 3822–3835.
26. Long, Q. X., et al., (2020). Antibody responses to SARS-CoV-2 in patients with COVID-19. *Nature Medicine*, 1–4.
27. Mallapaty, S., (2020). Will coronavirus antibody tests really change everything? *Nature, 580*(7805), 571, 572.
28. Vogel, G., (2020). *First Antibody Surveys Draw Fire for Quality, Bias.* American Association for the Advancement of Science.
29. Alm, E., et al., (2020). Geographical and temporal distribution of SARS-CoV-2 clades in the WHO European Region. *Eurosurveillance, 25*(32), 2001410.
30. Corman, V. M., et al., (2020). Detection of 2019 novel coronavirus (2019-nCoV) by real-time RT-PCR. *Eurosurveillance, 25*(3), 2000045.
31. Wang, W., et al., (2020). Detection of SARS-CoV-2 in different types of clinical specimens. *JAMA, 323*(18), 1843, 1844.
32. Zou, L., et al., (2020). SARS-CoV-2 viral load in upper respiratory specimens of infected patients. *New England Journal of Medicine, 382*(12), 1177–1179.
33. Loeffelholz, M. J., & Tang, Y. W., (2020). Laboratory diagnosis of emerging human coronavirus infections-the state of the art. *Emerging Microbes & Infections, 9*(1), 747–756.
34. Charlton, C. L., et al., (2018). Practical guidance for clinical microbiology laboratories: Viruses causing acute respiratory tract infections. *Clinical Microbiology Reviews, 32*(1).
35. Organization, W. H., (2020). *Laboratory Testing for Coronavirus Disease (COVID-19) in Suspected Human Cases: Interim Guidance.* World Health Organization.
36. Yang, X., et al., (2020). Clinical course and outcomes of critically ill patients with SARS-CoV-2 pneumonia in Wuhan, China: A single-centered, retrospective, observational study. *The Lancet Respiratory Medicine.*
37. Henry, B. M., et al., (2020). Hematologic, biochemical and immune biomarker abnormalities associated with severe illness and mortality in coronavirus disease 2019 (COVID-19): A meta-analysis. *Clinical Chemistry and Laboratory Medicine (CCLM), 58*(7), 1021–1028.
38. Chu, D. K., et al., (2020). *Molecular diagnosis of a novel coronavirus (2019-nCoV) causing an outbreak of pneumonia. Clinical Chemistry, 66*(4), 549–555.
39. Chua, F., et al., (2020). The role of CT in case ascertainment and management of COVID-19 pneumonia in the UK: Insights from high-incidence regions. *The Lancet Respiratory Medicine, 8*(5), 438–440.
40. Shi, H., et al., (2020). Radiological findings from 81 patients with COVID-19 pneumonia in Wuhan, China: A descriptive study. *The Lancet Infectious Diseases.*
41. Terpos, E., et al., (2020). Hematological findings and complications of COVID-19. *American Journal of Hematology.*
42. Mehta, P., et al., (2020). COVID-19: Consider cytokine storm syndromes and immunosuppression. *Lancet, 395*(10229), 1033. London, England.

43. Qin, C., Zhou, L., & Hu, Z., (2020). Dysregulation of immune response in patients with COVID-19 in Wuhan, China. [published online ahead of print, 2020 March 12]. *Clin. Infect. Dis.*
44. Henry, B. M., et al., (2020). Hyperinflammation and derangement of renin-angiotensin-aldosterone system in COVID-19: A novel hypothesis for clinically suspected hypercoagulopathy and microvascular immunothrombosis. *Clinica Chimica Acta.*
45. Bowles, L., et al., (2020). Lupus anticoagulant and abnormal coagulation tests in patients with Covid-19. *New England Journal of Medicine.*
46. Vickers, N. J., (2017). Animal communication: When I' m calling you, will you answer too? *Current Biology, 27*(14), R713–R715.
47. Tersalvi, G., et al., (2020). Elevated troponin in patients with Coronavirus disease 2019 (COVID-19): Possible mechanisms. *Journal of Cardiac Failure.*
48. Tian, S., et al., (2020). Characteristics of COVID-19 infection in Beijing. *Journal of Infection.*
49. Guo, T., Fan, Y., & Chen, M., (2020). Cardiovascular implications of fatal outcomes of patients with coronavirus disease 2019 (COVID-19) [e-pub ahead of print]. *JAMA Cardiol.*
50. Yang, W., et al., (2020). Clinical characteristics and imaging manifestations of the 2019 novel coronavirus disease (COVID-19): A multi-center study in Wenzhou city, Zhejiang, China. *Journal of Infection.*
51. Shi, S., et al., (2020). Cardiac injury in patients with coronavirus disease 2019. *JAMA Cardiol.*
52. Ruan, Q., et al., (2020). Clinical predictors of mortality due to COVID-19 based on an analysis of data of 150 patients from Wuhan, China. *Intensive Care Medicine, 46*(5), 846–848.
53. Januzzi, J., (2020). Troponin and BNP use in COVID-19. *Cardiology Magazine, 18.*
54. Chapman, A. R., Bularga, A., & Mills, N. L., (2020). High-sensitivity cardiac troponin can be an ally in the fight against COVID-19. *Circulation, 141*(22), 1733–1735.
55. Bansal, M., (2020). Cardiovascular disease and COVID-19. *Diabetes & Metabolic Syndrome: Clinical Research & Reviews.*
56. Chen, N., et al., (2020). Epidemiological and clinical characteristics of 99 cases of 2019 novel coronavirus pneumonia in Wuhan, China: A descriptive study. *The Lancet, 395* (10223), 507–513.
57. Guan, W. J., et al., (2020). Clinical characteristics of coronavirus disease 2019 in China. *New England Journal of Medicine, 382*(18), 1708–1720.
58. Cai, Q., et al., (2020). COVID-19: Abnormal liver function tests. *Journal of Hepatology.*
59. Fan, Z., et al., (2020). Clinical features of COVID-19-related liver damage. *Clinical Gastroenterology and Hepatology.*
60. Zhang, C., Shi, L., & Wang, F. S., (2020). Liver injury in COVID-19: Management and challenges. *The Lancet Gastroenterology & Hepatology, 5*(5), 428–430.
61. Bangash, M. N., Patel, J., & Parekh, D., (2020). COVID-19 and the liver: Little cause for concern. *The Lancet, Gastroenterology & Hepatology, 5*(6), 529.
62. Sun, J., et al., (2020). COVID-19 and liver disease. *Liver International.*
63. Chu, K. H., et al., (2005). Acute renal impairment in coronavirus-associated severe acute respiratory syndrome. *Kidney International, 67*(2), 698–705.
64. Zaim, S., et al., (2020). COVID-19 and multi-organ response. *Current Problems in Cardiology,* 100618.
65. Cheng, Y., et al., (2020). Kidney disease is associated with in-hospital death of patients with COVID-19. *Kidney International.*

66. Ge, S., et al., (2016). Epidemiology and outcomes of acute kidney injury in elderly Chinese patients: A subgroup analysis from the EACH study. *BMC Nephrology, 17*(1), 136.
67. Ronco, C., & Reis, T., (2020). Kidney involvement in COVID-19 and rationale for extracorporeal therapies. *Nature Reviews Nephrology*, 1–3.
68. Maxim, L. D., Niebo, R., & Utell, M. J., (2014). Screening tests: A review with examples. *Inhalation Toxicology, 26*(13), 811–828.
69. Park, T. J., et al., (2009). A self-assembled fusion protein-based surface plasmon resonance biosensor for rapid diagnosis of severe acute respiratory syndrome. *Talanta, 79*(2), 295–301.
70. Khan, S., et al., (2020). *Analysis of Serologic Cross-Reactivity Between Common Human Coronaviruses and SARS-CoV-2 Using Coronavirus Antigen Microarray.* BioRxiv.
71. D'Annessa, I., Marchetti, F., & Colombo, G., (2020). *Differential Antibody Recognition by Novel SARS-CoV-2 and SARS-CoV Spike Protein Receptor Binding Domains: Mechanistic Insights and Implications for the Design of Diagnostics and Therapeutics.* BioRxiv.
72. Abeshouse, A., et al., (2015). The molecular taxonomy of primary prostate cancer. *Cell, 163*(4), 1011–1025.
73. Che, X. Y., et al., (2004). Sensitive and specific monoclonal antibody-based capture enzyme immunoassay for detection of nucleocapsid antigen in sera from patients with severe acute respiratory syndrome. *Journal of Clinical Microbiology, 42*(6), 2629–2635.
74. Yang, X., & Sun, X., (2005). Chemiluminescent immunometric detection of SARS-CoV in sera as an early marker for the diagnosis of SARS. in *Bioluminescence and Chemiluminescence: Progress and Perspectives* (pp. 491–494). World Scientific.
75. Azhar, Z. I., et al., (2020). COVID-19 review: An epidemiological perspective and Malaysian scenario in handling the pandemic. *Journal of Clinical and Health Sciences, 5*(1), 26–41.
76. Organization, W. H., (2020). *Considerations for Quarantine of Individuals in the Context of Containment for Coronavirus Disease (COVID-19): Interim Guidance.* World Health Organization.
77. Xu, Z., et al., (2020). Pathological findings of COVID-19 associated with acute respiratory distress syndrome. *The Lancet Respiratory Medicine, 8*(4), 420–422.
78. Bowman, G. L., (2017). *Biomarkers for Early Detection of Parkinson Disease: A Scent of Consistency with Olfactory Dysfunction.* AAN Enterprises.
79. Erard, M., Dupré-Crochet, S., & Nüße, O., (2018). Biosensors for spatiotemporal detection of reactive oxygen species in cells and tissues. *American Journal of Physiology-Regulatory, Integrative and Comparative Physiology, 314*(5), R667–R683.
80. Del, R. J. S., et al., (2019). An antifouling coating that enables affinity-based electrochemical biosensing in complex biological fluids. *Nature nanotechnology, 14*(12), 1143–1149.
81. Yoo, Y. K., et al., (2020). Gold nanoparticles assisted sensitivity improvement of interdigitated microelectrodes biosensor for amyloid-β detection in plasma sample. *Sensors and Actuators B: Chemical, 308*, 127710.
82. Hall, D. A., et al., (2013). A 256 pixel magnetoresistive biosensor microarray in 0.18 μm CMOS. *IEEE Journal of Solid-State Circuits, 48*(5), 1290–1301.
83. Tort, N., Salvador, J. P., & Marco, M. P., (2017). Multimodal plasmonic biosensing nanostructures prepared by DNA-directed immobilization of multifunctional DNA-gold nanoparticles. *Biosensors and Bioelectronics, 90*, 13–22.

84. Bhalla, N., & Estrela, P., (2018). Exploiting the signatures of nanoplasmon-exciton coupling on proton sensitive insulator-semiconductor devices for drug discovery applications. *Nanoscale, 10*(28), 13320–13328.
85. Gibson, T., et al., (1992). Extended shelf life of enzyme-based biosensors using a novel stabilization system. *Biosensors and Bioelectronics, 7*(10), 701–708.
86. Yoo, E. H., & Lee, S. Y., (2010). Glucose biosensors: An overview of use in clinical practice. *Sensors, 10*(5), 4558–4576.
87. Block, I. D., Chan, L. L., & Cunningham, B. T., (2007). Large-area submicron replica molding of porous low-k dielectric films and application to photonic crystal biosensor fabrication. *Microelectronic Engineering, 84*(4), 603–608.
88. Talukder, S., Gabai, G., & Celi, P., (2015). The use of digital infrared thermography and measurement of oxidative stress biomarkers as tools to diagnose foot lesions in sheep. *Small Ruminant Research, 127*, 80–85.
89. Layqah, L. A., & Eissa, S., (2019). An electrochemical immunosensor for the coronavirus associated with the middle east respiratory syndrome using an array of gold nanoparticle-modified carbon electrodes. *Microchimica Acta, 186*(4), 224.
90. Li, Y., et al., (2012). Highly sensitive electrochemical immunoassay for H1N1 influenza virus based on copper-mediated amplification. *Chemical Communications, 48*(52), 6562–6564.
91. Ishikawa, F. N., et al., (2009). Label-free, electrical detection of the SARS virus N-protein with nanowire biosensors utilizing antibody mimics as capture probes. *ACS Nano, 3*(5), 1219–1224.
92. Mahari, S., et al., (2020). *eCovSens-Ultrasensitive Novel in-House Built Printed Circuit Board Based Electrochemical Device for Rapid Detection of nCovid-19 Antigen, a Spike Protein Domain 1 of SARS-CoV-2.* BioRxiv.
93. Takemura, K., et al., (2017). Versatility of a localized surface plasmon resonance-based gold nanoparticle-alloyed quantum dot nanobiosensor for immunofluorescence detection of viruses. *Biosensors and Bioelectronics, 89*, 998–1005.
94. Qiu, G., et al., (2020). Dual-functional plasmonic photothermal biosensors for highly accurate severe acute respiratory syndrome coronavirus 2 detection. *ACS Nano, 14*(5), 5268–5277.
95. Wei, Q., et al., (2013). Fluorescent imaging of single nanoparticles and viruses on a smart phone. *ACS Nano, 7*(10), 9147–9155.
96. Gray, E. R., et al., (2018). Ultra-rapid, sensitive and specific digital diagnosis of HIV with a dual-channel SAW biosensor in a pilot clinical study. *NPJ Digital Medicine, 1*(1), 1–8.
97. Urdea, M., et al., (2006). Requirements for high impact diagnostics in the developing world. *Nature, 444*(1), 73–79.
98. Xu, Y., et al., (2020). Characteristics of pediatric SARS-CoV-2 infection and potential evidence for persistent fecal viral shedding. *Nature Medicine, 26*(4), 502–505.
99. Medema, G., et al., (2020). Presence of SARS-Coronavirus-2 RNA in sewage and correlation with reported COVID-19 prevalence in the early stage of the epidemic in the Netherlands. *Environmental Science & Technology Letters*.
100. Yang, Z., et al., (2018). *Rapid veterinary diagnosis of bovine reproductive infectious diseases from semen using paper-origami DNA microfluidics. ACS Sensors,* 3(2), 403–409.
101. Men, D., et al., (2016). Fluorescent protein nanowire-mediated protein microarrays for multiplexed and highly sensitive pathogen detection. *ACS Applied Materials & Interfaces, 8*(27), 17472–17477.

102. Choi, J. R., et al., (2016). An integrated paper-based sample-to-answer biosensor for nucleic acid testing at the point of care. *Lab on a Chip, 16*(3), 611–621.
103. Chen, Y., et al., (2020). The presence of SARS-CoV-2 RNA in the feces of COVID-19 patients. *Journal of Medical Virology.*
104. Nguyen, T. H. V., et al., (2019). Structure and oligomerization state of the C-terminal region of the Middle East respiratory syndrome coronavirus nucleoprotein. *Acta Crystallographica Section D: Structural Biology, 75*(1), 8–15.
105. Lu, R., et al., (2020). Genomic characterization and epidemiology of 2019 novel coronavirus: Implications for virus origins and receptor binding. *The Lancet, 395*(10224), 565–574.
106. Xiao, A. T., Tong, Y. X., & Zhang, S., (2020). False-negative of RT-PCR and prolonged nucleic acid conversion in COVID-19: Rather than recurrence. *Journal of Medical Virology.*
107. Russo, K. I., et al., (2013). An overview of biological macromolecule crystallization. *International Journal of Molecular Sciences, 14*(6), 11643–11691.
108. Perera, R., Khaliq, M., & Kuhn, R. J., (2008). Closing the door on flaviviruses: Entry as a target for antiviral drug design. *Antiviral Research, 80*(1), 11–22.
109. Garcıa, R., & Perez, R., (2002). Dynamic atomic force microscopy methods. *Surface Science Reports, 47*(6–8), 197–301.
110. Hinterdorfer, P., & Dufrêne, Y. F., (2006). Detection and localization of single molecular recognition events using atomic force microscopy. *Nature Methods, 3*(5), 347–355.
111. Dufrêne, Y. F., et al., (2013). Multiparametric imaging of biological systems by force-distance curve-based AFM. *Nature Methods, 10*(9), 847–854.
112. Lin, S., et al., (2005). Surface ultrastructure of SARS coronavirus revealed by atomic force microscopy. *Cellular Microbiology, 7*(12), 1763–1770.
113. Yang, J., et al., (2020). Molecular interaction and inhibition of SARS-CoV-2 binding to the ACE2 receptor. *Nature Communications, 11*(1), 1–10.
114. Narayanan, K., & Makino, S., (2001). Cooperation of an RNA packaging signal and a viral envelope protein in coronavirus RNA packaging. *Journal of Virology, 75*(19), 9059–9067.
115. Fehr, A. R., & Perlman, S., (2015). Coronaviruses: An overview of their replication and pathogenesis. In: *Coronaviruses* (pp. 1–23). Springer.
116. Leila, M., & Sorayya, G., (2020). Genotype and phenotype of COVID-19: Their roles in pathogenesis. *Journal of Microbiology, Immunology and Infection, 10.*
117. Bhalla, N., et al., (2020). Opportunities and challenges for biosensors and nanoscale analytical tools for pandemics: COVID-19. *ACS Nano, 14*(7), 7783–7807.
118. Pokhrel, P., Hu, C., & Mao, H., (2020). Detecting the coronavirus (COVID-19). *ACS Sensors, 5*(8), 2283–2296.
119. Kang, J., et al., (2019). Development of a DNA aptamer selection method based on the heterogeneous sandwich form and its application in a colorimetric assay for influenza A virus detection. *New Journal of Chemistry, 43*(18), 6883–6889.
120. Tamura, H., et al., (1997). A dry phantom material composed of ceramic and graphite powder. *IEEE Transactions on Electromagnetic Compatibility, 39*(2), 132–137.
121. Ravi, N., et al., (2020). Diagnostics for SARS-CoV-2 detection: A comprehensive review of the FDA-EUA COVID-19 testing landscape. *Biosensors and Bioelectronics, 165*, 112454.
122. Markwalter, C. F., et al., (2018). Inorganic complexes and metal-based nanomaterials for infectious disease diagnostics. *Chemical Reviews, 119*(2), 1456–1518.

123. Li, H., et al., (2020). Coronavirus disease 2019 (COVID-19): Current status and future perspective. *International Journal of Antimicrobial Agents*, 105951.
124. Wölfel, R., et al., (2020). Virological assessment of hospitalized patients with COVID-2019. *Nature, 581*(7809), 465–469.
125. Bivins, A., et al., (2020). *Wastewater-Based Epidemiology: Global Collaborative to Maximize Contributions in the Fight Against COVID-19*. ACS Publications.
126. Sin, M. L., et al., (2014). Advances and challenges in biosensor-based diagnosis of infectious diseases. *Expert Review of Molecular Diagnostics, 14*(2), 225–244.
127. Claes, T., Bogaerts, W., & Bienstman, P., (2011). Vernier-cascade label-free biosensor with integrated arrayed waveguide grating for wavelength interrogation with low-cost broadband source. *Optics Letters, 36*(17), 3320–3322.
128. Pelling, A. E., et al., (2005). Nanoscale visualization and characterization of *Myxococcus Xanthus* cells with atomic force microscopy. *Proceedings of the National Academy of Sciences, 102*(18), 6484–6489.
129. Reimer, L., (2000). *Scanning Electron Microscopy: Physics of Image Formation and Microanalysis*. IOP Publishing.
130. Miao, J., et al., (1999). Extending the methodology of X-ray crystallography to allow imaging of micrometre-sized non-crystalline specimens. *Nature, 400*(6742), 342–344.
131. Jakhmola, S., et al., (2020). SARS-CoV-2, an underestimated pathogen of the nervous system. *SN Comprehensive Clinical Medicine,* 1–10.
132. Walls, A. C., et al., (2017). Tectonic conformational changes of a coronavirus spike glycoprotein promote membrane fusion. *Proceedings of the National Academy of Sciences, 114*(42), 11157–11162.
133. Ghosh, S., (2020). Virion structure and mechanism of propagation of coronaviruses including SARS-CoV 2 (COVID-19) and some meaningful points for drug or vaccine development. *Virology*. doi: 10.20944/preprints202008.0312.v1.
134. Cascella, M.; Rajnik, M.; Cuomo, A.; Dulebohn, S. C.; Di Napoli, R. Features, Evaluation and Treatment Coronavirus (COVID-19). In StatPearls; StatPearls Publishing, Treasure Island, FL, 2020.
135. Ferretti, L.; Wymant, C.; Kendall, M.; Zhao, L.; Nurtay, A.; Abeler-Dörner, L.; Parker, M.; Bonsall, D.; Fraser, C. Quantifying SARS-CoV-2 Transmission Suggests Epidemic Control with Digital Contact Tracing. Science 2020, 368, eabb6936 DOI: 10.1126/science.abb6936

PART II
Prevention Strategies

CHAPTER 5

Social Distancing and Quarantine as COVID-19 Control Remedy

ADEEL AHMAD,[1] MUHAMMAD HUSSAAN,[2] FATIMA BATOOL,[3] SAHAR MUMTAZ,[3] NAGINA REHMAN,[4] SAMINA YAQOOB,[5] and HUMAIRA KAUSAR[6]

[1]*Department of Agronomy, University of Agriculture Faisalabad, Pakistan, E-mail: adeelahmad772@gmail.com*

[2]*Department of Botany, Government College University Faisalabad, Pakistan, E-mail: mhussaan7866@gmail.com*

[3]*Department of Botany, Division of Science and Technology, University of Education, Lahore, Punjab, Pakistan*

[4]*Department of Zoology, Government College University Faisalabad, Pakistan*

[5]*School of Business and Economics, University of Management and Technology, Lahore, Pakistan*

[6]*Department of Chemistry, Lahore College for Women University, Lahore–54000, Pakistan*

ABSTRACT

Coronavirus 2019 (COVID-19) appeared in Wuhan, China, and has been reported all over the world. Human coronavirus was later renamed SARS-CoV-2 because it resembles the virus responsible for severe respiratory distress syndrome (SARS-CoV). Preventive measures are the most favorable and only way to tackle with the coronavirus outbreak. In these inevitable pandemic conditions, we have some preventive tools such as quarantine, social distancing, and isolation to avoid these circumstances. Understanding of these measures is very necessary and need of time. These precautionary measures carry some long-term impacts on human mental health. By following these preventive tools, a global movement is encouraged that supports healthy eating and physical activities to encourage people to return to a healthy life.

5.1 INTRODUCTION

Recently, the highly transmittable and pathogenic viral infection is Coronavirus (COVID-19) originally, reported from Wuhan city, China. Its genomic makeup has a strong link with the severe acute respiratory syndrome (SARS) and bat viruses, which are thought to be the primary reservoir of coronavirus disease. Coronaviruses (CoVs) belong to a large group of viruses' families, and SARS-CoV-2 is same as MERS-CoV and SARS-CoV with their origin in a bat. However, the reported clinical symptoms associated with coronavirus disease observed from mild to severe and even death, but severe illness is reported in only 16% of cases. Presently, there is no effective remedies/medicines/vaccines available for treating COVID-19. For this reason, implementation of preventive measures including quarantine, isolation, and social distancing have been used all over the world to halt the spreading of coronavirus disease. During the SARS outbreak in 2003, the quarantine measure was successfully implemented to avoid disease spread [1].

The isolation makes it easy to identify the infected persons with detail of their close contact [2]. Isolation can prevent hospital-acquired infections and response to emerging contagious disease threat globally [3]. However, these preventive tools are often a tedious experience for those who undergo it. People living in quarantine can feel a permanent state of mental distress, and other symptoms like depression, insomnia, anxiety, and loneliness. So, these tools are an unpleasant condition for people; however, it has public health benefits. In fact, current coronavirus outbreak is one of the leading causes of mental retardation in other groups of people [4, 5]. But during this outbreak, people and administrations have no choice other than to take these preventive measures. The WHO gave proper guidelines for the protections for people and medical personnel. The precautions must be adopted, otherwise, the chances of infection transmission will be greater.

5.2 THE BACKGROUND OF CORONAVIRUSES (COVS)

All over the world, people are responding to an immense respiratory disease (pneumonia) outbreak detected in Wuhan, China which is the central hub of cultural and economics of China comprising of 11 million people [6]. In the beginning, World Health Organization (WHO) notified 59 cases, and none of them were fatal and after 10 days of its first outbreak, WHO confirms 282 cases as four in Japan, Thailand, and South Korea [7]. Moreover, 6 more deaths were notified in Wuhan, with 51 people died and 12 in critical conditions. The pneumatic outbreak's responsible virus was isolated on the 7th of January and shared on the 12th of January [8]. This respiratory syndrome was due to SARS-CoV-2 and the disease spread by this has been named "severe acute respiratory syndrome coronavirus disease 2019" (COVID-19).

CoVs belong to a large group of viruses' family and SARS-CoV-2 is same like SARS-CoV with their origin in a bat. This sequence of origin was similar to that China initially posted regarding the emergence of this virus from animal resources. These two viruses, MERS-CoV, and SARS-CoV have been known for its severe illness, but the complete picture of clinical illness of COVID-19 is still not clear. However, the reported clinical symptoms associated with coronavirus disease ranged from mild to severe and even death, but serious illness is reported in only 16% of cases. The severity of COVID-19 is linked with the immune system and other health conditions (lungs, heart disease and diabetes). Those who compromise on their immunity are supposed to be at greater risk of illness [9]. The origin of coronavirus disease was observed at "wet market" in Wuhan city of China, and that market is the hub of selling live animals including dogs, cats, rabbits, bats, and fish. Researchers believed that humans are exposed to this new detected virus is most probably a mutated form of Coronavirus commonly found in those animals present in Wuhan's wet market.

Many studies were reported that Coronavirus infected many species, but no evidence was found regarding its infections in humans till mid of 1960s. It belongs to enveloped, single stranded RNA viruses in order of Nidovirales, family Coronaviridae and subfamily Coronavirinae. On the basis of genetic makeup and cross-reactivity of different antigens, 26 different species named alpha, beta, gamma, and delta were recognized. Among these, only two strains, i.e., alpha, and betacoronavirus, are pathogenic to humans [10]. The COVID-19 is thought to be originated from bats because of its close genetic match (96%) with bats CoVs. However, no tangible link is found for another host's existence before transmission to humans, although viruses share about 92% similarities to pangolin CoVs. Few evidences have suggested that SARS-CoV-2 might be that bat-borne virus which is transferred to pangolin then back to bats and then back to humans due to some incorporating homology of pangolin.

The very first isolation of avian infectious bronchitis coronavirus was done in 1973 that cause extensive damage to chicken. Tyrrell and Bynoe isolated the human Coronavirus in 1965 from the nasal cavity and spread on cilia of embryonic tracheal cells. Moreover, for at least 500–800 years, the first Coronavirus was found in humans with its origination in bats [11, 12]. These CoVs have recombination of genes, high genetic diversity, and increased interaction with human and animals [13]. This fact of Coronavirus, was further evident during late 2019 and in early 2020, when a COVID-19 was reported as a source of a widespread of disease in Wuhan city of China (WHO statement about mass pneumonia cases in Wuhan, China. Provisionally, this novel virus 2019-nCoV was designated and characterized as 7th discrete viral species capable of inducing human diseases) (Figure 5.1).

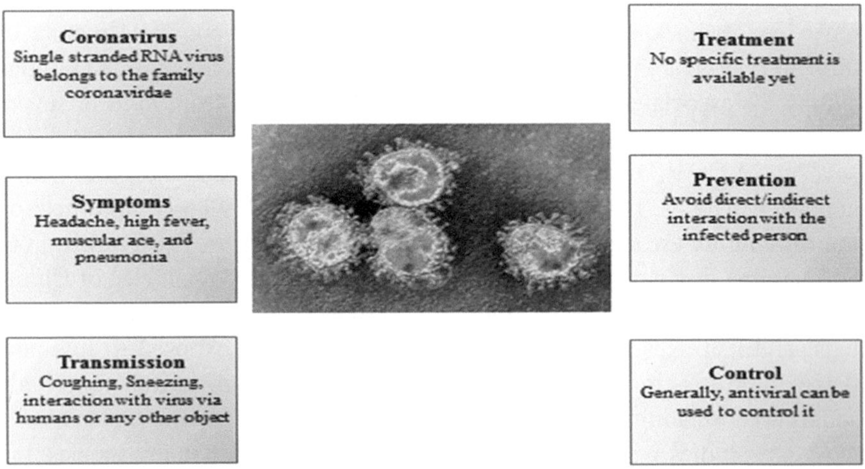

FIGURE 5.1 Image of human coronavirus particles.

5.2.1 *STRUCTURAL MORPHOLOGY AND REPLICATION OF CORONAVIRUS*

Coronavirus got the attention of virologists because of its unique spike-like appearance with round tips that give the look of the sun's atmosphere that is known as corona. This crown-like appearance was formed by peplomers of the spike composed of glycoprotein emerging from the virus lipid envelope [14]. Generally, viruses are made up of two major proteins S glycoprotein and transmembrane glycoprotein, involved in the binding and envelop formation [15, 16]. However, in Coronavirus, a third glycoprotein, i.e., *Hemagglutinin esterase* (HE) associated with the basic non-segmented phosphoprotein, single-stranded RNA of about 26–32 kb, 5' methylated cap and poly-A tail of 3' having 7–10 different open reading frames making it the longest RNA viral genome [15, 17]. One thing that is interesting about the CoVs is that, *in vivo*, these viruses have the ability to adapt new hosts through genetic recombination relying on RNA-dependent RNA polymerase (RdRp) for the replication of the viral genome. The intrinsic error rate of is about 1,000,000 mutation/site/replication inducing point mutation. An important thing to be noted is that this point mutation is not enough to produce new virus strains, and it is only possible when a single host is infected with two strains of CoVs for multiple times enables recombination of viral infection. The question is, when does a coronavirus can increase its ecological niche or to create a new genome? It happens when Coronavirus gain a genomic fragment of about hundreds or thousands base pair from another CoV strain and both infect the same host [11, 18, 19]. Moreover, this viral exposure empowers the appearance of three human CoVs species, i.e., MERS-CoV, SARS-CoV, and CoVn-2019 in about two decades (Figure 5.2).

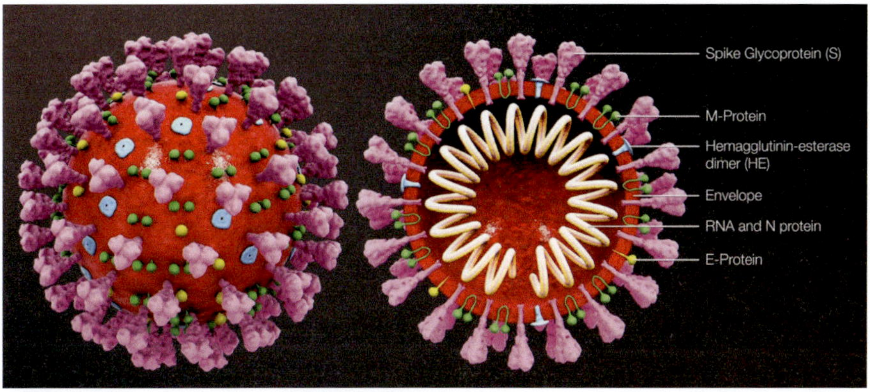

FIGURE 5.2 Structural morphology of Coronavirus.

Source: Reprinted from Mary Yandani M.S., 2019 Novel Coronavirus SARS-COV-2: The Emergence of COVID-19. Wednesday, February 19, 2020 https://www.prosci-inc.com/blog/2019_Novel_Coronavirus/.

5.3 HOW QUARANTINE METHOD IS BENEFICIAL IN CORONAVIRUS TREATMENT?

Nowadays, COVID-19 is dominating the news on all social media to keep struggling for the healthcare. So, it is essential to know the protective measures and their efficacy for COVID-19. Among various protective measures, it is important to know the effectiveness of quarantine method in controlling COVID-19.

5.3.1 WHAT IS THE MEANING OF QUARANTINE?

First of all, it is important to make sure that quarantine does not means a scary thing. However, it is an effective method to protect the public from the spreading of this contagious disease. Quarantine is designed for those groups who are not ill but exposed to this viral disease. Quarantine is adopted to keep others safe from those who are susceptible to COVID-19.

5.3.2 MEANING OF "EXPOSED" TO COVID-19?

Close interaction with the infected person for a long time period. It also means that if a person is sharing the same healthcare space with a COVID-19 infected person or sneezed or coughed on by someone who was the carrier of a disease. So, it is important to listen to the instructions of COVID-19 exposure from your healthcare department. Moreover, healthcare departments have authority to contact and inform you through contact tracing. You have been in contact with a confirmed COVID-19 patient and what you have to do for further precautionary steps. However, if you are a caretaker and came in contact with the confirmed case, reach out your healthcare department on immediate basis.

5.3.3 WHAT HAPPENS WHEN YOU ARE QUARANTINED?

Center for disease control (CDCP) recommends how to do best quarantine part as follows:

1. **Stay at Home:** Do not leave home unless it is very important, i.e., no work, school, or traditional celebrations.
2. **Call to Healthcare:** Call ahead in case you are having any symptoms to keep yourself updated regarding the preventive measures for yourself and to save others from getting infected.
3. **Avoid Pet Interaction:** Although there is no evidence reported regarding the transmission of COVID-19 with pet interaction, it is still good to use caution. If you are exposed to a COVID-infected person already, try to avoid close interaction with pets during the quarantine.

4. **Keep Your Stuff Separate:** Do not mix your dishes, bedding, towels, and utensils with others in your home.
5. **Keep Hygiene:** Keep yourself hygiene is the most integral part of this quarantine time. First-line defense should start with hand washing and then do not forget to keep your elbow on nose/mouth before sneezing or coughing or in case of tissue papers, through it immediately after using.

5.3.4 DIFFERENCE BETWEEN QUARANTINE AND ISOLATION

Although both the term isolation and quarantine serve the same meaning, as it is used for that situation in which the person who is confirmed sick is kept isolate to prevent others from being infected. Staying in isolation also keeps infected people from healthy persons to protect them.

5.3.5 SOCIAL DISTANCING

We usually do not think to avoid people unless and until we are strictly asked to do so as social distancing means to avoid gathering to limit the number of people. This will help in spreading the threat of COVID-19 around the community. Social distancing includes:

- Can talk to your boss/supervisor for the possibility to work from home;
- Switch to online classes or close schools;
- No outstation trips and gatherings and plan virtual meetings;
- Mandatory to keep a distance of 6 feet from each other.

By following the SOPs of quarantine, social distancing, and isolation, it will eventually stop the spreading of COVID-19. However, coping with COVID-19 is a real challenge of 2020 when no medical treatment is yet not reported.

5.3.6 EFFECTIVENESS OF QUARANTINE ALONG WITH OTHER PUBLIC HEALTH MEASURES IN CONTROLLING COVID-19

The quarantine measure with other healthcare tools is very crucial in reducing the spread of COVID-19 but still how these strategies can be best to adopt for how much time is a matter of concern.

Presently, there is no effective remedies/medicines/vaccines available for treating COVID-19. For this reason, implementation of isolating strategies including quarantine has been used worldwide to reduce the risk of virus spreading. Implementation of quarantine can be voluntary or enforced on the community by the administrations. Cochrane's organization conducted an immediate review to update the combating effects and impacts of COVID-19 based on following quick questions:

- An asymptomatic person who exposed to a confirmed COVID-19 should be quarantined?
- A group of individuals who have traveling history from a country with COVID-19 history should be quarantined?
- Is there any quarantine effectiveness when combined with other strategies, including isolation, school closure and antiviral drugs intake?
- And is there any change in the efficacy of quarantine during different isolating settings?

More than 29 different relevant studies were conducted focusing on COVID-19, SARS, and MERS studied the outbreak in various countries including the United Kingdom, China, and South Korea. These studies also reviewed the benefits of different quarantine strategies, both separately and combined for controlling COVID-19. Reviews concluding that:

- People who are exposed to COVID-19 patients have a high expectancy of infection and death as compared to non-exposed.
- The quarantine with other protective measures, including isolation, school closure, etc., greatly reduced the infected cases compared to the quarantine alone.
- Early implementation of protective measures might be more effective than late implementation and treatment against COVID-19 outbreak.
- Efficacy of quarantine of the travelers with a declared history of COVID-19 greatly reduced the chances of its spreading and death rate.

The researchers and reviewers still stress on the importance of basic adaptation of quarantine measures that how and when it should be implemented and lifted.

Karla Soares-Weiser, who is chief in editor Cochrane also added that, "The spread of COVID-19 gives a challenge to government globally." He also provided the best availability for policymakers to balance rigor with speed. That might be helpful in implementing the quarantine to get maximum results [20].

5.3.7 BENEFIT OF QUARANTINE

The "quarantine" is the most significant measures to control the spread of contagious diseases. Quarantine is used to limit the activities of people at risk of infectious diseases to determine if they are unhealthy and limit their risk of infecting others [21]. It limits the movements of people who are suspected of having an infection but they did not get sick because they were not infected or still in the incubation period [22]. This common health practice was widely used in Italy in the 14th century. At that time, ships arriving in Venice's city from the disaster-stricken city had to spend 40 days in separation (Italian: Quaranta for 40 days) [23]. This period provides sufficient time for the incubation of virus so, symptomatic persons could be identifying. The quarantine was a useful tool to reduce the transmission of disease during the SARS epidemic [1]. Quarantine can be carried out on an individual or group level and usually includes restrictions in the home or selected locations. Separation can be voluntary or coercive and has been described as a regulation to restrict people's movement, which can be considered an effective measure to control the spread of coronavirus disease globally [23]. During quarantine, everyone should be monitored for symptoms. If anyone does show some sign of infection, they should be immediately placed in an isolated area that is well-suited to respiratory infections. Approximately 3.9 billion people worldwide are being quarantined at home [24].

The current situation has closed educational institutes and restricted social activities. There is no suitable treatment available for coronavirus [2]. Human coronavirus transmission studies were reported to take place during an incubation period of approximately 2 to 10 days [25, 26]. Thus, we totally depend on public safety measures like quarantine to limit the contagious disease. Quarantine also includes the exclusion or limits the movement of people of other regions. In this situation, the persons with COVID-19 are separated from other community members, and this can be practiced in the hospital. Quarantine can stop the transmission of the virus to humans to prevent the spread of the disease [2].

Quarantine was implemented in 2003 to stop the spread of SARS [1]. This plays an important role in the problem of the disease. Separation is possible for individuals or in groups, usually including restrictions on family or specific groups. All necessary medical treatment should be used immediately to isolate the affected person at a designated location if any symptoms appear. The isolation makes it easy to identify the infected persons with detail of their close contact [2]. In addition, the quarantine proved to be significant in the following ways:

- The quarantine of people susceptible to reported cases will limit disease spread and mortality rate compared to non-quarantine control.
- Quarantine of migrants from a country where the disease has been reported to prevent disease and death is also effective.
- The combination of lockdown with other precautions (like social distancing, school closures and travel restrictions has had a significant effect on disease prevention, compared with quarantine alone. So, earlier, and systematic prevention may prove more effective [27].

After two months of lockdown, the number of cases in China has decreased. A clear explanation of the coronavirus outbreak and how China can control the spread of this disease. As the number of COVID-19 cases increases worldwide, China is gradually eradicating this infectious disease through complex methods and treatments. It was officially announced that on March 12, 2020, the country overcame the COVID-19 outbreak at the top of the mountain. It has been officially announced that on March 12, 2020, the country passed the COVID-19 peak shown in Figure 5.3 [28].

The lockdown in China with strict outdoor movement restriction combined with facility-based isolation and extensive contact tracing had significantly controlled the spread of Coronavirus [29]. However, less strict quarantine could also control the spread as compared to no quarantine [30].

Implementing the lockdown combined strict enforcement of physical distancing, contact tracing, and isolation was feasible for containing Coronavirus. It is notable, that in South Korea, through temporary quarantine time scheduling, and the use of news to technologies and isolate everyone as much as possible, the regulation of disease is lost. In some regions like Taiwan [31], Singapore [32] and Hong Kong, a flat curve of COVID-19 was maintained with testing, isolating the prompt cases outside the community, and early contact tracing.

5.4 ISOLATION METHOD IS USEFUL IN REDUCING THE RISK OF CORONAVIRUS

The separation of infected persons from people who are not infected to minimize disease transmission is known as Isolation [33]. This measure aims to protect non-infected persons from a person sick with a contagious disease. Isolation usually occurs in hospital under intense care settings. People who have no signs of disease but tested positive for Coronavirus will likely to go into isolation. Healthcare workers (HCWs) are advised to take special isolation preventive measures for COVID-19. Almost all the hospitals have special wards for sick persons, but doctors may also recommend the people to isolate at home for mild symptoms of coronavirus disease [34].

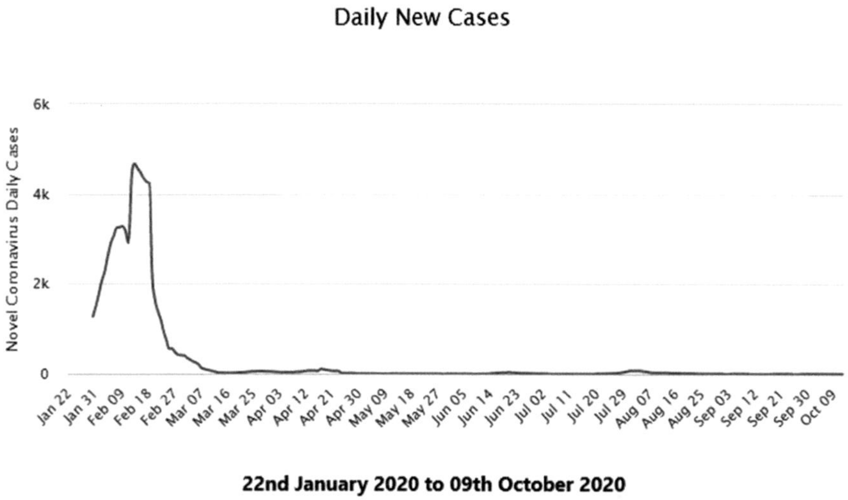

FIGURE 5.3 Cases in China from 22nd January 2020 to 09th October 2020 (Worldometers, 2020).

The transmission of contagious disease can occur through an infected person in worksite, home, and other crowded places. Even if someone takes all the preventive measures to protect oneself from disease, he or she can still have risk to get sick. This situation may cause problems if someone contracts the disease. Hence, Isolation is a key precaution practice to prevent the transmission of contagious disease to others. Isolation can prevent hospital-acquired infections and response to emerging contagious disease threat globally [35].

If a person is experiencing the mild signs of Coronavirus: cough, fever, tiredness, and unrest in-breath, take rest, stay home away from family members, and avoid contact with others until you feel completely better. Avoid sharing bedroom and bathroom with others. There is no vaccination or medication for COVID-19 disease, a person with mild symptoms is safer staying home than going to a place where you might expose others with this disease [36]. Always follow the recommendation from your healthcare department and your doctor about when you can end your isolation showed in Figure 5.4.

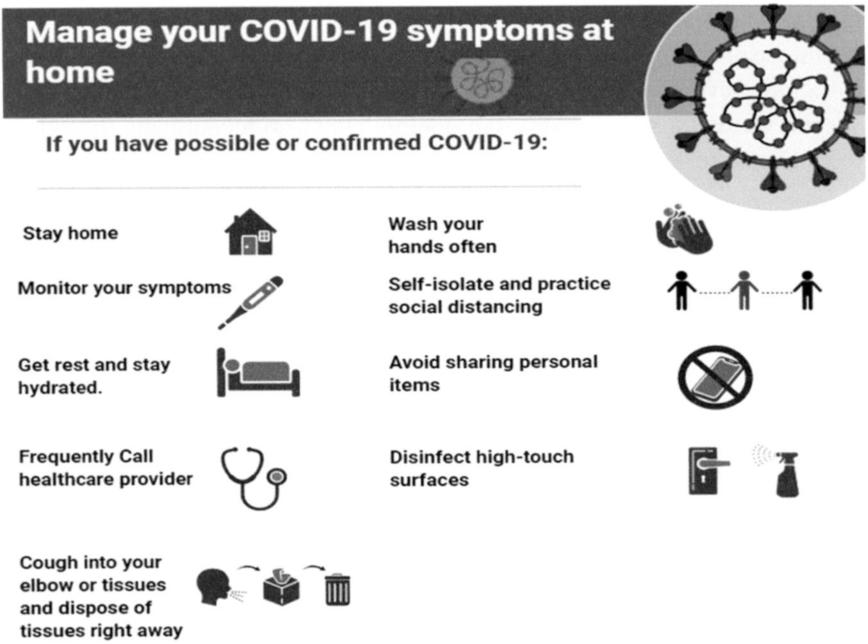

FIGURE 5.4 Possible steps to manage your Coronavirus at home source.

Source: Adapted from Centers for Disease Control and Prevention (CDCP). https://www.cdc.gov/coronavirus/2019-ncov/if-you-are-sick/steps-when-sick.html/

5.5 EFFECT OF QUARANTINE AND SOCIAL DISTANCING ON MENTAL HEALTH

Quarantine and isolation are often a tedious experience for those who undergo it. From a psychological point, people living in quarantine can feel a permanent state of mental distress, and other symptoms, i.e., anxiety, depression, insomnia, and loneliness (Figure 5.5). So, the quarantine is an unpleasant condition for people; however, it has public health benefits [4]. Current coronavirus outbreak is one of the leading causes of mental retardation in other groups of people. The quick spread of infection and deaths due to Coronavirus cause depression, anxiety, and mental stress [37]. Boredom, loss of freedom, separation from family and community and the uncertain pandemic can create a dramatic psychological impact.

The quarantine has a great influence on human mental health during this pandemic. Anxiety and depression symptoms were found among quarantined people [38]. A study found that 23.5% of medical students felt depressed and disheartened during COVID-19 pandemic. The research reported that quarantine negatively impacts mental health such as anger, confusion, and post-traumatic stress [4]. The psychology of quarantine and non-quarantine people were reported in many studies [39–42]. A study on HCWs was reported that the quarantine has a great impact on people's psychology and induced stress disorder [39].

The workers who were quarantined was founded with irritability, poor concentration in their work and exhaustive. The post-traumatic stress was also observed even after three years in quarantined persons [42]. A study comparing the symptoms of mental retardation of quarantined parents and children with non-isolated [41] reported that the quarantined children had an average stress score of four times higher than that of non-quarantined. Liu et al. [40] reported that 9% (48 of 549) of hospital staff found with high depressive symptoms three years after quarantine. Studies have widely reported psychological symptoms [43], emotional distress, depression [37], exhaustive, irritability, insomnia [43], acute post-traumatic stress disorder [44], irritation [32] and feelings of weakness. People were suppressed because of their close association with people who may be affected by SARS [44]. Studies also reported a number of other mental issues with quarantine, like confusion [45, 46]. Anger, sadness [46, 47] and depression caused by confusion during pandemic [48]. A study of people quarantines for possible exposure to SARS [44] revealed that 54% of detainees (524 out of 1057) avoided coughing or sneeze people, with 26% (255 people) avoiding closed places, and 21% (204) avoiding public places within a few weeks after the quarantine period. A study [47] observed some people with described long-term behavioral changes after quarantined, such as vigilance in handwashing and avoided crowds, and in some cases, return to the routine that was delayed by several months.

Quarantine also raises other problems, such as anxiety about affecting others, especially family members, and anxiety over the disease spread. These unpleasant mental states cause people to feel intimate, which is often associated with a lack of familiarity (such as attending gatherings) [44]. The main reason for the negative impact of quarantine on people's psychology is that they have to leave their friends, acquaintances, and family, are unable to move freely, doubts about the spread of the disease, and has a strong Emotion and response. The quarantine phase is a critical issue in public health management [49].

Considering this situation, long-term isolation is associated with mental stress, and people will be under more stress. In some cases, these stresses persist for several months after the retention period. Many people say that lack of information coverage is one of the reasons for the increased fear of this disease [4]. The spread of misinformation or lack of scientific evidence will exacerbate this situation, causing more and more anxiety and depression [50]. In life-threatening emergencies like coronavirus disease, suspicion, and distress stigma are common and are usually linked with resistance and objection to psychiatric treatment [37]. The disease is now exacerbated because it is an incurable virus. Moreover, due to contagious diseases, psychiatrists, and general practitioners should not be in interaction with people undergoing treatment (especially abandoned patients) to prevent certain viral infections. In this case, the medical team of physicians and medical professionals will be the main agent to improve the mental health of people infected with coronavirus [51, 52]. Furthermore, these forces might be insufficient may not be enough for the psychological treatment of persons who are ill because they are under a lot of stress to reduce the body's effects of the disease and withstand stress burden. In addition to these important elements, there is a lack of experts in the mental health [52].

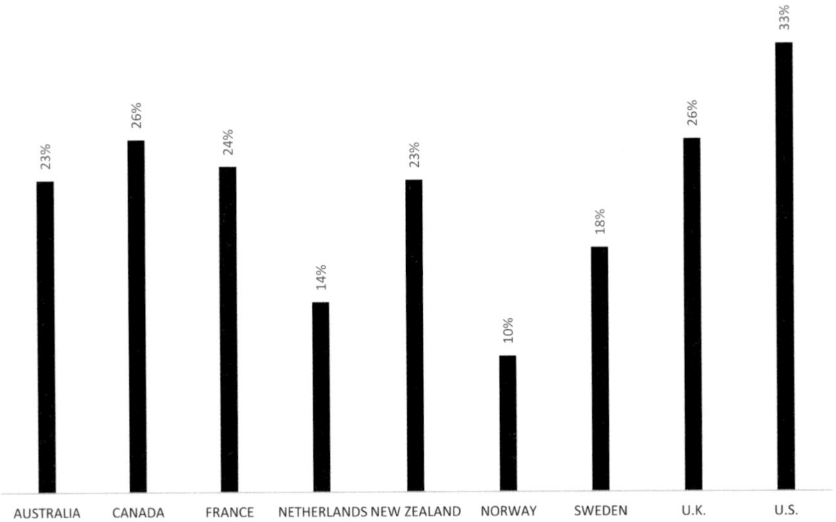

FIGURE 5.5 Anxiety, stress, and sadness in adults since the COVID-19 outbreak (Commonwealth Fund, 2020).

5.5.1 SOURCES OF STRESS DURING ISOLATION AND QUARANTINE

5.5.1.1 FEARS OF DISEASE

Participants in many studies stated concern with their health or concern for the well-being of others (Figure 5.6) [39, 47, 53–55], which appear to be likely to harm the members of their family [39]. They are also concerned about whether they have experienced physical symptoms that may be associated with the disease [53], and are concerned that symptoms may indicate that the infection is still associated with mental retardation in a few months later [55].

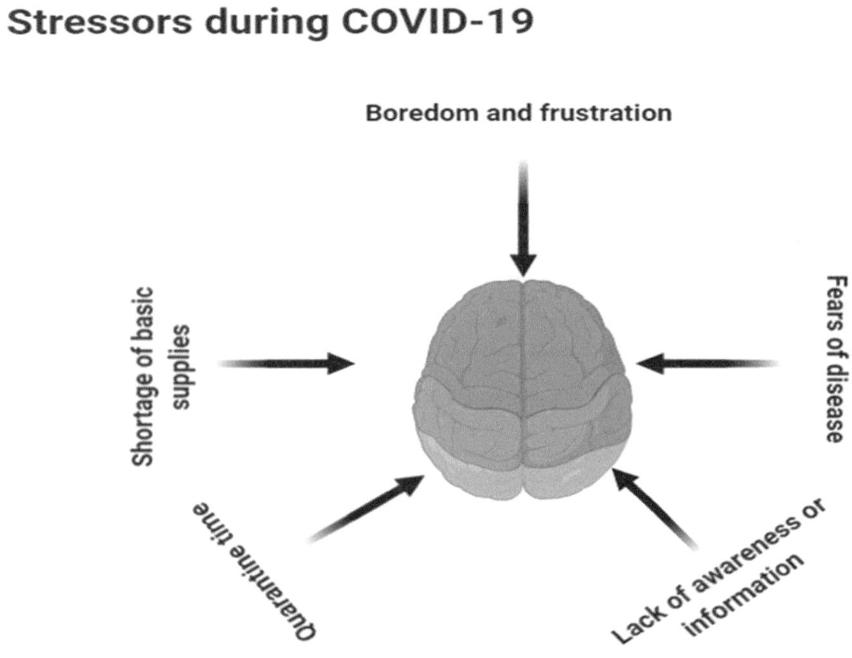

FIGURE 5.6 Stressors during quarantine.

Source: Adapted from Ref. [4].

5.5.1.2 QUARANTINE TIME

Studies have shown that prolonged quarantine time is linked with post-traumatic stress disorder [44] anger and avoidance [56]. Hawryluck et al. [54] showed that post-traumatic stress rate was higher in people who were left for more than 10 days as compared to others who were quarantined for less than 10 days.

5.5.1.3 BOREDOM AND FRUSTRATION OF DISEASE

It is often shown that stopping, losing daily habits, and reducing physical contact with others can lead to frustration, unhappiness, and isolation from other parts of the world, were feeling dissatisfied with people [45, 53, 58]. This is due to individuals' inability to participate in everyday activities (such as purchasing essentials goods or participating in social activities via telephone or the Internet) [55].

5.5.1.4 SHORTAGE OF BASIC SUPPLIES

Lack of basic food items and goods during the quarantine period is frustrating [58, 59] and continues to be associated with anger and anxiety [55]. The inability to access regular medical and prescription medications also appears to be a problem [59]. Food supply takes a long time to arrive [56]. Although people hospitalized during respiratory distress syndrome (SARS) in Toronto praised the public health department for supplying health supplies at the beginning of quarantine, they did not find the products or basic necessities required for everyday life [60].

5.5.1.5 LACK OF AWARENESS OR INFORMATION

Many of the participants stated lack of information from authorities, poor guidelines on actions, and uncertainty about the cause of the isolation [46, 60]. Following the onset of SARS in Toronto, participants believed that the cause of the confusion was the diversity of systems, methods, and contents in various health information systems [60]. In particular, a lack of understanding of the various risk factors caused participants to worry about the worst-case scenario [53]. Participants also reported that health and government agencies did not know the severity of the disease [45]. In one study, it may have been associated with a lack of clear instructions or reasons. He considers difficulty in complying with backup rules to be an important threat to mental illness after a crisis [44].

The Chinese National Health Commission (NHC) has issued an Emergency Response Plan for COVID-19, which guides the civil society to perform psychiatric treatments in pneumonia caused by a new virus. In this regard, the National Mental Health Association and the Academic Association have prepared a team of professors and promoted top-level content training courses in the form of videos and published articles. Sections, such as health professors, are present in the population-like adults. Moreover, digital numbers can be used to treat persons affected by the current disease [48]. Thus, it is clearly appropriate to construct an action to reduce the depression rate to fulfill people's requirements affected by coronavirus [37]. Therefore, it is indispensable for other countries to push for the issuance of regulations to regulate the implementation and distribution of mental health services to ensure individuals are supervised by experts, reducing the period of human integration at the time of leaving. The potential benefits of isolation and quarantine need to be weighed carefully against the possible mental costs. Successful use of quarantine measures as a public health measure requires us to limit the possible negative impacts of it.

5.6 DIFFERENT LEVEL OF CORONAVIRUS DISEASE TRANSMISSION

WHO states that viruses are emerging continuously and make a severe public health issue. Several viral pandemics were reported during the last 20 years, such as SARS-CoV in 2002–2003, H1N1 influenza in 2009 and MERS-CoV in 2012. However, the first case of human Coronavirus Wuhan's as found in sea-et of Wuhan by direct human-animal exposure which is presumed as the basic mechanism. However, further cases reported are not linked with this mechanism that is why it was thought that COVID-19 is transferred with human-to-human exposure. Considering the pathogenicity of respiratory diseases, transmission is believed to happen due to coughing and sneezing through respiratory droplets having size of less than 5–10 μm.

5.6.1 MODES OF TRANSMISSION OF COVID-19

5.6.1.1 DROPLET TRANSMISSION

Droplet transmission of respiratory diseases depends upon the size of droplets which varies in different sizes, i.e., respiratory droplets have size greater than 5–10 μm while droplet nuclei are less than 5 μm in diameter [61]. Currently, evidences proved that primarily COVID-19 transferred between two persons via respiratory droplets and contact routes [62–64]. Transmission through droplets does occur when a person comes in contact, closer to a distance of about 1 m with the one who is suffering from the symptoms of respiratory disorder like coughing, sneezing. It enhances mucosae's risk (either from nose or mouth) and conjunctiva (eyes) transmission through potentially infected respiratory droplets. Moreover, immediate transmission can occur when the person came across the fomites in an infected person's environment [65]. Hence, the transmission of CoVs can be occurred through direct (with the infected person) or indirect (with the infected objects in the immediate environment of infected person) contact like the thermometer, stethoscope, utensils, etc.

5.6.1.2 AIRBORNE TRANSMISSION

Airborne transmission is another possible source of COVID-19 transmission but this mode of transfusion is different from the previous one as it deals with the existence of microbes present inside the droplet nuclei that are about less than 5 μm in diameter and these particles can stay stable in air and later on can be transferred to others for a distance of about 1 m or greater than that. Moreover, in the context of COVID-19, it is reported that airborne transmission done under a specific environmental condition like those procedures which produce aerosols, i.e., open suctioning, bronchoscopy, endotracheal intubation, nebulization, disconnecting ventilator, manual ventilation before intubation, cardiopulmonary restoration, and tracheostomy, etc. However, there are some evidences regarding the transfusion of COVID-19 into intestine and feces, but very less data is available. Only one case study has erudite the presence of COVID-19 in stool specimens [66].

5.6.1.3 HUMIDITY LEVEL

It is believed that, the viability of viruses depends upon the modulation of humidity and temperature that affects the structural properties of viruses including lipid membrane and surface proteins level of humidity, i.e., equilibrium vapor state, greatly affects every type of contagious droplets including respiratory viruses without considering its source either from aerosolized or respiratory tract and **site** either airborne or surface settled. Therefore, relative humidity has dramatically influence. Moreover, measurements were taken of 40 housing apartments in New York and 6 commercial buildings in the Midwest of indoor humidity level revealed that there is a striking link exist on winter virus stability at a low relative humidity (20–50%). In contrast, the summer viruses' stability increased at a higher relative humidity (80%) [67].

Considering this available evidence, WHO still emphasizes the implementation of droplet and contact precautions with the person having symptoms or taking care of COVID-19 patients. Moreover, WHO still adds in airborne precautions in the infected circumstances in which aerosol-generating procedure and risk assessment was done [67]. These precautionary recommendations were also in accordance with the national and international guidelines of respiratory disorders that are compiled by the Society of Critical Care Medicine and European Society of Intensive Care Medicine that are also implementing in Canada, the United Kingdom, and Canada (Figure 5.7) [68].

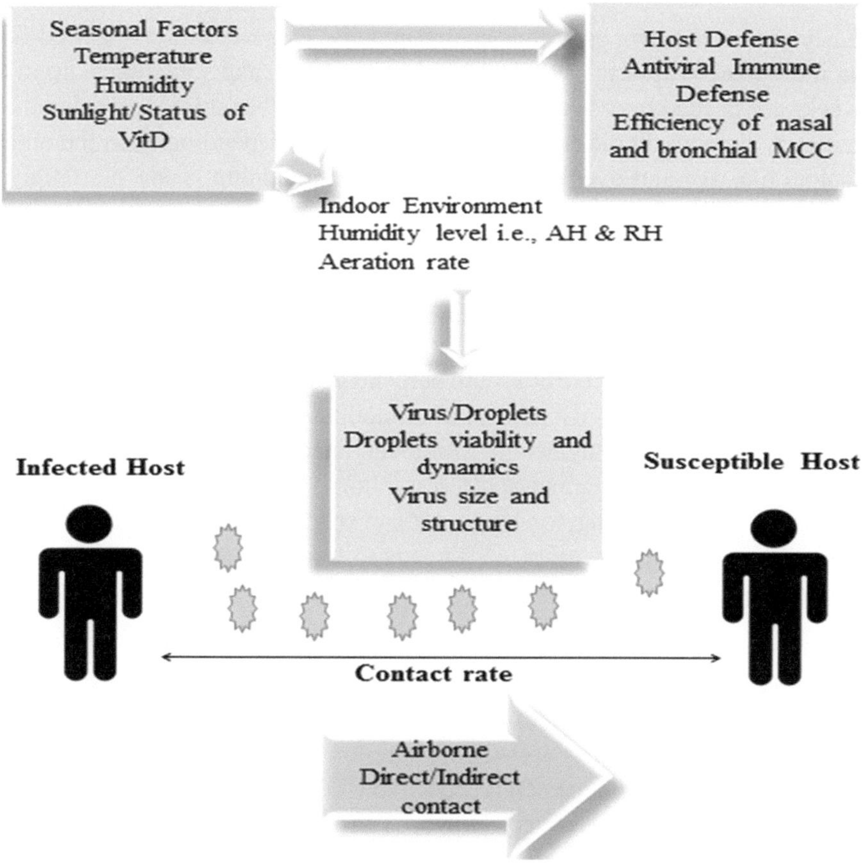

FIGURE 5.7 Factors affecting the transmission of respiratory viruses.

5.7 RECOVERY TIME OF CORONAVIRUS INFECTED PATIENTS

Scientists and researchers are constantly working on tracking information regarding COVID-19 infections and their recoveries. But recovery data is only available in confirmed cases of infected persons of COVID-19 but no data counting found in those who are not tested. However, based on early estimation, it is believed that the overall recovery rate of COVID-19 ranges between 97–99.5% [69].

5.7.1 WHAT IS THE APPROXIMATE RECOVERY TIME OF CORONAVIRUS INFECTION?

Early researches proposed that approximately, two weeks are required for an individual to appear COVID-19 mild symptoms, and sometimes, up to 6 weeks are needed in case of severity. Moreover, further studies revealed that recovery time might differ in different individuals depending upon the other factors like age and overall health conditions, including headache, fatigue, shortness of breathing that may linger on.

5.7.2 RECOVERY AFTER A SEVERE ILLNESS OF COVID-19

Studies revealed that, there is a small percentage of people with the symptoms of COVID-19 need to visit a hospital to facilitate breathing depending upon their age and overall body health. Moreover, in case of severe complications, a term is being used named acute respiratory distress syndrome (ARDS), which is very damaging for lungs and severe breathing problems. In that case, the intensive care unit (ICU) needs to treat that may result in weight loss and body strength.

5.7.3 RECOVERY STANCE

Researchers and scientists are still working on the recovery stance that how the immune system of a person responds to COVID-19 or is it possible to get infected again after first recovery. However, an early study on monkeys revealed no evidence of re-infection after first recovery. Still, few studies revealed that a person might lose antibodies after a couple of months. Furthermore, the person may have viruses in the body for weeks, but this fact endorsed the frequent hand wash practice and staying at home whenever possible.

5.7.4 RECOVERY STAGES

The recovery process from COVID-19 depends upon the level of illness, i.e., either mild, moderate to a severe case of illness.

5.7.5 RECOVERY FROM MILD COVID-19 ILLNESS

According to Dr. Septimus, about 80% of the population may experience mild symptoms or remain completely asymptomatic in first-time infection. About one week to 10 days' recovery time is needed in case of mild symptoms, and recovery will be similar as like other respiratory infections, e.g., flu [70].

5.7.6 RECOVERY FROM MODERATE COVID-19 ILLNESS

People who are having moderate or alarming symptoms of COVID-19 like the patient is warrant to visit the hospital, in that case, recovery time may take longer duration than mild symptoms. During recovery from a moderate stage of COVID-19, the patient may feel fatigue, shortness of breath, and cough, and several weeks are required to recover from such prolonged symptoms [70].

5.7.7 RECOVERY FROM SEVERE COVID-19 ILLNESS

In severe illness, the person may be in ICU or even on a ventilator and takes few weeks to months to recover. Recovering from severe COVID-19 illness will take more time to regain the normal working of the pulmonary and immune system of the body. In addition, if a person is on a ventilator, the body takes some time to get its independence back, which also depends on body strength and the ratio of lung damage. It is evident that illness intensity varies from person to person either develop pneumonia or the immune system does efforts to eliminate the virus. As a result, inflammatory response produces that SARS causing lungs damage, even respiratory failure [70].

5.7.8 ONCE RECOVERED, STILL BE INFECTIOUS FOR SOME TIME

One thing to keep in mind is that, once the person is subsided with the symptoms and fever, the body is still contagious. If someone gets free from symptoms for 72 hours, the person still continues to shed respiratory droplets even through stool, although it is not clear for how long. Therefore, it is believed that after recovery, the person should wear a mask while moving out of home or to interact with other persons. It was also added that disinfection should keep on frequently doing for commonly used surfaces, i.e., bathroom surfaces, flusher, and especially wash your hands properly whenever use washroom [70].

5.7.9 *HOW TO FEEL BETTER?*

If you are staying in the hospital, there is no treatment for COVID-19 and some medicines may shorten the recovery. However, there are many things to do to speed up recovery of COVID-19:

- Healthy food takes vitamins, limit the intake of sugary foods such as soda and cookies. Do not force yourself for eating, if you are not feeling any appetite.
- Fluid's intake lot of fluids, even when you are not having appetite.
- Low down fever use acetaminophen/ibuprofen in case of fever and body but do not take 3,000 mg/24 hours.
- Rest take rest by isolating yourself or visit the hospital in case of severe symptoms [71].

5.8 IMPORTANCE OF SOCIAL DISTANCING TO OVERCOME THE CORONAVIRUS

Social distancing aimed to limit contacts among those people who are not yet identified as an infected persons and not isolated [72]. During the flu pandemic of 2009, the WHO described social distancing as reducing the social gatherings and maintaining at least an arm's length distance from others. The Centers for Disease Control and Prevention definite social distancing as maintaining six feet distance from others, avoid gatherings and remain out of crowded places [73].

Social distancing is a necessary step in limiting the COVID-19 spread. Social distancing is reducing the chances of spreading the virus by preventing the physical interaction among people. It is especially important during the coronavirus outbreak to protect persons who are at high risk of Coronavirus. It includes delay or postpone of mega-events, playgrounds, closure of school and markets. The entire city is isolated to restrict the interaction among people except limited interaction to give basic goods. These tools are the only way to limit disease spread in the absence of a suitable vaccine for COVID-19 disease [74].

During the coronavirus outbreak, many governments emphasized on the adoption of precautionary measures especially on social distancing as alternatives to an enforced quarantine of highly affected areas [75]. Over 100 countries announced closures of schools in response to coronavirus pandemic. The United Kingdom administration, advised their people to avoid cinemas, theaters, and public places [76]. In the United States of America, the government has issued guidelines for the public to avoid public gatherings of 10 or more people to contain the COVID-19. Schools, universities, playgrounds, and cultural events have been closed. Moreover, the government has also imposed restrictions on travel to minimize the external exposure of country to COVID-19.

The community-wide implementation of social distancing is a complex measure [25]. The social distancing is a practice where the connections among cases is unclear, where the human-to-human transfusion is believed to have occurred and where restrictions on a single person is insufficient to halt the spread of the virus (Figure 5.8) [33]. In this situation, many countries have issued guidelines and policies to adopt social distancing measures.

Research indicates that measures must be implemented immediately for effective control of disease [77]. These measures could be helpful in reducing the infectious disease [2]. The distance of 2 m should be maintained to avoid the further transmission of the virus.

5.9 ISOLATION OF CORONAVIRUS PATIENTS IN HOSPITALS

In the hospitals, special equipment like gowns, masks, gloves are used with mechanical barriers, laminar airflow, and positive and negative pressure rooms. Temporary or dedicated isolation units may be prebuilt in the response of epidemic emergency [78]. In the hospitals, the aerosols transmission of disease can be limited by designing an isolation ward with negative pressure. Early detection of disease in a patient might have effective results in controlling the spread of COVID-19. HCWs are also affected by infected persons even if they take all the necessary preventive measures to limit transmission. If a medical worker gets a contagious disease, the transmission may occur to coworkers and patients living in close contact. Hence, the Occupational Safety and Health Administration has developed guidelines [79]. The Centers for Diseases Control and Prevention has released guides for HCWs to limits their exposure to the disease.

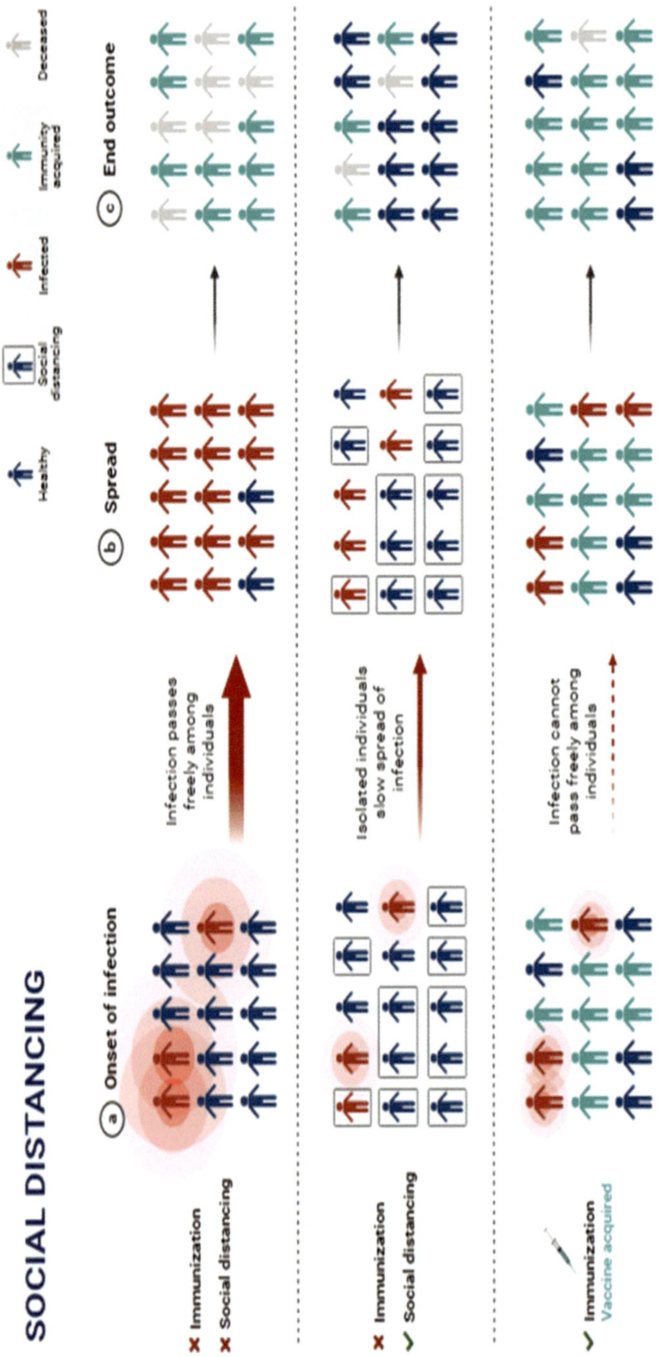

FIGURE 5.8 Impact of social distancing on disease spread [33].

Most hospitals are managing COVID-19 passively. They isolated the people in isolation units only if positive for COVID-19 and discharge the patients if they test negative for virus. Potential policies for disease control include the following:

- Screening all visitors for any respiratory disorders, including cough, fever, pharyngitis, rhinorrhea;
- Restricting medical workers to work if they have disease symptoms;
- Screening and testing of patients for all the respiratory viruses including COVID-19. Providing all the necessary and immediate care for COVID-19 positive patients [80].

A special staff that is minimally exposed to other patients should be assigned for patients diagnosed with Coronavirus. All of these measures are not easy. Hospital capacity in accommodation of serious patients, special staff for their care and supplies of goods are challenges for all the countries dealing with this pandemic.

5.10 SAFETY PRECAUTION IN CORONAVIRUS AND RECOMMENDATIONS

Currently, there is no suitable cure available for CoVs disease [2]. Prevention is the most favorable and only way to tackle with the coronavirus outbreak. Evidences confirmed that the infection of COVID-19 could be limited by avoiding the contact of infected people with others. For the effective precaution of coronavirus disease, two types of precautions are adopted: (i) general preventive measures, is meant for each member living in a society; (ii) specific preventive measures are meant for people those are ill, close contacts of Coronavirus, travelers, and healthcare staff (Figure 5.9). All the preventive measures are implemented to address the problems of three groups of the community as general, infected, and close contact persons and medical staff.

The prevention of disease is best accomplished by identifying, testing, and isolating the infectious cases as quickly as possible [81, 82]. Moreover, it is critical to trace all people living in close contact with infected person [83], so that they can be isolated and quarantined to halt the further spread of disease. These measures' prime objectives are the prevention of interpersonal transmission by isolating people living in close vicinity. The preventive measures we have are social distancing, isolation, and quarantine. All these measures are implemented in the world on a massive scale. The quarantining of close contacts reduces the further shedding of the virus before it appears on secondary cases. On average, the Coronavirus takes 5–6 days but sometimes takes 14 days to onset the symptoms of infection [84, 85]. Therefore, the quarantine period should be practice for 14 days from the last contact with an infected person. Social distancing can effectively limit the spread of coronavirus disease [2]. Meanwhile, the asymptomatic infected people can spread the virus; it is also significant to use the masks in public to restrict the further spread of disease. Fabric masks, can act as a barrier to control the transmission of virus if made and worn properly [83]. However, the comprehensive preventive measures, which include physical distancing, cleaning, and disinfecting the environment and frequent hand hygiene must be adopted with a face mask. The indoor crowding, especially where physical distancing is not possible, also includes recommended precautions of CoVs disease [86, 87].

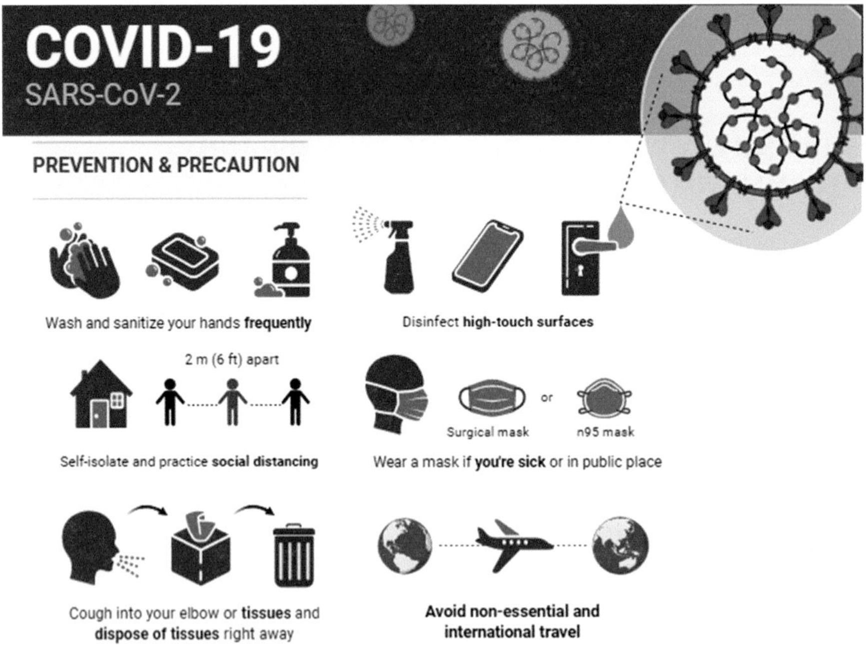

FIGURE 5.9 Preventive measures during coronavirus pandemic [21].

WHO recommend contact and droplet precautions for medical and paramedical staff when dealing with infected patients. WHO also recommends prevention from diseased persons by using a risk assessment approach [88]. These guidelines are in line with other international recommendations, including the Infectious Diseases Society of America [89], Society of critical care medicine and European Society of Intensive Care Medicine [90]. Additionally, WHO advice to caregivers and health care workers, to wear a medical mask during their routine activities in the clinics [8]. The United States Centers for Diseases Control and Prevention and the European Center for Disease Prevention and Control [91], also recommends airborne preventions for HCWs dealing with CoVs patients.

The WHO gave proper guidelines for the protections for people and medical personnel. The precautions must be adopted, otherwise, the chances of infection transfusion will be greater. Precaution is the finest course we can follow until we find a suitable vaccine or vaccine. Precautions can be taken to prevent people from triggering Coronavirus as follows:

- Maintain proper hygiene;
- Wash your hands with 70% alcohol-based soap or hand wash;
- Maintain proper social distance of 1 m;
- Stay at home, if you feel mild symptoms of a disease, seek medical attention;
- Always follow the medical guidelines;
- Medical staff must use personal protective equipment like face shield, sterile gloves, goggles, N95 masks;
- Healthcare staff should quarantine themselves for alternative weeks;
- Avoid close contact with others during the disease;
- Screen those who show the symptoms of disease;
- Use a disinfectant for cleaning environment and highly touching surfaces;
- Spreading awareness of disease through online videos;
- Overcrowding in the markets and on public places should be strictly avoided [57].

5.11 CONCLUSION

CoVs belong to the same like many viruses' family and SARS-CoV-2 is the same as MERS-CoV and SARS-CoV, their origin in a bat. Considering the pathogenicity of respiratory diseases, transmission is believed to happen due to coughing and sneezing through respiratory droplets having a size of less than 5–10 μm. Preventive measures are very important for public health. The aim is to reduce the number of human infections and deaths. In order to use resources efficiently, it is essential to implement these measures early and effectively. The combination of different preventive tools had the greatest impact on transmission, incident cases, and reduced mortality. To maintain the effective preventive measures, decision-makers must continuously monitor the impact of pandemics and implementation of measures. The potential benefits of isolation, quarantine, and social distancing must be carefully weighed against the possible psychological impact. The successful use of quarantine treatments as a measure of public health, reduced the possible negative impacts of it.

KEYWORDS

- **coronavirus transmission**
- **COVID-19**
- **isolation**
- **pandemic**
- **quarantine**
- **social distancing**

REFERENCES

1. Goh, K. T., & Chew, S. K., (2006). Epidemiology of emerging infectious diseases in Singapore, with special reference to SARS. *Popul. Dyn. Infect. Dis. Asia*, 287–304.
2. Wilder-Smith, A., & Freedman, D. O., (2020). Isolation, quarantine, social distancing and community containment: Pivotal role for old-style public health measures in the novel Coronavirus (2019-nCoV) outbreak. *J. Travel Med., 27*, 1–4.
3. Gammon, J., & Hunt, J., (2018). A review of isolation practices and procedures in healthcare settings. *Br. J. Nurs., 27*, 137–140.
4. Brooks, S. K., Webster, R. K., Smith, L. E., Woodland, L., Wessely, S., Greenberg, N., & Rubin, G. J., (2020). The psychological impact of quarantine and how to reduce it: Rapid review of the evidence. *Lancet, 395*, 912–920.
5. Li, Q., Guan, X., Wu, P., Wang, X., Zhou, L., Tong, Y., & Feng, Z., (2020). Early transmission dynamics in Wuhan, China, of novel Coronavirus-infected pneumonia. *N. Engl. J. Med.* doi: 10.1056/NEJMoa2001316.
6. World Health Organization, (2020a). *GCM Teleconference-Note for the Records*. Subject: Pneumonia in Wuhan, China. https://www.who.int/blueprint/10-01-2020-nfr-gcm.pdf?ua=1 (accessed on 5 August 2021).
7. World Health Organization, (2020b) *Teleconference of the R&D Blueprint GCM*. Pneumonia of unknown etiology in Wuhan China. https://www.who.int/blueprint/priority-diseases/key-action/20–01–2020-nfr-gcm.pdf (accessed on 24 August 2021).

8. World Health Organization, (2020c). *Novel Coronavirus (2019-nCoV)*. Situation Report-1. https://apps.who.int/iris/bitstream/handle/10665/330760/nCoVsitrep21Jan2020-eng.pdf?sequence=3&isAllowed=y (accessed on 24 August 2021).
9. (2019). *American Academy of Physical Medicine and Rehabilitation (AAPMR 2019) Physiatrist Member Support and Resource Center*. https://www.aapmr.org/news-publications/covid-19 (accessed on 5 August 2021).
10. Paules, C. I., Marston, H. D., & Fauci, A. S., (2020). Coronavirus infections—more than just the common cold. *JAMA, 323*, 707–708.
11. Chan, P. K., & Chan, M. C., (2013). Tracing the SARS-coronavirus. *J. Thorac. Dis., 5*, 118–121.
12. Berry, M., Fielding, B. C., & Gamieldien, J., (2015). Potential broad-spectrum inhibitors of the Coronavirus 3CLpro: A virtual screening and structure-based drug design study. *Viruses, 7*, 6642–6660.
13. Hui, D. S. C., Chan, M. C. H., & Wu, A. K. G. P. C., (2004). Severe acute respiratory syndrome (SARS): Epidemiology and clinical features. *Postgrad. Med., 80*, 373–381.
14. Chan, R. B., Tanner, L., & Wenk, M. R., (2010). Implications for lipids during replication of enveloped viruses. *Chem. Phys. Lipids, 163*, 449–459.
15. Song, Z., Xu, Y., Bao, L., Zhang, L., Yu, P., Qu, Y., & Qin, C., (2019). From SARS to MERS, thrusting coronaviruses into the spotlight. *Viruses, 11*, 59.
16. Tseng, Y. T., Wang, S. M., Huang, K. J., Amber, I., Lee, R., Chiang, C. C., & Wang, C. T., (2010). Self-assembly of severe acute respiratory syndrome coronavirus membrane protein. *J. Biol. Chem., 285*, 12862–12872.
17. Kilianski, A., & Baker, S. C., (2014). Cell-based antiviral screening against coronaviruses: Developing virus-specific and broad-spectrum inhibitors. *Antivir. Res., 101*, 105–112.
18. Raj, V. S., Farag, E. A., Reusken, C. B., Lamers, M. M., Pas, S. D., Voermans, J., & Haagmans, B. L., (2014). Isolation of MERS Coronavirus from a dromedary camel, Qatar. *Emerg. Infect. Dis., 20*, 1339.
19. Gralinski, L. E., & Baric, R. S., (2015). Molecular pathology of emerging coronavirus infections. *J. Pathol., 235*, 185–195.
20. Nussbaumer-Streit, B., Mayr, V., Dobrescu, A. I., Chapman, A., Persad, E., Klerings, I., & Gartlehner, G., (2020). Quarantine alone or in combination with other public health measures to control COVID-19: A rapid review. *Cochrane Database Syst. Rev., 9*, doi: 10.1002/14651858.CD013574.
21. Centers for Disease Control and Prevention (CDCP), (2020a) *Image of Coronavirus with Spike Protein*. https://www.cdc.gov/media/subtopic/images.htm (accessed on 5 August 2021).
22. Cetron, M., & Landwirth, J., (2005). Public health and ethical considerations in planning for quarantine. *Yale J. Biol. Med., 78*, 329–334.
23. Cetron, M., & Simone, P., (2004). Battling 21st-century scourges with a 14th-century toolbox. *Emerg. Infect. Dis., 10*, 2053.
24. Daily Mail, (2020). *Half the World in Lockdown: 3.9 billion People are Currently Called on to Stay in Their Homes due to Coronavirus*. https://www.dailymail.co.uk/news/article-8181001/3-9-billion-people-currently-called-stay-homes-coronavirus.html_(accessed on 5 August 2021).
25. Rothe, C., Schunk, M., Sothmann, P., Bretzel, G., Froeschl, G., Wallrauch, C., & Hoelscher, M., (2020). Transmission of 2019-nCoV infection from an asymptomatic contact in Germany. *N. Engl. J. Med., 382*, 970–971.

26. Sohrabi, C., Alsafi, Z., O'Neill, N., Khan, M., Kerwan, A., Al-Jabir, A., & Agha, R., (2020). World health organization declares global emergency: A review of the 2019 novel coronavirus (COVID-19). *Int. J. Surg., 76*, 71–76.
27. Science Daily, (2020). *How Effective is Quarantine Alone or in Combination with Other Public Health Measures to Control Coronavirus* (COVID-19)? https://www.sciencedaily.com/releases/2020/04/200408133253.htm (accessed on 5 August 2021).
28. Time, (2020). *China's Draconian Lockdown Is Getting Credit for Slowing Coronavirus. Would it Work Anywhere Else*? https://time.com/5796425/china-coronavirus-lockdown/ (accessed on 24 August 2021).
29. Lau, H., Khosrawipour, V., Kocbach, P., Mikolajczyk, A., Schubert, J., Bania, J., & Khosrawipour, T., (2020). The positive impact of lockdown in Wuhan on containing the COVID-19 outbreak in China. *J. Travel. Med., 27*, taaa037.
30. Anderson, R. M., Heesterbeek, H., Klinkenberg, D., & Hollingsworth, T. D., (2020). How will country-based mitigation measures influence the course of the COVID-19 epidemic? *Lancet, 395*, 931–934.
31. Wang, C. J., Ng, C. Y., & Brook, R. H., (2020b), Response to COVID-19 in Taiwan: Big data analytics, new technology, and proactive testing. *JAMA, 323*, 1341, 1342.
32. Lee, V. J., Chiew, C. J., & Khong, W. X., (2020). Interrupting transmission of COVID-19: Lessons from containment efforts in Singapore. *J. Travel. Med., 27*, taaa039.
33. Centers for Disease Control and Prevention (CDCP), (2020b). *Prevent Getting Sick*. https://www.cdc.gov/coronavirus/2019-ncov/prevent-getting-sick/social-distancing.html (accessed on 5 August 2021).
34. Mayo clinic, (2020). *COVID-19 Quarantine, Self-Isolation and Social Distancing*. https://www.mayoclinic.org/diseases-conditions/coronavirus/in-depth/coronavirus-quarantine-and-isolation/art-20484503_(accessed on 5 August 2021).
35. Swanson, J., & Jeanes, A., (2011). Infection control in the community: A pragmatic approach. *Br. J. Commun. Nurs., 16*, 282–288.
36. Phila Government, (2020). *Social Distancing, Isolation, and Quarantine During COVID-19 Coronavirus*. https://www.phila.gov/2020-03-31-social-distancing-isolation-and-quarantine-during-covid-19-coronavirus/_(accessed on 5 August 2021).
37. Xiang, Y. T., Yang, Y., Li, W., Zhang, L., Zhang, Q., Cheung, T., & Ng, C. H., (2020). Timely mental health care for the 2019 novel coronavirus outbreak is urgently needed. *Lancet Psychiatry, 7*, 228–229.
38. Röhr, S., Müller, F., Jung, F., Apfelbacher, C., Seidler, A., & Riedel-Heller, S. G., (2020). Psychosocial impact of quarantine measures during serious coronavirus outbreaks: A rapid review. *Psychiatr. Prax., 47*, 179–189.
39. Bai, Y., Lin, C. C., Lin, C. Y., Chen, J. Y., Chue, C. M., & Chou, P., (2004). Survey of stress reactions among health care workers involved with the SARS outbreak. *Psychiatr. Serv., 55*, 1055–1057.
40. Liu, X., Kakade, M., Fuller, C. J., Fan, B., Fang, Y., Kong, J., & Wu, P., (2012). Depression after exposure to stressful events: Lessons learned from the severe acute respiratory syndrome epidemic. *Compr. Psychiatry, 53*, 15–23.
41. Sprang, G., & Silman, M., (2013). Posttraumatic stress disorder in parents and youth after health-related disasters. *Disaster Med. Public Health Prep., 7*, 105–110.
42. Wu, P., Fang, Y., Guan, Z., Fan, B., Kong, J., Yao, Z., & Hoven, C. W., (2009). The psychological impact of the SARS epidemic on hospital employees in China: Exposure, risk perception, and altruistic acceptance of risk. *Can. J. Psychiatry, 54*, 302–311.

43. Lee, S., Chan, L. Y., Chau, A. M., Kwok, K. P., & Kleinman, A., (2005). The experience of SARS-related stigma at Amoy Gardens. *Soc. Sci. Med., 61*, 2038–2046.
44. Reynolds, D. L., Garay, J. R., Deamond, S. L., Moran, M. K., Gold, W., & Styra, R., (2008). Understanding, compliance and psychological impact of the SARS quarantine experience. *Epidemiol. Infect., 136*, 997–1007.
45. Braunack-Mayer, A., Tooher, R., Collins, J. E., Street, J. M., & Marshall, H., (2013). Understanding the school community's response to school closures during the H1N1 2009 influenza pandemic. *BMC Public Health, 13*, 1–15.
46. Caleo, G., Duncombe, J., Jephcott, F., Lokuge, K., Mills, C., Looijen, E., & Greig, J., (2018). The factors affecting household transmission dynamics and community compliance with Ebola control measures: A mixed-methods study in a rural village in Sierra Leone. *BMC Public Health, 18*, 1–13.
47. Cava, M. A., Fay, K. E., Beanlands, H. J., McCay, E. A., & Wignall, R., (2005). The experience of quarantine for individuals affected by SARS in Toronto. *Public Health Nurs., 22*, 398–406.
48. Li, H., Liu, S. M., Yu, X. H., Tang, S. L., & Tang, C. K., (2020). Coronavirus disease 2019 (COVID-19): Current status and future perspectives. *Int. J. Antimicrob. Agents, 55*, 105951.
49. Barbisch, D., Koenig, K. L., & Shih, F. Y., (2015). Is there a case for quarantine? Perspectives from SARS to Ebola. Disaster Med. *Public Health Prep., 9*, 547–553.
50. Bao, Y., Sun, Y., Meng, S., Shi, J., & Lu, L., (2020). 2019-nCoV epidemic: Address mental health care to empower society. *Lancet, 395*, e37, e38.
51. Liu, S., Yang, L., Zhang, C., Xiang, Y. T., Liu, Z., Hu, S., & Zhang, B., (2020a). Online mental health services in China during the COVID-19 outbreak. *Lancet Psychiatry, 7*, e17, e18.
52. Duan, L., & Zhu, G., (2020). Psychological interventions for people affected by the COVID-19 epidemic. *Lancet Psychiatry, 7*, 300–302.
53. Desclaux, A., Badji, D., Ndione, A. G., & Sow, K., (2017). Accepted monitoring or endured quarantine? Ebola contacts' perceptions in Senegal. *Soc. Sci. Med., 178*, 38–45.
54. Hawryluck, L., Gold, W. L., Robinson, S., Pogorski, S., Galea, S., & Styra, R., (2004). SARS control and psychological effects of quarantine, Toronto, Canada. *Emerg. Infect. Dis., 10*, 1206–1212.
55. Jeong, H., Yim, H. W., Song, Y. J., Ki, M., Min, J. A., Cho, J., & Chae, J. H., (2016). Mental health status of people isolated due to middle east respiratory syndrome. *Epidemiol. Health, 38*, 2016048.
56. Marjanovic, Z., Greenglass, E. R., & Coffey, S., (2017). The relevance of psychosocial variables and working conditions in predicting nurses' coping strategies during the SARS crisis: An online questionnaire survey. *Int. J. Nurs. Stud., 44*, 991–998.
57. World Health Organization, (2020j). *Prevention and Control of COVID-19 in Prisons and Other Places of Detention.* https://www.euro.who.int/en/health-topics/health-emergencies/coronavirus-covid-19/publications-and-technical-guidance/vulnerable-populations/prevention-and-control-of-covid-19-in-prisons-and-other-places-of-detention (accessed on 5 August 2021).
58. Wilken, J. A., Pordell, P., Goode, B., Jarteh, R., Miller, Z., Saygar, Sr. B. G., & Yeiah, A., (2017). Knowledge, attitudes, and practices among members of households actively monitored or quarantined to prevent transmission of Ebola virus disease--Margibi County, Liberia. *Prehosp. Disaster Med., 32*, 673–678.

59. Blendon, R. J., Benson, J. M., Desroches, C. M., Raleigh, E., & Taylor-Clark, K., (2004). The public's response to severe acute respiratory syndrome in Toronto and the United States. *Clin. Infect. Dis., 38*, 925–931.
60. DiGiovanni, C., Conley, J., Chiu, D., & Zaborski, J., (2004). Factors influencing compliance with quarantine in Toronto during the 2003 SARS outbreak. *Biosecurity and bioterrorism. Biosecur. Bioterror., 2*, 265–272.
61. World Health Organization, (2014). *Infection Prevention and Control of Epidemic- and Pandemic-Prone Acute Respiratory Infections in Health Care*. Geneva: World Health Organization. Available from: https://apps.who.int/iris/bitstream/handle/10665/112656/9789241507134_eng.pdf?sequence=1 (accessed on 5 August 2021).
62. Liu, J., Liao, X., Qian, S., Yuan, J., Wang, F., Liu, Y., & Zhang, Z., (2020b) Community transmission of severe acute respiratory syndrome coronavirus 2, Shenzhen, China-2020. *Emerg. Infect. Dis., 26*, 1320.
63. Huang, C., Wang, Y., Li, X., Ren, L., Zhao, J., Hu, Y., & Cao, B., (2020). Clinical features of patients infected with 2019 novel coronavirus in Wuhan, China. *Lancet, 395*, 497–506.
64. Burke, R. M., (2020). Active monitoring of persons exposed to patients with confirmed COVID-19—United States. *MMWR Morb. Mortal. Wkly. Rep., 69*, 245, 246.
65. Ong, S. W. X., Tan, Y. K., Chia, P. Y., Lee, T. H., Ng, O. T., Wong, M. S. Y., & Marimuthu, K., (2020). Air, surface environmental, and personal protective equipment contamination by severe acute respiratory syndrome coronavirus 2 (SARS-CoV-2) from asymptomatic patient. *JAMA, 323*, 1610–1612.
66. Zhang, Y., Chen, C., Zhu, S., Shu, C., Wang, D., Song, J., & Xu, W., (2020). Isolation of 2019-nCoV from a stool specimen of a laboratory-confirmed case of the coronavirus disease 2019 (COVID-19). *China CDC Weekly, 2*, 123, 124.
67. Moriyama, M., Hugentobler, W. J., & Iwasaki, A., (2020). Seasonality of respiratory viral infections. *Annu. Rev. Virol., 7*, 83–101.
68. *Coronavirus Disease (COVID-19): For Health Professionals.* https://www.canada.ca/en/public-health/services/diseases/2019-novel-coronavirus-infection/health-professionals.html (accessed on 5 August 2021).
69. Marfin, C., (2020). *How Long Does it Take to Recover from the Coronavirus?* Medical Express.
70. McCallum, K., (2020). *Recovering From Coronavirus: What to Expect During and After your Recovery.* Houston Methodist Leading Medicine on Health.
71. Webmd, (2020). *Coronavirus Recovery.* https://www.webmd.com/lung/covid-recovery-overview#1 (accessed on 24 August 2021).
72. The Washington Post, (2020). *Social Distancing Could buy US Valuable Time Against Coronavirus*. https://www.washingtonpost.com/health/2020/03/10/social-distancing-coronavirus/(accessed on 24 August 2021).
73. Hub, (2020). *What is Social Distancing and How Can it Slow the Spread of Covid-19?* https://hub.jhu.edu/2020/03/13/what-is-social-distancing/ (accessed on 24 August 2021).
74. Lewnard, J. A., & Lo, N. C., (2020). Scientific and ethical basis for social-distancing interventions against COVID-19. *Lancet Infect Dis., 20*, 631–633.
75. Stawicki, S. P., Jeanmonod, R., Miller, A. C., Paladino, L., Gaieski, D. F., Yaffee, A. Q., & Garg, M., (2020). The 2019–2020 novel coronavirus (severe acute respiratory syndrome coronavirus 2) pandemic: A joint American college of academic international

medicine-world academic council of emergency medicine multidisciplinary COVID-19 working group consensus paper. *J. Glob. Infect. Dis., 212*, 47–93.
76. BBC News, (2020). *Coronavirus: Odeon, Vue and Cineworld Shut UK Cinemas*. https://www.bbc.com/news/entertainment-arts-51925490 (accessed on 24 August 2021).
77. Maharaj, S., & Kleczkowski, A., (2012). Controlling epidemic spread by social distancing: Do it well or not at all. *BMC Public Health, 12*, 1–16.
78. Uys, L. R., (2003). Activity and stimulation need. In: *Fundamental Nursing* (pp. 163–201). essay, Maskew Miller/Longman, Pearson South Africa. ISBN: 978–0-636–04208–7.
79. OSHA, (2019). *United State Department of Labor, Safety and Health, Healthcare-Infectious Diseases*. Occupational Safety and Health Administration. https://www.osha.gov/SLTC/healthcarefacilities/infectious_diseases.html_(accessed on 5 August 2021).
80. Klompas, M., (2020). Coronavirus disease 2019 (COVID-19): Protecting hospitals from the invisible. *Ann. Intern. Med., 172*, 619, 620. doi: 10.7326/M20–0751.
81. World Health Organization (2020d). *Considerations in the Investigation of Cases and Clusters of COVID-19: Interim Guidance*. Geneva: Available at: https://www.who.int/publications/i/item/considerations-in-the-investigation-of-cases-and-clusters-of-covid-19 (accessed on 24 August 2021).
82. World Health Organization, (2020e). *Global Surveillance for COVID-19 Caused by Human Infection with COVID-19 Virus: Interim Guidance*. Available at: https://apps.who.int/iris/bitstream/handle/10665/331506/WHO-2019-nCoV-SurveillanceGuidance-2020.6-eng.pdf?sequence=1&isAllowed=y (accessed on 24 August 2021).
83. World Health Organization, (2020f). *Advice on the Use of Masks in the Context of COVID-19: Interim Guidance*. Available at: https://apps.who.int/iris/bitstream/handle/10665/331693/WHO-2019-nCov-IPC_Masks-2020.3-eng.pdf?sequence=1&isAllowed=y (accessed on 24 August 2021).
84. Lauer, S. A., Grantz, K. H., Bi, Q., Jones, F. K., Zheng, Q., Meredith, H. R., & Lessler, J., (2020). The incubation period of coronavirus disease 2019 (COVID-19) from publicly reported confirmed cases: Estimation and application. *Ann. Int. Med., 172*, 577–582.
85. Yu, P., Zhu, J., Zhang, Z., & Han, Y., (2020). A familial cluster of infection associated with the 2019 novel coronavirus indicating possible person-to-person transmission during the incubation period. *J. Infect. Dis., 221*, 1757–1761.
86. World Health Organization, (2020g). *Considerations for Public Health and Social Measures in the Workplace in the Context of COVID-19: Annex to Considerations in Adjusting Public Health and Social Measures in the Context of COVID-19*. Available at: https://apps.who.int/iris/rest/bitstreams/1277575/retrieve (accessed on 24 August 2021).
87. World Health Organization, (2020h). *Key Planning Recommendations for Mass Gatherings in the Context of the Current COVID-19 Outbreak: Interim Guidance*. Available at: https://www.who.int/publications/i/item/10665-332235 (accessed on 24 August 2021).
88. World Health Organization (2020i). *Infection Prevention and Control During Health Care when COVID-19 is Suspected: Interim Guidance*. Available at: https://www.who.int/publications/i/item/WHO-2019-nCoV-IPC-2020.4 (accessed on 5 August 2021).
89. Lynch, J. B., Davitkov, P., Anderson, D. J., Bhimraj, A., Cheng, V. C. C., Guzman-Cottrill, J., & Sultan, S., (2020). Infectious diseases society of America guidelines on infection prevention for health care personnel caring for patients with suspected or known COVID-19. *J. Glob Health Sci.* https://doi.org/10. 1093/cid/ciaa1063.

90. Alhazzani, W., Møller, M. H., Arabi, Y. M., Loeb, M., Gong, M. N., Fan, E., & Rhodes, A., (2020). Surviving Sepsis Campaign: Guidelines on the management of critically ill adults with Coronavirus Disease 2019 (COVID-19). *Intensive Care Med., 46*, 854–887.
91. European Centre for Disease Prevention and Control (ECDC), (2020). *Infection PREVENTION and Control and Preparedness for Covid-19 IN Healthcare Settings - Fourth Update*. Available at https://www.ecdc.europa.eu/sites/default/files/documents/Infectionprevention-and-control-in-healthcare-settings-COVID-19_4th_update.pdf (accessed on 5 August 2021).

CHAPTER 6

Face Masks and Hand Sanitizers

SHAHZAD SHARIF,[1] MAHNOOR ZAHID,[1] MAHAM SAEED,[1]
IZAZ AHMAD,[1] M. ZIA-UL-HAQ,[2] and RIZWAN AHMAD[3]

[1]*Department of Chemistry, GC University, Lahore–54000, Pakistan, E-mail: mssharif@gcu.edu.pk (S. Sharif)*

[2]*Office of Research, Innovation and Commercialization, Lahore College for Women University, Lahore–54000, Pakistan*

[3]*Natural Products and Alternative Medicines, College of Clinical Pharmacy, Imam Abdulrahman Bin Faisal University, Dammam, Kingdom of Saudi Arabia*

ABSTRACT

COVID-19 since its outbreak has affected the daily life of humans throughout the world. Virus causing COVID-19 transmission happens through droplets from one to another person with airflow. COVID-19 spread can be limited by taking into account simple as well as effective precautionary measures as well as adopting habits of using sanitizers and covering face with masks. Facemasks along with sanitizers help the humans to come back to their routine work during COVID-19 to control the harm at source by limiting the spread of the virus. This chapter has highlighted the use of different types of facemasks and hand sanitizers, their effect on the human health and environment, recommendations by WHO as well as formulation of more safe and efficient sanitizers.

6.1 COVID PANDEMIC

COVID-19 pandemic began in the Chinese city "Wuhan" as the number of cases were reported at the end of December 2019 [1]. COVID-19 is a disease like pneumonia occurs because of SARS-COV-2 (severe acute respiratory syndrome coronavirus 2) infection. The disease has similarity with Severe acute respiratory syndrome and Middle East Respiratory disease, also known as MERS [2]. As the spreading risk of coronavirus enhanced in China, WHO announced a Public Health Emergency of International Concern (PHEIC) on 30-01-2020. In the announcement, WHO reported about 170 deaths due to viral disease which was later named "COVID-19." As the COVID-19 spread continued, WHO referred to it a "Pandemic" [3].

To limit the COVID-19 spread, officially Government and stakeholders for public health has declared some precautionary steps. However, healthcare workers (HCWs) dealing with the SARS-CoV-2 patients are at the greatest risk of catching the infection. In 2003, when the SARS pandemic (Severe Acute Respiratory Disease) breakout, infected HCWs contributed to 21% of total reported cases globally. A report on 138 COVID-19 patients hospitalized in Wuhan indicated a total of 29%, i.e., 40 patients were health-care providers, which were infected in the hospital. On 11th February, 2020, a report by China's "Infectious Disease Information System" involved more than 1,500 infected health-care workers [4–6].

Coronavirus basically spreads through transmission of aerosols and droplets from the asymptomatic persons during the process of breathing and speaking. Method of transferring infection is altered through the size of droplets. The droplets which are greater than 20 micrometers have more tendency to stay on the objects due to gravitational force, while droplets smaller than 10 micrometers will remain in the air. Those with size of 1 micrometer can travel more than 20 feet after strong sneezing and coughing [7, 8]. An analysis was performed on the respiratory aerosols of COVID-19 patients without masks which were detected to contain coronavirus. But the respiratory droplets of the patients with masks were not tested positive for coronavirus [9–11].

In view of the above scenario among all the precautionary measures, the public was thoroughly advised to cover their faces and prefer to use some medical-grade masks, goggles, and other similar items. It helps a lot in reducing the risk of catching or transmitting the novel disease [12, 13]. Keeping in view all these circumstances, the precautionary measures are taken into account by using face masks and hand sanitizers to minimize its spread.

6.2 FACE MASKS

History of masks began with a polish surgeon named, Mikulicz Radecki who used it for the first time with his assistant in 1897 and made a publication on how the usage of face masks is helpful in minimizing the mouth droplets to spread [14]. That mask contained only one layer of gauze for the coverage of the mouth. As it was experienced in a year later that increase in number of gauze layers enhance the protecting capacity of masks so, in 1899 Fluge developed a type of mask which could give the coverage to mouth with the help of roller gauze strips [15, 16]. In 1905, to stop the spread of droplets of tuberculosis, usage of "Mouth Guard" was developed [17]. With the passage of time, requirements to make the masks better were taken under consideration as:

- They should be low in cost;
- They should be washable;
- They should be comfortable to wear, cover the area of nose and mouth properly;
- They should not be able to cause the fogging of spectacles, while wearing;
- They should not allow the passage of microorganisms across the product.

In recent times, deflector style masks have been developing by using materials of variable styles between the gauze. Further developments also include some masks based on paper and filter, but in comparison, masks based on filter came out to be highly efficient. In 1960, disposable masks were also developed as a prototype [18]. Later on, propylene-based masks, which are also called "Fiber Glass Filters" were also developed. This change in mask making was so effective that in 1970, usage of disposable masks made 75% of all the masks being used. Now days, usage of gauze masks and muslin is very uncommon.

6.3 EFFECTIVENESS AND FITTING

The efficacy of surgical and cotton-based masks was examined through an experiment in which face masks wearing patients of coronavirus coughed three to five times on a Petri-plate. It resulted in extremely less load of virus as compared to those not wearing a mask. When the experiment was performed with surgical masks, reduction from 3.53–3.26 log copies per ml had been seen, while in the case of cotton masks reduction of 2.27 log copies per ml had been observed. However, no clue of virus presence has been found at the inner surface of the masks, but 2.76 and 2.21 log copies per milliliter has been seen on the outer surface showing the inefficiency of both cotton and surgical masks against the virus. The performed research was criticized for many reasons; such as basically the masks have been specifically developed to restrict the viral transmission when a person is coughing, singing, breathing, speaking, and sneezing. Because it is always recommended to cover the mouth while sneezing or coughing, some other steps must be carried out in view of the above perspective to enhance their overall effectiveness [19].

It was observed that when a person coughed in a room with no mask and then covering the face could contaminate that area. The research paper with this experiment has been withdrawn as the number of patients involved were less. A separate research has also been performed in which a mask wearing patient was observed while coughing. The results showed the droplets could penetrate the mask and were able to travel to 1.2 meters. Overall initial efficiency of the masks was 91% [20]. In short, the study revealed that without face masks, the respiratory droplets are able to travel over 70 centimeters, but with mask they cover half of this distance. It indicates that droplets can penetrate the face mask, but their traveling distance gets limited. The above study only considers the "coughing" and the experiments while singing, speaking, breathing, and sneezing should also be performed to have a better idea of "Face-masks effectiveness." A comparison of surgical masks with N95 revealed that surgical masks are not able to filter submicron level particles, most probably due to their size [21].

However, the fact of designing the facial masks lies in protection of "healthy persons" surrounding the one which may have a viral infection. Surgical masks are designed in such a way that their void spaces are capable of protecting particles having a diameter more than 100-micron meter so wearing them for the protection against SARS-COV-2 is of no use as its diameter can be up to 140 nm [22]. However, they are efficient to avoid the spread of aerosols and respiratory droplets having large size. N95 respirators could stop the transmission of particles having a diameter of 100 nanometers but the particles less than this size are able to pass the respirator [23]. N95 respirators just like face masks are able to inhibit the passage of droplets formed after sneezing and coughing with 100 μm and 1 μm diameter, respectively.

In case of N95 masks, which can provide tight fitting as they are unable to allow the passage of air side-ways but it can pass through the mask [24]. Before using the respirators, the users should test its fitting so that it can be ensured that there is not any kind of leakage [25]. A study was also done to know the number of persons who can pass the fit tests with N100 masks, N95 masks (Ref1860) and N95 masks (Ref9210). The efficiency of their pass rates was 70%, 69% and 55% respectively. The experiments with the user seal check showed about passing of 71 to 75%. But the Quantitative Fit Testing incorrectly passed the 18 to 31% of the user seal checks. It indicates that for the overall effectiveness of the respirator, it should be fitted and worn properly. To check the fitting of the respirator, "Quantitative Fit testing" is more preferable than the user seal check. When surgical masks were checked, they came out with very poor fit factor and the fit factor of 13.7 was observed while wearing five surgical masks together. The respirator covering the half-face came out to have as low as 100 fit factors [19]. Qualitative tests on the face masks fitting revealed that almost all the 100% masks were failed while breathing normally. In the case of aided and non-aided Quantitative fit testing, fit factors from 2.8 to 9.6 and 2.5 to 6.9 were obtained, respectively [26]. These face masks cannot replace respirators as they have been designed in such a way that the space remains between the face and mask and thus also show less fit factor even when used in a multiple number together.

The term face masks comprise medical/surgical masks or N95 respirators which individuals use as precautionary measure against Coronavirus Disease. As the purpose of using face masks is to limit COVID-19 transmittance, still there are some countries which do not recommend it like USA, Australia, and Canada have not supported the idea that a specific area population can restrict the corona-virus by using masks. On the other hand, official Health Departments in Philippines, China, and Indonesia have given instructions for using face masks [13, 27–30].

A varying set of information has been obtained on face-masks from the health officials against COVID-19. This information has been collected from the web pages and news outlets as these are the primary platform to share information with the public. The interview of a former health secretary of Philippines which was aired on CNN Philippines states is as under:

"It cannot be said that face masks are highly effective to provide protection against COVID-19 as air can pass through the spaces but wearing it is preferable than not using it."

Further, he added; "Wearing face masks can be avoided in an area where a person is assured that there is no one present with coronavirus case. But if you are in a mall without knowing from where the rest of public belongs to, they may be from China and may have coronavirus." On January 30, 2020, a report said that wearing masks is mandatory for the public in at least the two provinces of China. In another interview with General of Environmental Health Directorate and Secretary of Health Ministry Disease Control in Indonesia, it was revealed that "Surgical/Medical mask is sufficient to provide protection against any viral or bacterial infection unless we use it rightly."

Another recommendation includes that the masks must be wore by persons during sickness to avoid the viral transfer at the time of cough or sneeze. On the other hand, people wearing it remain protective from the virus in gatherings or public points [27]. Thus, the above information indicates health ministry of China, Philippines, and Indonesia is in agreement that face mask may avoid coronavirus spread among those who are medically fit.

The British Columbia Center for Disease Control and Prevention (CDC) in Canada have provided instructions that the use of face masks is only for the sick persons. It also states that wearing the face mask by a healthy person is not much effective giving a wrong sense of protection as when a person is wearing a mask, he touches his face more times to fit it properly, etc. [27]. However, the Chief Medical Officer in Canada and Ontario has said that "Face masks are not supported because the public is unaware of its proper usage, as may touch beneath the mask which also may spread the germs."

N95 respirators are called so as they can inhibit 95% of the small sized particles from traveling to the mouth and nose. These respirators work accurately if they fit tightly and properly, but it is difficult in the case of individuals having hair on face [27]. A professor in the department of immunology (Canadian university) stated:

"The main problem of mask is that they are not well fitted and there is a chance that something can enter through the loosely fit areas."

The interviewee further added in the statement that as the COVID-19 spreads through the transmission of droplets by coughing or sneezing of an infected one so wearing a properly fit mask with the coverage of all the exposed areas reduces the risk of the viral spread [27]. Due to contradicted statements obtained from different health officials and countries, there is less clear understanding about wearing of masks for the medically fit persons. However, the risk lies in the fact that individuals with no medical diagnosis of coronavirus may got exposure to the virus and may be pre-symptomatic, a-symptomatic, or symptomatic. It is difficult to differentiate the three types of persons as they carry odds of viral spread in public points.

The National Center of Immunization and Respiratory Diseases (USA) briefed on 30th January 2020 that wearing face masks routine wise is not supported as it can lead to respiratory illness. And at this time of coronavirus spread, it is not recommended for the persons who do not get a direct exposure to the novel virus [27]. The statements got on the face masks from the countries like Canada, the USA, and Australia are mixed and mostly disfavor them for the persons who are not diagnosed with coronavirus.

6.4 FACE MASKS AND SIMILAR BARRIER

When COVID-19 is undertaken, masks effectiveness on reducing the viral transfer via respiration become a topic of discussion. Randomized Controlled Trials provided the evidence that covering the face with masks reduces the chances of influenza like illness by 6%. Study was done on their effectiveness through many ways. In a house, the infected persons lived together with the uninfected ones. When all the individuals of house and servants wore face masks, the chance of spreading illness to further members were reduced by 19%. On the other hand, when the uninfected members covered the face with mask as a precautionary measure, the risk reduced to 7% only. The impact matched with the observation when only the house individuals used face-mask and chances of viral spread reduced to 5%. From the observational studies, it can be said that face masks are considered more effective for the protection of respiratory related sickness in the less gatherings such as shops, working places, educational institutions, and public transport. At the places which include large gatherings, evidences found for the effectiveness of face masks are conflicting.

During this pandemic, the main focus was the "Hajj Pilgrimage," which was typically not a large gathering. Wearing face masks proved to be effective when the infected persons were already present in the home. The primary and secondary preventive measures at Hajj and households did not appear to be much effective because of more chances of contact and being infected. One reason is also that face masks might not be used at the right time because usually it takes less than 24 hours when a person becomes symptomatic and might be in the duration of 48 hours, he or she got infected [31].

The observations in this coronavirus breakout involved the fact that face-masks are designed for the protection of individuals wearing it from the infected ones and these masks get wet because of droplets on their surface during respiration [32–34]. However, proper wearing of face-masks for the certain period of time reduced the spread of small droplets in influenza up to 6 times. During randomized controlled trials, wearing of masks for ill or physically well individuals at the beginning did not matter much as the secondary attack rates were the same as observed during household settings. These points suggested that it is not only the matter of wearing face-masks or not, but the time period and contact type also have a huge impact for the transmission of infectious disease. It is also difficult that well wearing of masks is made for the multiple hours in a day because of breathing discomforts and much other impairment such as:

- Wearing of masks can cause discomforts in sleeping, eating, and problems of Oral hygiene [35, 36];
- Sometimes, wearing of masks may feel like anti-social and may become the reason of rashes/allergic reactions on the skin due to heat produced [37, 38].

Previous research on the "Efficacy of face-masks" has been performed either with the combination of other precautionary measures or a group including health/non-healthcare providers [39–41]. Randomized Controlled Trials are kept the main focus in case of community use of face-masks. However, conclusions from the research obtained are mixed such as; face masks may or may not be effective, obviously effective, greatly effective, or not satisfactorily effective [42, 43].

It is also the fact that randomized controlled trials cannot be considered to provide best evidences on the behavior of the public for the use of face-masks [44]. As many evidences were reported in which the population did not seriously follow the prescribed directions; a major group of participants only wore masks at the time of monitoring while intervening ones did not use the masks for the major portion of time [45–47]. As compared to these trials-based evidences, case-controlled study (observational research) can give better quality results for the beneficial use of facemasks to remain safe from influenza like illness. No doubt there may be some confusing factors in the observational study which may be avoided in randomized controlled trials.

The main problem in this analysis is the mixed-use of different face-masks like the randomized controlled trial-based study by Brainard et al. involves mostly surgical masks or P2 grade like respirators followed by the protocol on:

- How to properly wear face-masks;
- The time period for which face-masks are used;
- The hygienic process of disposing the face-masks.

In an observational study, mostly face-masks used were of surgical grade, which is in agreement with the evidences collected through recent photography in the cities of China, Korea, and Japan. Surgical style barriers are also recommended by some regular users of face-masks and survey analysis in the Eastern countries [48, 49]. In the future, more investigation regarding what type of face masks is used for which period of time and the procedure to prepare them for again use should be performed. Further, the analysis of intervention timing can produce more satisfactory results and the evidences obtained on the use of facemask in the pre-symptomatic period or rightly after the onset of symptoms can make the whole study a powerful one.

6.5 FACE-MASKS V/S RESPIRATORS

According to a report, in the health-care system, the main types of face-masks used are:

- Type-II surgical-mask;
- Type II-R splashes.

Surgical masks undergo through a standardized testing process before marketing and are basically used to avoid transmission of respiratory droplet bacteria by the team during surgery. To check the efficacy of surgical masks, *Staphylococcus aureus* is used as a pathogen which is larger in size than the SARS-COV-2. The coronavirus is almost 120 nanometer in size and present on the droplets exhaled so, its size has not a crucial role.

Surgical-masks which usually do not make a tight seal on the face and should be used for 8 hours maximum, but if it gets wet by droplets or damaged then must be changed as early as possible. It can be contaminated when wear around neck. As compared to them, respirators are known as filtering face-piecepieces (FFP) in Europe and as N95 masks in the United States. Three types of FFP are known on the basis of their performance. These respirators are FFP1, FFP2, FFP3, which can filter the particles above 0.3 micrometer with greater than 80%, 94%, and 99% efficiency, respectively.

FFP2 respirators can avoid the air particles inhaling. The procedure to analyze FFP2 respirators involves maximum contamination of microbes so that air can leak through it. That is the reason for which a tight fit is required on the carrier face, but some users also find it uncomfortable [50]. The respirators with valves for expiration are not supported as they are not safe for surrounding individuals. Detailed research emphasizes on the use of "FFP2" masks if superior protection is required and "Surgical-Masks" in case of confirmed or suspected coronavirus cases [51, 52].

6.6 RECOMMENDATION OF SURGICAL MASKS THROUGH INDIRECT EVIDENCES

Because there is no publication on COVID-19 before, the comparative analysis of surgical masks with respirators effectiveness is provided on the basis of discussion with experts and research from the influenza, MERS, and SARS-1 pandemic [51, 52].

Although the clinical samples contained infectious droplets of influenza but no evidence has been reported for the spread of SARS and Influenza during practice in the clinical system [53]. A recent randomized controlled trial study involving 6,418 infected persons showed that surgical masks are more effective to provide safety for health care providers as compared to respirators [54]. On the other hand, an observational analysis indicated the surgical masks have similar effectiveness as the respirators. Similar results were also obtained during the case-controlled study in SARS-1 and Influenza [55].

Other findings also report that 35 health care providers covered their faces with surgical masks while working on the extubation, intubation, and non-invasive ventilation (aerosol-generating process) and they remain safe with no transmission of virus [56]. A Meta-analysis performance as a comparison of different masks with no use of masks supported the fact that masks are better to provide protection against SARS, coronavirus, and MERS with 77 and 96% efficacy of surgical masks and FFP2, respectively [57]. However, in another study, FFP2 respirators performed better in a health-care system than in a community setting. It can be concluded from the above discussion that no evidence is reported to favor FFP2 over surgical masks but still, for the better understanding, they should be compared directly.

6.7 MATHEMATICAL MODELING

Mathematical modeling is mandatory to make a better understanding of mechanisms through which infections spread. In this way, theoretical knowledge is obtained regarding the development of health policy for the public [58, 59]. During this coronavirus pandemic, the mathematical models used are categorized as under:

- Susceptible infective recovered (SIR) type models;
- Agent based models (ABMs).

The first category focuses on probabilistic differential equations and is related to population, while the second one is related to the individuals who meet on a type of network and develop probability of transferring the infection [60–63]. However, many difficulties are there with both models. Models related to population (SIR) are too common to summarize the real-world complexities [64]. On the other hand, ABMs vary on the basis of time leading to the compromise in accuracy when constructed [65]. The point of issue basically decides the sequence of network based, dynamic, data driven and stochastic based methods [66].

SIR modeling was applied to know the ability of face-masks during the influenza breakout [67]. The model was constructed by effect of masks on the rate of infection and reproduction number. Results from this modeling showed that home-made and surgical masks reduced the reproduction rate of viral attack. Reports also suggested that mask use decreased the transfer of influenza virus, reducing the rate of attacks which may lead to pandemic.

Another SIR type model was based on "which individuals should use face-masks to avoid infections" whether they should be infected or medically safe ones. To know the transmission of viral disease on the physical interaction of people when the connection was interrupted in a complicated network, stochastic cellular automation and common differential equations were used. Simulation model states that when no of masks are finite, then infectious individuals are recommended to wear masks [68]. The difficulty resides in the identification of such persons. Another SEIR model was applied in determining the effect of masks in H1N1 breakout. For such analysis, the population was divided as wearing and not wearing masks. Scientific status characterized the persons in the groups as; Infective individuals, exposed, recovered, and susceptible.

Moreover, the cumulative no of cases also reduces when the percentage of public wearing masks rises [69]. In terms of percentage efficacy of masks, 20% effective make the infectious cases half while masks with 50% efficacy could terminate the pandemic when only 25% of population used them. Another report suggested that the use of face masks in household setting limitedly controlled the seasonal viral infection [45].

An investigation was performed to analyze the masks efficiency with reference to three respiratory viruses, i.e., rhinovirus, coronavirus, and influenza virus presence on droplets exhaled during breath. The modeling involved two groups; with and without masks. Detection frequency was examined by 2-sided Fisher's Exact Test and un-adjusted Tobit Regression model was applied to measure viral load. Results indicated the reduction in transfer of droplets on use of masks, thereby lowering the risk of disease spread through an infective individual. When samples were collected from the COVID-19 and influenza virus patients, no virus was detected on exhaled respiratory droplets, but the virus was shed on aerosols by >50% of patients with rhinovirus. The viral load on droplets/aerosol was not significant, suggesting that a very close contact will only lead to transfer of infection from the ill person.

During this pandemic, the simulation model study on the basis of death rates was conducted in New York and Washington. Figure considers 18 scenarios for the future death tolling in New York city.

The results obtained after simulation model-based study indicate that even mild effective masks can flatten the death curve. In summary, from 17 to 45% of deaths in New York could be avoided with 80% use of face masks which are 50% effective. To again analyze the impact of using face mask, 2 models were developed based on the SIR system. The models involved whether population adopted masking, growth-rate on daily basis and percentage decrease from the increased growth rates. The results provided a perfect relation between early adoption of masks and reduction rates of growth/death on a daily basis. Most of the researchers also emphasize on "Universal Masking" in order to inhibit the viral spread as lockdown of mouth and nose seems more suitable than the full body in the lock-down. No use of masks, even with proper social distancing can enhance the risk of half of the population getting infected with death rates crossing million [70].

So, the conclusion from mathematical modeling is that a greater number of individuals adopting masks with other standard operating procedures (SOPs) will cause a decrease in the transfer and death rates due to coronavirus or any similar disease/infection [45, 66, 67, 70].

6.8 RECENT ADVANCES

To enhance the efficiency of masks and respirators in opposition of airborne particles, pathogens, and viruses, several modifications have been done like employment of nano-fiber webs and nano-fibers. With the development of fabrication and nanoscience, materials like silver nanoparticles, titanium oxide, iodine, and copper oxide have been used on the mask surfaces to improve disinfection ability [71–75].

6.8.1 USE OF NANO-FIBERS

Nano-fiber usage in the mask and respirators is really preferable as they increase the surface area per mass, improving the phenomenon like catalysis/ion exchange and overall trapping efficacy [75, 76]. Nanofibers are characterized by less weight, smaller size of voids with improved interconnectivity and better permeability [77]. Decomposition of contaminants can be enhanced by using nano-fibers with other chemicals and agents for nucleation, which in turn lower the risk of getting infected with viruses or pathogens [78]. The most widely used technique for their fabrication is "Electrospinning" [79]. When a surgical mask fabricated with nanofiber was taken into account by Skaria et al.

it showed lower resistance against air flow and better filtration efficacy than unmodified masks [80]. Another analysis of N95 FPPR masks loaded with nanofibers showed that they possessed higher passing rates for fit tests and thus better capability for filtering pathogens. In another demonstration, it was revealed that partially gelled polypropylene nanofibers and a biocide layer (hydrophilic) in FFPR improve air permeability and capability to inactivate the infection causing microbes [81, 82].

When another layer of fibers is incorporated, then it makes the filtering ability of masks better. For example, electret fibers in the material enhance the retention ability for electrostatic charges with the improvement in overall efficacy. Wang et al. used the jet spinning process to synthesize the light weight nylon 6-Polyacrylo-nitrile nanofiber net from the fibers of polyamide 6–15 and poly-acrylonitrile. The nanofiber net was able to capture particles with 2.5 micrometer or lesser in diameter. It showed 99.9% efficiency when followed the deep bed filtration [83]. A recent research was carried out to construct nanofibers according to the N95 requirements. For this purpose, polypropylene nanofibers were coated with polyvinylidene fluoride and cellulose acetate. The first large bubble point with 5.7 micrometer void size was observed by using 16% weight/volume of cellulose acetate [84]. The double-layered coating of polyvinylidene fluoride was required to get thin fibers with smaller void as the filtration efficiency largely depended on void section and resistance for airflow.

Another study focuses on the incorporation of nanostructures with the fibers to improve the strength of 3 dimensional structures. When carbon nanotubes agglomeration was done on a fluidized bed filter for the filtration of aerosols, it showed high water repellent ability with enhanced quality factor in comparison to commercial filters [84, 85]. Moreover, a polyetherimide Silica fibrous membrane showed excellent filtration capability, which was attributed to the permanent dipole moment of silica causing more charges to be trapped with better stability and adsorbing ability for viruses/pathogens [86].

Recently, research was performed with loading of titanium dioxide, zinc oxide and silver nanoparticles on polyacrylonitrile membrane through electrospinning method. Filtration assessment was done by sodium chloride. Titanium dioxide-based filter showed 100% efficiency due to high charged surface having lower diameter while AgNPs based filter displayed greatest quality factor due to smaller drop of air pressure. TiO_2 based filter also showed enhanced antibacterial performance against Escherichia coli (gram-negative) [87]. As a whole, the quality factor of synthesized membranes was higher in comparison to regular nanofiber membranes.

Proper disposal of face-masks is necessary to avoid secondary transmissions, especially in the current pandemic. To recycle the filters, several sterilization procedures have been used like; Ethylene oxide, Bleaching, treatment with H_2O_2 and UV but these methods have some limitations as well [88]. Therefore, there is a need to develop a viral decontamination method with the potential to lower the threat of infection and transmission. Modification of filters with antigen specific antibody or incorporation of a disinfectant material is the most common method to resist the viral attacks. Nanoparticles cannot only consider helpful for viral capture but can also inhibit its attachment through membrane penetration. Moreover, they do not have any harmful effects like itching or inflammation on the human skin [89, 90].

For deactivation of virus, modification of face-masks was performed with sodium chloride functionalized through fibrous filtration unit [91]. This process followed the two steps as under;

- Dissolution of the salt with virus; and
- Recrystallization of salt through evaporation.

At the drying and recrystallization stage, virus in the saline solution (super-saturated) gets deactivated. This strategy would be effective to reduce the viral spread risk in a breakout.

6.8.2 USE OF SILVER (AG) BASED COMPOUNDS

Silver based materials and silver ions are very beneficial to provide protection from microorganisms. However, accurately the mechanism involved is not known but it is believed through different studies that Ag+ ions can cause cell death by destroying the membrane and cell wall of bacterium [92, 93]. A study was performed by coating of silver nitrate and titanium dioxide on the surgical-masks which displayed a 100% decrease in growth of *Escherichia coli* and *S. aureus* in two days but the unmodified masks displayed 25% and 50% enhancement in growth of respective bacteria. When the anti-bacterial activity of silver nanoparticles was tested by Hiragond et al., the mask coated with 100 ppm of Ag nanoparticles exhibited higher efficiency against bacteria. These nanoparticles are able to destroy the bacteria by crossing the lipid bilayer of the cell membrane [94]. A regular filter unit coated with silica-AgNPs showed excellent activity against MS2 bacteriophage and its efficiency seemed to be improved as the silica-AgNPs amount was increased [95].

This simple method of nanoparticles coating obviously increases the efficacy of masks, but care must be done regarding their leakage when applied practically.

6.8.3 USE OF COPPER OXIDE

As copper oxide has the ability of possessing the anti-bacterial and anti-viral activities so it was impregnated on a respiratory mask to provide safety from the droplets containing the virus. The efficacy determined with both copper oxide and control surgical masks was the same for human influenza A-virus and avian influenza-virus also known as H1N1 and H9N2, respectively. The modifications in the mask displayed zero viral retention for H1N1 and 5 times lesser than control face-masks for avian influenza virus (AIV).

6.8.4 USE OF GRAPHENE OXIDE

When research was conducted on *E. coli* using graphene oxide, it showed excellent antimicrobial properties due to higher defect density and mechanisms associated with small sized sheets [96, 97]. A combination of graphene oxide and silver was found to be effective against infectious Bursal disease virus and Feline coronavirus. Actually, the lipid membrane of the virus gets damaged when it is attracted by graphene oxide. It was considered that synergism produced due to silver and graphene oxide sheets was responsible for the excellent activity of composite [98].

A novel system comprising polyethylene-based nanofiber with modifications like thermal stability, self-ability to sanitize and re-usability was developed. System for thermal stability basically increases or decreases the dissipation of heat according to environmental requirements. Getting a silver layer into it, avoids the loss of heat when temperature is low. Due to high dispersal of heat from the human body, the material also exhibited an excellent cooling effect [99].

6.8.5 USE OF CLOTH MASKS

Respirators and surgical masks are demandingly high in this pandemic, but due to their shortage, people mostly rely on cloth masks in countries of less economy. Therefore, it is necessary to determine the efficacy of fabrics against viral infections [100, 101]. A research was carried out to evaluate the filtration ability of chiffon, cotton, silk, and other combinations [102]. Their efficiency was determined via sodium chloride containing aerosols. The idea of comfort and breathing ability was taken by differential pressure. Silk, cotton, and chiffon masks were found to be over 50% efficient depending on more number of threads/inch and tight weavings. As the cloth masks remain loose around the both sides, so this is also the reason for their lower efficiency in filtering the airborne particles.

In short, the modification on the filtering materials enhances their capability to capture the virus and other pathogens, there is still a lot more to explore regarding their efficiency, thermal management, and reusability.

6.8.6 HAND SANITIZERS (AS HAND WASH)

The use of hand wash and hand rub which is alcohol-based hand sanitizer is equally functional. If we talk about the efficiency of hand wash, we came to know that washing hands with soap effectively kills all disease-causing microorganisms. On the other hand, the functionality of hand rub is not only effective against disease causing germs but also appropriate and abrade less [103]. Besides the versatility of hand rubs, CDC recommend to wash hands with soap when hands are stained and oily because the functionality of hand rubs is reduced due to less perforation power to remove the stain and dirt but also kill germs. Washing hands with soap and water results in sound cleansing and increased possible latency to remove germs. Pathogens including *Cryptosporidium*, nor virus, and *Clostridium difficile* can only be killed by washing hands with soap/hand wash as hand rubs are not as effective as hand wash as they contain adequate amount of detergent which is helpful in thorough cleansing to remove dirt and kill germs. Considering the usefulness of hand wash it is not convenient to wash hands every time when they came in contact with different surfaces and with other individuals, especially at work, bus station and public places. It is impossible to arrange a set up at these places, so hand sanitizers are helpful to minimize the risk of disease-causing viruses and bacteria [104, 105]. The effectiveness of hand sanitizers can be enhanced when used accurately and choosing the correct vessel which distribute the correct amount every time [105]. But when hands are clearly muddy or stained, it is recommended to wash them properly using hand wash/soap [106–108].

6.8.7 SOAP/SANITIZERS

Different hand sanitizers containing different ingredients could be compared to analyze their efficacy. Preferable use of soap for washing hands than sanitizers is instructed by CDCP [109]. It is preferred by keeping in mind all the factors including disinfection activity, penetration in soiled and oily hands. A systematic way was adopted in a review article to conclude the debate about the use of soap and sanitizer and which is preferred for food preparation, disinfectant activity, and hand hygiene [110]. However, there is a need to compare inactivation efficiency against enveloped viruses by soap and sanitizer. For this purpose, three different suspensions of alcohol-based hand sanitizers and soaps was used against enveloped viruses and results of suspension test showed 99.99% or 4 log 10 reduction in number of viruses [111]. Direct comparisons have limited number of evidence, but many studies showed the effectiveness of hand sanitizer over soap against enveloped viruses [112, 113]. Human norovirus GI and MNV1 was effectively treated by washing hands with soap/water with 5 log 10 efficacy, but hand sanitizer is not found as effective to inactivate the same viruses as shown by finger pad testing [114]. The activity of alcohol-based hand sanitizers is considerable in treating bacteria, but efficacy in opposition to viruses without envelop is lower. Effectiveness of alcohol-based sanitizers lack firm evidences against norovirus inactivation [115, 116]. It is reported by scientific study that 80% of individuals hold some toxic bacteria after handwashing [117]. Frequent hand washing removes fatty acids of the body and result in damaged skin that allow pathogens to enter in the body [118].

Hand wash possesses limited application, so hand sanitizers are modified by the addition of emollient to overcome skin irritation and to be more effective for disinfectant activity [119].

6.8.8 EFFICACY OF SANITIZERS AGAINST

6.8.8.1 BACTERIA AND FUNGI

Generally, bacterial infections are classified in two classes' transient floras or temporary microorganism and resident flora or permanent microorganism. As their name refers transient floras, including *E. coli* and *S. aureus* found at the outer layer of the skin and can be removed using hand wash or hand sanitizer. They are mostly developed from hospitals, one received by a patient during a hospital visit. Resident floras or permanent floras attached deeply to the skin and are difficult to remove, such as *Staphylococcus aureus*, *Staphylococcus epidermidis*, and *Enterococcus faecalis* [120]. Bacteria can also be passed on from person to person in many other ways and cause infections.

Alcohol based hand sanitizers proved productive against disease causing Microorganisms. The CDC proved disinfectant activity of sanitizers having alcohol is very effective *in vitro*. It is not only productive against antimicrobial activity but can also kill them like; *Enterococcus* [109]. Effectiveness of these sanitizers depends on Ethanol amount used. The amount of ethanol ranges between 60–80% and Washing/rubbing time of 15–30 seconds produced satisfactory results against bacteria and fungi [121]. By contaminated hands disinfectant activity has also been studied *in vivo* [122, 123]. Kirby-Bauer method was used to examine the disinfectant activity of different gram positive and negative bacteria by different formulations of alcohol-based hand sanitizers [124]. In this method infused disc of antibiotic used to check vulnerability of genetic variant of microorganisms. To stop the bacterial growth or increase the disinfectant activity, Propanol containing alcoholic sanitizers is more efficient as compared to ethanol-based sanitizers. A national push of excessive sanitizers application has increased the permissiveness of bacteria. Tolerance of Current bacteria against lower concentrations of alcoholic sanitizers, studied *in vitro* reveal that they are more resistant than their antecedent [125]. With the passage of time, current pathogens becomes more resistant not only to the lower concentrations [126] of alcohols but for benzalkonium chlorides as well [127, 128]. The risk of adaptation of microorganisms against any change in environment cannot be ignored. Microbes are up lifted to adapt against change in the environment by increasing their tolerance level. Few strains of bacteria have evolved resistant against 0.1 to 0.4% concentration of benzalkonium chloride since 1960 [129, 130]. The efficiency of disinfectant activity will be reduced day by day for both alcohol and benzalkonium chloride containing sanitizers. It is the time to look for the mechanism of tolerance of pathogens. Hand hygiene protocols must need to be adopted, including required concentrations of disinfecting agent in sanitizers, as well as proper handwashing methods that include contact time of sanitizer with hands and their frequent use.

6.8.8.2 VIRUSES

Study of viruses in living organisms is relatively hard to do as compared to Bacteria. The study of effectiveness of hand sanitizers have tried to Authenticate countlessly. Sanitizers with alcohol proved to be efficient for the viruses causing zika virus, diarrhea, hepatitis C virus (HCV), murine-virus, and coronavirus [113, 131]. The quantitative Effectiveness of alcoholic hand sanitizers is shown by Carrier test for disinfectants. And result is found satisfactory in case of viruses with envelop like H1N1 and enteric virus but found ineffective against viruses without envelop excluding rotavirus [114].

Efficiency of hand sanitizers is studied many times by washing hands after finger pad test and efficiency against disinfectant studied [132]. The number of viral particles left at the hands surface was reduced. The viral finger pad test found really effective in studying the working of disinfectants against non-enveloped viruses. Non-enveloped viruses are considered to be having higher resistance to disinfectants as compared to viruses with envelop [133, 134]. The number of non-enveloped viruses has also been adequately reduced using disinfectants. Alcohol containing Hand sanitizers activity against viruses (without envelop) can be enhanced by increasing the concentration of ethanol. Hepatitis A, enteroviruses, and rotavirus required HIGH concentration of ethanol 60–80%, which is sufficient to reduce the masses of clinically relevant viruses within a contact time of 10 seconds. Satisfactory results can be obtained by increasing the contact time or concentration of alcohol [135, 136].

The efficacy of hand sanitizers against rapidly emerging COVID-19 was attempted to relate with previously known data of coronavirus. The organized review has showed statistically notable consequence on severe acute respiratory syndrome 2002–2004 suggested that washing hands properly or using sanitizers reduced the disease transmission from hospitals and by social interaction [137]. Studies regarding the efficiency of disease reduction via washing hands with soap and sanitizers are diversified. Virus inactivation inside the living body cannot be tested after using hand sanitizers. However, the effectiveness of hand sanitizers *in vitro* can be tested systematically which showed effectiveness by reduction in numbers. Different alcohol-based formulation was tested on Sputum culture of coronavirus affected patients [138]. All the formulation was effective to inactivate the masses of viruses to such a range that is below our detection limit. Infected person can spread coronavirus up to 10 days through nonliving surfaces, sneezing, coughing, direct contact with contaminated hands. An important thing that is considered is the transmission source as well as efficacy of disinfectant for different transmitted sources [139]. Alcohol-based hand sanitizers are widely used worldwide and recommended to use against severe acute respiratory syndrome as well as against middle east respiratory syndrome (MERS) related coronavirus [140].

Less reliable method of Data collection through past events or situations which is deficient in standardization, come to light disinfection and handwashing method. In hospitals, there is a large number of variables that affect dependent variables, including frequency, magnitude of contact with infectious person and using precautions as independently sanitizers efficacy cannot be calculated. An effective Hand disinfection system using an antimicrobial agent prevent infection rate.

6.8.9 FORMULATIONS OF SANITIZERS

Health protection disinfectant products containing active decontaminate and inactive medium are recently used. These are mostly alcohol containing products with some other products which complete the formulation by providing it consistency, enhance product thickness, pH maintaining agents, preventatives, aroma, and coloring agents [141]. Different methods are used for formulations in which concentrations of ingredients could be taken in w/w, v/v reported in literature. Different methods are used for preparation depending upon ingredients and quality of the product.

6.8.10 TYPES OF HAND-SANITIZERS

Hand sanitizers are classified into two categories depending upon the active ingredient used. Following are the two types:

- Non-Alcohol based sanitizers (other than alcohol as active ingredient); and
- Alcohol-containing hand sanitizers (alcohol as the active ingredient).

6.8.10.1 NON-ALCOHOL BASED SANITIZERS (OTHER THAN ALCOHOL AS ACTIVE INGREDIENT)

Alcohol-based hand sanitizers causes skin dryness when used excessively and considered less convenient as causes adverse effects on skin. Other than active ingredients, excipients are added that work as moisturizers or skin hydrants which not only work to protect skin but also increase drying time that ultimately enhances bactericidal activity. Although they are also considered cost-effective but their adverse effects on skin cannot be neglected. They are also considered unstable as they can catch fire. The active ingredients include in Alcohol-based sanitizers are ethanol, n-propanol, and iso-propyl alcohol [92]. And alcohols desirable concentration must be between 60% to 95% by volume for effective bactericidal activity. Excipients include moisturizing agents that prevent dehydration of skin [142] and thickening agents that gave them a semisolid finish or a firm look.

The active ingredient of non-alcoholic sanitizers is quaternary ammonium and benzalkonium chloride [143]. They are thought to be consumer-friendly as they are alcohol free [143]. While using non-alcohol-based sanitizers, one must not be anxious as they are inflammable [143] and harmless when come in contact with the skin.

1. **Emollients:** The excessive use of Alcohol containing Hand rubs results in lack of skin moisture. Use of emollient found effective in reducing skin dryness [144–146]. To reduce skin dryness, Glycerin is used preferably as a moisturizing ingredient in hand sanitizers. Although use of glycerin in hand rubs moisturize the skin [147] but reduces surface pH and enhance the content of oily secretions which produced from sebum glands as a result of perspiration. The other deleterious effects of using a higher concentration of glycerin in hand rubs include reduced effectiveness to prevent the microbe's growth and delayed drying time by producing adhesive impact [147, 148]. By keeping the concentration of glycerin less than 1% worked effectively well with hand sanitizers to prevent germs growth [149, 150] and protect skin by keeping it moisturized. Use of glycerin in hand rubs more than 1% make it less effective against pathogens [151], and frequent use of hand sanitizers without emollients causes dryness of skin. Emollient other than glycerin which were found effective [150, 151] to work with isopropanol-based hand rubs one can use Ethyl hexyl glycerin, Dexpanthenol, and Fatty alcohols. These humectants are not only functional with hand sanitizers and cosmetics to stop bactericidal activity but are also available in cheaper rates as compared to glycerin such as propylene glycol [152, 153].

   Natural humectants have been used to avoid deleterious effects that reduce the efficiency of hand sanitizers. Aloe Vera has found vast applications in pharmaceutical. It also found to work well as a skin hydrator in cosmetics for long and used along with glycerin and propylene glycol as a natural moisturizer in sanitizers. Aloe Vera gel not only balance drying effects causes by alcohol-based sanitizers but also give sanitizers thickness or a solidified texture [154] when used in excess. Natural products incorporation as moisturizers attracts consumer's attention [155, 156] as use of natural emollients in sanitizers may account for better marketing tactics.

2. **Viscosity Enhancers:** Two local preparation methods for hand-sanitizers containing alcohol have been proposed by WHO when commercially not accessible [156]. They contain ingredients that are runny or contain very little friction and lost or run out quickly while washing. These formulations do not match standard formulations and found ineffective against antimicrobial activity. Gel based formulations are preferred over liquid based formulations as they are more manageable due to their viscosity and easy to distribute the same amount every time [157, 158]. The rate of evaporation of alcohols also reduced when they brought in the form of gels that enhances their contact time and ultimately their effectiveness. Thickening agents can also be used as excipients that helps them to form gels. A variety of thickening agents are easily accessible depending upon the need. Authentic sources such as Federfarma provided by SIFAP pin down the need to search by providing the list of some specific viscosity enhancer for coronavirus. Some of these are discussed below in detail [106, 159].
3. **Carbomer:** Carboxy Poly Methylene is a synthetic polymer of cross-linked poly-acrylic acid. For the pharmaceutical and cosmetic industry, Semisolid gels, oral or liquid products of desired consistencies can be made using a variety of carbomers. Their high molecular weight (MW) increases their viscosity. These are productive agents to increase particle suspension and prevent break down of emulsion using a small concentration of 0.1 to 3%. Different types of carbomers obtained by varying densities, cross-linking property, linking type and solvent type used while polymerization. Its classification can be made depending upon cross-linking type and density that made them low, medium, and high polymers that provide different viscosities in aqueous-alcoholic solutions. Their categories include carbomer homopolymer, carbomer copolymer and carbomer interpolymers. Traditional carbomers cannot be used for pharmaceutical applications as they are prepared in poisonous solvent benzene. For pharmaceutical purposes carbomers of mere ethyl acetate or its combined form and cyclohexane (C_6H_{12}) are used. In order to clear the selection of copolymers, suffix [106] are given to carbomers which are representing numbers such as 910, 934, 940, 941. These suffix or representing numbers indicate MW and constituent of polymers. Carbomers regularity of distribution

decreases if the pH range exceed from 6.5 to 7.5, which is appropriate for neutralization. Neutralizing agents includes a number of substances which are chosen carefully to prevent the precipitation, such as NaOH, NH_4OH, tetra hydroxyl propyl ethylene diamine, triethanolamine, tromethamine, PEG-15 cocamine, di isopropanol amine and tri-isopropanol amine. Carbomers obtained regularity, consistency, and adequate dispersion when thickeners are added. In the hydroalcoholic mixture containing 20% ethanol and triethanol amine-containing 50–60% ethanol, a small amount of NaOH and KOH are suggested to use. The neutralizers recommended to be used when the percentage of ethanol in hand sanitizers ranges between 60–95%, are tetra hydroxyl propyl ethylene diamine, aminomethyl propanol and tri-isopropanol amine (up to 80–90% of ethanol) [160]. Viscosities of carbomers are more in comparison to cellulose derivatives, with the requirement of five to nine pH. When 0.5% carbomers solution (weight by weight) at a neutralization point of 7.5 pH was made. It shows viscosities of 4,000–11,000, 29,400–39,400 and 40,000–60,000 mPa•s with a numeric code of 971P, 974P and 980, respectively. These standards are used for topical products such as creams, lotions, moisturizers, and gels [106]. Ethanol affects the regularity of hydrogels, a comparison must need to be made on consistencies of hydrogels prepared in alcohol and pure water. A study made on the comparison of consistency of sanitizers made in aqueous medium of 0.1–5% w/w solution and in alcoholic medium 15–30% w/v solution, showed that gels consistency decreases in ethanol [161]. That decrease was found to be more when a solution of 0.1–0.5% w/w concentration [162] with an acidic pH of 4. A guideline was also provided to make hydro alcoholic gels by constructors. Some recommended to use Ultrez™ because of smooth preparation and more clarity [106, 161] while others recommended 72% w/w concentration [106] of ethanol with a gel concentration of 0.35%. From these recommendations and experiences, it is concluded to use carbomers of 0.3–0.6% or 0.5–1% thickness along with neutralizing agents such as aminomethyl propanol for alcoholic sanitizers preparation.

4. **Hydroxy Ethyl Cellulose:** It is synthesized from ethylene oxide and cellulose, in an alkaline medium using NaOH with controlled experimental conditions. A cellulose polyether with partial substitution and non-ionic nature, available with brand name of Natrosol™. Glucose is the structural unit of cellulose-containing three hydroxyl

groups that involve in reaction. When all the three hydroxyl groups of glucose are involved in reaction three will be the degree of substitution (DS) which is not achievable. Hydroxyethyl groups introduced at free ethylene oxide provided the basic conditions which produce the side chain, which vary in number of hydroxyl ethyl groups. The number of ethylene oxide molecules attached with glucose sketches the total number of substitutions. Natrosol ™250 accessible in various thickness ranges with molecular grades known as low (L), medium (M), high (H) and very high thickness (HH).

They have grades/standards for pharmaceutical and cosmetics denoted by pharm and CS, respectively [106, 163]. Although, all other cellulose derivatives are soluble in inorganic solvent but hydroxyl ethyl cellulose is insoluble in inorganic solvents but soluble in hot and cold water. Low or medium grades of MW easily dissolved in glycerol and hydroalcoholic media with 60% ethanol [106] also dispersible in hydroxyl ethyl cellulose. The constructors denoted that water and ethanol with 70:30 ratio dispersible in hydroxyl ethyl cellulose at 25°C. If the ratio of water and ethanol changed into a new ratio of 40:60 hydroxyethyl cellulose becomes sparingly soluble at 60°C [106]. Mostly used viscosity enhancer is Natrosol 250 which is lyophilic colloid (completely dissolve in solvent) and keep lyophobic colloids to precipitate, viscosity modifier, prevent breakdown of emulsion and promote dispersion.

Viscosity of hydroxyethyl cellulose in aqueous medium increases with the increase in MW. Lower-grade MW polymers carry viscosity of 20 mPa.s and viscosities of very higher MW is up to 100,000 mPa•s. The manufacturer has not given any idea about the thickness of hydroxyethyl cellulose when dissolved in hydroalcoholic mixtures [163]. The resistance for dispersion of 3% hydroxyethyl cellulose in water and alcoholic mixture containing 60% ethanol was measured using elastic modulus. Elastic modulus showed G' 354 Pa in water. Maximum dispersion rate observed with 30% concentration of ethyl alcohol (ethanol) and start decreasing with increasing the concentration of ethanol from 30% to 40% and so on. Thickness decreases by increasing the concentration of ethanol, when 60% ethanol added viscosity decreases to 229 Pa due to lack of hydration [163]. Hydroxyethyl cellulose with high MW used for hand sanitizers' preparation with 50–60% ethanol. Gel formulation of hydroxyethyl cellulose-containing more than 60% ethanol are not suggested because they form cloudy solution and are not properly dispersed. More concentration of ethanol, i.e., 60–95% effective against disinfectant activity so hydroxy methylcellulose does not work well as thickener with alcohol-based sanitizers.

5. **Hydroxy Propyl Cellulose:** It is water dispersible, non-ionic, and ether derivative of cellulose that gives thickness in aqueous solution. Hydroxypropyl cellulose is commercially available with brand name Klucel™ by Ash land manufacturers. It is manufactured by derivatives of cellulose in an alkaline medium with propylene oxide at high temperature and pressure. An ether linkage is constructed between propylene and one or more –OH groups of glucose. DS can be three but not more than three, when secondary hydroxyl group reacts with propylene oxide in the side chain [106]. Hydroxyl propyl cellulose is dispersible in a wide range of solvents, including water, alcohols, polar organic solvents, polyethylene glycol, and propylene glycol. Their standards are available for food, pharmaceutical applications and cosmetics with grades F, F Pham, and CS, respectively.

   Hydroxypropyl cellulose is also distinguishable into different grades (E, H, L, EL, J, G, and M) depending on MW [164]. Hydroxyl propyl cellulose with 2% weight used to enhance viscosity rages from 10 to 10,000 mPa.s. In pure water thickness increases by increasing the concentration of hydroxyl propyl cellulose. Maximum thickness of 10,000 can be achieved by using w/w concentration range of 0.5–5%.

   Intermediate MW grades denoted by (J, L) used in 8–10% w/w concentration to achieve maximum thickness of 10,000 mPa.s. Low MW grades denoted by (E, EL) used when maximum viscosity of 100–1,000 mPa.s required. The manufacturer has not provided any knowledge about the impact of ethanol (C_2H_5OH) on thickness of hydroxypropyl cellulose. Clear solutions of hydroxyl propyl cellulose with ethanol can be made using 100% ethanol concentration, with low MW standards. Gel prepared in 100% water is more viscous than gel prepared in 100% ethanol concentration. But the viscosity difference is very slight. The decrease in viscosity is more noticeable when 100% ethanol is used with high and intermediate concentration grades than with low MW concentration standards. Hydroxyl propyl cellulose for intermediate MW polymers, when used in gel manufacturing is more viscous in hydroalcoholic system than with 100% water or any other pure solvent. Pure water and ethanol have viscosity of 270 and 210 mPa.s, respectively which is lower than the viscosity of (30: 70) ratio of ethanol and water when 2% hydroxypropyl cellulose gel added, 500 mPa.s viscosity observed. Same comparison was made with different combination ratio of water and ethanol, i.e., 50: 50 reported in literature [165] which shows same tendency of higher viscosities with hydroalcoholic systems than for pure solvents. The manufacturer reported when a hydro alcoholic gel with 72% w/w ethanol concentration used along with higher grade of 1.1% hydroxypropyl cellulose shows interesting viscosity that is interchangeable with commercially available alcohol-based hand rubs. Therefore, hydro alcohols with 1–1.5% hydroxypropyl cellulose are recommended for hand rubs preparation.

6. **Hydroxy-Propyl Methyl Cellulose:** This cellulose is a derivative used in pharmaceutical, cosmetic, food, and paints. Its main structure is made up of cellulose with methyl and hydroxypropyl substitutions. It is produced on commercial scales which vary in substituents (hydroxyl propyl, methyl) percentage and MW. According to Colorcon 4 numbers code is used to represent the abundance of substituting species. Such as a code 2910 of E type used according to colorcon, for the indication of 28–30% methoxy substitution and 7–12% hydroxyl propyl substitutions. For another 4-digit code 2208 or K type represents abundance of methoxy substitution 19–24% and abundance of hydroxypropyl substitution 7–12% [166, 167]. A code 2906 also known as F type carries 27% to 30% methoxy substitution and hydroxyl propyl substitution with 4% to 7%. Numeric codes followed by viscosities of 2% aqueous solution. As an example, Hypromellose with numeric code 22084 carries methoxy 19–24% abundance and hydroxyl propyl 7–12% abundance, with thickness of 4 mPa.s at 2% in aqueous medium. Hydroxypropyl methyl cellulose work well with aqueous solutions, as a large number of cases found in literature. Manufacturers used different kinds of mutually soluble solvents that work in a more efficient way; it is not recommended for non-aqueous solvents. Elastic response of 5% hydroxy methyl propyl cellulose in water-ethanol medium with 20:80% reported in literature. A bell-shaped curve is obtained for hydroxypropyl methyl cellulose for hydroalcoholic solution with a maximum value at approximately 50% ethanol concentration. When the concentration of ethanol was increased up to 80%, the viscosity of solution decreases as it is in pure water [168]. A similar observation was reported in literature when a 40% ethanol concentration in gel formulation used against

2% hydroxypropyl methyl cellulose with 2208 M numeric code [169]. The consistency of a numeric code of hydroxypropyl methyl cellulose 22084 M in combination with 10–40% hydroalcoholic mixture [169] shows appreciable resemblance with commercially available hand rubs. Another commercially available product "Biotè scudo gel" showed amazing resemblance in thickness when 1.5% hydroxypropyl methyl cellulose numeric code 2208 was made in 72% w/w alcohol. Hydroxypropyl methyl cellulose with 10 M 1.5% or 4M with 2–2.5% abundance recommended for alcohol-based hand rubs preparation which shows viscosity resemblance with commercially available product.

7. **Sodium Carboxy Methyl Cellulose:** It is lyophilic colloid (completely dissolve in solvent) and keep lyophobic colloids to precipitate, viscosity modifier, prevent breakdown of emulsion, film-forming agent and promote dispersion. Carboxymethyl cellulose made up of cellulose and sodium mono chloroacetate in alkaline medium created using NaOH in controlled conditions [82] which are not interrupted by any independent factor. It is commercially accessible with a brand name of Aqualon™ and Blanose™ carboxy methylcellulose. Their trade name depends upon the type of manufacturing and manufacturer, e.g., Tylose CB and Walocel C. Different derivatives of cellulose possess different physical properties as change in MW effect physical properties by changing viscosity. Carboxymethyl cellulose showed different DS such as 7, 9, and 12 for DS of 0.7, 0.9 and 1.2. They showed MW ranges between low, medium, and high. They have grades according to Japan, United States and European (EU) pharmacopeia for foods, cosmetics, and pharmaceutical compliance denoted by letters F, CS, PH, respectively [83]. Carboxy methylcellulose is easily dissolved in water at all temperatures and results in clear solutions when dispersed in 1–6%. They showed viscosity range of 10 to 10,000 mPa.s. They are not dissolved in organic solvents, including higher concentrations of ethanol. By reducing the concentration of ethanol to 40% and by using a combination of water and ethanol, carboxy methylcellulose can be made dispersible but form unclear solutions. Carboxy methylcellulose with low MW and low viscosity work in a better way as compared to carboxy methylcellulose with high viscosity grades that result in poor dispersion and opaque system. The information about the effect of ethanol concentration on dispersion is unclear as not provided by the manufacturer [170]. A comparison of viscosity

of 10% carboxymethyl cellulose in pure water and hydro alcohols available in literature. Formulation in pure water results in excellent viscosity of 432 Pa, decrease to 1186 Pa when hydro alcohols used with 30% ethanol concentration which further dropped down to 671 pa at 40% ethanol concentration and poor dispersion of carboxy methylcellulose. According to previous experimental knowledge, it is concluded that carboxy methylcellulose work well with 50% ethanol concentration in combination with water to form alcohol-based gels. More than 50% concentration of ethanol when work with carboxy methylcellulose results in precipitation and made system unclear. It is not preferable to use carboxy methylcellulose with alcohol-based hand rubs when ethanol concentration is as more as 60%.

6.8.10.2 ALCOHOLIC HAND SANITIZER

6.8.10.2.1 Mechanism of Action of Alcoholic Hand Sanitizers

Mostly used alcohol-based compound is n-propanol for antibacterial activity [106]. Mechanism accurately involved in this is not properly understood but involves membrane lysis or disconnect mRNA, stop protein synthesis by effecting ribosomes and RNA polymerase [171], and related to protein transformation [106]. For maximum bactericidal activity 60–90% concentration of alcohol is needed [172]. Or more precisely pure alcohol or with less than 1% water but its disinfection activity is lower than the previously mentioned range [172]. The presence of water is critical as it affects proteins denaturation process. Alcohols based chemical reaction taking place in living body affects all the process involve in bacterial membrane lysis that leads to loss of cell membrane. Alcohols based product is effective only against propagating bacteria or bacteria involved in binary fission. It is ineffective against bacterial spores [173].

6.8.10.2.2 Efficacy Against COVID

The genetic material of coronavirus showed resemblance with SARS Coronavirus that is why named SARS-CoV-2 [174, 175]. The beta coronavirus possesses the same genome which is enveloped single-stranded RNA [176, 177]. Inactivation of mentioned viruses can happen by using solvents containing lipid-like 75% ether, ethyl alcohol, chloroform, and disinfectants with chlorine [177]. Ethyl alcohol with 60–80% concentration is a very efficient chemical disinfectant against all lipophilic viruses including influenza, vaccinia, and herpes virus and against numerous lipophilic viruses including entero-virus, adenovirus, rhino-virus, and rotaviruses but unproductive against polio-virus and hepatitis A virus [178]. The World Health Organization (WHO) proposed a disinfectant category list for hand rubs with 80% and 75% concentration (volume/volume) of ethyl alcohol and isopropyl alcohol, respectively [179]. Comparison of different solvents concentration showed that ethanol with 60–85% is most efficient as compared to isopropanol and n-propanol with 60–80% [180]. WHO proved alcohol-based products most strongly deactivating against prominent viruses such as EBOV, ZIKV, SARS-CoV, etc. [113]. A more evidence found as per literature proved; ethyl alcohol with as much as 42.6% (w/w) concentration was found effective against SARS coronavirus and MERS coronavirus within half minute time [112]. The disinfectant activity of Alcohol-based hand sanitizers using different concentrations were found in literature.

6.8.10.2.3 Synthetic Methods for Alcohol-Based Sanitizers

The following methods can be used for the synthesis of alcoholic sanitizers:

1. **Direct Addition Method:** This method is considered as the simplest method as all the components are dissolved at once in universal solvent water or alcoholic mixture. When they are soluble completely thickening agents are added gradually in the whirl of strongly disconcerted alcoholic solution with continuous Magnetic or Mechanical stirring. Neutralizing agents are needed along with carbomers which are used as thickeners. Buffers are used for this purpose, and their pH is monitored using pH meters/indicators. At first, thickeners are treated in a way they become homogeneously dispersed in the solution, neutralizing agents are added gradually at regular intervals and pH monitored during the complete process. For thick solutions pH Electrodes are preferably used. This method is preferred for gel Preparation. Gels are prepared using surface processing grades of carbomers that fastens the process. Carbomer thickeners such as Carbopol, Ultrez grades, Natrosol R-grades for hydroxypropyl cellulose are modified for surface treatment and fastly dispersed due to less irregularity. The pH-dependent viscosity of carbomers made their dispersion rate fasten and regularity. This method is also

advantageous as during the process, it is found in a liquid state that made their rate of solvent evaporation and polymer hydration very quick. This system remained throughout in liquid state and converted into gel as neutralization point reached. Cellulose gels like Hydroxymethyl/propyl are difficult to handle using the direct addition method due to aptness of aggregates formation. Overall, this method is very quick, economical and well organized when attached with a proficient stirring system.

2. **Reverse Addition Method:** An organic solvent which is Unmixable with water was required in this technique to pre-soak the thickeners. Glycerol and propylene glycerol could be the best choice as miscible organic solvent for wetting purposes when used in 1:1 to 1:4 ratios of polymer and thickener, respectively. For pre-wetting purpose, mortar, and pestle is used to mix solvents with polymer. After mixing it is brought in the form of uniform sludge. On the other hand, hydroalcoholic solution with all other constituents separately made and slowly added with continuous stimulating using pestle. Carbomers are added in the same manner as in direct addition method. Carbomers addition required to maintain pH by adding neutralizing agents and measured using pH meters or pH strips. This method is suggested to use at small scale or for spontaneous mixing, as magnetic or mechanical stirrers are not used in this method. This technique is preferably suited in pharmaceutical applications when limited amount is needed.
3. **Other Methods:** Hydroxypropyl cellulose and hydroxypropyl methylcellulose gels are strenuous to make as they readily form lumps. Mostly used technique to overcome such trouble without reducing the speed of reaction can be done by using hot/cold technique. This technique is not preferred for alcohol-based gels due to possible loss of ethanol by evaporation during the formation. Roberts et al. modified this technique so it can be used for ethanol gel. The procedure is modified in way volatile components are cooled and added with continuous stirring. The following amount of solvents are added 40% ethanol, 2% hydroxypropyl methyl cellulose gel and 4 molar hydro alcoholic gels. Although, this technique can be used as an alternative but increasing the concentration of ethanol made this technique ineffective for alcoholic gels. A new technique is used which is a combination of both direct and reverse addition method. This hybrid method is similar to the direct addition method in a way continuous stirring with gradual addition of all the components

employed and shows resemblance with reverse addition method as wet slurry is used.

6.8.10.2.4 Adverse Effects

1. **Human Health:** Hand sanitizers are poisonous that can cause death if taken in the body accidentally [181] through skin contact [182] and self-poisoning [183].

   i. **Ethanol Toxicity:** Ethanol is used worldwide extensively as an efficient disinfectant as well as depleted as liquid refreshment. Its rate of causing skin cancer and its level of toxicity by accidental ingestion through skin is not found in literature [184]. Ethanol based hand sanitizers when came in contact with skin spread minimum toxicity [185]. Ethanol tolerance level is different for different people this made it complicated to measure the exact amount that fall in the extent of toxicity. Alcohol based hand rubs with 74.1% ethanol concentration applied for 10 min revealed 1 to 1.5 mg per liter serum-ethanol concentration used in hand rubs as detection limit is 0.5 mg per liter of ethanol is negligible [186]. A study was conducted with a group of 12 members as reported in literature; they are directed to use hand rubs containing different w/w ethanol concentrations [187]. After every 20 minutes, a quantity of 4 ml was used for 30 seconds, maximum absorptions was obtained to be 20.95 mg/l, 11.45 mg/l and 6.9 mg/l for 95, 85 and 55% concentrations of ethanol, respectively. The maximum value observed in blood acetaldehyde was observed to be 0.57 mg/l. It is not intensely toxic but performance is affected when concentration reaches up to 200–300 mg/l [188]. It is found in literature that the actual values of intensity of toxicity is less than the calculated values. Severe toxicity occurred by repeated application of hand sanitizer [184, 188]. A case is reported in literature where 33% skin was badly affected by the 70% v/v concentration of ethanol [189]. Blood containing 0.046 g concentration of ethanol per 100 ml of blood is considered to be as similar as absorption of 30% surgical spirit. Immature skin is more sensitive when exposed to ethanol cause systematic contamination. Previously a study [190, 191] was made on 30 children under 33 months of age, showed toxicity of ethanol that effected skin through absorption. Many cases of premature babies were studied with state of intoxication, increase in alcohol concentration in blood, and skin necrosis where infant's skin is not affected by alcohol [192, 193]. Ethanol based products are prohibited to use on wounded or sensitive skin. Contact of skin with ethanol given rise to skin irritation, allergy, dryness of skin and red spots with itching. Skin irritation caused by ethanol is also reported in German study. A study related to excessive use of hand sanitizer reported an increase in concentration of urinary ethyl glucuronide [194] than observed in normal conditions when alcohol-based products are not in use. In spite of all the studies reported about the toxicity of ethanol, still many instructions are there to use alcohol containing hand rubs [194]. To calculate the amount of absorption of alcohol through skin during hand disinfection; a study was directed, and their results indicated that the concentration of absorption of alcohol through skin is safe for human life. Alcohol cause serious health and severe toxicity issues when orally alcohol-based products [195] was taken accidentally. The concentration of alcohol in blood that is considered to be fatal is ingestion of alcohol-based product containing 360 ml of ethanol. Life-threatening dose of ethanol in blood is 400 ml or more, i.e., almost 80% concentration [196, 197]. Absorption of ethanol was observed to take place in the lower portion of digestive tract starting from stomach 70% followed by duodenum 25%. Ethanol absorbed through skin metabolized into acetaldehyde and then into acetyl CO-A (acetyl coenzyme A). Absorption of ethanol by human body shows symptoms within 60 min by a hospitalized patient. Total number of solute particles per kilogram measured after 16–22 hours of hemodialysis. In severe condition when concentration of ingestion is high it causes central nervous system (CNS) depression, nausea, vomiting, and pain in upper abdominal area. High concentration of ethanol in blood causes respiratory depression leads to loss of respiratory response, change in heat beat due to change in electrical impulses that may lead to failure in blood flow, hypoglycemia that leads to ketoacidosis or hypotension. The concentration of ethanol is more for cardiac arrest, which is 500 or more mg/dl, as compared to respiratory arrest which is 300 mg/dl. Absorption of alcohol through the skin may also cause hypocalcemia, hypophosphatemia, hypomagnesemia, hypokalemia, hepatic disease [198] and water diuresis (reduced secretions of antidiuretic hormones) [199]. This debate can be concluded, excess use of ethanol is dangerous for health. It causes dryness and irritation as well as dermal absorption can lead to serious heart and respiratory diseases when used for several months as used in recent days. Frequent use of hand rubs and hand sanitizers without proper guidelines and preventive measures can be fatal for human health [199, 200].

ii. **Isopropyl Alcohol Toxicity:** The MW of Isopropyl alcohol is higher and considered to be more toxic as compared to Ethanol [198]. Accidental ingestion of Isopropyl alcohol-based product results in toxicity as these products are used for rectum and dermal application. In literature, the toxicity level of isopropyl alcohol is considered to be 160–240 ml [201] or at some places 250 ml was mentioned [202]. Many cases were reported in which dermal applications proved to cause unconsciousness [203–205]. Halloa Enterprises presented material safety data in which level of severe toxicity was mentioned LD50 > 2,000 mg/kg and the range of toxicity through skin absorption LD50 > 2,000 mg/kg and inhalation of isopropyl also becomes toxic up to LC50 > 5 mg/l. About 1 g/l concentration of isopropyl alcohol in blood is also reported as poisonous for health. The level of concentration that may cause death in up to 250 ml [202]. The use of isopropyl alcohol in small amounts is not considered to be fatal as it showed very minor symptoms when a concentration of 50% or 20–30 ml is used [206]. A case study on a group of children under the age of six-yearyears as they are affected by the ingestion of dose of I ounce of isopropanol [207]. The toxic level of Alcohol-based hand sanitizers is containing 70% isopropyl with 0.1–5 ml amount [208]. It is reported that consumption of 240 ml is fatal for adults [209].

Accidentally ingested isopropyl alcohol absorbed in the body within two hours and further processing was completed by liver and stomach to convert it into acetone [183] and its removal from the body. The conversion of isopropyl alcohol into acetone may also cause CNS depression, hypotension, and respiratory illness [209, 210]. Isopropyl alcohol cause irritation in the lining of various cavities including gastrointestinal (GI) tract and inflammation of the lining of stomach [211]. This may lead to hypoglycemia, respiratory depression, raise level of ketone [210] and serum creatinine in the body [211].

Myocardial depression results due to higher concentration and frequent use that may lead to myoglobinuria, rhabdomyolysis, and acute renal failure in severe conditions. Ingestion of 100–200 ml with 70% concentration of isopropyl alcohol solution is lethal which raises plasma concentration level. Isopropyl alcohol ingestion causes hypotension and restlessness as reported in a 43 years old person [185]. The absorption of isopropyl alcohol results in dermal exanthem, irritation, and loss of moisture from the skin.

iii. **Hydrogen Peroxide Toxicity:** The intake of hydrogen per oxide in high concentration can be toxic [212]. The lower concentration of hydrogen per oxide can cause minor health issues [213] as 3% (lower concentration) solution of hydrogen per oxide [214] is not toxic to cause serious health issues. Narrowing or blockage of portal vein which supplies blood to the liver, GI lining inflammation and vomiting. Minor health issue includes bowel dilation is reported by 3% concentrated solution of hydrogen peroxide [213, 215]. The toxic level of hydrogen per oxide may cause tissue injury by interconnecting with catalase, which is found in tissues to prevent tissue by peroxides, and spoil it by converting it into water and oxygen. Amount of oxygen produced may vary by varying the concentration of hydrogen per oxide as 10 ml oxygen is produced at STP by 1 ml of 3% hydrogen peroxide. This may cause enlargement of stomach and blockage of artery and vein by air bubble that could be fatal when this air bubble travels to heart and brain. Higher amount of oxygen in small opening or in central space of organ or tissue such as stomach, the air bubble travels through internal epithelial lining. Gas embolus is observed in many organs due to presence of excess tissue catalase which is available for hydrogen peroxide to decompose into oxygen and water. A case of 670 persons were reported to study the ingestion of 3% hydrogen per oxide. Results disclosed that out of 670 cases, more than 70% cases were of ingestion, including half children cases below six years of age. Most of the individuals showed mild symptoms such as vomiting and nausea, gas emboli rarely found. A child was observed with severe symptoms of duodenal erosion, mucosal irritation, and gastric ulcer that is exposed to 2–4 oz of 3% hydrogen peroxide. A very few cases were observed when ingestion of sanitizers containing 3% of hydrogen per oxide caused death. Air embolism was observed to cause death by ingestion of 8 oz of hydrogen peroxide with 3% concentration. Hydrogen peroxide absorption from skin is not observed to cause severe health issues, just mild irritation of mucous membrane and skin reported [214].

Availability of sanitizers in market in bright and beautiful bottles that have very attractive and sweet smell and found successful in grabbing the attention of children. This is the thing we need to worry about if children ingest these alcohol containing sanitizers due to its appealing smell that could be toxic if more amount is ingested [214]. Young life is more likely to be at risk than adults by alcohol poisoning. The amount of stored glycogen is reduced in children that may cause hypoglycemia and may involve other pharmacokinetic factors that made the children more susceptible to alcohol poisoning. Serious health issues have been reported in children by sanitizers ingestion including alcohol such as coma [181] as per National Poison Data System report (2011–2014). This study was conducted with 70,669 number of children belonging to the age group of (0–5) and (6–12) years of age. Out of 70,669 cases, 92% of children were exposed to alcohol containing sanitizers and left-over percentage with no alcohol hand-sanitizers [181].

In recent pandemic situation from December-2019, precautionary measure has been taken for disinfectant activity to prevent microorganisms to spread. WHO recommended to use hand sanitizers as a protective measure against corona-virus, which led to high usage of alcohol containing products. Excessive usage of alcohol-based products causing alcohol poisoning, 9504 cases reported in American Association of Poison Control Center under 12 years age.

Small amount of alcohol effecting children under 12 years of age by alcohol poisoning causing vomiting and nausea, which may leads to fatal respiratory infections [181].

2. **On Environment:**

   i. **Ethanol:** Extensive use of ethanol in the form of alcohol-based products in home and industries left impair able effects on environment [216]. Water bodies directly affected by ethanol exposure. Ethanol causes different effects on various species [214]. New England Interstate Water Pollution Control assessed the effects of ethanol usage on water quality. The benchmark level calculated for aquatic invertebrates calculated to be 564 mgL^{-1} and 63 mgL^{-1} for Daphnia species, fathead minnow, and rainbow trout. Environmental protection agency of the United States created a Database, ECOTOX (ecotoxicology database), for collecting single chemical toxicity data of aquatic life with additional information other than provided earlier by NEIWPCC. ECOTOX provided us with very little information about above mentioned aquatic invertebrates. It was reported in literature, Daphnia Magna when exposed for 21 days to 0.05% of ethanol, i.e., 5,000 mg/l it had no effect on descendant production of males. Hazardous Substances Data Bank showed accumulation of octanol to water coefficient KOW for 0.49 ethanol in fatty tissues is not likely to be true due to fat metabolism [214]. New England Interstate Water Pollution Control Commission calculated contamination of water with ethanol. A decrease in oxygen level observed 55 mg/l for small stream, 32 mg/l for average River and 13 mg/l for large size river. The chance of exposure of ethanol for terrestrial animals is improbable as it evaporates rapidly in air and quickly degrades in water bodies and soil. Unintentional leakage of ethanol in water bodies is found to be toxic for invertebrates and microorganisms [217]. Environmental protection agency of USA reported the effect of different percentages of ethanol on wildlife. Exposure of different concentration of ethanol is more devastating for aquatic life as compared to terrestrial life. Ethanol containing food is improbable to cause toxic effects due to volatility and highest fatty tissues biodegradation rate.

ii. **Iso Propyl Alcohol:** Groundwater can be contaminated by accidental leakage of isopropanol that gets penetrate in the soil. Isopropanol is unable to exist for long in the atmosphere due to Oxidation reaction by absorption of ultraviolet (UV) light and fast biodegradation prevents its accumulation. Contamination of aquatic environment by exposure of isopropanol may result in oxygen depletion that ultimately affect aquatic life [214]. Water samples are collected from industrial areas to check the [217] amount and toxicity of propanol in drinking water. Quantities in traces are reported in drinking water. Accidental leakages may cause adverse effects on aquatic life, but normal usage has no harmful impacts. Isopropanol is not involved in ozone and photochemical smog formation as other volatile compounds are involved.

iii. **Hydrogen Peroxide:** Agency for toxic substances and disease registry reported hydrogen peroxide as harmless due its reactivity [214]. It does not accumulate in soil and water due to highest rate of biodegradation. Abiotic half-life is not observed by the presence of hydrogen peroxide in soil and water as reported by European risk assessment. Hydrogen per oxide is very reactive hence a short-lived substance with a half-life of 24 hours. Acute toxicity was observed in fish, invertebrates, and algae by a short-term exposure of hydrogen per oxide. The toxicity below an unacceptable effect was observed by a test known as No Observed Effect Concentration for algae was found 0.1 mg/l. Long term data is also available for zebra mussels. The risk of toxicity of hydrogen per oxide was estimated for aquatic life and microorganism. The evaluation was completed successfully on hydrogen per oxide no further testing is required [214].

6.8.11 RECOMMENDATIONS TO MINIMIZE ADVERSE EFFECTS

Hazardous impacts of hand sanitizers can be minimized by taking precautions such as selecting less irritating agents containing products, to avoid dullness of skin moisturizers need to be used after every use of hand sanitizer and changing habits which enhance skin irritation [218–220]. Health care workers are affected more by frequent exposure of hand sanitizers. So, they are recommended to select such products which are not only efficient against disinfectant activity but also safe to use for their skin. The use of alcohol-based products causing skin dryness and irritation may reduce its use and acceptance among consumers [221]. This problem was reduced by using emollients and humectants in alcohol-based hand sanitizers [222]. Nonalcoholic hand rubs such as benzethonium chloride which is water-based antiseptic lotion which not only cut down cutaneous adverse effect but also found more effective against viruses. Nonalcoholic sanitizers are also preferred as they are not flammable as compared to alcoholic sanitizers [223]. Skin issues including irritation, redness, sore, and sometimes blisters after use of alcohol-based sanitizers affected by two factors temperature and humidity. In tropical and humid places, skin moisture retain for a longer time as compared to dry and cold places that effect skin as skin moisture is not retained for longer. Environmental and climate conditions must need to be kept in mind while formulating sanitizers. As dry and cold regions need a varying amount of emollients with alcohol-based sanitizers [223]. An older person and health care workers suffer more by dry skin. It is recommended for such individuals to moisturize their skin using humectants, oils, and fats that protect the skin to efficiently perform the function of the skin barrier [223].

6.8.12 RISK OF OTHER VIRAL DISEASES SPREAD

Frequent use of sanitizers containing alcohol is prescribed by health experts to prevent microbe infections including coronavirus. But exposure of alcohol increased the risk of dermatitis. Excess use of sanitizers containing alcohol against pneumonia virus affected skin badly and made it vulnerable for other viral infections. Hand sanitizers are used in excess all over the world as disinfectant considering the risk of viral infections. Skin dullness and dryness caused by excessive application of alcohol-based sanitizers that affected the function of skin as well as skin barrier by increasing its permeability [214]. Dry skin increased the risk for viral and bacterial infection as it is quite easy for microbes to infect a person with damaged skin [214]. It is reported in literature that frequent exposure to alcoholic sanitizers increases viral infection risk. The outbreak of norovirus risk is also increase by excess use of alcohol-based products as reported in literature [116]. The correlation of alcohol containing sanitizers and norovirus outbreak was studied by arranging 160 care facilities. They were observed to apply hand sanitizers 6 times in comparison to soap/water, and 91 were countered positively, 73 were infected in these cases, and 29 were confirmed for norovirus [115].

6.8.13 EXCESSIVE APPLICATION OF SANITIZERS

In recent situation of pandemic government, scientists, and doctors are active to educate the public about hand hygiene [214]. Sanitizers based on alcohol are excessively applied in the last few decades to prevent microbial infection [224]. Frequent use of alcohol-based sanitizer developed resistance against disinfectants and situation become worst for doctors and health care professionals (HCPs). By mutation microorganisms developed resistant by natural process due to frequent use of disinfectants, hand rubs, and antibiotics. A study on antimicrobial-resistant against disinfectant in *Enterococcus faecium* has been reported in 2018. Enterococcus faecium was isolated from 139 hospitals from 1997 to 2015 and was found 10 times more resistant to alcoholic antimicrobe products after 2010. Escalating the amount of hand sanitizers in Australian hospitals resulted in an increased rate of enterococcal infections. Other infection causing microbes also developed resistance after frequent exposure of sanitizers, as reported in other parts of the world [214]. The resistance of *E. coli* against all types of available sanitizers was found to be 48% and for Pseudomonas aeruginosa 64%. Sunshine hand sanitizer was found ineffective against *Pneumonia aeruginosa* and *Micrococcus leutusbutit* as both of these microbes developed resistance. It is reported that sanitizers including Cool n cool, Insta foam, Safeguard, Fresh up become less effective against all Gram-negative bacteria [225].

6.8.14 HAND HYGIENE RECOMMENDATIONS BY CDC (US)/WHO

With the purpose of reducing viral count on hands, alcohol-based hand rubs and sanitizers are recommended. Washing hands properly or hand hygiene is also very necessary to restrict the transfer of microorganisms including SARS-CoV-2. Five examples are coated for hand hygiene, including contact patients directly with medical devices used for patient care, later on contact with another person's body fluid, contact with objects of patient vicinity and while practicing contamination prevention techniques [226]. The CDC suggested to wash hands with soap to prevent the risk of all microorganisms [105]. In case of unavailability of this, it is recommended to use hand sanitizer with 60% ethanol concentration or 70% isopropyl alcohol concentration for effective disinfectant activity.

Pathogens can be removed from hands by washing hands with soap and using sanitizers but effectiveness of antimicrobial agents (synthetic substance that can kill pathogen) is greater than ordinary soaps and sanitizers [226]. The CDC, WHO, and infection control Ministry of Health Malaysia recommended standard of 7 steps method with 40–60 seconds hand washing duration. Alcoholic sanitizers with 60% concentration of alcohol were found more effective to kill microbes as compared to antimicrobial soaps [164]. Washing hands with soap/water instead of sanitizer is recommended when unclean and greasy because of less penetration power of sanitizers. The approximate duration of 20–30 seconds is recommended for hand rubs using sanitizers.

6.9 CONCLUSION

The spreading risk of COVID-19 virus through aerosol droplets can be limited by using face masks on regular self-basis. For this purpose, hand sanitization is also a preliminary protective measure that is why; it is challenging to maintain its demand according to its current needs. By using alcohol-based hand sanitizers, an individual has the least risk, having greater quality of product and ease to use. On the other hand, the use of poorly formulated products may be inappropriate. To lower the risk factor, there should be counseling of the customer by pharmacists to select the suitable product for the control of the infection. The individuals should not purchase these products online from unknown or unreliable e-commerce sites. There should be seminars and conferences to inform the public about products for general hygiene as well as control of COVID-19 infection. Moreover, there should be visits of the regulatory authorities on a regular basis for better protection of the consumers. Due to high demand of sanitizers for a long time to prevent the infection by COVID-19 pandemic, it is our foremost duty to get the public aware of the importance of hand hygiene throughout the world to use sanitizers not only in this pandemic situation but routinely, thus creating a new norm of self-hygiene.

KEYWORDS

- **COVID-19**
- **facemasks**
- **hand sanitizers**
- **precautionary measures**
- **recommendations**
- **severe acute respiratory syndrome coronavirus 2**

REFERENCES

1. Zheng, Y. Y., et al., (2020). COVID-19 and the cardiovascular system. *Nature Reviews Cardiology, 17*(5), 259, 260.
2. Sohrabi, C., et al., (2020). World Health Organization declares global emergency: A review of the 2019 novel coronavirus (COVID-19). *International Journal of Surgery.*

3. Brainard, J. S., et al., (2020). *Facemasks and Similar Barriers to Prevent Respiratory Illness Such as COVID-19: A Rapid Systematic Review.* medRxiv.
4. Johnston, B. L., & Conly, J. M., (2004). Severe acute respiratory syndrome: What have we learned two years later? *Canadian Journal of Infectious Diseases and Medical Microbiology, 15.*
5. Novel, C. P. E. R. E., (2020). The epidemiological characteristics of an outbreak of 2019 novel coronavirus diseases (COVID-19) in China. *Zhonghua Liu xing bing xue za zhi= Zhonghua Liuxingbingxue Zazhi, 41*(2), 145.
6. Wang, D., et al., (2020). Clinical characteristics of 138 hospitalized patients with 2019 novel coronavirus-infected pneumonia in Wuhan, China. *JAMA, 323*(11), 1061–1069.
7. Prather, K. A., Wang, C. C., & Schooley, R. T., (2020). Reducing transmission of SARS-CoV-2. *Science.*
8. Anderson, E. L., et al., (2020). Consideration of the aerosol transmission for COVID-19 and public health. *Risk Analysis.*
9. Leung, N. H., et al., (2020). Respiratory virus shedding in exhaled breath and efficacy of face masks. *Nature Medicine, 26*(5), 676–680.
10. Zia-Ul-Haq, M., et al., (2021). *Alternative Medicine Interventions for COVID-19.* Springer, Cham: Springer Nature Switzerland AG 2021. XII, 284.
11. Zia-Ul-Haq, M., Dewanjee, S., & Riaz, M., (2021). *Carotenoids: Structure and Function in the Human Body* (Vol. XVI, p. 859). Springer Nature Switzerland AG: Springer International Publishing.
12. Wu, H. L., et al., (2020). Facemask shortage and the novel coronavirus disease (COVID-19) outbreak: Reflections on public health measures. *EClinicalMedicine*, 100329.
13. MacIntyre, C. R., & Chughtai, A. A., (2015). Facemasks for the prevention of infection in healthcare and community settings. *BMJ, 350*, h694.
14. Tunevall, T. G., (1991). Postoperative wound infections and surgical face masks: A controlled study. *World Journal of Surgery, 15*(3), 383–387.
15. Spooner, J. L., (1967). History of surgical face masks. *AORN Journal, 5*(1), 76–80.
16. Rockwood, C. A., & O'donoghue, D. H., (1960). The surgical mask: Its development, usage, and efficiency: A review of the literature, and new experimental studies. *AMA Archives of Surgery, 80*(6), 963–971.
17. Belkin, N. L., (1997). The evolution of the surgical mask: Filtering efficiency versus effectiveness. *Infection Control & Hospital Epidemiology, 18*(1), 49–57.
18. Adams, L. W., et al., (2016). Uncovering the history of operating room attire through photographs. *Anesthesiology, 124*(1), 19–24.
19. Bae, S., et al., (2020). Effectiveness of surgical and cotton masks in blocking SARS–CoV-2: A controlled comparison in 4 patients. *Annals of Internal Medicine.*
20. Dbouk, T., & Drikakis, D., (2020). On respiratory droplets and face masks. *Physics of Fluids, 32*(6), 063303.
21. Derrick, J. L., & Gomersall, C., (2005). Protecting healthcare staff from severe acute respiratory syndrome: Filtration capacity of multiple surgical masks. *Journal of Hospital Infection, 59*(4), 365–368.
22. Smereka, J., et al., (2020). Role of mask/respirator protection against SARS-CoV-2. *Anesthesia and Analgesia.*
23. Bar-On, Y. M., et al., (2020). Science Forum: SARS-CoV-2 (COVID-19) by the numbers. *Elife, 9*, e57309.

24. Kim, M. N., (2020). What type of face mask is appropriate for everyone-mask-wearing policy amidst COVID-19 pandemic? *Journal of Korean Medical Science, 35*(20).
25. Lam, S., et al., (2011). Sensitivity and specificity of the user-seal-check in determining the fit of N95 respirators. *Journal of Hospital Infection, 77*(3), 252–256.
26. Oberg, T., & Brosseau, L. M., (2008). Surgical mask filter and fit performance. *American Journal of Infection Control, 36*(4), 276–282.
27. Marasinghe, K. M., (2020). *Concerns around Public Health Recommendations on Face Mask Use Among Individuals Who are Not Medically Diagnosed with COVID-19 Supported by a Systematic Review Search for Evidence.*
28. Greenhalgh, T., et al., (2020). Face masks for the public during the covid-19 crisis. *BMJ, 369.*
29. Qualls, N., et al., (2017). Community mitigation guidelines to prevent pandemic influenza—United States. *MMWR Recommendations and Reports, 66*(1), 1.
30. Shen, M., et al., (2020). *Modelling the Epidemic Trend of the 2019 Novel Coronavirus Outbreak in China.* BioRxiv, (2020).
31. Wang, W., et al., (2020). Detection of SARS-CoV-2 in different types of clinical specimens. *JAMA, 323*(18), 1843–1844.
32. Huang, P. H., (2020). *Pandemic Emotions: The Good, the Bad, and the Unconscious—Implications for Public Health, Financial Economics, Law, and Leadership* (pp. 14–20). U of Colorado Law Legal Studies Research Paper.
33. Geggel, L., (2020). Can wearing a face mask protect you from the new coronavirus. *Live Science.*
34. Hendrick, C., et al., (2020). *Recruitment of African American Men into a Community-Based Exercise Training Trial: The ARTIIS Study.* SAGE Publications Ltd.
35. Simmerman, J. M., et al., (2011). Findings from a household randomized controlled trial of hand washing and face masks to reduce influenza transmission in Bangkok, Thailand. *INFLUENZA and other Respiratory Viruses, 5*(4), 256–267.
36. Süß, T., et al., (2011). Facemasks and intensified hand hygiene in a German household trial during the 2009/2010 influenza A (H1N1) pandemic: Adherence and tolerability in children and adults. *Epidemiology & Infection, 139*(12), 1895–1901.
37. Al Badri, F. M., (2017). Surgical mask contact dermatitis and epidemiology of contact dermatitis in healthcare workers: Allergies in the workplace. *Current Allergy & Clinical Immunology, 30*(3), 183–188.
38. Donovan, J., et al., (2007). Skin reactions following use of N95 facial masks. *Dermatitis, 18*(2), 104.
39. Saunders-Hastings, P., et al., (2017). Effectiveness of personal protective measures in reducing pandemic influenza transmission: A systematic review and meta-analysis. *Epidemics, 20*, 1–20.
40. Jefferson, T., et al., (2008). Physical interventions to interrupt or reduce the spread of respiratory viruses: Systematic review. *BMJ, 336*(7635), 77–80.
41. Wong, V. W., Cowling, B. J., & Aiello, A. E., (2014). Hand hygiene and risk of influenza virus infections in the community: A systematic review and meta-analysis. *Epidemiology & Infection, 142*(5), 922–932.
42. Bin-Reza, F., et al., (2012). The use of masks and respirators to prevent transmission of influenza: A systematic review of the scientific evidence. *Influenza and Other Respiratory Viruses, 6*(4), 257–267.

43. Barasheed, O., et al., (2016). Uptake and effectiveness of facemask against respiratory infections at mass gatherings: A systematic review. *International Journal of Infectious Diseases, 47*, 105–111.
44. Alfelali, M., et al., (2019). *Facemask Versus no Facemask in Preventing Viral Respiratory Infections During Hajj: A Cluster Randomized Open-Label Trial.* doi.org/10.2139/ssrn.3349234.
45. MacIntyre, C. R., et al., (2009). Face mask use and control of respiratory virus transmission in households. *Emerging Infectious Diseases, 15*(2), 233.
46. MacIntyre, C. R., et al., (2016). Cluster randomized controlled trial to examine medical mask use as source control for people with respiratory illness. *BMJ Open, 6*(12).
47. Cowling, B. J., et al., (2009). Facemasks and hand hygiene to prevent influenza transmission in households: A cluster randomized trial. *Annals of Internal Medicine, 151*(7), 437–446.
48. Wada, K., Oka-Ezoe, K., & Smith, D. R., (2012). Wearing face masks in public during the influenza season may reflect other positive hygiene practices in Japan. *BMC Public Health, 12*(1), 1065.
49. Burgess, A., & Horii, M., (2012). Risk, ritual and health responsibilization: Japan's 'safety blanket' of surgical face mask-wearing. *Sociology of Health & Illness, 34*(8), 1184–1198.
50. MacIntyre, C. R., et al., (2013). A randomized clinical trial of three options for N95 respirators and medical masks in health workers. *American Journal of Respiratory and Critical Care Medicine, 187*(9), 960–966.
51. Sommerstein, R., et al., (2020). Risk of SARS-CoV-2 transmission by aerosols, the rational use of masks, and protection of healthcare workers from COVID-19. *Antimicrobial Resistance & Infection Control, 9*(1), 1–8.
52. Wang, Z., et al., (2020). Transmission and prevention of SARS-CoV-2. *Biochemical Society Transactions, 48*(5), 2307–2316.
53. Bartoszko, J. J., et al., (2020). Medical masks vs N95 respirators for preventing COVID-19 in healthcare workers: A systematic review and meta-analysis of randomized trials. *Influenza and other Respiratory Viruses.*
54. Milton, D. K., et al., (2013). Influenza virus aerosols in human exhaled breath: Particle size, culturability, and effect of surgical masks. *PLoS Pathog., 9*(3), e1003205.
55. Smith, J. D., et al., (2016). Effectiveness of N95 respirators versus surgical masks in protecting health care workers from acute respiratory infection: A systematic review and meta-analysis. *CMAJ, 188*(8), 567–574.
56. Ng, K., et al., (2020). COVID-19 and the risk to health care workers: A case report. *Annals of Internal Medicine.*
57. Chu, D. K., et al., (2020). Physical distancing, face masks, and eye protection to prevent person-to-person transmission of SARS-CoV-2 and COVID-19: A systematic review and meta-analysis. *The Lancet.*
58. Tuite, A. R., Fisman, D. N., & Greer, A. L., (2020). Mathematical modelling of COVID-19 transmission and mitigation strategies in the population of Ontario, Canada. *CMAJ, 192*(19), E497–E505.
59. Griffin, J. T., et al., (2016). Potential for reduction of burden and local elimination of malaria by reducing Plasmodium falciparum malaria transmission: A mathematical modelling study. *The Lancet Infectious Diseases, 16*(4), 465–472.
60. Toda, A. A., (2020). *Susceptible-Infected-Recovered (sir) Dynamics of Covid-19 and Economic Impact.* arXiv preprint arXiv:2003.11221.

61. Bastos, S. B., & Cajueiro, D. O., (2020). *Modeling and Forecasting the Covid-19 Pandemic in Brazil.* arXiv preprint arXiv:2003.14288.
62. Chang, S. L., et al., (2020). *Modeling Transmission and Control of the COVID-19 Pandemic in Australia.* arXiv preprint arXiv:2003.10218.
63. Liu, D., et al., (2020). *A Machine Learning Methodology for Real-Time Forecasting of the 2019-2020 COVID-19 Outbreak Using Internet Searches, News Alerts, and Estimates from Mechanistic Models.* arXiv preprint arXiv:2004.04019.
64. Mejía, S., & Wong, R., (2018). Empirical issues in the study of cognitive aging through population-based studies. *Innovation in Aging, 2*(Suppl 1), 245.
65. Kiesling, E., et al., (2012). Agent-based simulation of innovation diffusion: A review. *Central European Journal of Operations Research, 20*(2), 183–230.
66. Eikenberry, S. E., et al., (2020). To mask or not to mask: Modeling the potential for face mask use by the general public to curtail the COVID-19 pandemic. *Infectious Disease Modeling.*
67. Brienen, N. C., et al., (2010). The effect of mask use on the spread of influenza during a pandemic. *Risk Analysis: An International Journal, 30*(8), 1210–1218.
68. Schimit, P., & Monteiro, L., (2010). Who should wear mask against airborne infections? Altering the contact network for controlling the spread of contagious diseases. *Ecological modelling, 221*(9), 1329–1332.
69. Tracht, S. M., Del, V. S. Y., & Hyman, J. M., (2010). Mathematical modeling of the effectiveness of facemasks in reducing the spread of novel influenza A (H1N1). *PloS One, 5*(2), e9018.
70. Kai, D., et al., (2020). *Universal Masking is Urgent in the Covid-19 Pandemic: Seir and Agent-Based Models, Empirical Validation, Policy Recommendations.* arXiv preprint arXiv:2004.13553.
71. Li, Y., et al., (2006). Antimicrobial effect of surgical masks coated with nanoparticles. *Journal of Hospital Infection, 62*(1), 58–63.
72. Borkow, G., et al., (2010). A novel anti-influenza copper oxide containing respiratory face mask. *PLoS One, 5*(6), e11295.
73. Ratnesar-Shumate, S., et al., (2008). Evaluation of physical capture efficiency and disinfection capability of an iodinated biocidal filter medium. *Aerosol and Air Quality Research, 8*(1), 1–18.
74. Lee, J. H., et al., (2008). Efficacy of iodine-treated biocidal filter media against bacterial spore aerosols. *Journal of applied microbiology, 105*(5), 1318–1326.
75. Pini, M., et al., (2017). Assessment of environmental performance of TiO_2 nanoparticles coated self-cleaning float glass. *Coatings, 7*(1), 8.
76. Akduman, C., & Kumbasar, E. A., (2018). Nanofibers in face masks and respirators to provide better protection. In: *IOP Conference Series: Materials Science and Engineering.* IOP Publishing.
77. Thavasi, V., Singh, G., & Ramakrishna, S., (2008). Electrospun nanofibers in energy and environmental applications. *Energy & Environmental Science, 1*(2), 205–221.
78. Ramaseshan, R., et al., (2006). Functionalized polymer nanofibre membranes for protection from chemical warfare stimulants. *Nanotechnology, 17*(12), 2947.
79. Zhu, M., et al., (2017). Electrospun nanofibers membranes for effective air filtration. *Macromolecular Materials and Engineering, 302*(1), 1600353.
80. Skaria, S. D., & Smaldone, G. C., (2014). Respiratory source control using surgical masks with nanofiber media. *Annals of occupational hygiene, 58*(6), 771–781.

81. Suen, L., et al., (2020). Comparing mask fit and usability of traditional and nanofibre N95 filtering facepiece respirators before and after nursing procedures. *Journal of Hospital Infection, 104*(3), 336–343.
82. Tong, H. W., Kwok, S. K. C., & Kwok, H. C., (2019). *Protective Masks with Coating Comprising Different Electrospun Fibers Interweaved with Each Other, Formulations Forming the Same, and Method of Producing Thereof.* Google Patents.
83. Wang, N., et al., (2015). Ultra-light 3D nanofibre-nets binary structured nylon 6–polyacrylonitrile membranes for efficient filtration of fine particulate matter. *Journal of Materials Chemistry A, 3*(47), 23946–23954.
84. Akduman, C., (2019). Cellulose acetate and polyvinylidene fluoride nanofiber mats for N95 respirators. *Journal of Industrial Textiles*, 1528083719858760.
85. Wang, C., et al., (2014). A high efficiency particulate air filter based on agglomerated carbon nanotube fluidized bed. *Carbon, 79*, 424–431.
86. Li, X., et al., (2015). Electreted polyetherimide-silica fibrous membranes for enhanced filtration of fine particles. *Journal of Colloid and Interface Science, 439*, 12–20.
87. Canalli, B. A. C., et al., (2019). Composites based on nanoparticle and pan electrospun nanofiber membranes for air filtration and bacterial removal. *Nanomaterials, 9*(12), 1740.
88. Rubino, I., & Choi, H. J., (2017). Respiratory protection against pandemic and epidemic diseases. *Trends in Biotechnology, 35*(10), 907–910.
89. Kerry, R. G., et al., (2019). Nano-based approach to combat emerging viral (NIPAH virus) infection. *Nanomedicine: Nanotechnology, Biology and Medicine, 18*, 196–220.
90. Coronavirus, N. S., (2020). *Nanotech Surface Sanitizes Milan with Nanomaterials Remaining Self-Sterilized for Years| STATNANO.*
91. Quan, F. S., et al., (2017). Universal and reusable virus deactivation system for respiratory protection. *Scientific Reports, 7*(1), 1–10.
92. Abbasinia, M., et al., (2018). Application of nanomaterials in personal respiratory protection equipment: A literature review. *Safety, 4*(4), 47.
93. Elechiguerra, J. L., et al., (2005). Interaction of silver nanoparticles with HIV-1. *Journal of Nanobiotechnology, 3*(1), 1–10.
94. Hiragond, C. B., et al., (2018). Enhanced anti-microbial response of commercial face mask using colloidal silver nanoparticles. *Vacuum, 156*, 475–482.
95. Park, D. H., Joe, Y. H., & Hwang, J., (2019). Dry aerosol coating of anti-viral particles on commercial air filters using a high-volume flow atomizer. *Aerosol and Air Quality Research, 19*(7), 1636–1644.
96. Bhattacharjee, S., et al., (2019). Graphene modified multifunctional personal protective clothing. *Advanced Materials Interfaces, 6*(21), 1900622.
97. Perreault, F., et al., (2015). Antimicrobial properties of graphene oxide nanosheets: Why size matters. *ACS Nano, 9*(7), 7226–7236.
98. Chen, Y. N., et al., (2016). Antiviral activity of graphene-silver nanocomposites against non-enveloped and enveloped viruses. *International Journal of Environmental Research and Public Health, 13*(4), 430.
99. Yang, A., et al., (2017). Thermal management in nanofiber-based face mask. *Nano Letters, 17*(6), 3506–3510.
100. Rengasamy, S., Eimer, B., & Shaffer, R. E., (2010). Simple respiratory protection—evaluation of the filtration performance of cloth masks and common fabric materials against 20–1000 nm size particles. *Annals of occupational hygiene, 54*(7), 789–798.

101. Shakya, K. M., et al., (2017). Evaluating the efficacy of cloth facemasks in reducing particulate matter exposure. *Journal of Exposure Science & Environmental Epidemiology, 27*(3), 352–357.
102. Konda, A., et al., (2020). Aerosol filtration efficiency of common fabrics used in respiratory cloth masks. *ACS Nano, 14*(5), 6339–6347.
103. Edmonds, S. L., Macinga, D. R., & Jarvis, W. R., (2013). Reply to letter to the editor on "comparative efficacy of commercially available alcohol-based hand rubs and World Health Organization-recommended hand rubs." *American Journal of Infection Control, 41*(5), 474–475.
104. Yip, L., et al., (2020). Serious adverse health events, including death, associated with ingesting alcohol-based hand sanitizers containing methanol—Arizona and New Mexico. *Morbidity and Mortality Weekly Report, 69*(32), 1070.
105. Hadaway, A., (2020). Handwashing: Clean hands save lives. *Journal of Consumer Health on the Internet, 24*(1), 43–49.
106. Berardi, A., et al., (2020). Hand sanitizers amid CoViD-19: A critical review of alcohol-based products on the market and formulation approaches to respond to increasing demand. *International Journal of Pharmaceutics*, 119431.
107. Edmonds, S. L., et al., (2012). Comparative efficacy of commercially available alcohol-based hand rubs and World Health Organization-recommended hand rubs: Formulation matters. *American Journal of Infection Control, 40*(6), 521–525.
108. Monegro, A. F., Muppidi, V., & Regunath, H., (2020). *Hospital Acquired Infections.* StatPearls [Internet].
109. Gerberding, J. L., O'Grady, N. P., & Pearson, M. L., (2002). *Guidelines for the Prevention of Intravascular Catheter-Related Infections.*
110. Foddai, A. C., Grant, I. R., & Dean, M., (2016). Efficacy of instant hand sanitizers against foodborne pathogens compared with handwashing with soap and water in food preparation settings: A systematic review. *Journal of Food Protection, 79*(6), 1040–1054.
111. Steinmann, J., et al., (2012). Comparison of virucidal activity of alcohol-based hand sanitizers versus antimicrobial hand soaps in vitro and in vivo. *Journal of Hospital Infection, 82*(4), 277–280.
112. Kampf, G., (2018). Efficacy of ethanol against viruses in hand disinfection. *Journal of Hospital Infection, 98*(4), 331–338.
113. Siddharta, A., et al., (2017). Virucidal activity of World Health Organization-recommended formulations against enveloped viruses, including zika, Ebola, and emerging coronaviruses. *The Journal of Infectious Diseases, 215*(6), 902–906.
114. Tuladhar, E., et al., (2015). Reducing viral contamination from finger pads: Handwashing is more effective than alcohol-based hand disinfectants. *Journal of Hospital Infection, 90*(3), 226–234.
115. Blaney, D. D., et al., (2011). Use of alcohol-based hand sanitizers as a risk factor for norovirus outbreaks in long-term care facilities in northern New England. *American Journal of Infection Control, 39*(4), 296–301.
116. Vogel, L., (2011). *Hand Sanitizers May Increase Norovirus Risk.* Can Med Assoc.
117. Tambekar, D., et al., (2007). Prevention of transmission of infectious disease: Studies on hand hygiene in health-care among students. *Continental J. Biomedical Sciences, 1*, 6–10.
118. Larson, E. L., et al., (1998). Changes in bacterial flora associated with skin damage on hands of health care personnel. *American journal of infection control, 26*(5), 513–521.

119. Lauharanta, J., et al., (1991). Prevention of dryness and eczema of the hands of hospital staff by emulsion cleansing instead of washing with soap. *Journal of Hospital Infection, 17*(3), 207–215.
120. Jain, V. M., et al., (2016). Comparative assessment of antimicrobial efficacy of different hand sanitizers: An in vitro study. *Dental Research Journal, 13*(5), 424.
121. Fendler, E., et al., (2002). The impact of alcohol hand sanitizer use on infection rates in an extended care facility. *American Journal of Infection Control, 30*(4), 226–233.
122. Di Muzio, M., et al., (2015). Hand hygiene in preventing nosocomial infections: A nursing research. *Annali di Igiene: Medicina Preventiva e di Comunità, 27*(2), 485.
123. Ramasethu, J., (2017). Prevention and treatment of neonatal nosocomial infections. *Maternal Health, Neonatology and Perinatology, 3*(1), 5.
124. Gold, N. A., & Avva, U., (2018). *Alcohol Sanitizer*. In StatPearls [Internet]. StatPearls Publishing.
125. Pidot, S. J., et al., (2018). Increasing tolerance of hospital *Enterococcus faecium* to handwash alcohols. *Science Translational Medicine, 10*(452), eaar6115.
126. Islam, R., et al., (2009). Influence of initial cellulose concentration on the carbon flow distribution during batch fermentation by *Clostridium thermocellum* ATCC 27405. *Applied Microbiology and Biotechnology, 82*(1), 141.
127. Minarovičová, J., et al., (2018). Benzalkonium chloride tolerance of *Listeria monocytogenes* strains isolated from a meat processing facility is related to the presence of plasmid-borne bcrABC cassette. *Antonie Van Leeuwenhoek, 111*(10), 1913–1923.
128. Bore, E., et al., (2007). Adapted tolerance to benzalkonium chloride in *Escherichia col*i K-12 studied by transcriptome and proteome analyses. *Microbiology, 153*(4), 935–946.
129. Malizia, W. F., Gangarosa, E. J., & Goley, A. F., (1960). Benzalkonium chloride as a source of infection. *New England Journal of Medicine, 263*(16), 800–802.
130. Adair, F. W., Geftic, S. G., & Gelzer, J., (1969). Resistance of *Pseudomonas* to quaternary ammonium compounds. I. Growth in benzalkonium chloride solution. *Applied Microbiology, 18*(3), 299–302.
131. Steinmann, J., et al., (2010). Virucidal activity of 2 alcohol-based formulations proposed as hand rubs by the World Health Organization. *American Journal of Infection Control, 38*(1), 66–68.
132. Ansari, S., et al., (1989). In vivo protocol for testing efficacy of hand-washing agents against viruses and bacteria: Experiments with rotavirus and *Escherichia coli. Applied and Environmental Microbiology, 55*(12), 3113–3118.
133. Sattar, S. A., et al., (2000). Activity of an alcohol-based hand gel against human adeno-, rhino-, and rotaviruses using the finger pad method. *Infection Control & Hospital Epidemiology, 21*(8), 516–519.
134. Kampf, G., Grotheer, D., & Steinmann, J., (2005). *Efficacy of three ethanol-based hand rubs against feline calicivirus, a surrogate virus for norovirus. Journal of Hospital Infection, 60*(2), 144–149.
135. Kampf, G., et al., (2002). Spectrum of antimicrobial activity and user acceptability of the hand disinfectant agent sterillium® gel. *Journal of Hospital Infection, 52*(2), 141–147.
136. Boyce, J., & Pittet, D., (2002). Society for health care epidemiology of America. Association for professionals in infection control. infectious diseases society of America. Hand hygiene task force. Guideline for hand hygiene in health-care settings: Recommendations of the health care infection control practices advisory committee and the HICPAC. *MMWR Recomm. Rep., 51*, 1–45.

137. Fung, I. C. H., & Cairncross, S., (2006). Effectiveness of handwashing in preventing SARS: A review. *Tropical Medicine & International Health, 11*(11), 1749–1758.
138. Rabenau, H., et al., (2005). Efficacy of various disinfectants against SARS coronavirus. *Journal of Hospital Infection, 61*(2), 107–111.
139. Peeri, N. C., et al., (2020). The SARS, MERS and novel coronavirus (COVID-19) epidemics, the newest and biggest global health threats: What lessons have we learned? *International Journal of Epidemiology*.
140. Kampf, G., et al., (2020). Persistence of coronaviruses on inanimate surfaces and their inactivation with biocidal agents. *Journal of Hospital Infection, 104*(3), 246–251.
141. Todd, E. C., et al., (2010). Outbreaks where food workers have been implicated in the spread of foodborne disease. Part 10. Alcohol-based antiseptics for hand disinfection and a comparison of their effectiveness with soaps. *Journal of Food Protection, 73*(11), 2128–2140.
142. Bush, L., Benson, L. M., & White, J. H., (1986). Pigskin as test substrate for evaluating topical antimicrobial activity. *Journal of Clinical Microbiology, 24*(3), 343–348.
143. La Fleur, P., & Jones, S., (2017). *Non-Alcohol Based Hand Rubs: A Review of Clinical Effectiveness and Guidelines*. PMID: 29266912.
144. Ahmed-Lecheheb, D., et al., (2012). Prospective observational study to assess hand skin condition after application of alcohol-based hand rub solutions. *American Journal of Infection Control, 40*(2), 160–164.
145. Harbarth, S., et al., (2002). Interventional study to evaluate the impact of an alcohol-based hand gel in improving hand hygiene compliance. *The Pediatric Infectious Disease Journal, 21*(6), 489–495.
146. Kramer, A., Bernig, T., & Kampf, G., (2002). Clinical double-blind trial on the dermal tolerance and user acceptability of six alcohol-based hand disinfectants for hygienic hand disinfection. *Journal of Hospital Infection, 51*(2), 114–120.
147. Houben, E., De Paepe, K., & Rogiers, V., (2006). Skin condition associated with intensive use of alcoholic gels for hand disinfection: A combination of biophysical and sensorial data. *Contact Dermatitis, 54*(5), 261–267.
148. Greenaway, R., et al., (2018). Impact of hand sanitizer format (gel/foam/liquid) and dose amount on its sensory properties and acceptability for improving hand hygiene compliance. *Journal of Hospital Infection, 100*(2), 195–201.
149. Menegueti, M. G., et al., (2019). Glycerol content within the WHO ethanol-based handrub formulation: Balancing tolerability with antimicrobial efficacy. *Antimicrobial Resistance & Infection Control, 8*(1), 109.
150. Suchomel, M., Weinlich, M., & Kundi, M., (2017). Influence of glycerol and an alternative humectant on the immediate and 3-hours bactericidal efficacies of two isopropanol-based antiseptics in laboratory experiments in vivo according to EN 12791. *Antimicrobial Resistance & Infection Control, 6*(1), 72.
151. Suchomel, M., et al., (2013). Glycerol significantly decreases the three hour efficacy of alcohol-based surgical hand rubs. *Journal of Hospital Infection, 83*(4), 284–287.
152. Barel, A. O., Paye, M., & Maibach, H. I., (2014). *Handbook of Cosmetic Science and Technology*. CRC press.
153. Flick, E. W., (2014). *Cosmetic and Toiletry Formulations,* 3. Elsevier.
154. Meadows, T. P., (1980). Aloe as a humectant in new skin preparations. *Cosmetics and Toiletries, 95*(11), 51–56.

155. Javed, S., (2014). Aloe vera gel in food, health products, and cosmetics industry. In: *Studies in Natural Products Chemistry* (pp. 261–285). Elsevier.
156. Wilkinson, M., et al., (2017). Dose considerations for alcohol-based hand rubs. *Journal of Hospital Infection, 95*(2), 175–182.
157. Fu, L., et al., (2020). Different efficacies of common disinfection methods against *Candida auris* and other candida species. *Journal of Infection and Public Health.*
158. Howes, L., (2020). What is hand sanitizer, and does it keep your hands germ-free. *Chem. Eng. News, 98.*
159. Ordini, S. G. S. T. G., & Superiori, A. *Nimbus Gocce 50ML.* ViaFarmaciaonline, https://www.viafarmaciaonline.it/nimbus-gocce-50-ml.html (accessed on 24 August 2021).
160. Asare-Addo, K., et al., (2013). Aqueous and hydro-alcoholic media effects on polyols. *Colloids and Surfaces B: Biointerfaces, 111*, 24–29.
161. Fresno, M., Ramırez, A., & Jiménez, M., (2002). Systematic study of the flow behavior and mechanical properties of carbopol® ultrez™ 10 hydroalcoholic gels. *European Journal of Pharmaceutics and Biopharmaceutics, 54*(3), 329–335.
162. Osei-Asare, C., et al., (2020). Managing vibrio cholerae with a local beverage: Preparation of an affordable ethanol based hand sanitizer. *Heliyon, 6*(1), e03105.
163. Guo, J. H., et al., (1998). Pharmaceutical applications of naturally occurring water-soluble polymers. *Pharmaceutical Science & Technology Today, 1*(6), 254–261. doi: 10.1016/s1461–5347(98)00072–8.
164. Picker-Freyer, K. M., & Dürig, T., (2007). Physical mechanical and tablet formation properties of hydroxypropyl cellulose: In pure form and in mixtures. *AAPS Pharmscitech, 8*(4), 82.
165. Ramachandran, S., Chen, S., & Etzler, F., (1999). Rheological characterization of hydroxy-propyl cellulose gels. *Drug Development and Industrial Pharmacy, 25*(2), 153–161.
166. Company, D. C., (2002). *Methocel Cellulose Ethers Technical Handbook.* The Dow Chemical Company USA.
167. Li, C. L., et al., (2005). The use of hypromellose in oral drug delivery. *Journal of Pharmacy and Pharmacology, 57*(5), 533–546.
168. Brown, A., Jones, D., & Woolfson, A., (1998). *The effect of alcoholic solvents on the rheological properties of gels composed of cellulose derivatives. Journal of Pharmacy and Pharmacology, 50*(S9), 157–157.
169. Roberts, M., et al., (2007). Influence of ethanol on aspirin release from hypromellose matrices. *International Journal of Pharmaceutics, 332*(1, 2), 31–37.
170. Eyler, R., Klug, E., & Diephuis, F., (1947). Determination of degree of substitution of sodium carboxymethylcellulose. *Analytical Chemistry, 19*(1), 24–27.
171. Haft, R. J., et al., (2014). Correcting direct effects of ethanol on translation and transcription machinery confers ethanol tolerance in bacteria. *Proceedings of the National Academy of Sciences, 111*(25), E2576–E2585.
172. Morton, H. E., (1950). The relationship of concentration and germicidal efficiency of ethyl alcohol. *NYASA, 53*(1), 191–196.
173. Thomas, P., (2012). Long-term survival of *Bacillus* spores in alcohol and identification of 90% ethanol as relatively more spori/bactericidal. *Current Microbiology, 64*(2), 130–139.
174. Wu, F., et al., (2020). A new coronavirus associated with human respiratory disease in China. *Nature, 579*(7798), 265–269.
175. Zhou, P., et al., (2020). A pneumonia outbreak associated with a new coronavirus of probable bat origin. *Nature, 579*(7798), 270–273.

176. Cascella, M., et al., (2020). *Features, Evaluation and Treatment Coronavirus (COVID-19)*. In Statpearls [internet]. StatPearls Publishing.
177. Goldsmith, C. S., et al., (2004). *Ultrastructural Characterization of SARS Coronavirus. Emerging Infectious Diseases, 10*(2), 320.
178. PHARMACOLOGIST'S, N., (2020). Recommendations for compounded hand sanitizers during COVID-19. *Contemporary Pediatrics, 26.*
179. Organization, W. H., (2015). *The Selection and Use of Essential Medicines: Report of the WHO Expert Committee, 2015 (Including the 19th WHO Model List of Essential Medicines and the 5th WHO Model List of Essential Medicines for Children)* (p. 994). World Health Organization.
180. Jing, J. L. J., et al., (2020). Hand sanitizers: A review on formulation aspects, adverse effects, and regulations. *International Journal of Environmental Research and Public Health, 17*(9), 3326.
181. Santos, C., et al., (2017). Reported adverse health effects in children from ingestion of alcohol-based hand sanitizers—United States, 2011–2014. *MMWR. Morbidity and Mortality Weekly Report, 66*(8), 223.
182. Leeper, S., et al., (2000). Topical absorption of isopropyl alcohol-induced cardiac and neurologic deficits in an adult female with intact skin. *Veterinary and Human Toxicology, 42*(1), 15–17.
183. Zaman, F., Pervez, A., & Abreo, K., (2002). Isopropyl alcohol intoxication: A diagnostic challenge. *American Journal of Kidney Diseases, 40*(3), e12. 1–e12. 4.
184. Lachenmeier, D. W., (2008). Safety evaluation of topical applications of ethanol on the skin and inside the oral cavity. *Journal of Occupational Medicine and Toxicology, 3*(1), 26.
185. Emadi, A., & Coberly, L., (2007). Intoxication of a hospitalized patient with an isopropanol-based hand sanitizer. *New England Journal of Medicine, 356*(5), 530–531.
186. Kirschner, M. H., et al., (2009). Transdermal resorption of an ethanol-and 2-propanol-containing skin disinfectant. *Langenbeck's Archives of Surgery, 394*(1), 151–157.
187. Kramer, A., et al., (2007). Quantity of ethanol absorption after excessive hand disinfection using three commercially available hand rubs is minimal and below toxic levels for humans. *BMC Infectious Diseases, 7*(1), 117.
188. Singer, M. V., & Teyssen, S., (2005). *Alkohol und Alkoholfolgekrankheiten: Grundlagen-Diagnostik-Therapie*. Springer.
189. Jones, A. W., & Rajs, J., (1997). Appreciable blood-ethanol concentration after washing abraised and lacerated skin with surgical spirit. *Journal of Analytical Toxicology, 21*(7), 587–588.
190. Edwards, W. H., et al., (2004). The effect of prophylactic ointment therapy on nosocomial sepsis rates and skin integrity in infants with birth weights of 501 to 1000 g. *Pediatrics, 113*(5), 1195–1203.
191. Gim, E. R., et al., (1968). Percutaneous alcohol intoxication. *Clinical Toxicology, 1*(1), 39–48.
192. Harpin, V., & Rutter, N., (1982). Percutaneous alcohol absorption and skin necrosis in a preterm infant. *Archives of Disease in Childhood, 57*(6), 477–479.
193. Al-Jawad, S., (1983). Percutaneous alcohol absorption and skin necrosis in a preterm infant. *Archives of Disease in Childhood, 58*(5), 395.
194. Salomone, A., et al., (2018). Occupational exposure to alcohol-based hand sanitizers: The diagnostic role of alcohol biomarkers in hair. *Journal of Analytical Toxicology, 42*(3), 157–162.

195. Vonghia, L., et al., (2008). Acute alcohol intoxication. *European Journal of Internal Medicine, 19*(8), 561–567.
196. Archer, J. R., et al., (2007). Alcohol hand rubs: Hygiene and hazard. *BMJ, 335*(7630), 1154, 1155.
197. Sanap, M., & Chapman, M. J., (2003). Severe ethanol poisoning: A case report and brief review. *Critical Care and Resuscitation, 5*(2), 106.
198. Wilson, M., Guru, P., & Park, J., (2015). Recurrent lactic acidosis secondary to hand sanitizer ingestion. *Indian Journal of Nephrology, 25*(1), 57.
199. Bouthoorn, S. H., et al., (2011). Alcohol intoxication among Dutch adolescents: Acute medical complications in the years 2000–2010. *Clinical Pediatrics, 50*(3), 244–251.
200. Gormley, N. J., et al., (2012). The rising incidence of intentional ingestion of ethanol-containing hand sanitizers. *Critical Care Medicine, 40*(1), 290.
201. Ashkar, F., & Miller, R., (1971). Hospital ketosis in the alcoholic diabetic: A syndrome due to isopropyl alcohol intoxication. *Southern Medical Journal, 64*(11), 1409.
202. McBay, A. J., (1973). Toxicological findings in fatal poisonings. *Clinical Chemistry, 19*(4), 361–365.
203. McFadden, S. W., & Haddow, J. E., (1969). Coma produced by topical application of isopropanol. *Pediatrics, 43*(4), 622–623.
204. Moss, M. H., (1970). Alcohol-induced hypoglycemia and coma caused by alcohol sponging. *Pediatrics, 46*(3), 445.
205. Vermeulen, R., (1966). Isopropyl alcohol and diabetes. *Pennsylvania Medicine, 69*(4), 53.
206. Fuller, H., & Hunter, O., (1927). Isopropyl alcohol—An investigation of its physiologic properties. *J. Lab. Clin. Med., 12*, 326–349.
207. Stremski, E., & Hennes, H., (2000). Accidental isopropanol ingestion in children. *Pediatric Emergency Care, 16*(4), 238–240.
208. Olson, K. R., et al., (2007). *Poisoning & Drug Overdose* (Vol. 13). Lange Medical Books/McGraw-Hill.
209. Gosselin, R., (1984). Hydrogen sulfide. *Clinical Toxicology of Commercial Products*, 198–202.
210. Trummel, J., Ford, M., & Austin, P., (1996). Ingestion of an unknown alcohol. *Annals of Emergency Medicine, 27*(3), 368–374.
211. Slaughter, R., et al., (2014). Isopropanol poisoning. *Clinical Toxicology, 52*(5), 470–478.
212. Food and Drug Administration, (1988). Oral health care drug products for over-the-counter human use: Tentative final monograph: Notice of proposed rulemaking. *Federal Register, 53*, 2436–2461.
213. Moon, J. M., Chun, B. J., & Min, Y. I., (2006). Hemorrhagic gastritis and gas emboli after ingesting 3% hydrogen peroxide. *The Journal of Emergency Medicine, 30*(4), 403–406.
214. Mahmood, A., et al., (2020). COVID-19 and frequent use of hand sanitizers; human health and environmental hazards by exposure pathways. *Science of the Total Environment, 742*, 140561.
215. Henry, M. C., et al., (1996). Hydrogen peroxide 3% exposures. *Journal of Toxicology: Clinical Toxicology, 34*(3), 323–327.
216. Pendlington, R., et al., (2001). Fate of ethanol topically applied to skin. *Food and Chemical Toxicology, 39*(2), 169–174.
217. Moser, S., et al., (2009). *The Future is Now: An update on Climate Change Science Impacts and Response Options for California.* California Energy Commission Public Interest Energy Research Program CEC-500-2008-071.

218. Winnefeld, M., et al., (2000). Skin tolerance and effectiveness of two hand decontamination procedures in everyday hospital use. *British Journal of Dermatology, 143*(3), 546–550.
219. Organization, W. H., (2009). *WHO Guidelines on Hand Hygiene in Health Care: First Global patient Safety Challenge: Clean Care is Safer Care Geneva, Switzerland.* World Health Organization.
220. Larson, E. L., et al., (2001). Assessment of two hand hygiene regimens for intensive care unit personnel. *Critical Care Medicine, 29*(5), 944–951.
221. Anderson, R. L., (1989). Iodophor antiseptics: Intrinsic microbial contamination with resistant bacteria. *Infection Control & Hospital Epidemiology, 10*(10), 443–446.
222. Kantor, R., & Silverberg, J. I., (2017). Environmental risk factors and their role in the management of atopic dermatitis. *Expert Review of Clinical Immunology, 13*(1), 15–26.
223. Wilhelm, K. P., (1996). Prevention of surfactant-induced irritant contact dermatitis. In: *Prevention of Contact Dermatitis* (pp. 78–85). Karger Publishers.
224. Pittet, D., Peters, A., & Tartari, E., (2018). Enterococcus faecium tolerance to isopropanol: From good science to misinformation. *The Lancet Infectious Diseases, 18*(10), 1065, 1066.
225. Hayat, A., & Munnawar, F., (2016). Antibacterial effectiveness of commercially available hand sanitizers. *Int. J. Biol. Biotech., 13*(3), 427–431.
226. Monks, K. M., (2000). *Pocket Guide to Home Health Care*. Elsevier Health Sciences.

CHAPTER 7

Lockdown as a Strategy to Control COVID-19

NAHEED BANO,[1] RIZWAN AHMAD,[2] ZAHID KHAN,[3] and MAJID KHAN[4]

[1]*Faculty of Veterinary and Animal Sciences, MNS-University of Agriculture, Multan, Pakistan, E-mail: naheed.bano@mnsuam.edu.pk*

[2]*Natural Products and Alternative Medicines, College of Clinical Pharmacy, Imam Abdulrahman Bin Faisal University, Dammam, Kingdom of Saudi Arabia*

[3]*Department of Pharmacognosy, Faculty of Pharmacy, Federal Urdu University, Karachi, Pakistan*

[4]*Department of Pharmacy, Shaheed Benazir Bhutto University, Sheringal, Pakistan*

ABSTRACT

The pattern of spread and rate of deaths remain different among different areas of one country. These different responses are significant for pandemic control as these responses have a positive or negative effect on the prevalence of corona and deaths of infected people. The most suitable and essential method in controlling the spread of corona infections among people in quarantine. The most effective strategy for controlling the pandemic remains lockdown, but it is also suggested as neither a good nor bad strategy. As when the world was coming out of lockdown as ad hoc or illogical exit strategies, the number of infected confirmed cases still flooding and we feel lack of planning in some countries of the world and smells terrible. The primary weapon against the coronavirus remains care and effective communication with strict follow-up SOPs against the virus. Here smart lockdown also remains effective for lives. Continuous public messages kept people alert and attentive to changing environment. After the lockdown, the scenario changed and back to work adopted with strict safety measures including mask-wearing, sit apart during traveling and escalators quarantine. At that time, it was estimated that isolation rate improvement remains excellent to end the epidemic. The lockdown strategy also was helpful for the invention of a vaccine.

7.1 INTRODUCTION

Infectious pneumonia by coronavirus become threatens to human globally. It was first identified in Wuhan. This epidemic outbreak remains changed in different parts of the world. An association between the wholesale market of Wuhan and the coronavirus was reported in primary reported cases [1]. And the possible source of this virus in that market was supposed to be the bat. In December 2019, the transmission of this virus from human to human was confirmed after the World Health Organization (WHO) announced the name of this virus as COVID-19. The disease was named coronavirus disease in February 2020. If we look at the early reported number of cases, the total confirmed cases in Hubei were equal to the total cases in the rest of China [2]. And the pattern of spread and rate of deaths were also different among different areas of one country. These different responses are significant for the control of pandemic as these responses have a positive or negative effect on the prevalence of corona and deaths of infected people. China has faced the most considerable quarantine history of human with controlling the pandemic.

This is not the first time that a human is facing a zoonotic or infectious disease. In the past also human has encountered such problems which also affected the economy of the countries. And a massive death rate was reported, which ranges from 30 to 45% worldwide. This entire pass-through different channels, and different people participated as reported in documents, education, labor, economics, income, and civil wars. All forces participated in the process [3, 65]. We can simply say that COVID like communicable diseases have a higher rate of indisposition and transience worldwide. We can also say that this kind of disease affects the labor market, and economic performance is damaged [4–5, 66]. Most countries provide health care facilities publicly and in such an outbreak period, there is a need for divergent resources and policies towards health resources.

Researchers are working, and a lot of epidemiology and economic-related literature with analysis methods, mathematical implications, and dynamic forces of transmittable diseases has been established from the last two decades. The characterization of any disease becomes more manageable by using mathematical modeling and epidemiology, whereas the economic structuring and epidemiology make the mechanisms understandable for policy-making and treatment [5, 67]. But most scientists and researchers also not tried to focus on macro-economic implications. The chaos may probably be created by cracks in health risks and economic interrelationship during epidemics. There are both short and long-run effects of epidemics on the economy. Still, what is needed is to find the treatment and preventive measures policies efficiency. The epidemic dynamics may be characterized by modeling susceptible-infected-susceptible design, which is the most effective epidemiological mathematical model [4, 68].

The COVID-19 has recently prompted the sympathetic communal associations of disease with health, economy, and their outcomes. This disease has proved itself a highly infectious viral disease transmitted through close contacts with objects carrying the virus, droplets, contacts between infective animals or people and infectors. This transmission is high-speed among humans as humans transfer and spread fast, especially from the cough or respiratory droplets and sneezes. Other carriers may be clothes, furniture, handles, and utensils [8, 69]. There are different implemented policy plans and SOPs which different countries have adopted. Nearly 13,500 policies instigated in almost 200 countries, in addition to the traditionally applied preventive measures and treatments. The aim of social distancing and lockdown remains to reduce the transmission rate of any disease like COVID by controlling the exposure of man to a potential infection source. Thus, social distancing and lockdown stay the most effective method of controlling COVID without using drugs (in the absence of a vaccine).

Lockdown not only helped in lowering the peak of infestation but also helped truly in sparing the general community from contagion. Suppose we look at the best strategies for controlling the spread of infection, which strategy is best dependent upon the lowest cost, various predictable parameters. Different parameters check the strategy and their performance qualitatively, even they are very different from each other. For example, skibob thresholds are well known for judgment and comparison, like how the lockdown remains effective in saving lives and creating jobs after lockdown. When two communities or different populations adopt different policies, they must further understand or face different strengths of the outbreak; its spread may be diverse, and even economically effects will be other.

7.1.1 PRIMARY MEANS IN CONTROLLING MORTALITY

After the global spread of COVID-19 different countries responded differentially, and these different levels of responses from other civilizations resulted in different intensities of epidemics. Researchers tried to find the best method to control the spread of corona and estimated the mortality and infected person ratio during quarantine [3]. It was observed that by taking active measures, isolation or quarantine, the causalities due to corona were under control (Figure 7.1). From all studies, it may be concluded that COVID-19 may be under control if people are aware and prepared. But if early preventive measures and intrusion are missed, it will lead to severe conditions that disturb the health system, with 20% severe cases. The result will be an increase in the death ratio [4]. The most suitable and essential method of controlling the spread of corona infections is quarantine. Some scientists also suggested that detection of cases on a large scale, correct diagnosis, early detection, and integrated management is necessary to control the epidemic.

We can determine the effect of strict quarantine on the spread and mortality rate. In most countries, lockdown started as a low level and was uncompromising in the second phase. As the outbreak began from Wuhan, their quarantine measures were strictly followed by the government in the start (early stage) to reduce the movement of potentially infected persons. China faced immense isolation in history [5]. This activity proved to be partially successful in spreading this disease out of China. But this makes the city (Wuhan) a concentrated area for corona, which pressurized the health system of that area. That pressure was mainly from unadorned cases, which require equipment for monitoring and support [6]. The care of medical and paramedical staff is also necessary as they have to work in the front line.

Likewise, adjustment, strengthening, and release of lockdown are not outrageous. During a lockdown, many unusual behaviors in terms of the adoption of policy arose. Always there were great ways and ideas to work further. But some of the silent limitations are present, which may be ignored. One of the limitations is control modeling for vigorous testing and contact tracing [5–7]. The reason may be that if the infected number of people are controlled and are less, then tracing and aggressive testing may keep the spread in control even after lockdown when everyone goes back to their work. This strategy also helped to use aggressive lockdown for a long time, and we do not need to sustain it until the vaccine development remains successful [8]. There is no doubt that this strategy will be helpful worldwide, but the cost will be a prolonged economic pain.

Another leeway may be the migration from one near the geographic area to the other which may be nearby and where the degree of prevalence is lower than the home region [9, 10]. But this could create problems for the low prevalence region, so this led to the restrictions on movement, traveling, and border closures, as was seen in mid of 2019. And similar was observed since the Soviet Union collapsed. This is also very important to know if the border closure strategy was indeed required. Two-dimensional heterogeneity is related to the infection rate among different age groups [11–13]. As the pandemic remains fatal for two groups of people, one is the old age group, and the other has some preexisting health issues. So, there is a quid pro quo among economic losses and health stress.

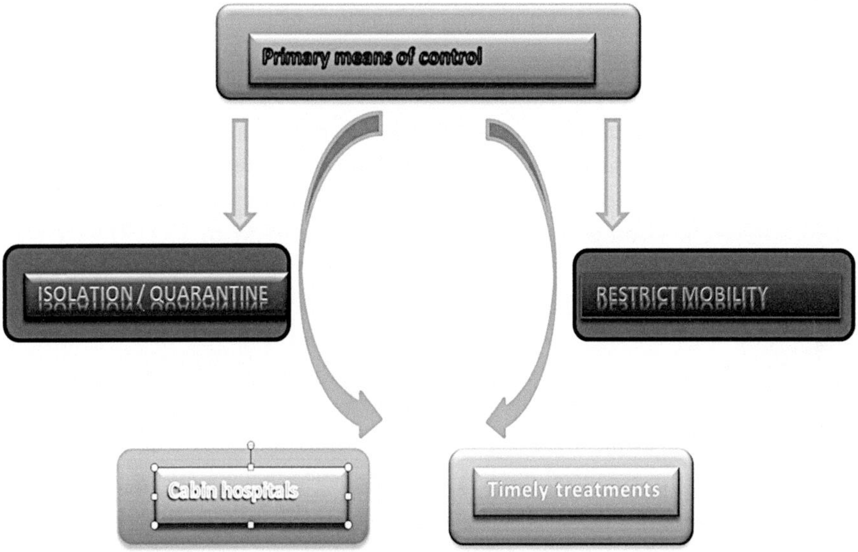

FIGURE 7.1 Primary means adopted for controlling COVID-19.

The reported death rate for severe cases is nearly 61.5%. This may be why the high death rate at Hubei compared to other regions, as the number of severe cases was reported low in other parts. Some people not show prominent symptoms of infection, and some minor display symptoms and recover naturally. It was reported that the disease confirmed cases rose in the start but, after isolation strategy, decreased. However, this may be due to the underestimation of actual infections [7]. This may result in a large number of mortalities, and different recent publications also supported this.

One more thing is selection bias which must also be not ignored. We usually face some limitations; these include hospital capacity, medical staff, and training regarding outbreak and detection kits. It was also observed that only severe cases were reported, and the mild infection goes unnoticed and unidentified [8]. The presence of those infected but not showing symptoms is observed all over the world.

Although governments of each country took necessary measures to control the spread of corona and strict mobility measures were adopted. People were informed about taking distance and avoiding close contacts, but many people traveled everywhere like young and middle-aged labor who returned home cities or countries [9]. Some people also take part in spring festivals, so their movement also may not be underestimated. We may take the fatality rate as an example to understand the primary means of controlling mortality from the coronavirus. As under the strict observations in different provinces of chins, the mortality rate remains 0.3%.

The number of severe confirmed cases becomes low in Hubei compared to other areas of China [10]. This credit goes to the hospitals as Hubei hospitals raise the standards of significant severe cases whereas other sites reported cases because of limitations of resources which was 20%. Different strategies for controlling the spread of COVID-19 were adopted (Table 7.1), which affected differentially. One crucial innovation is related to public gloominess that is also directly related to the duration and strength of lockdown. So, we can consider it as the fifth variable of state, which also put away amenableness of distancing, leading to a lower infection rate.

Another important strategy was cabin hospitals. In China, 14 cabin hospitals play an essential role in quarantine and restrictions in mobility [11]. This was usually for the treatment of mild infections and provided treatment to 10,000 people. This also helped reduce family transmission by isolating mild confirmed cases at home [12]. One more benefit of this mobile hospital was that if the mild infected case becomes severe and needs specialized facilities, he can quickly transfer to the hospital and get timely treatments. Lockdown as a strategy remain complex and qualitative its extent is different. The forcefully derived lockdown increased the stress among people but lowered the infection rates and proved to be a good strategy as a hurdle against the extreme spread of COVID. Lockdown helped reduce the peak of infection and helped truly in sparing the general community from contagion.

TABLE 7.1 Effective Control Strategies Adopted Against COVID-19

SL. No.	Effective Control Strategies	Effectiveness		
		Low	Medium	High
1.	Lockdown			✓
2.	Aggressive testing	✓	✓	
3.	Quarantining			✓
4.	Policies development			✓
5.	Distancing			✓
6.	Effective communication			✓
7.	Following guidelines			✓
8.	Strict follow of SOPs			✓
9.	Smart lockdown		✓	
10.	Availability of testing kits		✓	
11.	Mobile hospitals		✓	
12.	Isolation			✓
13.	Self-quarantine/quarantine			✓
14.	Health care facilities		✓	✓
15.	Training of health care workers		✓	✓
16.	Restricted traveling		✓	✓
17.	Sanitizers		✓	✓
18.	Mass gathering restriction		✓	✓

7.1.2 STRICT ISOLATION AND QUARANTINE MEASURES

To understand the effect of isolation and quarantine, we can again take China experiences as an example. It was February 4th when the curve of mortality rate decreased, and it was concluded that this pandemic could be managed and preventable. Human learns from experiences, same is the case with the virus [13]. From the fight against one disease of the virus, we experience many things that can help in fighting against others. China also learnt from SARS in 2003, and timely action against the present outbreak did not let it out of control slightly.

South Korea also faced a brutal hit of coronavirus during the early days. South Korea succeeded in fighting against COVID-19 by viral testing on a large scale, restricting the gathering and different rallies, which resulted in remarkable success against coronavirus [14]. Mobile hospitals were also adopted in South Korea, and the mildly infected person was isolated here to limit the cluster spread in the family.

Europe, however, has seen a massive coronavirus outbreak as compared to South Korea. In Europe, the number of confirmed patients remain close to the origin province, i.e., Hubei. The reason may be a vast number of people at a place, non-restricted traveling, inadequate testing for viral genome, home quarantine of non-serious cases and mass gathering [15]. These reasons led the situation worse, and the number of cases got close to the Hubei, where the death rate was getting higher, and the medical facility was skeptical. Above all, the situation helps us emphasize that timely active measures help control the epidemic.

Antagonistic viral tests, quick isolation measures, face mask, quarantine of people with a mild infection, popularization of face mask, sanitizers, inhibition of large gatherings were proved to be powerful tool in controlling the spread of coronavirus [16]. When the testing kits remain insufficient, clinical diagnosis may be well thought out as a problem-solving benchmark. Model mobile cabins are likewise valued erudition. The truth is, markets may be closed instantaneously. Still, reopening may not be an easy task as, by the orders of policymakers, the business cannot become at a peak, and unemployment levels cannot be returned to the previous levels. As job creation is complex compared to destruction, the employment levels and economy must be treated as a national variable.

Media also played an essential role in spreading information regarding the controlling strategies faster than the spread of the virus (Figure 7.2). This communication media not only helped in the spread of information but also obviously relaxed the government and help in publicizing the information regarding epidemic prevention [17, 18]. No doubt media also fortified rumors to blow out swiftly. Each man agrees that COVID-19 is among the absolute disaster of current years; nevertheless, numerous dishonest stories created excessive panic among people. These even resulted in discrimination and defamation against affected regions in other areas [19]. The main point is this virus is controllable by preparations, but it does not mean that we should take this lightly. We must take it seriously and make all necessary preparations to fight against it [20, 21]. Other countries may follow the quarantine and isolation methods of China and Korea.

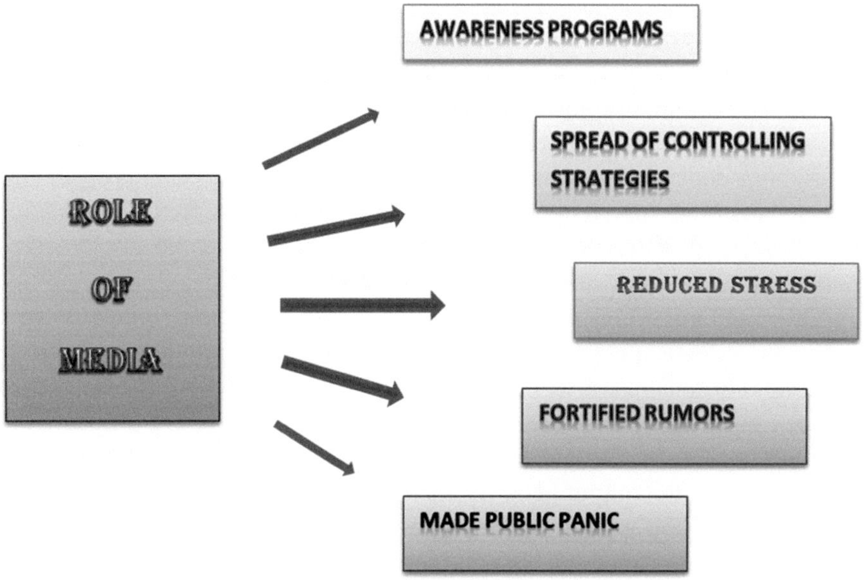

FIGURE 7.2 The role of media during lockdown.

7.2 EFFECTIVE CONTROL STRATEGIES

The most effective strategy considered controlling the pandemic remains lockdown, but it is also suggested as neither good nor bad. As now world is coming out of lockdown as ad hoc or illogical exit strategies, the number of infected confirmed cases still flooding, and we feel a lack of planning in some countries of the world and smells bad [22, 23]. The main reason behind the lockdown was that the health crisis was turning into an economic crisis. So many developing countries decided to open the lock with necessary precautionary measures and SOPs. The lack of aggressive testing, quarantining, and treating asymptotic and sympatric testing during lockdown is also associated with incomplete data of infected people [24, 25].

Some countries do not follow the WHO call of testing, testing, and testing. South Korea proves itself a benchmark, and the credit goes to its strategy of massive aggressive testing. After all the situations get exciting, the disease shifted from China to G7 countries [26, 27]. Different countries adopted social distancing differently; it ranges from isolation to quarantine, mobility, or traveling restrictions to lockdown. The other important safety measure remains wearing a face mask, keeping social distance, strict restraints on single human (person) conduct, closure of workplace or reduction of employees and workforce, reducing interaction [28, 29, 69].

However, limiting the man force also devastated the economy, increased unemployment, and dropped GDP (gross domestic product). The countries and areas that remain more affected by social distancing and traveling restrictions depended on sectors like tourism and manufacturing. So, this also affected the other linked industries. Policymakers also worked for managing pandemic, and different researchers tried to investigate the implemented policies and economic allegations of COVID-19 [30, 68].

Other scientists also analyze the self-motivated epidemiological system so that the infected person recovered and a permanent immunity is produced. Comparative analysis also helped show extenuation energies also helped reduce transmission of disease and rate of affection. There is a link between expenses, economy, and pandemic with policies related to lockdown, which help determine the output [31]. By focusing on the social charter, optimization, duration, and type of lockdown may be determined. This also makes it convenient to implement austere lockdown after the outburst and slowly release and opening.

During the present pandemic condition, the conditioning of epidemiology and lockdown with its effects on different age groups, especially on old, middle age, and young groups, is essential. Duration and intensity of lockdown in various areas where the outbreak was initial than new areas remain different. It is important to note that health and life become safe, but the lockdown affected the economy, income generation, and reduced consumption of various goods [32, 33, 69]. This also increases the trade-off between economic outcome and health. The effectiveness of policies related to the intensity of lockdown was also analyzed by fundamental changing aspects and rigorous altitudes of the pandemic.

The tackling of COVID-19 was challenging for all governments and what needed is institutions and policy. The main focus was given to the hot spots and faced success at different levels [28, 29]. Now we can say that policies and their responses improve mitigation and relief not only to human's life but also the economic catastrophe before getting late. Among the world's most powerful countries, Pakistan, with a weak economy, also stands as a role model in the COVID-19 challenge. The primary weapon against coronavirus remains care and effective communication with strict follow-up SOPs against viruses [30]. Here smart lockdown also remains effective. Continuous public messages kept people alert and attentive to changing environment.

The number of infected persons decreased with time, and the implementation of different policies remain important in this regard [31]. If we thoroughly look at the trend, we may find that other approaches were implemented with different strategies, and it works well. And with time, it was suggested that coronavirus reaches the fourth generation with the aerosol transmission. Internationally the forecasts always remain important, and public security and health can be improved [32]. Domestic news and international outcomes both are of importance when we have to overcome a pandemic situation.

One other problem was under-reporting and delayed diagnosis tics, especially during the start of the outbreak. The actual infected reported cases were higher than the confirmed cases, and the reason behind this was a preliminary diagnosis and un-reported cases [33, 34]. The primary cause may be non-availability of testing kits, errors in results, unclear, and un-differentiated signs, and symptoms. As the number of test kits increased and detection capacity was enhanced by the efforts of different policies, the detection dimensions also improved. So, the number of reported and confirmed cases increased, and there was a sharp rise in affection.

Interventions like self-quarantine, vacations, and isolation of high-risk population helped in controlling the corona [35]. The primary response from many countries was the first-level response, and mainly people not responded. And in the start, people not responded positively and not isolated themselves. Still, after some time, they responded, and the number of self-quarantine adoption increased, which helped control the pandemic [36, 37]. Some other problems were a shortage of hospital beds and medicine [38, 39].

No doubt that all countries made significant decisions in controlling the coronavirus, but this is the fact that complete control is not yet achieved. To stop the second outbreak of epidemic, it is essential to maintain the quarantine level [40]. Community screening is also vital after CT scan and testing kits. Furthermore, better monitoring of quarantine areas is also essential for managing infected people and preventing infection with improved health of conformed patients. As the infectivity of the coronavirus is high, and the global spread is still increasing, the countries need more active mobilization and medical equipment with risk assessments [41].

There is need of characterization of policies with a sequential planning for the welfare of mankind facing the pandemic [41–43]. The myth that was in circulation is actually without evidences and most of people understand and believed that once recovered from disease will not be secured and recently many people are reported positive after vaccination. As the antibodies produced by immune system will not be for life time. But all over the world people have learnt the management of pandemic [44–46]. As mostly all the saving can be entirely consumed in lower-income countries. Some scientists take the time horizon as infinite during studies, but a finite time for the investigation of intensity and policy optimization is also good.

Some other problems must also be considered and centralized as the outbreak response remains the regulations for public safety and government rules but not the changes in behavior [45–47]. What the social planners do is also important; social distancing adoptions also work for treatment. In that case, therapeutic measures and facilities are directly provided to the general public, which is financed by the taxes; for example, income tax collected from the public may be utilized. So, the problem of shortage of funds can be overcome, and the spread of pandemic is also reduced [48]. Many social planners also focused on lockdown results with minimum cost and disease prevalence with solid management tools related to policy. However, a different approach may be adopted, like analytical determination instead of numerical mockup. During studies, it is also important to not rely on existing work entirely. Still, analysis of early epidemic and late interventions with their long-term impact on health and economic consequences must also be analyzed [48–51].

7.2.1 TRAVEL RESTRICTIONS IN CONTROL OF TRANSMISSION

In response to corona, many countries respond by implementing travel restrictions and community interaction. The detailed actions were different, but commonly, all governments adopted restrictions of premises like schools and office remained close worldwide with the lockdown of recreational areas and worship places [41]. All countries also try to provide necessary basic needs to the public like health care, washing, cleaning, food, and supply chain services were not banned and this help in the sustainability of economy with the welfare of the community. Travel restrictions and lockdown successfully reduced the spread and growth of the epidemic. People were informed about taking distance and avoiding close contacts, but many people traveled everywhere like young and middle-aged labor who returned home cities or countries. Some people also take part in spring festivals, so their movement may not be underestimated [42, 43]. We may take the fatality rate as an example to understand the primary means of controlling mortality from the coronavirus.

An irregular lockdown system was proposed by initiating and then gradual closing of places until 2022. It will avoid extreme cases spread and limit the cases so that the hospital capacities will also be satisfied. There is a need for long-term management to settle economic disruption with healthy social and mental consequences. It was also noted that lockdown and travel restrictions with social distancing created a positive effect. Isolation facilities and health care measurements are important to be considered during all phases from lockdown start to end, and it is necessary to maintain standards of healthcare [16, 44].

The maintenance of all standard will help reduce fatality rates. With all standards, extensive education is also essential. Because people must learn and follow distancing, wearing masks, preventive measures, and other hygiene practices [17]. The same rules were followed in Singapore, and it was the 10th of March 2020 when social distancing was implemented there with gradual strictness in regulations related to travel. After 7th April there were a complete lockdown and circuit breaks as the cases increased. Singapore remains successful in controlling the spread of the epidemic by this lockdown and school closure.

Similar strategies were followed in New Zealand even though it is geographically isolated from another land. But here comes many students and tourists in this country during summer, especially from China and Europe. The policy adopted by New Zealand was to delay the arrival of the pandemic in the country by border control, and hospitals were prepared to control the flood of patients. The first case in New Zealand was reported on 26th February, and this was when the WHO reported that COVID is behaving more like SARS than influenza, so its control was probable [19, 45]. The adoption of community transmission was reported, and the government switched to an elimination strategy, and the decision was to lock down the country. New Zealand, in just 103 days, came to a post-elimination period. It was possible only by travel restrictions with all other control measures. It is important to note that the total cases of infections and death remain the lowest in New Zealand.

7.2.2 LONG TERM STRATEGIES

In underdeveloped, low, or middle earning countries, lockdown, and social distancing strategies against COVID are unsustainable in the long term as these have an adverse psychological and socio-economic effect. Long term strategies must be safe, which can balance both economy and health globally

[46]. Safe reopening and epidemiological plans with low surveillance and diagnostic setup is the need of time. These strategies include zonal lockdown, constant alleviation and safely planned prerequisite with limitations measure. Long-term strategies will also differ in different geographical areas, economic conditions, and nationwide [20, 47].

Zonal isolation and local areas lockdown are suitable and may be feasible in real-time where a new outbreak is identified. Long term strategy must include zonal management and comprehensive testing. WHO also suggested a rolling lockdown strategy that may succeed in epidemic control in the long run [21, 25]. But for adopting this strategy, needful must be done for economy and supply chain modification. From the past review, we can say those nations learned many lessons with economic disturbances after losing more than 600,000 people worldwide. Now they know we need a long-term strategy after opening international travel and lockdown. Control measures must be related to physical distancing, population-level, and nationwide [48]. Lockdown has been reported among the chief tactic against COVID-19, and the lockup of region and zones helped in the reduction of interactions, gathering, and communicable conduction. Various republics and states aggressively adopted a lockdown policy and gradually opened the economy, workplaces, and schools. Reopening of markets impelled contamination rates, spread, and also lock down fatigue.

No doubt, in the absence of effective treatment and vaccine, the use of mask, social distance, and different types of lockdown strategies effectively control the spread. But must also be taken into consideration that there is high population density and interaction among people in low income and economically weak countries, which increases the risk of transmission [49]. These countries also face problems related to hygiene and the availability of drinking water. Another problem in most countries is that the public health areas are mostly less equipped and limited resources. There are limitations in access to healthcare, and most people in these areas remain out of pocket [26, 30]. Social distance remains unsuitable in the long run as it affects the economy, social behaviors, and psychology. In this scenario, three strategies may be helpful: persistent extenuation, zone-specific lockdown, and vibrant actions (systematic lockdown).

Economically strong or developed countries like Italy, Switzerland, and France adopted isolation, social distancing, masks, and banned gatherings [50]. However, this extenuation strategy depends on other factors like lockdown situation, mitigation approaches, fatality rates, contact tracing, test kits, and population of an area. Among all, contact tracing may remain less effective in areas where community spread is higher. Some other strategies plans include physical distances, quarantine situation, and hygiene [33, 51].

Among long term strategies also include special attention, ICU, and care centers or hospitals. Care centers and hospitals are essential for long term strategic management. Other managements include personal protective apparatus like masks and sanitizers. Training of staff working in hospitals or health care centers is also vital with an excellent working hygiene environment. It will improve efficiency and reduce transmission of infection among workers and ordinary people [52]. During the lockdown, most of the people who become jobless were of a young age group, whereas the old age group and retired persons benefit from health benefits. There are heterogenic activities of people related to social or during the other viral disease scenario. Some people remain socially isolated, and some are very social and considered butterflies. Some remain social in close premises where there is no fresh airflow, and even recirculation of air is low. So, the infection rate among those people will also be different from other people.

People worldwide will agree that less restriction than complete lockdown with all necessary measures is significant. It will also reduce socio-economic issues primarily related to finance and combat the reduction in production by social distances. Sweden adopted a similar approach. They adopted the strategy to keep restaurants, bars, and workout places open with strict physical distancing rules [53]. One important point that must be taken in mind while dealing with long-term strategies that the age group that is vulnerable to COVID needs more attention due to comorbid environment like other physical issues: hypertension, diabetes, and obesity.

Furthermore, the most challenging for a country is reducing disease dispersal with up liftmen in the local economy. Therefore, it is crucial to give equal value to life and livelihood during planning. So, the survey, tests, treatments, social, economic issues, implementations of all needful must be implemented with each necessary measure [45, 54].

To overcome the adverse effects on the economy, the government must implement supporting programs that will help small businesses, unemployed, and daily wages employees. It is reported that policy is deficient regarding the workplace and a poor supply of equipment, increasing the stress among workers [55]. So, it is important and must be the priority of organizations and government to safeguard the employee and public, respectively. Every government has to follow WHO guidelines as these guidelines are both for non-health and health workers. All the workplaces other than hospitals or health care, six points are important to be followed: first is the cleaning of surroundings, second is protection and handwashing habit adoption, third breath safe air by using a mask and respiratory hygiene, fourth is traveling safety, or following the travel safety rules, fifth is isolation strict if having symptoms similar to flu or feeling fever and last sixth one is arrangements of events and meetings by following all recommended safety instructions [56].

WHO published important information about the prevention and spread of the coronavirus. Safety measures and health-related rules were also provided by the European agency, which was supposed to be followed by all workers working in any working environment [57]. Other organizations like the Canadian center of health and international labor organization also emphasized following these safety rules. These safety measures include management of conformed cases, face mask, cleaning body parts, workplace guidelines, traveling, and meeting rules [55, 58]. No doubt, the previous experience of 2003 with SARS also helped prepare guidelines and policy for coronavirus. Most of the stress observed in workers was related to worries about the spread of pandemic among family members. Means people remain less worried about themselves as compared to their family. Furthermore, the public was also confused about their government policies for the control of COVID. Meanwhile, they were also not confident for health workers [59].

Personal hygiene and workplace safety were of significant importance for the control of COVID-19. For long-term management, social distancing and mask use was also reported critical with personal hygiene and safety workplace measures. Workplace safety may be divided into two groups. One of the first groups is micro safety (workplace safety measures and public health guidelines), and the second is macro safety (government or international policies). There is a need for stress management, reduced workload, social distancing, and guidelines related to protective measures and safety [48, 60]. Macro security includes adopting policies like accepting borders close, awareness not to hide travel history, work from home, use of face mask, and financial assistance. We can conclude that policies are fundamental for public health and to control COVID spread. Undoubtedly, policy implementation and awareness need some time for restructuring of cultures and organizations (duty hours and social activities) and reducing mental stress [61].

7.2.3 ANTIBODY TESTING

Antibody testing is another intervention; it was adopted as antibody testing on a large scale. The two reasons for the adoption and support of antibody testing are: the extent of infection, mortality rate, immunity period, strength, and the a-symptomatic people's details can be understood easily by antibody survey or testing [62–64]. Different countries have adopted this method, including China, so; others can have an epidemiological model and policies. The second reason is, this antibody testing activity supports the facilitation of the economy after lockups. The issues of immunity certificates may facilitate this. Some other researchers found some other reasons for the support of antibody testing on a large scale. These include: the vulnerable people and individuals without any symptoms have developed immunity or not, when is supported by antibody test, this also reduces socialization of those people, and the risk of transmission of infection is also reduced [65, 74].

Most people with low immunity levels or without imitating their state of health response to the pandemic. They do not bother the information regarding symptoms and do not believe that more than 50% of people are infected without showing signs [66, 35–38]. Those people are playing with the lives of their family and friends and harming all the community. Other than 50% of asymptomatic people, among healthy people, many shows mild symptoms. Even in France, the UK, and Spain, nearly 80% of people have been reported as immune and were not found infected or show any signs. Most people do not know what is there: they are immune, susceptible, or asymptomatic [45–48, 67, 75]. And vigorous antibody testing ends this uncertain situation, and each person can understand their health by the antibody presence. As the test reveals, either a man is immune or susceptible.

Similarly, a model was designed to check the relation of immunity with antibodies. The forecasted results showed that there might be different agents related to the lifetime with health care conditions [68, 69]. These agents may adopt social activity, which is directly related to social and economic concerns. Besides this, the selected model agents may be symptomatic, recovered, symptomatic, or may die. The vital point is that the susceptible will not contain antibodies against the virus, leading to the risk of viral infection. At the same time, the person with or without any symptoms may be able to spread the disease [70, 71].

7.3 IMPACT OF LOCKDOWN

The best strategy in controlling the spread of COVID remains lockdown, and after a strict lockdown, the smart lockdown was introduced. Many countries adopted different lockdowns, and many kinds of distancing were introduced. There was a positive effect of lockdown in controlling the spread of the coronavirus. No doubt, as there was no vaccine, social distancing and lockdown positively impacted transmission and spread measures [62, 72]. As we can understand, the first social distancing was adopted by the Chinese government. Many control measures were implemented to control the epidemic and, in the absence of any knowledge about this virus, remain successful. The traveling was also restricted with lockdown, which also helped control the spread of the virus intracity and intercity and likewise inter-country and nationwide [34, 62].

Lockdown remains successful in the pandemic spread, but it affected the public's customs, culture, behaviors, mental, and physical conditions (Figure 7.3). A complete lockdown was strictly followed by some relaxation strategies that helped release stress among the public. As the outside activities were not allowed, indoor games and activities adaptation also changed some traditions [63]. These lockdown strategies reduced or somewhat declined the spread and helped control corona, and scientists could get some time for the invention of a vaccine. There is a need for a strict policy for older adults as their immune response is weak. Likewise, with lockdown, there is a need for concentrated care units with all health care facilities. As the number of infected persons increases with the critical situation needing health care, the chances of death rate may exceed if the emergency health facilities are limited and the infected person remains unsuccessful in receiving appropriate care.

According to an estimation, the lockdown strategy reduced the chances of spread and transmission of the virus by nearly 90%. An overall decline in fossil fuel use also showed a positive effect on global warming [64]. What was needed to study the epidemic is a model that may be calibrated. National, international, and regional policies may be individualized, where primary and secondary stages of epidemic models may be related. This also illustrates the early stage and passage of epidemic operations in actual domain situations. All countries adopted a different degree of lockdown, but one challenge remains open for all the optimum or best degree of lockdown that a government may adopt.

These lockdown strategies also affected the economy of each country. Undoubtedly, underdeveloped or economically weak countries were strongly affected, but highly developed countries also faced economic loss [64]. It was also noted that after the release of lockdown, the infection rate increased, and the renewal of lockdown was adopted. This again outbreak was in some areas severe and sometimes more severe than the previous. There has been a non-trivial percentage of the resident public that suffered from infection, and after passing through it, there comes a recovered state. This remains uncertain that the recovered state with immunity may be momentary, like in response to seasonal flu or life long as in chickenpox. Different researchers remain able to model and present the impacts of lockdown in other cities of the world. These also reported and confirmed that restrictions in people's movement remain helpful in preventing virus spread and helped in control [22, 64].

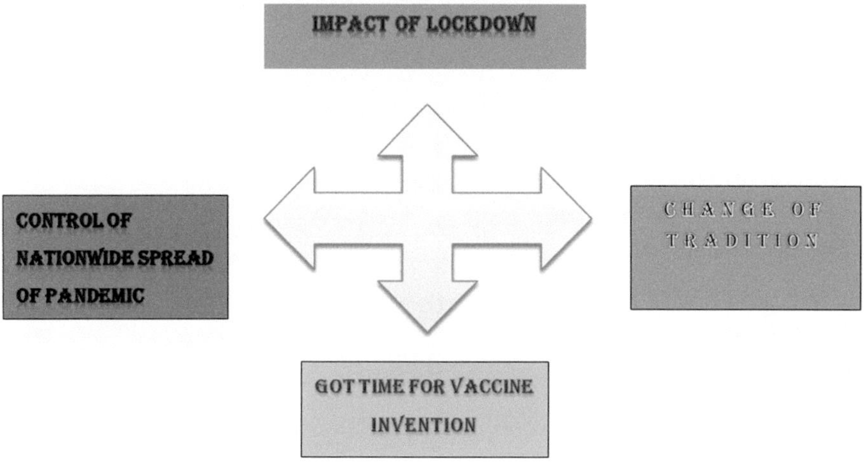

FIGURE 7.3 Impact of lockdown.

7.4 AFTER LOCKDOWN STRATEGIES

After controlling the spread of COVID by lockdown strategy, it was vital to plan further (Figure 7.4). What may be the best way which humanity may adopt after lockdown strategies? This was very important to adopt preventive measures and open workplaces to stop the collapse of any country's economy [65]. The first thing after the lockdown was a ban on mass gatherings. This was the way by which corona can become uncontrollable. After that, the next step was the education of the public to strictly follow the distancing of six feet, wear mask and hand wash. This was the best way globally corona spread, and the key factors were the reduction in new infections and cured of the disease [54, 66].

It was also noted that after the release of lockdown, the infection rate increased. So, the renewal of lockdown was adopted that made the outbreak severe in some areas and sometimes more severe than the previous. There has been a non-trivial percentage of the resident public that suffered from infection, and after passing through it, there comes a recovered state. It was also noted in many areas of world that after release of lockdown pandemic spread ratio was more than previous observations. To control that situation, again lock down strategy was necessary which created tension among people. But that tension was released after the reports of recovery This remains uncertain that the recovered state with immunity may be momentary, like in response to seasonal flu or life long as in chickenpox [66, 69].

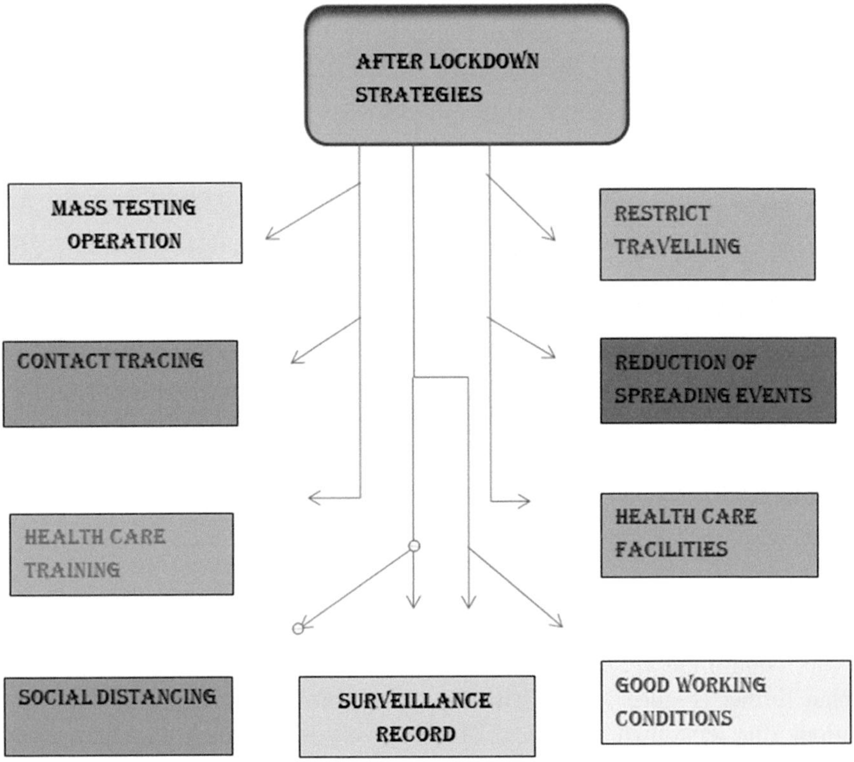

FIGURE 7.4 The best strategies after lockdown.

Many researchers worked to find evidence that physical distancing is effective in controlling the spread of COVID. Many other measures were also taken like school closure, work from home concept, social distancing, wearing a mask, bans on public gathering, traveling, and national events [35, 66]. Many countries take active steps, but some do not take it seriously. Many workers made models to establish relations with different events. Many researchers collected all data, worked with cases reported daily from other independent countries.

There is a need for a strict policy for older people as their immune response is weak. Likewise, with lockdown, there is a need for concentrated care units with all health care facilities. As the number of infected persons increases with the critical situation needing health care, the chances of death rate may exceed if the emergency health facilities are limited and the infected person remains unsuccessful in receiving appropriate care. However, we can say that exhibiting lockdown was not very difficult, and optimization maybe only for a period, not for intensity. But some people also try to use modeling of rigorous aptitude of care with different durations and strictness of lockdown. With all this, fatigue study was also critical, and the memories associated with pandemic, lockdown, and isolation also affect the lockdown efficiency.

Preferences of different policy adoption show the need difference, not the disagreeing with a specific policy. There is a need to analyze the reason for adopting a particular approach by talking with the government or authorities related to the generosity and unassuming nature [68, 70–72]. As the number of lockdowns, their length and strength are associated with disease and transfer rate intensity. Some people think that the lockdown is an ideal way out, and according to the degree of a pandemic, it may be adopted as smart, reinstituting, and a strict lockdown compared to the previous one. Hence, when a country adopts a lockdown strategy and goes towards the second phase, it does not prove anything about the failure of the previous one, or it may be wrong to criticize policymakers for the inability of lockdown [73, 74] as this is not the proof of the failure of policy.

7.4.1 AN OPTIMIZATION OF LOCKDOWN

Social distancing was introduced at the global level to control the spread of COVID-19. The control of corona was achieved by adopting lockdown and after lockdown strategies. After that, optimization of lockdown was required. There was a need for isolation and distancing to pledge COVID-19, which was adopted in different countries and remained successful. As the complete lockdown have adverse economic, psychological, and cultural effects. Smart lockdown, complete lockdown, and strict lockdown were introduced according to the situation, but optimization was necessary [45, 67].

This is important to optimize the lockdown timing, intensity, and duration so that its beneficial effects on health and the economy can be balanced. Without any doubt, we can reduce the disease spread and incidence by social distancing and interaction or mobility restriction. But it may also lead to the decline of prolific economic dimensions. Therefore, it is proposed to focus on minimizing two essential levels: the prevalence levels of pandemic and the reduction in productivity due to isolation policy [68]. All countries adopted a different degree of lockdown, but one challenge remains open for all the optimum or best degrees of lockdown that a country may adopt. To address this, a best optimum model to control was needed to design. The model may be a classic differential equation addressing the vulnerable to infested-recuperated conditions.

The disease's lethality depends on the instantaneous contagion types and the rate that serious overhaul measurements remain infested. Some necessary leeway is required to balance three deliberations: the first one is health (improvement in health and immunity-related to COVID and decrease in mortality), second is economy (overcome economic loss, unemployment, and decrease in financial loss), the third one is modification and regulation cost, i.e., effects of severe fluctuating lockdown intensities on the general public and occupational adaptation [67–70, 75].

A variety of work has been done to investigate the corona consequences and macroeconomic consequences. Many scientists have also determined optimal duration and intensity of lockdown and social distance, and they designed linear differential equations that may provide the outbreak early stages and disease dynamics. After the early stage, the guesstimate cannot be crescendos and may exclude the possibility of reasoned explanations. The epidemiology of each disease varies vastly, and the optimization of lockdown and social distancing remains possible by using numerical mockups. For example, the flu in changing seasons needed a strict distance policy compared to standard cold because the previous had a more significant infection rate [69].

With all necessary measures, contact reduction policies are required to be designed and strictly must be followed. Optimization of lockdown and following of SOPs will remain helpful in flattening the curve and help in amenability. Social isolation and distancing will be effective in lowering the number of cases, public health and will moderate the adverse effects of isolation. Commonly adopted social distancing includes restriction of public gatherings, events, education place closure, limited transportation, and physical contacts [67–69]. Different researchers also proposed that the decline in infected cases is possible by networking of inter-personal contacts with management and optimization.

7.5 MACROECONOMICS AND LOCKDOWN

The work and literature related to COVID-19 and its effects on the economy coupled to change in social behavior and lockdown are developing. Although there is still a need for more investigation, the literature does not provide sufficient data regarding optimization, timing, extent, strength, length, and duration of lockdown. Some researchers designed a simple epidemiological model to find the optimal intensity and time of lockdown with the effect on macro-economy and health consequences [71–73]. At the same time, some used the standard model and focused on the fractions of the community facing lockdown. This traditional model was derived both without and with control variables as the lockdown was started after a week of disease occurrence and was released nearly one month later. Test for COVID-19 and lockdown strategies are interrelated, resulting in an average lockdown, which is also connected with epidemiology [74].

The COVID-19 has recently prompted the sympathetic communal associations of disease with health, macro-economy, and outcomes. This disease has proved itself a highly infectious viral disease that can be transmitted through close contacts with objects carrying virus, droplets, contacts between infective animals or people and infectors. Scientists and researchers have also not tried to focus on macro-economic implications [35, 73]. The chaos may probably be created by cracks in health risks and economic inter relationships during epidemics. There are both short and long-run effects of epidemics on the economy.

Some researchers also analyzed the impact of social distancing and locking down on the rate of infections. Their work helped in finding the relationship between immune systems, death rate, and infected groups. This work and literature also help minimize the fatality within the population and its economic cost. These are also crucial in finding different lockdown conditions for other people belonging to a different sex, age, and work types. So, lockdown may be different for students, health workers, housekeepers, labors, kids, young, old, middle-aged people. According to this hypothesis, different preventive measures may perform differentially, leaving behind the concept of uniform policies [72–74].

Still, what is needed is to find the treatment and preventive measures policies efficiency. The testing and lockdown are both linked with the epidemiology of outbreak as the recovered population with time increases, the amplification of lockdown shrinks, and the recovered people may also be quarantined or lockdown. When a state adopts lockdown and the economy of that country also is shut down, meta-observation can be seen. The trade-off value becomes complex, and state dynamics also become complex [69–73, 75]. As we hope COVID-19 will be the last pandemic in our life, the analysis is done using different models and is inspired by corona. There are some tensions related to the outbreak, and also some considerations and adoption are the innovation of the pandemic duration. We can deal by adopting these not only during current crises but also for humans prepared for the future.

7.6 CONCLUSION

The best strategy in controlling the spread of COVID remains lockdown, and after a strict lockdown, the smart lockdown was introduced that was also proved to be a good strategy. Many countries adopted different lockdowns, and any distancing was introduced. There was a positive effect of lockdown in controlling the spread of coronavirus. So we can say that three deliberations are needed to be balanced which are health improvement (strong immune population), improvement in finances and the last one is modified adaptations during different lockdown intensities. There is need of creation of some models on which basis, policy can also be characterized. All these process can be assisted by social planning and welfare. Experiences also showed that such models will also be useful in finding the optimum intensity of lockdown. But no doubt personal immunity of each person varies. So, we cannot say that once a person if get recovered will remain immune in future. This statement was also proved by different observations and data according to which after recovery people were again infected and even died. Social planning is most important prospect that can help in fight against corona. During this fight, the main issues were related to economy as a person cannot stay at home and may not have enough savings to consume. This issue is more prominent in low income or underdeveloped countries. There are some other problems also which need to be addressed like regulations for public safety, government rules and policies, changing behavior.

No doubt, as there was no vaccine, social distancing and lockdown positively impacted transmission and spread measures.

KEYWORDS

- **contact tracing**
- **epidemiology**
- **global warming**
- **health care**
- **lockdown**
- **quarantine**
- **World Health Organization**

REFERENCES

1. Ahmed, F., Zviedrite, N., & Uzicanin, A., (2018). Effectiveness of workplace social distancing measures in reducing influenza transmission: A systematic review. *BMC Public Health, 18*, 518.
2. Al-Najjar, H., Al-Rousan, N., Al-Najjar, D., Assous, H. F., & Al-Najjar, D., (2021). Impact of COVID-19 pandemic virus on G8 countries' financial indices based on artificial neural network. *Journal of Chinese Economic and Foreign Trade Studies, 14*(1), 89–103. doi.org/10.1108/JCEFTS-06-2020-0025.
3. Deng, S. Q., & Peng, H. J., (2020). Characteristics of and public health responses to the coronavirus disease 2019 outbreak in China. *Clinical Medicine*, 9.
4. World Health Organization, (WHO). *Coronavirus Disease (COVID-2019) Situation Reports-88*. Available at: https://www.who.int/news-room/feature-stories/detail/more-backing-for-who-to-counter-the-pandemic-across-the-world (accessed on 24 August 2021).
5. *The Central People's Government of the People's Republic of China*. Available at: http://www.gov.cn/xinwen/2020-01/22/content_5471437.htm (accessed on 6 August 2021).
6. Guan, W. J., Ni, Z. Y., & Hu, Y., et al., (2020). Clinical characteristics of Coronavirus disease 2019 in China. *The New England Journal of Medicine*.
7. Yang, Y., Lu, Q., & Liu, M., et al., (2020). *Epidemiological and Clinical Features of the 2019 Novel Coronavirus Outbreak in China.* medRxiv 2020:2020.02.10.20021675.
8. Kretzschmar, M. E., Rozhnova, G., & Van, B. M. E., (2020). *Isolation and Contact Tracing Can Tip the Scale to Containment of COVID-19 in Populations with Social Distancing*. medRxiv 2020:2020.03.10.20033738.
9. Zhou, X., Wu, Z., & Yu, R., et al., (2020). *Modeling-Based Evaluation of the Effect of Quarantine Control by the Chinese Government in the Coronavirus Disease 2019 Outbreak*. medRxiv 2020:2020.03.03.20030445.
10. Liu, K., Ai, S., & Song, S., et al., (2020). *Population Movement, City Closure in Wuhan and Geographical Expansion of the 2019-nCoV Pneumonia Infection in China, 71*(16), 2045–2051. doi: 10.1093/cid/ciaa422.
11. National Health Commission of the People's Republic of China and National Administration of Traditional Chinese Medicine. *The National Clinical guidelines for COVID-19* (6th edn.). At http://www.nhc.gov.cn/xcs/zhengcwj/202002/8334a8326dd94d329df351d7da8aefc2.shtml (accessed on 6 August 2021).
12. Viboud, C., Bjørnstad, O. N., Smith, D. L., Simonsen, L., Miller, M. A., & Grenfell, B. T., (2006). Synchrony, waves, and spatial hierarchies in the spread of influenza. *Science, 312*, 447–451. New York, NY.
13. Huang, C., Wang, Y., & Li, X., et al., (2020). Clinical features of patients infected with 2019 novel coronavirus in Wuhan, China. *Lancet, 395*, 497–506.
14. Adhanom, T., (2020). *WHO Director-General's Opening Remarks at the Media Briefing on COVID-19.* https://www.who.int/dg/speeches/detail/who-director-general-s-opening-remarks-at-the-media-briefing-on-covid-19---11-march-2020 (accessed on 6 August 2021).
15. Jonathan, P. C., Dieter, G., Gustav, F., Richard, F. H., Peter, M. K., Alexia, P., Andrea, S., & Stefan, W., (2021). The optimal lockdown intensity for COVID-19. *Journal of Mathematical Economics, 93*, 102489. https://doi.org/10.1016/j.jmateco.2021.102489.
16. Jackson, C., Vynnycky, E., Hawker, J., Olowokure, B., & Mangtani, P., (2013). School closures and influenza: Systematic review of epidemiological studies. *BMJ Open, 3*(2).

17. Ahmed, F., Zviedrite, N., & Uzicanin, A., (2018). Effectiveness of workplace social distancing measures in reducing influenza transmission: A systematic review. *BMC Public Health, 18*(1), 518.
18. Soumyajyoti, B., & Amit, K. M., (2021). Parallel Minority Game and its application in movement optimization during an epidemic. *Physica A, 561*, 125271. https://doi.org/10.1016/j.physa.2020.125271.
19. Hatchett, R. J., Mecher, C. E., & Lipsitch, M., (2007). Public health interventions and epidemic intensity during the 1918 influenza pandemic. *Proc. Nat. Acad. Sci. USA, 104*, 7582–7587.
20. Arastoo, N., Domenik, P., Cornelia, D., Sebastian, A., Alexandru, M., Stefan, H., & Harald, K. W., (2021). *Impact of Lockdown During the COVID-19 Pandemic on Number of Patients and Patterns of Injuries at a Level I Trauma Center, 133*(7, 8), 336–343. doi: 10.1007/s00508–021–01824-z.
21. Jackson, C., Mangtani, P., Fine, P., & Vynnycky, E., (2014). The effects of school holidays on transmission of varicella-zoster virus, England and Wales, 1967–2008. *PLoS One, 9*, e99762.
22. Ciavarella, C., Fumanelli, L., Merler, S., Cattuto, C., & Ajelli, M., (2016). School closure policies at municipality level for mitigating influenza spread: A model-based evaluation. *BMC Infect. Diseases, 16*, 576.
23. Wells, C. R., Sah, P., & Moghadas, S. M., et al., (2020). Impact of international travel and border control measures on the global spread of the novel 2019 coronavirus outbreak. *Proc. Nat. Acad. Sci. USA, 117*, 7504–7509.
24. Wicklin, R., (2020). *Estimates of Doubling Time for Exponential Growth*. https://blogs.sas.com/content/iml/2020/04/01/estimate-doubling-time-exponential-growth.html (accessed on 6 August 2021).
25. Ritchie, H., & Roser, M., (2019). *Gender Ratio*. https://ourworldindata.org/gender-ratio (accessed on 6 August 2021).
26. World Population, (2020). https://countrymeters.info/en/World (accessed on 6 August 2021).
27. Mills, K. T., Bundy, J. D., & Kelly, T. N., et al., (2016). Global disparities of hypertension prevalence and control: A systematic analysis of population-based studies from 90 countries. *Circulation, 134*, 441–450.
28. Luís, G., (2021). Antibody tests: They are more important than we thought. *Journal of Mathematical Economics, 93,* 102485. https://doi.org/10.1016/j.jmateco.2021.102485.
29. Ward, A., (2020). *Sweden's Government has Tried a Risky Coronavirus Strategy; It Could Backfire.* https://www.vox.com/2020/4/9/21213472/coronavirus-sweden-herd-immunity-cases-death (accessed on 6 August 2021).
30. Kaplan, J., Frias, L., & McFall-Johnsen, M., (2020). *A Third of the Global Population is on Coronavirus Lockdown—Here's Our Constantly Updated List of Countries Locking Down and Opening Up.* https://www.businessinsider.com/countries-on-lockdown-coronavirus-italy-2020-3#many-countries-have-also-closed-borders-to-prevent-international-travelers-from-spreading-the-virus-35 (accessed on 6 August 2021).
31. Crimmins, E. M., & Beltran-Sanchez, H., (2011). Mortality and morbidity trends: Is there compression of morbidity? *The Journal of Gerontology: Series B, Psychological Sciences and Social Sciences, 66,* 75–86.
32. Lewnard, J. A., & Lo, N. C., (2020). Scientific and ethical basis for social-distancing interventions against COVID-19. *Lancet Infectious Diseases, 20*(6), 631–633.

33. Prem, K., Liu, Y., & Russell, T. W., et al., (2020). The effect of control strategies to reduce social mixing on outcomes of the COVID-19 epidemic in Wuhan, China: A modeling study. *Lancet Public Health.*
34. Guan, W. J., Liang, W. H., & Zhao, Y., et al., (2020). Comorbidity and its impact on 1590 patients with Covid-19 in China: A nationwide analysis. *European Respiratory Journal, 55*, 2000547. 10.1183/13993003.00547-2020.
35. CDC COVID-19 Response Team, (2020). Severe outcomes among patients with Coronavirus disease 2019 (COVID-19)-United States. *Morbidity and Mortality Weekly Report, 69.*
36. Cabrera, J. M. L., & Kurmanaev, A., (2020). *Ecuador Gives Glimpse into Pandemic's Impact on Latin America*. https://www.nytimes.com/2020/04/08/world/americas/ecuador-coronavirus.html (accessed on 6 August 2021).
37. Roy, A., & Kalra, A., (2020). *Three Private Hospitals in South Mumbai Close to New Patients Amid Coronavirus Scare*. https://www.reuters.com/article/health-coronavirus-india-hospital/three-private-hospitals-in-south-mumbai-close-to-new-patients-amid-coronavirus-scare-idUSL3N2BX3BQ (accessed on 6 August 2021).
38. Saintvilus, R., (2020). *Coronavirus Market Volatility: Have We Reached the Bottom?* Nasdaq.
39. Cohen, P., & Hsu, T., (2020). *'Sudden Black Hole' for the Economy with Millions More Unemployed.* The New York Times.
40. Corkery, M., & Yaffe-Bellany, D., (2020). *U.S. Food Supply Chain Is Strained as Virus Spreads*. The New York Times.
41. Shah, J., Karimzadeh, S., Al-Ahdal, T. M. A., Mousavi, S. H., Zahid, S. U., & Huy, N. T., (2020). COVID-19: The current situation in Afghanistan. *Lancet Glob Health, 8*, E771–772.
42. Guled, A., & Nor, M. S., (2020). *In Somalia, Coronavirus Goes from Fairy Tale to Nightmare*. The Associated Press.
43. Ofner-Agostini, M., Wallington, T., & Henry, B., et al., (2008). Investigation of the second wave (phase 2) of severe acute respiratory syndrome (SARS) in Toronto, Canada. What happened? *Canada Communicable Disease Report, 34*, 1–11.
44. Walker, P., Whittaker, C., Watser, O., Baguelin, M., Ainslie, K., & Bhatia, S., et al., (2020). *The Global Impact of COVID-19 and Strategies for Mitigation and Suppression.* Imperial College London. doi: https://doi.org/10.25561/77735.
45. Makoni, M., (2020). Africa prepares for coronavirus. *The Lancet, 395*, 483. doi: https://doi.org/10.1016/S0140-6736(20)30355-X.
46. Ionnidis, J. P., (2020). Coronavirus disease 2019: The harms of exaggerated information and nonevidence-based measures. *European Journal of Clinical Investigation, 50*(4). doi: https://doi.org/10.1111/eci.13223.
47. Vigdor, N., (2020). *Man Fatally Poisons Himself While Self-Medicating for Coronavirus, Doctor Says*. The New York Times.
48. Ezeh, A., Oyebode, O., Satterthwaite, D., Chen, Y., Ndugwa, R., & Sartori, J., et al., (2017). The history, geography, and sociology of slums and the health problems of people who live in slums. *The Lancet, 389*, 547–558. doi: https://doi.org/10.1016/S0140-6736(16)31650-6.
49. Johnstone-Robertson, S., Mark, D., Morrow, C., Middelkoop, K., Chiswell, M., & Aquino, L., et al., (2011). Social mixing patterns within a South African township community: Implications for respiratory disease transmission and control. *American Journal of Epidemiology, 174*, 1246–1255. doi: https://doi.org/10.1093/aje/kwr251.

50. Waroux, O. L. P., Cohuet, S., Ndazima, D., Kucharski, A., Juan-Giner, A., & Flasche, S., et al., (2018). Characteristics of human encounters and social mixing patterns relevant to infectious diseases spread by close contact: A survey in Southwest Uganda. *BMC Infectious Diseases, 18*. doi: https://doi.org/10.1186/s12879-018-3073-1.
51. Winter, S., Dzombo, M., & Barchi, F., (2019). Exploring the complex relationship between women's sanitation practices and household diarrhea in the slums of Nairobi: A cross-sectional study. *BMC Infectious Diseases, 19*(242). doi: https://doi.org/10.1186/s12879-019-3875-9.
52. Snyder, R., Boone, C., Cardoso, C. A., Aguiar-Alves, F., Neves, F., & Riley, L., (2017). Zika: A scourge in urban slums. *PLoS Neglected Tropical Diseases, 11*(3). doi: https://doi.org/10.1371/journal.pntd.0005287.
53. Borges, A., Moreau, C., Burke, A., Santos, O. D., & Chofakian, C., (2018). Women's reproductive health knowledge, attitudes and practices in relation to the Zika virus outbreak in northeast Brazil. *PLoS One, 13*(1). doi: https://doi.org/10.1371/journal.pone.0190024.
54. Wolf, M., Serper, M., Opsasnick, L., O'Conor, R., Curtis, L., & Benavente, J., et al., (2020). Awareness, attitudes, and actions related to COVID-19 among adults with chronic conditions at the onset of the US outbreak: A cross-sectional survey. *Annals of Internal Medicine*. doi: 10.7326/M20-1239.
55. Zhong, B., Luo, W., Li, H., Zhang, Q., Liu, X., & Li, W., et al., (2020). Knowledge, attitudes, and practices towards COVID-19 among Chinese residents during the rapid rise period of the COVID-19 outbreak: A quick online cross-sectional survey. *International Journal of Biological Sciences, 16*(10), 1745–1752. doi: 10.7150/ijbs.45221.
56. Geldsetzer, P., (2020). Knowledge and perceptions of COVID-19 among the general public in the United States and the United Kingdom: A cross-sectional online survey. *Annals of Internal Medicine*. doi: 10.7326/M20-0912.
57. Wu, Z., & McGoogan, J., (2020). Characteristics of and important lessons from the Coronavirus disease 2019 (COVID-19) outbreak in China. *JAMA Network, 323*, 1239–1242. doi: 10.1001/jama.2020.2648.
58. Chou, W., Oh, A., & Klein, W., (2020). Addressing health-related misinformation on social media. *JAMA, 320*, 2417–2418. doi: doi: 10.1001/jama.2018.16865.
59. Tidwell, J., Gopalakrishnan, A., Lovelady, S., Sheth, E., Unni, A., & Wright, R., et al., (2019). Effect of two complementary mass-scale media interventions on handwashing with soap among mothers. *Journal of Health Communication,* 1–13. doi: 10.1080/10810730.2019.1593554.
60. Fehr, A. R., & Perlman, S., (2015). Coronaviruses: An overview of their replication and pathogenesis. *Methods Mol. Biol., 1282*, 1–23. doi: 10.1007/978-1-4939-2438-7_1.
61. Lu, H., Stratton, C. W., & Tang, Y. W., (2020). The Wuhan SARS-CoV-2 - what's next for China [published online ahead of print, 2020 March 1]. *J. Medical Virology*. doi: 10.1002/jmv.25738.
62. Rothan, H. A., & Byrareddy, S. N., (2020). The epidemiology and pathogenesis of coronavirus disease (COVID-19) outbreak [published online ahead of print, 2020 Feb. 26]. *J. Autoimmun.*, 102433. doi: 10.1016/j.jaut.2020.102433.
63. Tang, B., Bragazzi, N. L., Li, Q., Tang, S., Xiao, Y., & Wu, J., (2020). An updated estimation of the risk of transmission of the novel coronavirus (2019-nCov). *Infectious Diseases Modeling, 5*, 248–255. doi: 10.1016/j.idm.2020.02.001.

64. Mouchtouri, V. A., Christoforidou, E. P., & An Der, H. M., et al., (2019). Exit and entry screening practices for infectious diseases among travelers at points of entry: Looking for evidence on public health impact. *International J. Environ. Res. Public Health, 16*, 4638. doi: 10.3390/ijerph16234638.
65. Tang, S., Tang, B., & Bragazzi, N. L., et al., (2020). Analysis of COVID-19 epidemic traced data and stochastic discrete transmission dynamic model (in Chinese). *Science China Mathematics, 50,* 1–16.
66. Special Expert Group for Control of the Epidemic of Novel Coronavirus Pneumonia of the Chinese Preventive Medicine Association, (2020). The Chinese Preventive Medicine Association. An update on the epidemiological characteristics of novel coronavirus pneumonia (COVID-19). *Chinese Journal of Epidemiology, 41*, 139–144.
67. Kong, I., Park, Y., Woo, Y., Lee, J., Cha, J., & Choi, J., et al., (2020). Early epidemiological and clinical characteristics of 28 cases of coronavirus disease in South Korea. *Osong Public Heal. Res. Perspect., 11*(1), 8–14.
68. Qiu, H., Wu, J., Hong, L., Luo, Y., Song, Q., & Chen, D., (2020). Clinical and epidemiological features of 36 children with coronavirus disease 2019 (COVID-19) in Zhejiang, China: An observational cohort study. *Lancet Infectious Diseases-2019*, 1–8. http://www.sciencedirect.com/science/article/pii/S1473309920301985 (accessed on 6 August 2021).
69. Verity, R., Okell, L. C., Dorigatti, I., Winskill, P., Whittaker, C., & Imai, N., et al., (2020). Estimates of the severity of coronavirus disease 2019: A model-based analysis. *Lancet Infectious Diseases, 3099*(20), 1–9.
70. Russell, T. W., Hellewell, J., & Jarvis, C. I., et al., (2020). Estimating the infection and case fatality ratio for coronavirus disease (COVID-19) using age-adjusted data from the outbreak on the Diamond Princess cruise ship. *Euro Surveillance, 25*(12), pii=2000256. https://doi.org/10.2807/1560-7917.ES.2020.25.12.2000256.
71. Bernal, J. L., Cummins, S., & Gasparrini, A., (2017). Interrupted time series regression for the evaluation of public health interventions: A tutorial. *International Journal of Epidemiology, 46*, 348–355.
72. Samantha, K. B., Rebecca, K. W., Louise, E. S., Lisa, W., Simon, W., Neil, G., & Gideon, J. R., (2020). The psychological impact of quarantine and how to reduce it: Rapid review of the evidence. *The Lancet, 395*, 912–920. doi: https://doi.org/10.1016/S0140-6736(20)30460-8.
73. Davide, L. T., Danilo, L., & Simone, M., (2021). Epidemics and macroeconomic outcomes: Social distancing intensity and duration. *Journal of Mathematical Economics, 93*, 102473. https://doi.org/10.1016/j.jmateco.2021.102473.
74. Simon, L., & Ellen, V. M., (2021). Road to recovery: Managing an epidemic. *Journal of Mathematical Economics, 93*, 102482. https://doi.org/10.1016/j.jmateco.2021.102482.
75. Aditya, G., Lin, L., & Manh-Hung, N., (2021). SIR economic epidemiological models with disease induced mortality. *Journal of Mathematical Economics, 93*, 102476. https://doi.org/10.1016/j.jmateco.2021.102476.

CHAPTER 8

Vaccines Against COVID-19

MAJID KHAN,[1] MUHAMMAD FAHEEM,[2] NAJMUR RAHMAN,[1] RIZWAN AHMAD,[3] M. ZIA-UL-HAQ,[4] and MUHAMMAD RIAZ[1]

[1]*Department of Pharmacy, Shaheed Benazir Bhutto University, Sheringal, Pakistan, E-mail: pharmariaz@gmail.com (M. Riaz)*

[2]*Department of Pharmacy, University of Swabi Anbar, Pakistan*

[3]*Natural Products and Alternative Medicines, College of Clinical Pharmacy, Imam Abdulrahman Bin Faisal University, Dammam, Kingdom of Saudi Arabia*

[4]*Office of Research, Innovation and Commercialization, Lahore College for Women University, Lahore–54000, Pakistan*

ABSTRACT

The disastrous effects of COVID-19 on health, education, and economy prompt for the development of an effective vaccine candidate in order to this global issue. The vaccine candidature against COVID-19 depends on the virus spike (S) protein engrained with the property of pathogenicity. Previously, a number of vaccines have been developed utilizing the envelope (E) protein, nucleocapsid (N) protein, and the non-structural proteins. The imminent vaccine candidates for COVID-19 may be divided into 10 types: mRNA-based, DNA, viral vector-based, subunit protein-based, inactivated whole virus (IWVV), replicating/non-replicating, live attenuated (LAV), VVr + Antigen-presenting cell, and VVnr + Antigen-presenting cell vaccines. This literature work exclusively discusses the available vaccine platforms and candidates' status, pandemic progress, targets, and challenges in vaccine development, the proposed designs in the pipeline (pre-clinical and clinical trials with ethical principles), and global access to COVID-19 vaccines. The traditional/classical versus vaccine candidates for COVID-19 is also a part of the intensive discussion.

8.1 INTRODUCTION

Vaccines are biological preparations to enhance the acquired immunity against particular diseases/infections. Vaccines are prepared either from attenuated/killed microorganisms or their specific parts administered into the body to stimulate an individual's immune system. Vaccine is derived from the Latin word "Vacca," which means "cow," referring to the first-ever smallpox vaccine introduced by British scientist Edward Jenner after the colossal death toll in 1796 [1]. In 1980, a successful eradication for smallpox was achieved due to the vaccine's therapeutic power as reported by WHO. The Jenner concept was further adopted for numerous diseases like polio, mumps, measles, whooping cough, rubella, tetanus, yellow fever, typhoid, hepatitis B, etc. [2].

The vaccine has splendid therapeutic potential in low doses with a high safety profile. The basic sources for vaccine development are the killed or attenuated forms of bacteria and viruses. Mechanistically when vaccines are administered to the body in later life, the body's immune system will identify and kill the pathogens. During the immunity developing process, the body generates antibodies against a particular type of microorganisms that create a defense system. These antibodies defy the system when microorganisms attack next time, thus preventing the disease known as prophylaxis. Vaccines are more economical therapeutic agents for protection against deadly diseases. Studies showed that vaccines are much better affordable therapeutic agents [3]. The importance of vaccines may be realized from the global mortality rate of malaria, AIDS, and tuberculosis due to lack of any vaccine [4, 5]. The death rate was further raised when the deadly virus CORONA appeared in Wuhan, China during December 2019, named COVID-19. It was declared as the first-generation virus because of its association with human to animal transmission [6]. It was January, 2020 where the second generation of virus with transmission from human to human was confirmed, followed by a third and fourth generations, recently identified on February 4 and thus declared a pandemic by "WHO." In the initial stage, the virus's transmission was highly crucial to restrict the spread but uncontrolled due to a lack of scientist's quick response, knowledge, and controlling manner [7].

Coronavirus, a single positive-stranded (RNA) virus belongs to coronaviridae. Numerous fatal coronavirus cases have been reported, including middle east respiratory syndrome (MERS), severe acute respiratory syndrome (SARS), and the recently COVID-19. The history of dates back to the 1960s where it was considered a common cold virus till an outbreak occurred in 2002 (Guangdong province, China), which quickly escalated worldwide. The causative agent for an episode of the common cold in Saudi Arabia in 2012 was identified as coronavirus and subsided with several deaths. Due to the heavy toll of deaths in the COVID-19 pandemic, apart from other treatment alternatives [8, 9], vaccines' master role in disease prevention cannot be overlooked. Various projects are underway for an effective vaccine candidate [10, 11], and few of the vaccine's studies are in clinical Phases however, a number of challenges still exist. An effective and secure vaccine product is utmost necessary to alleviate the negative effects of current COVID-19 pandemic. Presently, eight primary forms of COVID-19 vaccines are under development which include DNA-based, RNA-based, viral-like particles VLP, live attenuated, non-replicated, replicated, subunit, inactivated, VVr + antigen-presenting cell (APC), and VVnr + APC vaccines as shown in Figure 8.1 [12, 13].

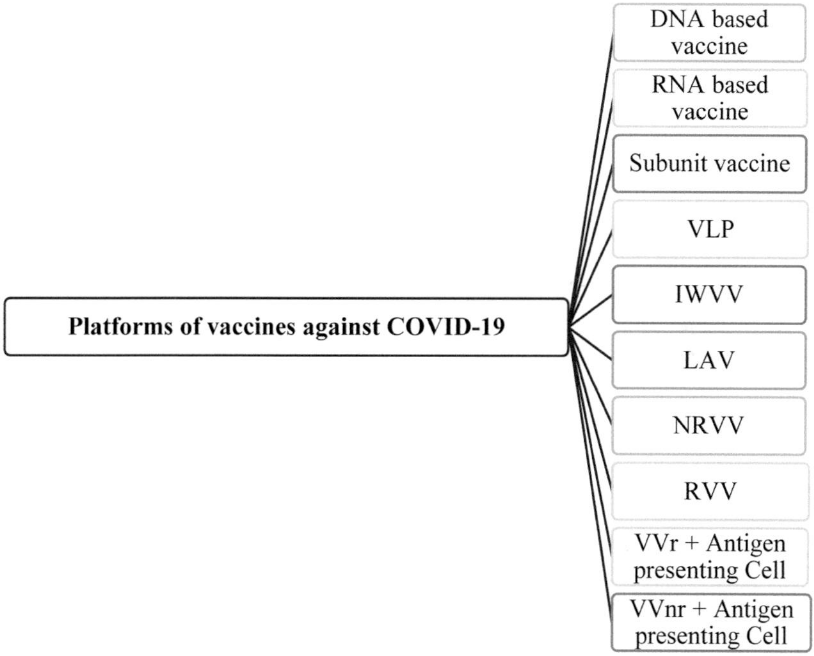

FIGURE 8.1 Platforms of the vaccine against COVID-19.

8.1.1 TYPES OF VACCINES

8.1.1.1 DNA BASED VACCINES

Scientists mainly target the synthetic DNA vaccines by targeting Spike (Protein) of MERS coronavirus. The S portion is the major antigen at the surface for a clinical study. Synthetic DNA based vaccine also targets the S protein of SARS-CoV-2 as reported in mice and guinea pigs where the results showed a binding between Spike (S) protein with ACE2 receptor and targeting antibodies in the lungs. This type of vaccine was immediately designed on January 11, 2020. The expression of the DNA vaccine candidate's immunogenicity was determined in several animal models and mice utilized for humoral and T cell responses where S protein binding to ACE2 was noted [14]. This type of vaccine comprises of the plasmid encoding immunogens and usually shows a direct access into the host cells via injection, electroporation, and/or gene gun. DNA vaccines are considered superior in two ways over protein-based or subunit vaccine, i.e., ease of manipulation and being economical. The main target for DNA vaccines is the S-proteins of coronavirus, neutralizing the antibodies with an improved cell-mediated immunity in camels, macaques, and mice. There are three DNA-based candidate vaccines currently in clinical trials under the supervision of GeneOne Life Science, Korea. The Phase-I clinical studies have been conducted to evaluate the safety of healthy volunteers with success in the Walter Reed Army Institute of Research (WRAIR), US NIH. Currently, phase I and II clinical trials are underway in the Korean International Vaccine Institute to validate the immunogenicity, safety, and efficacy of GLS-5300 by using an electroporation device [15]. The experiment showed that the DNAs encoding the spike S-proteins (mostly S1) were neutralizing antibodies in corona strains of both camel and human origins. The S-domain is considered more superior to the full-length S-protein. A potential risk with less probability in this type of vaccine is spontaneous plasmid integration into host genomes [15].

8.1.1.2 mRNA-BASED VACCINE

The messenger RNA-based vaccines are considered quickly developing tools to alleviate infectious diseases. This type of vaccine contains mRNAs encoding which are translated by vaccination into the host cellular machinery. mRNA-vaccines are more advantageous over traditional vaccines due to lack of genome integration, modification of immune reactions, fast development, and the presence of multimeric antigens. Moderna commenced clinical trials for messenger RNA vaccines encoded with viral S-proteins of the SARS. This study was financed by the National Institute of Allergy and Infectious Diseases (NIAID). A cell culture system is used for the manufacturing of these vaccines. Moderna mRNA type of vaccine is manufactured in-silico for potential quick development and high efficacy. Moderna phase I study was supported by CEPI [14].

8.1.1.3 SUBUNIT VACCINE

Subunit vaccines present the safest profile compared to currently available vaccines due to their fewer immunogenicities. The developer should be highly vigilant in developing this type of spiked-based protein vaccine in order to prevent the production of non-neutralizing antibodies which contribute to undesirable pathological consequences. Subunit vaccines' safety and effectiveness with numerous conformational neutralizing epitopes, imparts it the property of being a promising candidate for developing the COVID-19 vaccine over full length S-proteins [15].

Generally, these S-domain-based vaccines necessitate a conjunction or adjuvant with an immune-activator to increase the immunogenicity. Numerous studies in mice purports that fusion in vaccinated mice showed a potent systemic neutralizing antibody along with a cellular immune response. Interestingly, smallpox was the first eradicative vaccine produced via subunit concept [12, 16, 17]. Moreover, the pipelined projects for successful immunization plan against COVID-19 are mostly based on subunit protein vaccine [18]. The comparative advantages subunit vaccine is the safety, lesser adversities, potentiating immune system with enhanced T-cell immune response, high titer of neutralizing antibodies with lack of prone of immune system to auxiliary viruses. The Clover Biopharmaceuticals and the University of Queensland have utilized GSK's adjuvant protocol and on the clinical studies for subunit vaccines are in in-continuation [18, 19].

8.1.1.4 VIRUS-LIKE PROTEIN (VLP) BASED VACCINE

This type of vaccine is similar to the native virus but deficient in pathogenic genetic materials. These vaccines are comprised of repetitive viral structures (proteins) with intrinsic self-assembly properties and may be produced via expression of the structural proteins of the virus in a desirable expression system. VLPs vaccines resembles IWV, i.e., to alter the viral protein's immunogenicity and antigenicity however, VLPs may be produced in in a less-restraint manufacturing conditions. VLPs are involved in expressing the E, S, and M proteins of COVID-19. This type of vaccine is observed indistinguishable under an electron microscope from the genuine viral particle. The research on immune response in rodents indicated an excellent response of antibodies for these agents in the presence of adjuvants like alum. A significantly higher titer of neutralizing antibodies was observed [15].

8.1.1.5 INACTIVATED WHOLE VIRUS VACCINE (IWVV)

Inactivated whole virus vaccine (IWVV) are developed from physical or chemically inactivation of the pathogenic virion. The IWVV offers various advantages of relatively low production cost, less laborious genetic manipulation, and a good safety profile [16] however, the production of IWVV requires a fully grown (peak level) live virus, and the antigenicity may alter during inactivation step of the virus [20]. IWV can be combined with alum like adjuvants to enhance immunity against COVID-19. This reveals the compatibility of such vaccines with adjuvants, but the challenge of hypersensitivity-type lung immunopathologic reactions is associated with it [21].

Currently, four main types of IWVV vaccines are under clinical trials: Sinovac (i); Sinopharm (ii); and Institute of Medical Biology (Chinese Academy of Medical Sciences) (iii) [18].

8.1.1.6 LIVE ATTENUATED VACCINE (LAV)

Live attenuated vaccines LAV is a highly effective vaccine that may persuade an immunity similar to natural immunity. LAV are developed through the removal of virulence genes using reverse genetic tool. LAV are highly immunogenic, no adjuvant is required for optimal efficacy, and a single-dose immunization is achieved however, still few serious risks of reversion to virulent strain, the need for a cold chain, unsuitable for infants/geriatric/, and immunocompromised population do exist [22]. The vaccine was introduced by removing the E-gene for absence of infectivity, and replication occurs in a single cycle. The biosafety problems are also associated with live attenuated vaccines due to reversion risk, thus need a safe alternative. Currently, there are many LAVs in pre-clinical trials [15, 18].

8.1.1.7 NON-REPLICATED VIRAL VACCINE (NRVV)

NRVV vectors are the modern approach for developing vaccines, targeting the mucosal inductive sites. NRVV is stable both, physically and genetically; no integration is possible and are considered safe. NRVV is non-pathogenic, high immunogenic, and resistant to acids. Such vaccines are produced more nowadays, and approximately four candidates are in the clinical trials stage by AstraZeneca, CanSino Biological Inc, Gamaleya Research Institute, and Janssen Pharmaceuticals. The main drawbacks associated with NRVV are the applications of high doses for potent immunity and obstacles in production [18, 23].

8.1.1.8 REPLICATED VIRAL VACCINE (RVV)

RVV vectors is a novel, rare approach in vaccine's development for COVID-19. The distinct feature for such vaccine's includes low dose, induction of persistent immunity, and safe via oral route along with a genetically stable and excellent immunogenicity in smallpox history. No integration is required and they are conveniently produced. Currently, Institute Pasteur/Them is conducting clinical studies on RVV against COVID-19. Yet again, RVV poses safety concerns and are potentially neurovirulent [18, 23]. VVr + Antigen-presenting Cell and VVnr + Antigen-presenting Cell are rare types of vaccines nowadays.

8.2 VACCINE PLATFORMS

The development and manufacturing of SARs vaccines were principally focusing the Spike protein of coronavirus. In the recent era, the subunit vaccine got a wide attention for developing vaccines against COVID-19, mainly focusing on S protein and RBD produced in heterologous expression systems [24, 25].

At the latest, World Health Organization (WHO) reported 87 vaccine candidates in human trials consisting of; DNA (10), RNA (12), inactivated (12), NRVV (120), subunit (28), RVV (4), VLP (4), LAV (2), VVr + APC (2), and VVnr + Antigen-presenting (1) vaccines [18]. Figures 8.2–8.4 show that subunit vaccine's development against COVID-19 is at the pinnacle.

8.3 STATUS OF VACCINE CANDIDATES

Vaccine is a crucial strategy for preventing infectious diseases as they are economical and decreases morbidity and mortality without prolonging effects. Prophylactic and therapeutic vaccines are the meaningful way to protect and provide quality health globally [15]. WHO has identified more than 184 promising vaccines candidates against COVID-19 in the pre-clinical stage and 102 in the clinical with an almost 8 vaccines approved for full use until May 2021 [18, 26].

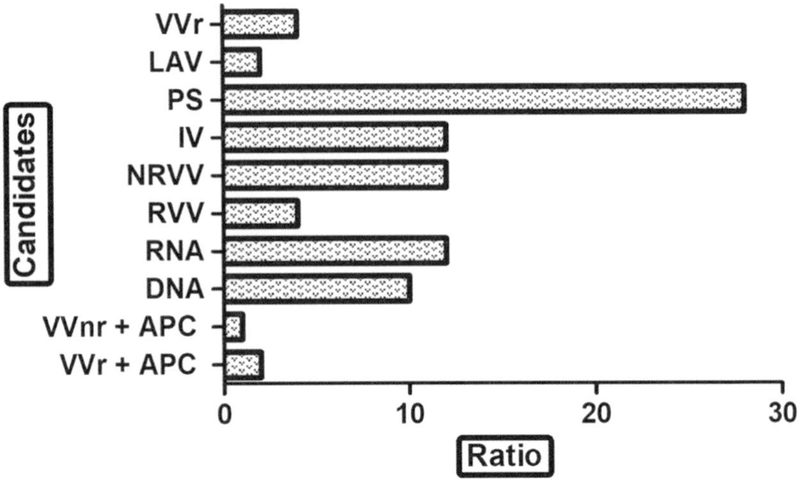

FIGURE 8.2 WHO current reports of vaccine candidates, April 9, 2021.

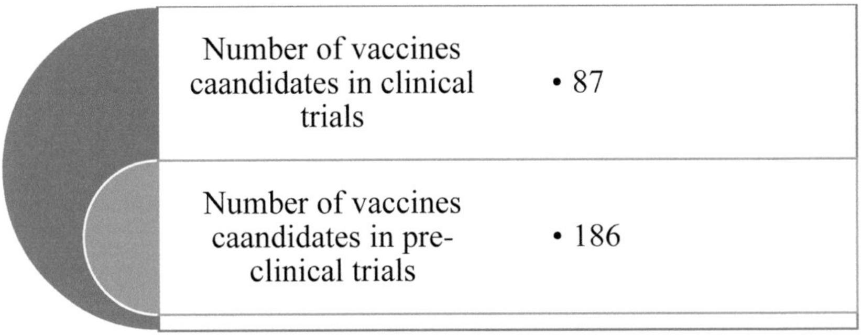

FIGURE 8.3 WHO candidates landscape until April 9, 2021.

These projects produced a written exploration for preclinical data, but it was the Unites States (Inovio, Moderna), Hong Kong (CanSino), and Chinese projects (2) to take the lead for clinical studies. These clinical trials began in March 2020 and produced a successful outcome. The United Kingdom have reported many pre-clinical studies but one vaccine Vaxzervria got authorization for emergency use in UK, EU, and Brazil. Moderna uses several genetic engineering technologies, such as *CureVac* uses mRNA technology and Inovio uses DNA technology with expected successful outcomes and got authorization of use in the US, EU, and other countries [26].

Among the large pharmaceutical industries, Johnson and Johnson, Pfizer, and Sanofi who are participating in vaccine development against COVID-19.

GlaxoSmithKline GSK and Merck are on a quiet side of the scenario, although GSK has a crucial role in adding adjuvants to boost immunity [26].

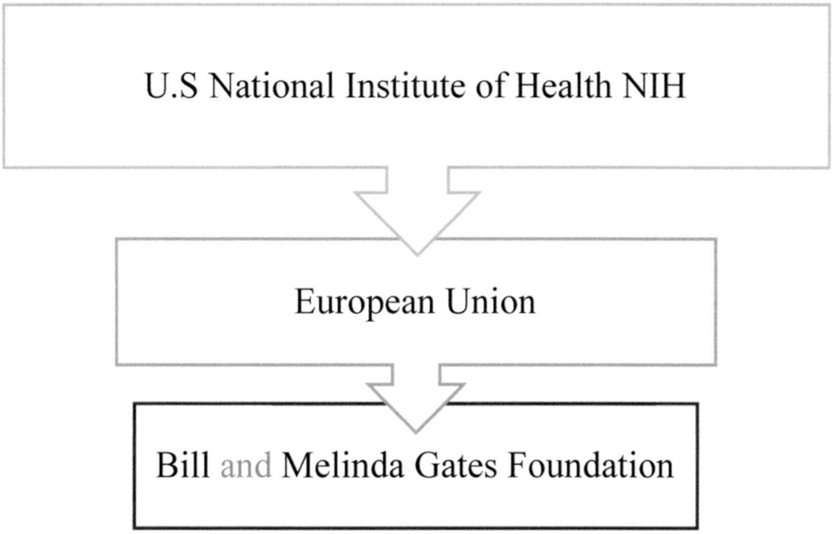

FIGURE 8.4 Prominent funders for COVID-19 vaccines development.

8.4 VACCINES DEVELOPMENT IN PANDEMIC

The development of a vaccine pattern/design is significantly different in a pandemic rather than in a traditional/classical vaccine design due to the time constraints observed in both cases (Figure 8.8). Most studies on MERs and SARs vaccine candidates were kept out because they were carried out in cell or animal models [27].

8.5 CHALLENGES IN VACCINES DEVELOPMENT

The world needs vaccines to mitigate current pandemic and normalize the human health, education as well as economy. Though its tiresome to produce an effective vaccine, yet not impossible. Many challenges pose hindrances in the vaccine development for COVID-19. It seems exhaustive to developing a vaccine due to the cost and complexity (target), strain variation, length of time required, probability of trial success: failure, and adverse effects involved [26].

8.5.1 COST AND COMPLEXITIES

Most of the studies revealed that optimistically, after six months, the most frequent probability to develop a vaccine is around 18 months. The pipelined COVID-19 vaccines were supposed to ensures vaccines' availability sooner however, due to the economic obstacles, a delay has been observed [13]. Likewise, a higher mutation rates compared to other viruses resulting in significant genetic diversity, is another considerable factor for the vaccine delay (primarily in DNA vector) [26].

8.5.2 TIME

It takes years (approximately 9–10 years) to develop a vaccine in a traditional or classical way. For COVID-19 vaccine, though the time frame is slightly different, yet it is impossible to introduce its vaccine in a matter of few months as the estimated time per WHO requirement is 18 months for the development of an effective and safe vaccine. This long duration of time is also one of the biggest challenges in developing effective vaccine candidates [13, 15, 26].

8.5.3 TRIALS FAILURE

COVID-19 vaccine seems a huge challenge and an extremely vigilant approach is required before and between the trials. Most of the trials fail in the pre-clinical stage due to the complex morphology and homology of the virus. Besides, animal selection in the pre-clinical trial is exceptionally confusing as different animal models of macaques, marmosets, chimpanzees, dromedary camels, mice, and rabbits have been reported by the researchers [15]. As previously reported, it was realized after the trials that despite the use of any animal model, it was macaques and marmosets which gave more desirable results [15, 28, 29].

8.5.4 ADVERSE EFFECTS

A vaccine against COVID-19 shows severe adversities, in particular the hypersensitivity reactions where fatal bronchial constriction has been observed. For the same reason, adverse effects are among the mega-challenge in developing effective vaccine candidates [15]. Several approaches have been introduced to develop adversities-free vaccine candidates. For instance, the nucleocapsid (N) protein may be a useful substitute to alleviate the associated adversities. N (nucleocapsid) protein is not a surface protein, rather it is found inside the virus however, it induces antibodies alike incited by the vaccine. DNA candidate vaccines targeting SARs N-protein may produce cellular and N humoral immunogenic responses [30, 31].

Antigenicity of vaccine candidate purports numerical criteria for the vaccine's ability to bind any T- and B-cells' receptors and aggravate the immunogenic response in the host cells. VaxiJen is a technique used for the analysis of antigenicity. Allergen proteins release IgE antibodies, which cause allergic reactions; the candidate should be designed to avoid allergic reactions in the body [30]. These loopholes are associated with significant disputes in the development of an effective and safe vaccine.

8.6 POTENTIAL VACCINE TARGETS

Development and manufacturing of effective and safe vaccines are urgently required to prevent infections of coronavirus. Structurally this virus is RNA-positive-strand covered with a nucleocapsid underneath membrane and envelope. Such nuclear materials (Spike (S) protein) neutralize antibodies and the RBD found in spike particularly in the S1 subunit, which bears numerous epitopes for neutralization (Figure 8.5). This morphology purports that the recombinant proteins in RBD and vectors (responsible for the encoding of RBD sequence) can be utilized for developing effective and safe coronavirus vaccines [32].

Precise mechanisms between the host receptors and the virus surface proteins are crucial for understanding host tropism, cross-species diffusion, and establishing animal models to develop vaccines [32]. The S-protein of coronaviruses (CoVs) is an essential target for developing a vaccine because it joins the infection mechanism via receptor binding of the host cells. Spike protein of coronavirus identifies different host receptors (SARs utilizes ACE2 as a receptor). The S1-subunit possesses a receptor-binding domain whereas, the S2 is essential for fusion with the membrane of viruses and host cells [31, 32].

The primary strategy to design a novel multi-epitope protein form is COVID-19 based responses to humoral and cellular immune systems. The candidate is better selected with low immunogenicity of the epitope and domains with a diverse response. The candidate should have the potential to enhance T cell response. These cells are crucial for identifying and killing cells, mainly found in infected individuals' lungs. Other cells include CD4 helper T-cells which generates definite antibodies. The CD8 T-cytotoxic cells are better identified in this scenario [31, 32].

The size of the coronavirus genome is about 30 kb and encodes both structural and non-structural proteins. Structural proteins comprise S (Spike) protein either S1 or S2, N (Nucleocapsid) protein, E (Envelope) protein, and M (Membrane) protein [32].

Nucleocapsid (N) is associated with replica-transcriptase complexes and binds with the RNA in the coronavirus's genome. N protein is related to the transcription, replication, and packaging of coronavirus proteins. The protein is a suitable candidate because of its conserved multifunctional antigens. Literature supports N-proteins to be better for vaccine candidates against COVID-19 because they induce potent antibodies and triggers cytokines' production. Besides, M-protein has a major role in virions assemblage. The M-protein, via interaction with N-protein, produces a network with the genomics. Several studies preferred S, N, and M proteins to be targeted against COVID-19 for their epitopes. Cellular and humoral immunity have been identified to play a vital role in the protective response against COVID-19. Recently multi-epitope novel fusion proteins were designed mainly with N- and M-proteins as well as a richer antigenic epitopic domains [30]. Due to an increased mortality and morbidity rate, safe, and specific vaccine candidates are quite essential [31].

Mechanistically, human coronavirus enters the cell through the receptor of ACE2 (angiotensin-converting enzyme-2). SARS corona primarily attacks the lower airways of the lungs and attaches to the ACE2 on the epithelial cells of alveoli. These can induce inflammatory cytokines—the "cytokine storm," which leads to the organ damage. Both viruses trigger the immune system cells, secretes inflammatory chemokines and cytokines inside lungs vascular endothelial cells [14], as shown in Figure 8.5.

It is essential to understand the morphology and desired targets while developing vaccines against COVID. More importantly, it is necessary to identify the virus target, retrieve protein sequence, evaluate antigenicity, and predict T- and B-cell epitope-rich domains. Certain factors like antigenicity, allergenicity, and pre-formulation factors should be considered while preparing vaccine candidates. The multi-epitope vaccine candidate is much essential against COVID-19 [31].

The S-protein-based vaccines are more convenient to produce due to its more fusion-liability, binding, and entrance to the immune system to neutralize antibodies. Spike protein comprises a signal peptide and three domains of intracellular, transmembrane, and extracellular environment. The ECD is further divided into spike-1 and spike-2 subunits. The spike-1 subunit is liable to recognize and bind the virus to the receptor (ACE-2) and spike-2 subunit is responsible for viral and target cell membrane fusion as it contains putative fusion peptides [30].

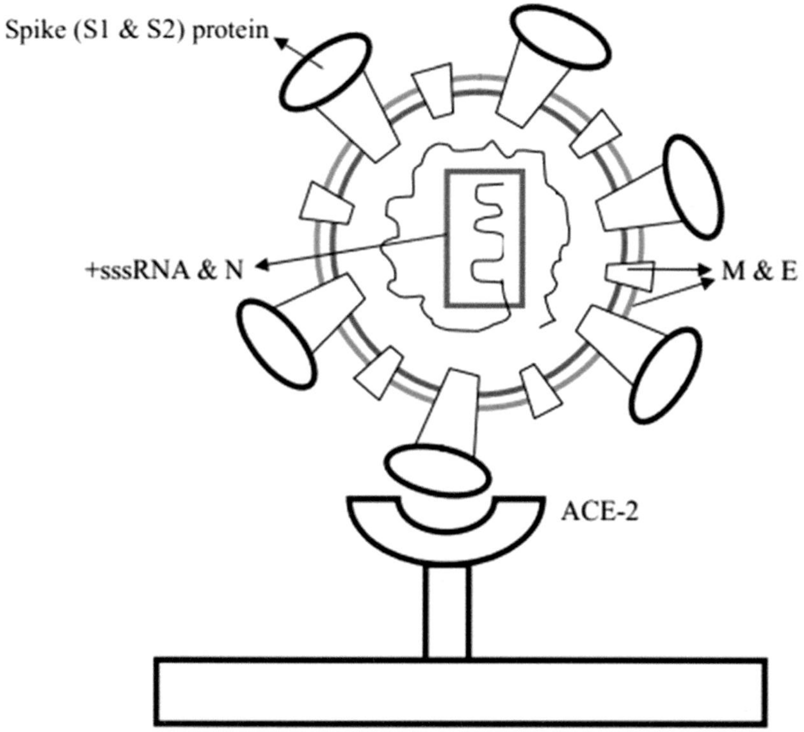

FIGURE 8.5 Strategy for designing vaccines for COVID-19. This virus expresses numerous structural proteins like (+sssRNA): Positive single-strand RNA, (M): membrane, (N): nucleocapsid, (E): envelope, (ACE-2): angiotensin-converting enzymes-2.

Several recombinant vaccines contain S-proteins based on vectors assessed in pre-clinical studies. The DNA vaccine candidate encoding S-protein has been reported and utilized for neutralizing antibodies found in rabbits. The most recently conducted animal study showed that the monoclonal and polyclonal antibodies against the Spike protein of COVID-19 neutralized infection and different deadly virus strains. These findings purport that the full-length S-protein has more safety and efficacy in vaccine development [31, 32].

8.7 VACCINE DESIGN

Ideally, each vaccine development completes in two main phases of pre-clinical and clinical studies. The pre-clinical was conducted on animals to determine safety [33, 34], as shown in Figure 8.6. Different types of animals were used to conduct studies as per the ethical principle's adherence. The most common animals used in these trials were macaques, marmosets, chimpanzees, rabbits, mice, and dromedary camels. It is suggested that the most effective results for COVID pre-clinical trials in macaques and marmosets may be due to genetic similarities with humans [15].

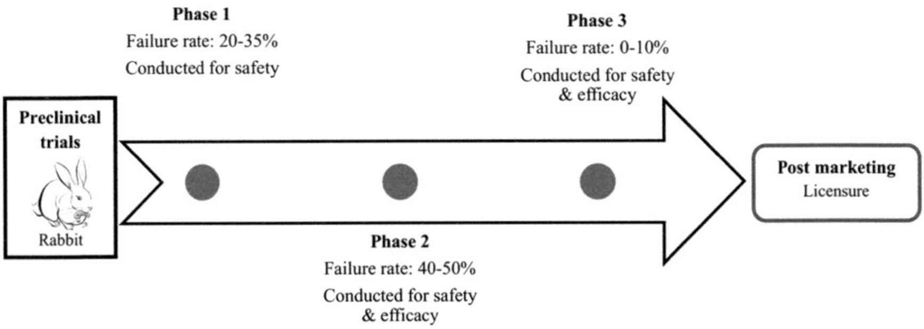

FIGURE 8.6 Typical patterns for vaccine design.

8.7.1 PRE-CLINICAL TRIALS

Preliminary, new drug/vaccine development commence from animal studies and the selection of animals is based on different parameters. Mostly an organism is preferred/chose upon the more genetic similarities to the human genome. Up till now, several pipelined studies for vaccines against COVID-19 used different animal models [16]. The traditional or classical pre-clinical trials are slightly different from emergency or pandemic vaccine development (Figure 8.8), yet each stage of these trials may firmly adhere with FDA or other standards and ethical guidelines [27].

8.7.2 CLINICAL TRIALS

Following a successful preclinical model, the vaccines are subjected to clinical studies in human beings. Clinical trials are further divided into different phases (Phase-I to V) Phase-1 commences directly upon the successful completion of pre-clinical trials, which requires 10–100 healthy human volunteers till post market surveillance. Though it may take approximately 30 months to complete Phase-I, for COVID-19, the time was constrained to six months with the same number of volunteers, due to emergency situations. FDA verifies each phase of vaccine development to ensure safety and efficacy [27, 35]. Each clinical trial phase should comply with ethical principles, including Helsinki, Belmont, and Nuremberg ethics principles in Figure 8.7.

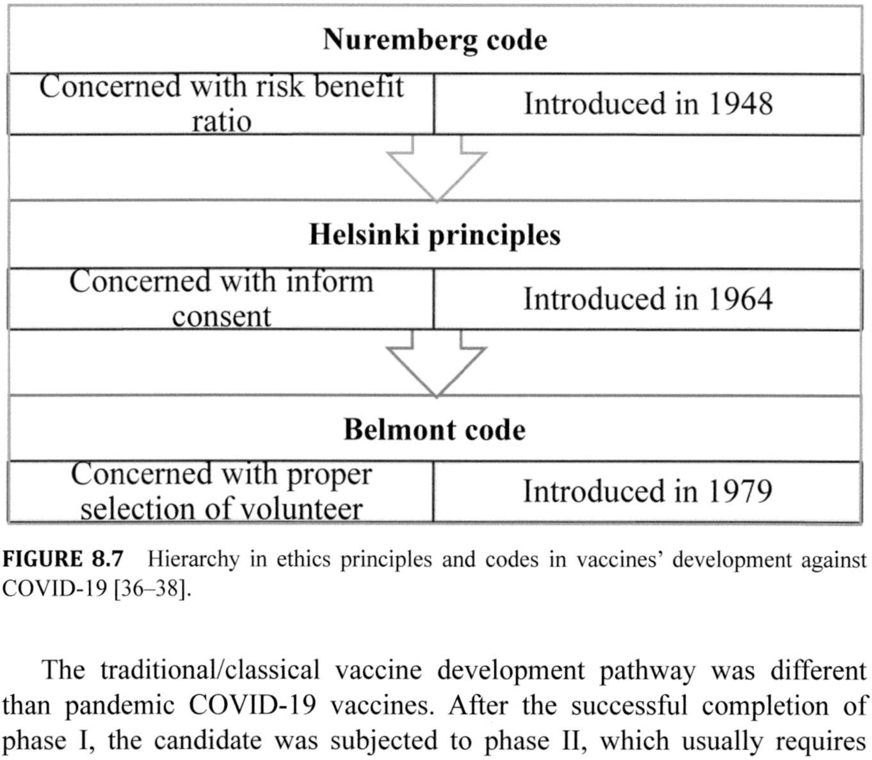

FIGURE 8.7 Hierarchy in ethics principles and codes in vaccines' development against COVID-19 [36–38].

The traditional/classical vaccine development pathway was different than pandemic COVID-19 vaccines. After the successful completion of phase I, the candidate was subjected to phase II, which usually requires more than 100 healthy human volunteers with a duration of approximately 32 months but for COVID-19 pandemic, the time duration is a few months only. Following successful outcomes of Phase-II, a Phase-III study with 100–1,000 healthy human volunteers in a time frame of around 30 months is conducted which again was reduced for COVID-19. The classical/traditional vaccines subjected for approval after successful completion of clinical phases for vaccination and marketing requires a duration of 1–2 years which was approximately six months in the case of COVID-19 [27] as shown in Figure 8.8.

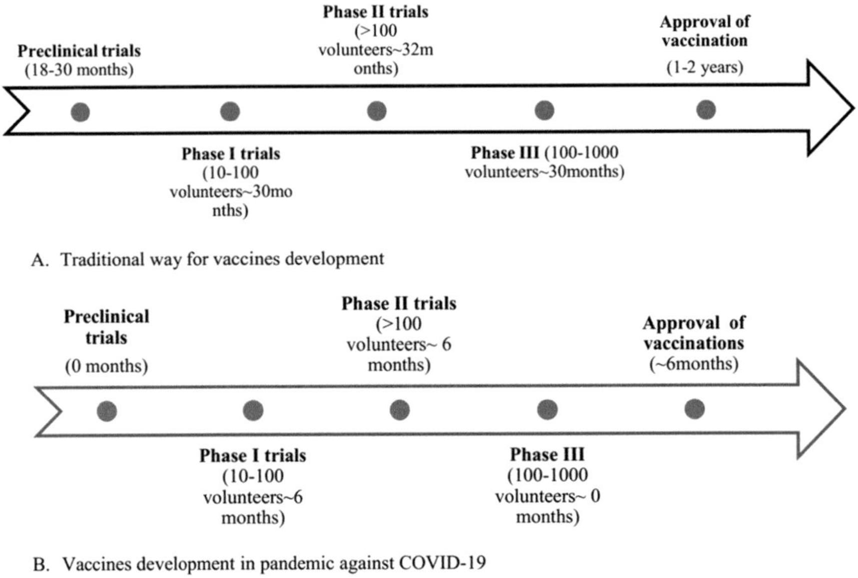

FIGURE 8.8 Traditional versus pandemic vaccines development.

8.8 GLOBAL ACCESS TO COVID-19 VACCINE

The existing response to the pandemic of COVID-19 required truculent strategies for suppression of symptoms, case identification, uses of sanitizers, isolation, quarantine, and social distancing. WHO alerts the public globally regarding sudden outbreaks of coronavirus [39]. Therefore, the vaccine development for COVID-19 may be an effective source to end the pandemic for this novel virus. The vaccine development should comprise three peremptory of speed, manufacturing, and formation scale along with a global access. Earlier, February 2020, the CEPI and World Bank released funds for developing vaccines focusing the primary purpose to launch and grow a vaccine with a quick global access. According to CEPI, an estimated budget of US $2 billion is required to develop three vaccines in forthcoming one and a half years [40].

Currently, eight vaccine candidates are in phase-1 clinical trials, and the progression of almost six candidates via phase-2 and 3 trials may be completed soon. Besides, three vaccines may need a regulatory requirement along with a global production. This estimate excluded the price of manufacturing and carriage. The developmental process is quit fast, and the clinical trial for vaccine candidate (phase-1), financially supported by the NIH (US) and CEPI, started on March 16, 2020 [41] whereas, a clinical trial was started in China just right after two days [42]. With a proper support of the existing financing systems, a cost-effective vaccine may be produced with ease. CEPI is financially supported by the World Bank's monetary fund which in turn links the public, philanthropists, and other private funding worldwide [43]. Using these funds, CEPI is mechanistically financing the vaccine development till licensing or testing procedures and provision for emergency use.

Due to the vast health and socio-economical consequences of the novel coronavirus, substantial investment is needed on behalf of each and individual governments. Besides, governmental contributions, innovative finance offices need to support this process as previous [44]. The international finance facility for immunization (IFFIm) put up funds with vaccine bonds, which turned on long-term financial aids by the donors into accessible cash. The IFFIm was shaped to support Gavi, the Vaccine Alliance, but should finance CEPI's vaccine efforts against COVID-19. With a highly developed market, the donors make funding promise to vaccine manufacturers. In exchange for this commitment, the companies may present a signed agreement to ensure vaccines availability for both low and middle-income countries at affordable prices.

Gavi's board agreed to use IFFIm and prior market agreements to synergize the concept of vaccine production, development, and access [45]. The urgent need for vaccines against COVID-19 with an appropriate distribution within populations is essential around the globe. Vaccines should be a top priority for health care providers and other individuals who are at the front line to the risk of severe morbidities and mortalities. The financially active countries should not monopolize the supply of vaccines for COVID-19 around the globe. This risk was observed in the influenza pandemic in 2009. Most prosperous nations negotiated advanced orders for vaccines whereas, overcrowded developing countries remained un-accessed [46]. The consequences resulted in a sub-optimal distribution of an initially inadequate resource. The responsibility for healthier solution comes upon the government's shoulders to ensure a fair allocation system around the world.

With copious political interest and public sector funding, a system should be created using existing institutions and instruments. The system's rudiments would need a global procurement agent, a considerable but limited-term advanced purchase pledge, and access to financial tools (through the system) such as concessional loans and indemnification from responsibility to compensate the risks by involving partners of private sectors. Vaccines acquired through this way should be free for the care of prioritized populations worldwide, with national allocations outlined through a fair procedure.

On March 16, 2020, a commitment was made by the G7 to support the commence of joint research ventures for vaccines against COVID-19 [47]. High-level dialog is required to make sure global access to vaccines against COVID-19. Investments should be made to make national systems for relief of potential vaccines like domestic and external funds from the World Bank Group's $14 billion COVID-19 Fast Track Facility and re-allocations from the Global Fund Fight Malaria AIDS and tuberculosis. Gavi, and Global Financing Facility grants for delivery services [48].

8.9 CONSIDERING PREGNANCY IN COVID-19 VACCINE TRIALS

During vaccines trials for COVID-19, pregnant women have been systemically excluded. For the reversal of this exclusion, appeals have been made to the national institute of health (NIH) and FDA, USA [49]. In earlier epidemics of other CoVs like SARS and MERS, severe problems were observed in pregnant women [50, 51]. In 2009, influenza H1NI pandemic, 5% of the US deaths were reported in women with pregnancy [52]. Nevertheless, despite above 18 million COVID-19 cases throughout the world [53], there is incomplete information on the effect of SARS-COV-2 on fetuses, infants, and pregnant women [54].

Three main queries are there to include pregnant women in COVID-19 vaccines. What is the short-term and long-term burden of COVID-19 in the fetus, infant, and pregnant women? Do pregnant women want to be part of such trials? What vaccine candidate is appropriate for pregnant women? [54].

8.10 ECONOMIC CONSIDERATIONS FOR THE DEVELOPMENT OF GLOBAL VACCINES

WHO had approved global vaccination action plan (GVAP) back in 2012. The plan primary purpose was to develop a decade of vaccine vision and access to immunization universally [55]. In its assessment report (2014), the GVAP administrations asked the WHO Scientific Advisory Group of Expert (SAGE) some questions: Are the circumstances most favorable for research and development of vaccines to progress as quickly as possible? Is there any obstacle in the road to success for vaccine? [56].

In 2002, more than 10 vaccine manufacturers were there in the US, about 40 in the 1960s. The reason for this decline is multifactorial, enlisted as below:

- High investment obsessed with stringent quality standards of manufacturing and regulation;
- Prolonged timeline for development mainly due to regulatory requirements;
- To facilitate efficient vaccine commercialization, a broad worldwide relationship and distribution networks the target governments, tender agencies, and some other organizations (like WHO, UNICEF, etc.);
- Complexity in manufacturing because of long production time, the delicateness of supply, and unpredictability of the demand (e.g., COVID-19 pandemic), frequently force the purchasers to agree with the recognized players [56].

The pharmaceutical industries generally have a minimal development budget and a varied set of investment opportunities. These investments are not merely allocated for vaccines but for an extended therapeutic area, development phases, geography, etc. This results in additional complexity and raises difficulty in deciding the allocation of budgets. Due to this reason, pharmaceutical companies mostly opted for valuation metrics, used to seek for combining assumptions for critical program trait-like costs, revenue, risk profile, timelines, etc., for the quantification of opportunity's expected values. The expected net present value (NPV) is one of the valuations metrics usually used by industry to analyze project/investment profitability. It is a risk-adjusted variation between current values of cash inflow and outflow. These valuation metrics are exceptional tools for investment decisions. It is essential to communicate that these metrics cannot cover all the strategic tones linked with a meticulous investment opportunity. Hence, management's judgment must always supplement these metrics. Few examples of such strategic elements are corporate social goals of responsibility, diversity, balance in the portfolio's objectives, and the need to keep the portfolio alignment along with the corporate mission, vision, and strategy [56].

8.11 MONITORING OF VACCINE SAFETY

As vaccines are administered to healthy as well as susceptible populations in special instances such as elderly, infant, and pregnant women thus the safety requirements for vaccine are much high. Moreover, vaccines are authorized and requisite by many governments, further increasing their safety expectations. The vaccine's safety is assessed in the development stages, even after its approval and during extensive use.

When the safety and efficacy are shown in clinical trials, the vaccine manufacturer applies to national regulatory authorities (NRA) for registration or licensure of vaccine. This application is termed a biological license application (BLA) whereas, known as marketing authorization application in Europe and submitted to the submitted to the FDA in the US and European Medicines Agency (EMA) in Europe. The countries with a lack of existence of NRA, WHO provides licensure for vaccine production. Nevertheless, such vaccines still need licensure in a state where it has to be used.

After the issuance of licensure, vaccines' safety monitoring depends upon the blend of active and passive surveillance. The passive type of surveillance is a sort of database where adverse events following immunization (AEFI), are collected spontaneously. Examples of passive surveillance systems are vaccine adverse event reporting system (VAERS) in the US and Eudra Vigilance (EV) in the European Union. In these systems, statistical analysis perceives the disproportionality amongst the number of reports observed and the number of reports expected of a solo adverse incident for a solitary vaccine, pursued by case assessment validation clinically. On the other hand, active surveillance seeks to assure all reports of already specified AEFIs from a prototypical sample. This is pursued by incidence analysis comparatively in sub-population that has not been given the vaccine. There is a vaccine safety datalink (VSD) in the US and the EU. The system is called accelerated development of vaccine benefit-risk collaboration in Europe [57].

8.12 ETHICAL CONSIDERATIONS IN VACCINE TRIALS IN RESOURCE-LIMITED SETTINGS

The trials for vaccines have a lot of ethical complications that stalk from many features including: vaccines trials are mostly international projects, includes high-income countries in work and settings with low income having undeveloped healthcare facilities, multicenter across and within the countries, and complex design of trials [58]. Moreover, vulnerable volunteers are hired for these trials, which increases the risk and weaken the consent. Sometimes the volunteers of the trials are more susceptible, like children and infants [59].

The ethics promote the volunteers' rights and well-being enrolled in vaccine trials [60, 61]. Many ethical resources are present that help the vaccine stakeholders respond to complexities of ethical concern in the trials of vaccines. These resources include ethical guidelines, ethical principles, ethical models, or frameworks, etc. [62].

The Research Ethics Committees (RECs) must review the trials of vaccines within the ethical-legal framework of a particular country. The participants enrolled in the trials must be "healthy yet at risk," getting the medical condition, which is the vaccine target [60, 61]. Last but not least, vaccine trials often need thousands of volunteers for a lengthy time of years in some cases, to undergo many trials, and to attend various procedures which may be troublesome at times [58]. Such trials must be conducted following standard guidelines described in Helsinki's declaration, international ethical guidelines of the Council of International Organization of Medical Sciences (CIOMS), and Joint United Nations Program on HIV/AIDS (UNAIDS) guidelines [61].

The vaccine trials must provide potentially crucial scientific information; the trials' volunteers are at potential risk [63]. Every trial of the vaccine shall make sure the fair recruitment of the volunteers for the trials. There are several examples in history where some vulnerable groups of the population, such as mentally ill persons and prisoners, etc., were recruited for the trials, which is recognized as a violation of the proper selection procedure [64]. Volunteers' choice for vaccine trials must be on a scientific basis with minimum risk [63]. A vaccine trial must present a balance of risks Vs benefit ratio, i.e., identify, and minimize the risk to the volunteers before vaccine trials.

Moreover, identify, and maximize such trials' potential benefits for the participants and society [58]. The investigators of vaccine trials should address the volunteers' medical requirements identified during trials of the vaccine [65]. Volunteers/their representatives (authorized legally in case of children) should give proper informed permission for participation in vaccine trials [58, 66]. There must be a constant effort to enhance the volunteers [58, 63, 67]. After the submission of the protocol, the proposed concerns should be evaluated [68]. Also, payment to the vaccine trial volunteers must be considered [69]. The ethical appropriateness should be reviewed by review bodies (like the research ethics committee) having independent, competent, and diverse members [70].

8.13 NEED FOR COVID-19 VACCINE

Vaccine design is the primary concern of scientists nowadays to encounter the COVID-19 pandemic [71, 72]. There are numerous reasons for vaccine designing and development against COVID-19. Some of them are discussed below.

8.13.1 CONTROL OF INFECTIONS

The globally faster spread and appearance of COVID-19 is mainly credited to many international travels, rapid globalization, immigration, and severe environmental changes [73, 74]. Vaccination is one of the essential parts of overcoming different infectious diseases. In medical history, vaccination has saved several lives. Moreover, vaccination is capable of prophylactic use against viral attacks [75]. This vaccination campaign also pushes back different prevention events like quarantine, social distancing, tracing, and history of contact, etc. [72, 76]. The main vaccination objective is to get inborn immunity against very high spreading pathogens like SARS-CoV-2 [74, 75].

8.14 EMERGENCE IN FUTURE

COVID epidemics dangerously affected humans' culture, lifestyle, natural human behavior, and economy worldwide [77]. The COVID vaccine development determinants have as the MERS and SARS are very rare after the 2013 and 2004 epidemic, respectively [76]. Nevertheless, there is an intense demand to develop vaccines [73]. Different six CoV are known for human infection, whereas no single vaccine has been approved against COVID-19 [71]. The SARS-CoV-2 is recently rising seventh CoV and likelihood for other remerging 8th mutated novel CoV [73, 76]. That is why the COVID-19 vaccine development is an urgent requirement to overcome today and emerging future CoV outbreak [73, 74].

8.15 DRUG REPURPOSING

Till now, no drug has been approved against COVID-19. Drug repurposing is one of the COVID-19 therapeutic strategies based on the mechanism of antiviral therapy and analysis of *in-vitro* inhibition [75, 77]. Nevertheless, random medications for COVID-19 may result in the resistant pathogen, lethal side effects, etc., that confine the direct application of antiviral drugs and knock the vaccine designing door [75].

8.16 HOMOLOGY IN GENE SEQUENCING

At the first stages of the novel COVID-19 outbreak (January 2020), there was very little information regarding the novel SARS-CoV-2 virus. The main challenge was to learn about the molecular biology, actual structure, genetic sequencing, and phylogenetic relationship of the virus [74, 78]. The phylogenetic study also revealed an 80% homology in the gene sequence of SARS-CoV and SARS-CoV-2 viruses [79]. This will open another way of hope toward rapid vaccine development [73, 80].

8.17 VIRAL MUTATION

Generally, there is a faster rate of mutation in RNA viruses. This may lead to an unsure immune system response during mutated strains of virus emergence [79]. On the other hand, in the case of infection of SARS-CoV-2 slower rate of mutation was observed. Therefore, we may say that, hopefully, vaccination may control SARS-CoV-2 infection [81].

8.18 TRAINED IMMUNITY-BASED VACCINES (TIBV)

The conventional vaccines result in pathogen-specific protection as it stimulates the acquired immunity. On the other hand, TibV results in inborn immunity stimulation, resulting in protection from non-related pathogens [82, 83]. Currently, the BCG (Bacille-Calmette-Guerin) vaccine is under clinical assessment for the capability to provoke immunity against COVID-19, which will require time for confirmation [84]. The main challenge of this approach is the variation in the standard of manufacturing of BCG vaccines in various countries, and it is uncertain if some quality criterion should be essential to produce fortification against COVID-19 [85].

8.19 OTHER POTENTIAL FACTORS OF THE COVID-19 VACCINE DEVELOPMENT

Many additional factors are accountable for quick vaccine designing and development such as; testing on animal models, determination of administration route, and adjuvant use are the three vital factors for the release of vaccine candidates on time.

8.20 APPROPRIATE ANIMAL MODEL SELECTION

Some of the fundamental objectives for selecting animal models are describing the pathogeneses of disease/virus, describing immunogenicity, evaluating ant-viral vaccine responses' progress, and monitoring symptoms clinically. Moreover, for a preclinical assessment of the efficiency of vaccines, animal models are used. This includes dose, safety, formulation, and route of administration of vaccines [33, 86]. Advanced computational bio-analytical techniques are utilized for the determination of a suitable animal model, which may reduce the cost and time of experiments on needless animal models [86, 87]. For COVID-19 vaccines development, different animal models were included in preclinical evaluation of the efficacy which consisted of mice [88, 89], hACE2 (human angiotensin-converting enzyme) Tg mice [90], BALB/c mice [90, 91], C57BL/6 mice [92], 129s6/SvEv mice [93], Wistar rate [94], golden Syrian hamster [95], rabbit [96], rhesus monkey [97, 98], and African green monkey [24].

To properly design a vaccine, the animal model has a critical position in providing details of both humoral and cellular immune responses [87]. Nevertheless, in some situations, animals' immune response is not predictable in humans [33]. Therefore, appropriate animal model selection is challenging for pandemic control [87, 99]. Moreover, SARS-CoV2 is an animal origin virus and can have various animal response types compared to human beings [100]. Therefore, animal model selection has a great significance required to be screened so that the immunogenic response of both animal models and human beings is near related to one another [79].

8.21 ADMINISTRATION ROUTE

The route of vaccine administration also affects efficacy. Usually, the administration route for vaccine is selected on the basis of minor impact in terms of adverse reactions with rapid and efficient immunogenicity [79]. COVID-19 is a respiratory tract disease, so it seems more beneficial to stimulate memory response at the site of the respiratory tract [101]. Hu et al. studied the induction of immunogenicity comparatively through various routes of drug administration and reported a better immunogenicity via the oral route however, the oral-intramuscular combination approach might impact the humoral and cellular immune response generation [102]. Gai et al. studied the effects of different immunization protocols for the SARS-CoV (inactivated) virus that indicated more IgG antibodies via intraperitoneal than intra-nasal immunization [103]. In recent times, Zhao et al. noted that intra-nasal administration provides a more effective cellular immunity response in mice [104]. Leyva et al. direct administration of vaccine into the respiratory tract showed efficient immunization [105]. Thus, various responses have been noted with the use of different vaccine administration routes that require proper screening, and make it more complex with an unnecessary delay to develop a vaccine faster [79]. Some of the vaccine administration routes are described in Table 8.1.

TABLE 8.1 Vaccines and Their Routes of Administration

SL. No.	Vaccine Type	Administration Route	References
1.	Live attenuated vaccine	Intranasal	[24]
2.	Inactivated vaccine	Subcutaneous	[106, 107]
		Intranasal	[103, 108]
		Intraperitoneal	[103]
		Intramuscular	[97, 98]
3.	Protein subunit vaccine	Intradermal	[93]
4.	Vector-based vaccine	Intranasal	[89, 94]
		Intramuscular	[89]
		Subcutaneous	[94]
5.	Nucleic acid vaccine	Intramuscular	[96, 104]
		Intradermal	[93]
6.	Nano based vaccine	Intramuscular	[109]
		Intranasal	[101, 109]

8.22 EFFICIENT ADJUVANT SELECTION

Some scientists reported that adjuvant augments antibodies production [91, 93]. However, some others did not observe any significant effect of adjuvant on antibodies' production in designing CoV vaccines [108]. Moreover, adjuvant use must be optimized in designing vaccines as some problems were reported while adjuvant usage like eosinophilic immune-pathology [110], the toxicity of lungs [111], cytotoxicity [112], pyrexia, rashes, myalgia, an allergic reaction, and sometimes neuro-toxicity. Different adjuvants approved by FDA are commercially available with a high level of purity which may be used safely and selectively for designing/improving vaccine performance [79].

Few researchers reported that adjuvant augments antibodies production [91, 93] whereas, other reported a lack of any significant effect of adjuvant on antibodies' production in designing COVID vaccines [108]. Moreover, the use of any adjuvant may be optimized in designing vaccines as some problems were reported during adjuvant usage like eosinophilic immune-pathology [110], the toxicity of lungs [111], cytotoxicity [112], pyrexia, rashes, myalgia, an allergic reaction and sometimes neuro-toxicity. Different adjuvants approved by FDA are commercially available with a high level of purity and can be safely and selectively used in designing for improving vaccine performance [79].

8.23 mRNA BASED VACCINE

Messenger RNA vaccines are quickly developing technologies to mitigate infectious illnesses. This type of vaccine contains mRNAs encoding and translated by vaccination into the host cellular machinery. mRNA vaccines are more advantageous over traditional vaccines by lack of genome integration, modification of immune responses, fast evolution, and the presence of multimeric antigen. Moderna began clinical trials for messenger RNA vaccines with encoding viral S proteins of SARS. The NIAID financially supported this project.

In contrast to traditional vaccines, mRNA vaccines are manufactured in a cell culture system. In Moderna's, this type of vaccine is manufactured in silico for potential quick development and high efficacy [83]. Moderna phase I study was supported by CEPI [15, 17].

Lipid nanoparticles (LNPs) are used for transcription as their efficiency is higher than naturally occurring mRNA. The classical formulation of LNP comprises a lipid that condenses RNA to produce complexes with mRNA molecule, lipids (helper) for structural stringency, and coating of lipidized polymer to modify surface characteristics of the molecule. After phagocytosis by the cell, LNPs to a lower pH environment within the endosome, followed by endosome puncturing by RNA condensing lipid, resulting in RNA's release into the cytosol. Hence, the main component of this platform is RNA condensing lipid [113].

8.24 CONCLUSION

Vaccine candidature against COVID-19 depends on the S-protein due to its key role in the viral infectivity yet, other studies reported and worked on proteins such as the nucleocapsid (N) protein, envelope (E) protein, and non-structural proteins. The possible vaccine candidates for COVID-19 can be divided into 10 types: DNA-based, mRNA-based, viral vector-based, subunit protein-based, inactivated whole virus (IWVV), replicating, and non-replicating viral vaccine, live attenuated vaccine (LAV), VVr + Antigen-presenting cell and VVnr + Antigen-presenting cell. There should be an essential step-change in developing a traditional vaccine that would take a longer duration. In contrast, Vaccine development against COVID-19 required the most urgent measures to overcome the pandemic.

KEYWORDS

- **COVID**
- **DNA**
- **platforms**
- **RNA**
- **severe acute respiratory syndrome**
- **vaccine**
- **World Health Organization**

REFERENCES

1. Behbehani, A. M., (1983). The smallpox story: Life and death of an old disease. *Microbiological Reviews, 47*(4), 455.
2. Plotkin, S., (2014). History of vaccination. *Proceedings of the National Academy of Sciences, 111*(34), 12283–12287.
3. Organization, W. H., (2012). *International travel and Health 2012: Situation as on 1 January 2012*. World Health Organization.
4. Katz, S. L., et al., (1960). Studies on an attenuated measles-virus vaccine: VIII. General summary and evaluation of the results of vaccination. *American Journal of Diseases of Children, 100*(6), 942–946.
5. Takahashi, M., (1975). Development of a live attenuated varicella vaccine. *Biken's Journal, 18*(1), 25–33.
6. Gross, A. E., & MacDougall, C., (2020). Roles of the clinical pharmacist during the COVID-19 pandemic. *Journal of the American College of Clinical Pharmacy, 3*(3), 564–566.
7. Li, Q., et al., (2020). Early transmission dynamics in Wuhan, China, of novel coronavirus-infected pneumonia. *New England Journal of Medicine*.
8. Zia-Ul-Haq, M., et al., (2021). *Alternative Medicine Interventions for COVID-19* (Vol. XII, p. 284). Springer, Cham: Springer Nature Switzerland AG.

9. Zia-Ul-Haq, M., Dewanjee, S., & Riaz, M., (2021). *Carotenoids: Structure and Function in the Human Body* (Vol. XVI, p. 859). Springer Nature Switzerland AG: Springer International Publishing.
10. World Health Organization, (2020). *Coronavirus Disease (COVID-2019) Situation Reports, 208*, 1–16.
11. Wang, C., et al., (2020). A novel coronavirus outbreak of global health concern. *The Lancet, 395*(10223), 470–473.
12. Ahn, D. G., et al., (2020). Current status of epidemiology, diagnosis, therapeutics, and vaccines for novel coronavirus disease 2019 (COVID-19). *J. Microbiol. Biotechnol., 28, 30*(3), 313–324. doi: 10.4014/jmb.2003.03011.
13. Jiang, F., et al., (2020). Review of the clinical characteristics of coronavirus disease 2019 (COVID-19). *Journal of General Internal Medicine*, 1–5.
14. Liu, C., et al., (2020). *Research and Development on Therapeutic Agents and Vaccines for COVID-19 and Related Human Coronavirus Diseases*. ACS Publications.
15. Yong, C. Y., et al., (2019). Recent advances in the vaccine development against Middle East respiratory syndrome-coronavirus. *Frontiers in Microbiology, 10*, 1781.
16. Organization, W. H., (2019). Hepatitis B vaccines: WHO position paper, July 2017–Recommendations. *Vaccine, 37*(2), 223–225.
17. Organization, W. H., (2016). *Global Health Sector Strategy on Viral Hepatitis 2016–2021. Towards Ending Viral Hepatitis*. World Health Organization.
18. Organization, W. H., (2020). *DRAFT Landscape of COVID-19 Candidate Vaccines.* World.
19. CEPI, (2020). *CEPI to Fund Three Programs to Develop Vaccines Against the Novel Coronavirus, nCoV-2019*. Available from: https://cepi.net/news_cepi/cepi-to-fund-three-programmes-to-develop-vaccines-against-the-novel-coronavirus-ncov-2019/ (accessed on 6 August 2021).
20. DeZure, A. D., et al., (2016). Whole-inactivated and virus-like particle vaccine strategies for chikungunya virus. *The Journal of Infectious Diseases, 214*(suppl_5), S497–S499.
21. Deng, Y., et al., (2018). Enhanced protection in mice induced by immunization with inactivated whole viruses compare to spike protein of middle east respiratory syndrome coronavirus. *Emerging Microbes & Infections, 7*(1), 1–10.
22. Lauring, A. S., Jones, J. O., & Andino, R., (2010). Rationalizing the development of live attenuated virus vaccines. *Nature Biotechnology, 28*(6), 573–579.
23. Robert-Guroff, M., (2007). Replicating and non-replicating viral vectors for vaccine development. *Current Opinion in Biotechnology, 18*(6), 546–556.
24. Bukreyev, A., et al., (2004). Mucosal immunization of African green monkeys (Cercopithecus aethiops) with an attenuated parainfluenza virus expressing the SARS coronavirus spike protein for the prevention of SARS. *The Lancet, 363*(9427), 2122–2127.
25. Yang, Z. Y., et al., (2004). A DNA vaccine induces SARS coronavirus neutralization and protective immunity in mice. *Nature, 428*(6982), 561–564.
26. Veugelers, R., & Zachmann, G., (2020). Racing against COVID-19: A vaccines strategy for Europe. *Policy Contribution*, (7), 1–19.
27. Calina, D., et al., (2020). Towards effective COVID-19 vaccines: Updates, perspectives and challenges. *International Journal of Molecular Medicine, 46*(1), 3–16.
28. Munster, V. J., De Wit, E., & Feldmann, H., (2013). Pneumonia from human coronavirus in a macaque model. *The New England Journal of Medicine, 368*(16).
29. Yu, P., et al., (2017). Comparative pathology of rhesus macaque and common marmoset animal models with Middle East respiratory syndrome coronavirus. *PLoS One, 12*(2), e0172093.

30. Enayatkhani, M., et al., (2020). Reverse vaccinology approach to design a novel multi-epitope vaccine candidate against COVID-19: An in silico study. *Journal of Biomolecular Structure and Dynamics*, 1–16.
31. Abdelmageed, M. I., et al., (2020). Design of a multiepitope-based peptide vaccine against the e protein of human COVID-19: An immunoinformatics approach. *BioMed Research International, 2020.*
32. Jiang, S., He, Y., & Liu, S., (2005). SARS vaccine development. *Emerging Infectious Diseases, 11*(7), 1016.
33. Gerdts, V., Griebel, P. J., & Babiuk, L. A., (2007). Use of animal models in the development of human vaccines. *Future Microbiology, 2*(6), 667–675.
34. Gerdts, V., et al., (2015). Large animal models for vaccine development and testing. *ILAR Journal, 56*(1), 53–62.
35. Goldstein, S. A., & Weiss, S. R., (2017). *Origins and Pathogenesis of Middle East Respiratory Syndrome-Associated Coronavirus: Recent Advances, 6.* F1000Research.
36. Code, N., (1949). *Reprinted from Trials of War Criminals Before the Nuremberg Military Tribunals under Control Council Law No. 10*(2), 181, 182. Washington, DC: US Government Printing Office.
37. Levine, R. J., (1988). *Ethics and Regulation of Clinical Research.* Yale University Press.
38. Association, W. M., (1989). *Inc: World Medical Association Declaration of Helsinki, as Amended by the 41st World Assembly, Hong Kong* (pp. 1, 2). Ferney-Voltaire, France.
39. Ferguson, N. M., et al., (2020). Imperial college COVID-19 response team. *Impact of Non-Pharmaceutical Interventions (NPIs) to Reduce COVID-19 Mortality and Healthcare Demand.*
40. Ahmed, K., (2020). *World's Most Vulnerable in "Third Wave" for COVID-19 Support, Experts Warn.* The Guardian.
41. National Institutes of Health, (2020). *NIH Clinical Trial of Investigational Vaccine for COVID-19 Begins.* Taken from: https://www.nih.gov/news-events/newsreleases/nih-clinical-trial-investigational-vaccine-covid-19-begins (accessed on 6 August 2021).
42. Biologics, G. J. C., *China Announces First Human Trials of COVID-19 Vaccine.* Market Screener.
43. Bank, W., (2020). *Financial Intermediary Funds (FIFs).* Available from: https://fiftrustee.worldbank.org/en/about/unit/dfi/fiftrustee (accessed on 6 August 2021).
44. Kickbusch, I., et al., (2018). Banking for health: Opportunities in cooperation between banking and health applying innovation from other sectors. *BMJ Global Health, 3*(Suppl 1).
45. Zerhouni, E., (2019). GAVI, the vaccine alliance. *Cell, 179*(1), 13–17.
46. Fidler, D. P., (2012). Negotiating equitable access to influenza vaccines: Global health diplomacy and the controversies surrounding avian influenza H5N1 and pandemic influenza H1N1. In *Negotiating and Navigating Global Health: Case Studies in Global Health Diplomacy* (pp. 161–172). World Scientific.
47. Meagan Byrd and the G7 Research Group, (2021). *2020 G7 Virtual Summit Final Compliance Report.* http://www.g7.utoronto.ca/evaluations/2020compliance-final/07–2020-G7-final-compliance-research.pdf (accessed on 6 August 2021).
48. Yamey, G., et al., (2020). Ensuring global access to COVID-19 vaccines. *The Lancet, 395*(10234), 1405–1406.
49. Whitehead, C. L., & Walker, S. P., (2020). Consider pregnancy in COVID-19 therapeutic drug and vaccine trials. *The Lancet, 395*(10237), e92.

50. Lam, C. M., et al., (2004). A case-controlled study comparing clinical course and outcomes of pregnant and non-pregnant women with severe acute respiratory syndrome. *BJOG: An International Journal of Obstetrics & Gynaecology, 111*(8), 771–774.
51. Omrani, A. S., Al-Tawfiq, J. A., & Memish, Z. A., (2015). Middle East respiratory syndrome coronavirus (MERS-CoV): Animal to human interaction. *Pathogens and Global Health, 109*(8), 354–362.
52. Siston, A. M., et al., (2010). Pandemic 2009 influenza A (H1N1) virus illness among pregnant women in the United States. *JAMA, 303*(15), 1517–1525.
53. Hopkins, J., (2020). *Center for Systems Science and Engineering. Coronavirus resource center: COVID19 dashboard by the Center for Systems Science and Engineering (CSSE) at Johns Hopkins University (JHU)*. Available from: https://coronavirus.jhu.edu/map.html (accessed on 6 August 2021).
54. Heath, P. T. Le Doare, K., & Khalil, A., (2020). Inclusion of pregnant women in COVID-19 vaccine development. *The Lancet Infectious Diseases*.
55. World Health Organization, (2020). *Global Vaccine Action Plan 2011–2020, Immunization, Vaccines and Biologicals.* Available from: http://www.who.int/immunization/global_vaccine_action_plan/GVAP_doc_2011_2020/en/ (accessed on 6 August 2021).
56. Bakken, D., Boyce, D., & Jodar, L., (2016). Economic considerations for the development of global vaccines: A perspective from the vaccine industry. In: *The Vaccine Book* (pp. 465–482) Elsevier.
57. Chandler, R. E., (2020). Optimizing safety surveillance for COVID-19 vaccines. *Nature Reviews Immunology, 20*(8), 451, 452.
58. Slack, C. M., (2016). Ethical considerations in vaccine trials in resource-limited settings. In: *The Vaccine Book* (pp. 447–462). Elsevier.
59. UNAIDS/WHO guidance document, (2012). *Ethical Considerations in Biomedical HIV Prevention Trials*. Available from: https://files.unaids.org/en/media/unaids/contentassets/documents/unaidspublication/2012/jc1399_ethical_considerations_en.pdf (accessed on 6 August 2021).
60. Emanuel, E. J., et al., (2008). *The Oxford Textbook of Clinical Research Ethics*.: Oxford University Press.
61. Tarantola, D., et al., (2007). Ethical considerations related to the provision of care and treatment in vaccine trials. *Vaccine, 25*(26), 4863–4874.
62. Grady, C., et al., (2008). Research benefits for hypothetical HIV vaccine trials: The views of Ugandans in the Rakai District. *IRB: Ethics & Human Research, 30*(2), 1–7.
63. Emanuel, E. J., Wendler, D., & Grady, C., (2000). What makes clinical research ethical? *JAMA, 283*(20), 2701–2711.
64. Grady, C., (2004). Ethics of vaccine research. *Nature Immunology, 5*(5), 465–468.
65. Richardson, H. S., (2007). Gradations of researchers' obligation to provide ancillary care for HIV/AIDS in developing countries. *American Journal of Public Health, 97*(11), 1956–1961.
66. Mamotte, N., et al., (2010). Convergent ethical issues in HIV/AIDS, tuberculosis and malaria vaccine trials in Africa: Report from the WHO/UNAIDS African AIDS vaccine program's ethics, law and human rights collaborating center consultation, Durban, South Africa. *BMC Medical Ethics, 11*(1), 1–5.
67. Emanuel, E. J., (2004). Ending concerns about undue inducement. *The Journal of Law, Medicine & Ethics, 32*(1), 100–105.
68. Ellenberg, S., (2007). Data Monitoring Committee. *Wiley Encyclopedia of Clinical Trials*, 1–8.

69. Grady, C., (2005). Payment of clinical research subjects. *The Journal of Clinical Investigation, 115*(7), 1681–1687.
70. Rid, A., et al., (2014). Placebo use in vaccine trials: Recommendations of a WHO expert panel. *Vaccine, 32*(37), 4708–4712.
71. Corman, V. M., et al., (2018). Hosts and sources of endemic human coronaviruses. In: *Advances in Virus Research* (pp. 163–188). Elsevier.
72. Sanche, S., et al., (2020). *The Novel Coronavirus, 2019-nCoV, is Highly Contagious and More Infectious Than Initially Estimated.* arXiv preprint arXiv:2002.03268.
73. Dhama, K., et al., (2020). COVID-19, an emerging coronavirus infection: Advances and prospects in designing and developing vaccines, immunotherapeutics, and therapeutics. *Human Vaccines & Immunotherapeutics*, 1–7.
74. El-Aziz, T. M. A., & Stockand, J. D., (2020). Recent progress and challenges in drug development against COVID-19 coronavirus (SARS-CoV-2)-an update on the status. *Infection, Genetics and Evolution*, 104327.
75. Sautto, G. A., et al., (2019). *Next-Generation Vaccines for Infectious Diseases*. Hindawi.
76. Choi, J., et al., (2017). Progress of middle east respiratory syndrome coronavirus vaccines: A patent review. *Expert Opinion on Therapeutic Patents, 27*(6), 721–731.
77. Badgujar, K. C., et al., (2020). Hydroxychloroquine for COVID-19: A review and a debate based on available clinical trials/case studies. *Journal of Drug Delivery and Therapeutics, 10*(3), 304–311.
78. Lu, R., et al., (2020). Genomic characterization and epidemiology of 2019 novel coronavirus: Implications for virus origins and receptor binding. *The Lancet, 395*(10224), 565–574.
79. Badgujar, K. C., Badgujar, V. C., & Badgujar, S. B., (2020). Vaccine development against coronavirus (2003 to present): An overview, recent advances, current scenario, opportunities and challenges. *Diabetes & Metabolic Syndrome: Clinical Research & Reviews.*
80. Kumar, V., Jung, Y. S., & Liang, P. H., (2013). Anti-SARS coronavirus agents: A patent review (2008–present). Expert *Opinion on Therapeutic Patents, 23*(10), 1337–1348.
81. Guo, X., et al., (2020). *Long-Term Persistence of IgG Antibodies in SARS-CoV Infected Healthcare Workers.* medRxiv.
82. Sánchez-Ramón, S., et al., (2018). Trained immunity-based vaccines: A new paradigm for the development of broad-spectrum anti-infectious formulations. *Frontiers in Immunology, 9*, 2936.
83. Quintin, J., et al., (2012). Candida albicans infection affords protection against reinfection via functional reprogramming of monocytes. *Cell Host & Microbe, 12*(2), 223–232.
84. Cirillio, J., (2020). *BCG Vaccine for Health Care Workers as Defense Against COVID 19 (BADAS)[Internet].* clinicaltrials.gov. (accessed on 6 August 2021).
85. Angelidou, A., et al., (2020). Licensed bacille Calmette-Guérin (BCG) formulations differ markedly in bacterial viability, RNA content and innate immune activation. *Vaccine, 38*(9), 2229–2240.
86. Orme, I. M., (2005). The use of animal models to guide rational vaccine design. *Microbes and Infection, 7*(5, 6), 905–910.
87. Griffin, J. F. T., (2002). A strategic approach to vaccine development: Animal models, monitoring vaccine efficacy, formulation and delivery. *Advanced Drug Delivery Reviews, 54*(6), 851–861.
88. Kapadia, S. U., et al., (2005). Long-term protection from SARS coronavirus infection conferred by a single immunization with an attenuated VSV-based vaccine. *Virology, 340*(2), 174–182.

89. Ababneh, M., & Mohammad. K. M. A., (2019). Recombinant adenoviral vaccine encoding the spike 1 subunit of the middle east respiratory syndrome coronavirus elicits strong humoral and cellular immune responses in mice. *Veterinary World, 12*(10), 1554.
90. Netland, J., et al., (2010). Immunization with an attenuated severe acute respiratory syndrome coronavirus deleted in E protein protects against lethal respiratory disease. *Virology, 399*(1), 120–128.
91. Tang, L., et al., (2003). Preparation, characterization and preliminary in vivo studies of inactivated SARS-CoV vaccine. *Chinese Science Bulletin, 48*(23), 2621–2625.
92. Zakhartchouk, A. N., et al., (2007). Optimization of a DNA vaccine against SARS. *DNA and Cell Biology, 26*(10), 721–726.
93. Zakhartchouk, A. N., et al., (2007). Immunogenicity of a receptor-binding domain of SARS coronavirus spike protein in mice: Implications for a subunit vaccine. *Vaccine, 25*(1), 136–143.
94. Liu, R. Y., et al., (2005). Adenoviral expression of a truncated S1 subunit of SARS-CoV spike protein results in specific humoral immune responses against SARS-CoV in rats. *Virus Research, 112*(1, 2), 24–31.
95. Roberts, A., et al., (2010). Immunogenicity and protective efficacy in mice and hamsters of a β-propiolactone inactivated whole virus SARS-CoV vaccine. *Viral Immunology, 23*(5), 509–519.
96. Li, J., et al., (2005). Immunogenicity of DNA vaccine that express spike gene fragment of SARS coronavirus. *Chinese Journal of Microbiology and Immunology, 25*(4), 297–301.
97. Zhong, Q., et al., (2005). Immunogenicity and safety of an inactivated SARS-associated coronavirus vaccine in rhesus monkeys. *Chinese Journal of Microbiology and Immunology, 25*(4).
98. Zhou, J., et al., (2005). Immunogenicity, safety, and protective efficacy of an inactivated SARS-associated coronavirus vaccine in rhesus monkeys. *Vaccine, 23*(24), 3202–3209.
99. Riese, P., et al., (2015). Rodents as pre-clinical models for predicting vaccine performance in humans. *Expert Review of Vaccines, 14*(9), 1213–1225.
100. Qin, E., et al., (2006). *Immunogenicity and protective efficacy in monkeys of purified inactivated Vero-cell SARS vaccine. Vaccine, 24*(7), 1028–1034.
101. Raghuwanshi, D., et al., (2012). Dendritic cell-targeted chitosan nanoparticles for nasal DNA immunization against SARS CoV nucleocapsid protein. *Molecular Pharmaceutics, 9*(4), 946–956.
102. Hu, H., et al., (2009). Comparative analysis of the immunogenicity of SARS-CoV nucleocapsid DNA vaccine administrated with different routes in mouse model. *Vaccine, 27*(11), 1758–1763.
103. Gai, W., et al., (2008). Effects of different immunization protocols and adjuvant on antibody responses to inactivated SARS-CoV vaccine. *Viral Immunology, 21*(1), 27–37.
104. Zhao, J., et al., (2016). Airway memory $CD4^+$ T cells mediate protective immunity against emerging respiratory coronaviruses. *Immunity, 44*(6), 1379–1391.
105. Leyva-Grado, V. H., et al., (2015). Direct administration in the respiratory tract improves the efficacy of broadly neutralizing anti-influenza virus monoclonal antibodies. *Antimicrobial Agents and Chemotherapy, 59*(7), 4162–4172.
106. Takasuka, N., et al., (2004). A subcutaneously injected UV-inactivated SARS coronavirus vaccine elicits systemic humoral immunity in mice. *International Immunology, 16*(10), 1423–1430.

107. Tsunetsugu-Yokota, Y., et al., (2007). Formalin-treated UV-inactivated SARS coronavirus vaccine retains its immunogenicity and promotes Th2-type immune responses. *Japanese Journal of Infectious Diseases, 60*(2, 3), 106.
108. Spruth, M., et al., (2006). A double-inactivated whole virus candidate SARS coronavirus vaccine stimulates neutralising and protective antibody responses. *Vaccine, 24*(5), 652–661.
109. Shim, B. S., et al., (2010). Intranasal immunization with plasmid DNA encoding spike protein of SARS-coronavirus/polyethylenimine nanoparticles elicits antigen-specific humoral and cellular immune responses. *BMC Immunology, 11*(1), 1–9.
110. Honda-Okubo, Y., et al., (2015). Severe acute respiratory syndrome-associated coronavirus vaccines formulated with delta inulin adjuvants provide enhanced protection while ameliorating lung eosinophilic immunopathology. *Journal of Virology, 89*(6), 2995–3007.
111. Wang, X., et al., (2014). Use of coated silver nanoparticles to understand the relationship of particle dissolution and bioavailability to cell and lung toxicological potential. *Small, 10*(2), 385–398.
112. Raetz, C. R., & Whitfield, C., (2002). Lipopolysaccharide endotoxins. *Annual Review of Biochemistry, 71*(1), 635–700.
113. Wang, J., et al., (2020). The COVID-19 vaccine race: Challenges and opportunities in vaccine formulation. *AAPS PharmSciTech, 21*(6), 1–12.

PART III
Treatment

CHAPTER 9

Medicinal Plants Against COVID-19

BINISH KHALIQ,[1] NAILA ALI,[1] AHMED AKREM,[2] M. YASIN ASHRAF,[1] ARIF MALIK,[1] ARIFA TAHIR,[3] and M. ZIA-UL-HAQ[4]

[1]*Institute of Molecular Biology and Biotechnology, The University of Lahore, Lahore, Pakistan, E-mail: beenish.khaliq@imbb.uol.edu.pk (B. Khaliq)*

[2]*Institute of Pure and Applied Biology, Bahauddin Zakariya University, Multan, Pakistan*

[3]*Environmental Science Department, Lahore College for Women University, Lahore–54000, Pakistan*

[4]*Office of Research, Innovation and Commercialization, Lahore College for Women University, Lahore–54000, Pakistan*

ABSTRACT

COVID-19 is catastrophic widespread in world history. There are many efforts and investments to develop the medicines as far the immune or treat this disease. However, drug and medication are paying to pivot the consideration; it seems from the results of different studies that have been done on plant-originated medicines. These medicines could also be potent candidates for the formulation and development of drugs that inhibit the activity of this virus and control the disease. In this study was discussed the antiviral capability of medicinal isolated natural products and phytochemicals from herbs and plant take part to prohibit the activity of many strains of coronaviruses (CoVs) that cause the diseases in the human. It shows that antiviral plant compounds or molecules is being used for the development of medicines against the CoVs which are responsible for the COVID-19 disease.

9.1 INTRODUCTION

The COVID-19 coronavirus infection has been announced widespread in the world and caused the number of human deaths of the unprotected peoples in 209 countries of the world. Even though many medicinal molecules or compounds are being used, no effective vaccines or antiviral medicine have been prepared. Since the outbreak of COVID-19, many conventional plant-derived compounds with heartening results used unattended or mix with antiviral medicines to cure people. In this chapter, demonstrate the use of natural substances or molecules to inhibit or cure the disease of coronavirus in the human. The plants extracts and isolated compounds have the antiviral potential by inhibited the viral replication and stop the entry. Herbal conventional remedies have been used to cure the COVID-19 from the first day of disease in China. In fact, these conventional remedies were shown 90% recovery of COVID-19 patients [1]. This chapter gives the attention on the possible uses of herbal, plant conventional originated remedies and natural substances in the anticipation and cure infection caused by COVID-19.

9.2 COVID-19

COVID-19 belongs to family Coroaviridae. COVID-19 has the enveloped, positive single-stranded RNA and nucleocapsid with symmetric helical [2]. There are 20 type proteins encode in the COVID-19 virus and four major proteins, i.e., nucleocapsid, spike, envelope, and membrane protein. Instead of these main structural proteins, there are many nonstructural proteins, i.e., papain-like protease, RNA dependent RNA polymerase and coronavirus main protease [3]. In human and bat cells the angiotensin-converting enzyme-2 (ACE2) receptor is responsible to allow entry and attach with coronavirus and then replicate the virus inside the cell [4, 5]. COVID-19 virus binds to host cell through the spike protein receptor and angiotensin-converting enzyme-2 receptor of the host cell. This binding between the virus and host cell receptors triggers the changes S2 subunits at the C terminal of the spike protein. A complex between virus spike protein and ACE2 of host cell catalyzed by transmembrane serine proteases and as the result of this process the ACE2 break and viral nucleic acid enter into the host cell [6]. The viral RNA is translated into pp1a and pp1ab polyproteins after entry and uncoating. These proteins go through a proteolytic breakdown and synthesized 15 to 16 nonstructural proteins. Following the vesicle is produced by the nonstructural proteins and cellular membrane rearrangement. However, RNA nucleic acid is coded into subgenomic RNA where its synthesis of structural and other associative proteins. At last, nucleocapsids are gather in the endoplasmic reticulum and Golgi apparatus complex and after this it free through secretory pathway [7]. COVID-19 has the many genetical and clinical similarities with β genus such as SAR coronavirus and NL63 of the coronaviruses (CoVs) [8]. For cause of disease, these viruses need their reaction with the ACE2 receptor. COVID-19 and SARS coronavirus genome has high nucleotides homology [9].

9.3 NATURAL PRODUCTS AGAINST THE COVID-19

A mixture of 11 medicinal species was used to treat COVID-19 and showed the inhibitory effect and anti-inflammatory activity. This is the Chinese herbal remedies called Lianhua quingwen [10]. Conventionally, This Chinese herbal remedy has been used to cure the pneumonia, cough, influenza, fever, early stage of measles and bronchitis [11]. The anti-COVID-19 assessment was observed in Vero E6 cells through cytopathic effect (CPE) prohibition assays. The herbal extract with IC_{50} of 0.4112 mg/ml concentration inhibited COVID-19 replication in a dose dependent pattern. Moreover, this herbal mixture was shown ability to put down the free of proinflammatory cytokines in a dose-dependent manner [10]. This result shown that cytokine is lethal to the COVID-19. The herbal remedies have the 61 molecules that showed the antiviral potential with IC_{50} from 4.9 ± 0.1 to 47.8 ± 1.5 μM [12]. Recently, Lung and his coworkers in 2020 reported that theaflavin can be used to formulate the COVID-19 drug. In addition, theaflavin has shown the positive docking affinities with COVID-19 virus catalytic pocket [13]. However, the bioavailability of this compound could limit the use of relevant amount and resist to breakdown by the microorganism [14]. The herbal medicines potency was checked against the H1N1 influenza and SARS virus by using the single cohort. *Glycyrrhiza glabra*, *Saposhnikovia divaricate*, *Atractylodes lancea, Lonicera japonica*, *Astragalus mongholicus* and *Forsythia suspense* herbal species were used frequently against the COVID-19. Yupingfeng powder that is conventional Chinese remedy was made by using these species [15]. The list of medicinal plants described in Table 9.1 which have the antiviral activity against the COVID-19.

TABLE 9.1 The List of Medicinal Plants which Have the Antiviral Activity Against the COVID-19

Plants	Compound	Strain	References
Alnus japonica Steud	Hirsutenone (ethanol extract)	CoV-PLpro	[16]
Angelica keiskei, Koidz	Xanthoangelol E (ethanol extract)	CoV-PLpro CoV-3CL	[17]
Aglaia perviridis Hiern	Myricetin	ACE (rabbit lung)	[18]
Cibotium barometz	Ethanol and methanol extracts	SARS-CoV	[19]
Cullen corylifolium Medik	Psoralidin (ethanol extract)	CoV-PLpro	[20]
Ecklonia cava	Dieckol (ethanol extract)	CoV-3CL(pro)	[21]
Paulownia tomentosa (Thunb) Steud.	Tomentin E (methanol extract)	CoV-PLpro	[22]
Rheum sp. *Polygonum* sp.	Emodin	Vero cells	[23]
Salvia miltiorrhiza Bunge	Cryptotanshinone (n-hexane extract)	CoV-PLpr	[24]
Sambucus javanica subsp.	Caffeic acid	HCoV-NL63	[25]
chinensis (Lindl.) Fukuoka	Chlorogenic acid		
	95% ethanol extract		
Scutellaria baicalensis Georg	Scutellarein	*In vitro*	[18]
Torreya nucifera Siebold and Zucc	Amentoflavone (ethanol extract)	*In vitro*	[26]
Tribulus terrestris	Terrestrimine (methanol extract)	CoV PLpro	[27]
	Lianhua Qingwen (herbal mixture)	CoV-2 virus	

9.4 ROLE OF MEDICINAL PLANTS AS ACE2 BLOCKERS

COVID-19 genome penetrates into cells of the host and spike proteins of this virus bind to the ACE2 host receptors [28]. Different animals like sheep, cats, and pigeons are the important intermediate hosts to transfer this virus [29]. Hoffman et al. [30] reported that ACE2 is responsible to enter this virus into the human cells. However, TMPRSS2 can be used as the inhibitor for the formulation of drug to COVID-19 [30]. TMPRSS2 belongs to proteases family and transmembrane serine protease which involved cleaving the ACE2 and the S protein of coronavirus. Recently, in 2020, Ortega, and his colleagues was used in silico techniques to sort out the changes in S protein of coronavirus and ACE2 host receptor [31]. They found the better affinity of spike protein of coronavirus with human ACE2 receptor as compared to spike protein and ACE2 receptor of Bat coronavirus.

COVID-19 used the ACE2 receptor as a bridge for transmission in humans. In 2020, Chen, and his colleagues demonstrated that spike glycoprotein of SARS-Coronavirus and COVID-19 has 72% structural similarities but SARS Coronavirus-2 RBD showed the better interaction with ACE2 as compare to the COVID-19 coronavirus [3]. ACE2 inhibitors take part to alter the binding site of RBD and mass infection caused by COVID-19. In addition, Wrapp and his colleagues [32] confirmed that spike protein of COVID-19 showed a higher similarity with ACE2 than SARS-Coronavirus [32]. Anti SARS drugs were used for blocking of SARS-Coronavirus with ACE2 inhibitors [33]. However, recent research has been shown that high blood pressure and diabetes remarkably provoked the infection chance of COVID-19 in the face of using Angiotensin-converting enzyme 2 (ACE2) inhibitors [34–36]. Ibuprofen, angiotensin II type-I receptor stoper, and Angiotensin-converting enzyme 2 (ACE2) inhibitors given on to ACE2 upregulation, which is need to use alternative ACE2 blockers [37].

Compound originated from medicinal plants have the potential to block the Angiotensin-converting enzyme 2 receptor, and these compounds will not inhibit the enzymes' function. Therefore, these medicinal compounds may be helpful to cure the COVID-19 widespread in humans. These compounds do not affect with ACE2 expression in infected people and therefore enhance the chance for COVID-19. The sequences of ACE and ACE2 have the similarities. Substances which showed the blockage effects toward ACE which have the same effect for ACE2 and stop the entry of virus [38]. In 2016, Patten, and his colleagues demonstrated the blockage effects of medicinal herbs and plants on ACE2. They reported the inhibitory potential of 141 medicinal plants, 73 families and 49 isolated natural substance on the ACE [39]. In addition, 16 medicinal plant species were accounted to slice the angiotensin type 1A receptor *in vitro* analysis. Sharifi and his colleagues in 2013 reported that four Iranian medicinal plants species, i.e., *Quercus infectoria*, *Berberis integerrima*, *Onopordum acanthium*, and *Crataegus laevigata* exhibited the more than 80% inhibitory activity against the ACE during the *in vitro* study [40]. *Quercus infectoria* at 330 µg/ml concentration showed 94% inhibition of ACE. The inhibitory activity of this medicinal plant might be due to its higher phenolic contents and increased antioxidant potent. In addition to phenolic contents and antioxidant potential showed by this plant extract, the condensed tannins present in its and these interfere with the ACE functions.

9.5 PAPAIN-LIKE PROTEINASE (PLPRO) ARE TARGETING BY NATURAL PRODUCTS

COVID-19 genome encoded the nonstructural Papain-Like Proteinase (PLpro) protein because it is important in the virus replication and it is involved in the slicing of viral polyproteins into effector proteins [6]. PLpro works antagonistically of the host's innate immunity [42, 43] In fact, Papain-Like Proteinase was exhibited to identify the interferon production by signaling pathways like nuclear translocation, dimerization, and IRF3 phosphorylation [44]. Same effects were showed in 3 receptors of Tol like and retinoic acid-path. This result was shown that COVID-19 Papain-Like Proteinase stop the TLR7 pathway through appease the signaling of TRAF3/6-TBK1-IRF3/NF-kB/AP1 path [42]. FDA approved drug that had the potential to inhibit PLpro protein. FDA-approved 16 drugs, i.e., Pethidine, Biltricide, Procainamide, Tetrahydrozoline, Terbinafine, Cinacalcet, Amitriptyline, Labetalol, Naphazoline, Levamisole, Ticlopidine, Ethoheptazine, Chlorothiazide, Chloroquine, Formoterol, and Benzylpenicillin showed binding affinity to PLpro of COVID-19 and are effective as anti-COVID-19 agents. In addition, an alcohol unpleasant medicine (Disulfiram) was accounted a merciless blocker of Papain-Like Proteinase of COVID-19 [45].

9.5.1 CINNAMIC AMIDES FROM TRIBULUS TERRESTRIS

Inhibitory effect for PLpro was found in many natural amalgams. Cinnamic amides including Feruloyloctopamine, Feruloyltryamine, Coumaroyltyramine, Caffeoyltryamine, Terrestrimine, and Terrestriamide in the fruits have a tendency to inhibit the PLpro of SARS Coronavirus activity which increases with increasing dose of amides, while, the value of inhibitory activity (IC_{50}) ranged from 15.8–70.1 μM [27]. Among them, the IC_{50} of Terrestrimine was 15.8 ± 0.6 μM proved to be the best amide working against PLpro of SARS coronavirus activity. The presence of the methylene groups containing ketone or alcohol (C8' and C7') is a reason of enhanced prohibition activity.

9.5.2 FLAVONOIDS IN CULLEN CORYLIFOLIUM

The effect against SARS coronavirus PLpro was observed in the ethanolic seed extract of *C. corylifolium* whose IC_{50} value was 15 μg/ml (Figure 9.1).

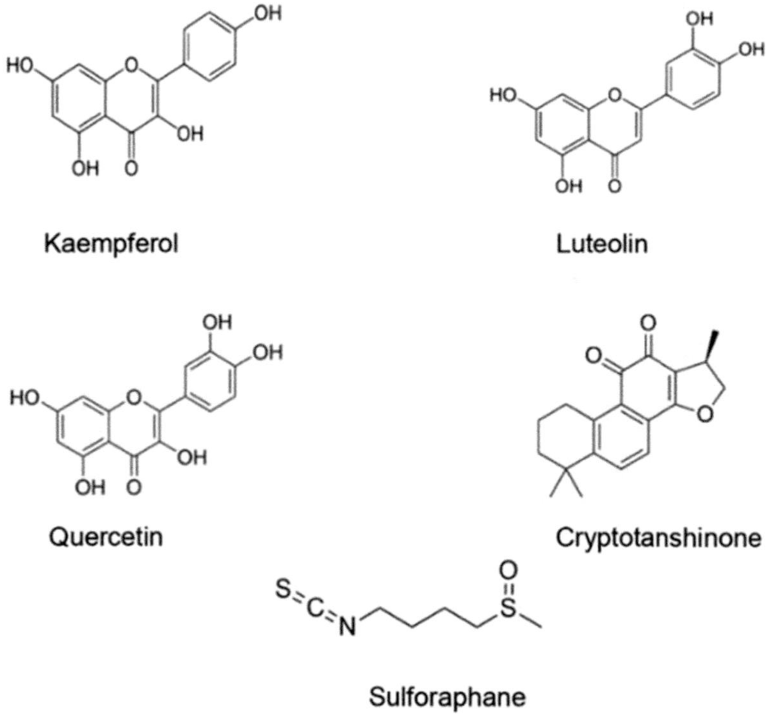

FIGURE 9.1 Natural compounds as TMPRSS2 prohibitors.

There were six flavonoids, i.e., corylifol, 40-O-methylbavachalcone, Bavachinin, isobavachalcone, neobavaisoflavone, and psoralidin in the extract whose effect against SARS-Coronavirus PLpro action was in accordance to plant extract concentration, when concentration increases the activity also increases and vice versa, although, the IC_{50} ranged from 4.2 to 38.4. The maximum effect was exhibited by isobavachalcone (IC_{50} = 7.3 ± 0.8 μM) followed by psoralidin with an IC_{50} value 4.2 ± 1.0 μM [20].

9.5.3 FLAVONOIDS IN *PAULOWNIA TOMENTOSA*

The extract of *P. tomentosa* fruits in ethanol showed 12 flavonoids, of which 5 are geranylated flavonones including tomentin A, B, C, D, and E. These all flavonoids were reversible and mixed inhibitors showing activity (IC_{50} = 5.0–14.4 mM) against SARS-CoV papain-like protease in a dose-reliance mode, while, Tomentin E flavonon showed the maximum (IC_{50} = 5.0 ± 0.06 μM) inhibitory effect. The molecules containing 3,4-dihydro-2H pyran rings showed greater prohibition value (Figure 9.2) [22].

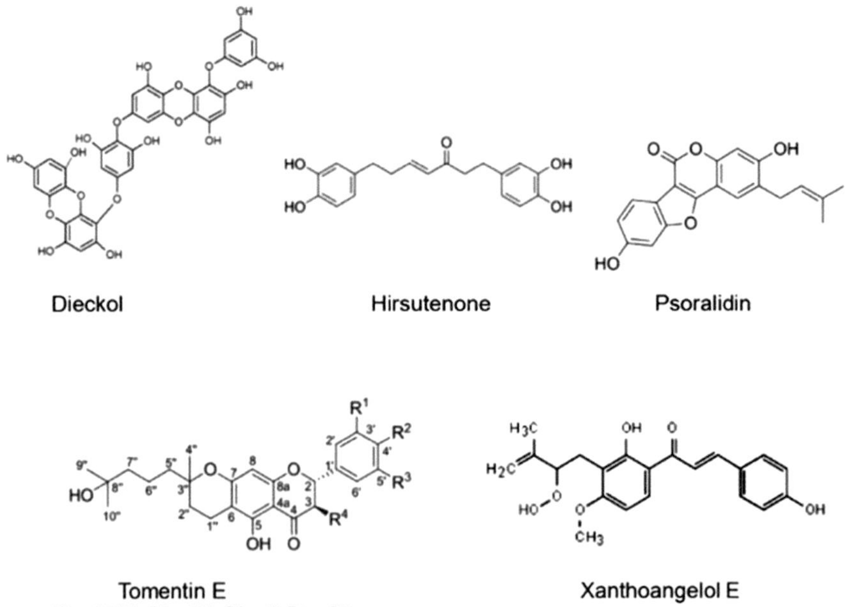

FIGURE 9.2 Natural flavonoids from the medicinal plants.

9.5.4 CHALCONES IN *ANGELICA KEISKEI*

The ethanolic extract of *A. keiskei* consisted of nine alkylated chalcones including xanthoangelol, 4-hydroxyderricin, A, B, D, E, F, G, four coumarins and isobavachalcone. Among them, chalcones containing alkyl groups repressed SARS coronavirus PLpro play function in a substantial manner depending on dose (IC_{50} = 1.2 ± 0.4 to 46.4 ± 7.8 μM), while the coumarins did not express the prohibitive effect on SARS-CoV papain-like protease activity. Among the chalcones isobavachalcone was an assorted inhibitor, while, the rest of them were uncompetitive. The silico studies showed that xanthoangelol E chalcone, exhibited 40 folds higher (IC_{50} = 1.2 ± 0.4 μM), inhibitory effect as compared to others [17].

9.5.5 TANSHINONES FROM SALVIA MILTIORRHIZA BUNGE

There were seven bioactive tanshinones, i.e., rosmariquinone, tanshinone IIA, IIB, dihydrotanshinone I, methyl tanshinonate, tanshinone I and cryptotanshinone known in the ethanolic extract of *S. miltiorrhiza* at the concentration of 30 μg/ml by n-hexane fraction which showed 88% suppressive activity towards SARS-CoV PLpro evaluated by fluorometric analysis. The inhibitory effect of these molecules was time-dependent ranging from IC_{50} = 0.8 to 30 μM, while, cryptotanshinone was the most effective inhibitor (IC_{50} = 0.8 ± 0.2 μM) of SARS-CoV PLpro. Kinetic investigations verified that all the transhinones were noncompetitive except rosmariquinone which was an assorted inhibitor of SARS-CoV PLpro [24].

9.5.6 DIARYLHEPTANOIDS IN ALNUS JAPONICA

There were nine diarylheptanoids including rubranoside B, and A, platyphyllenone, platyphyllonol-5-xylopyranoside, rubranol, oregonin, platyphyllone, hirsutanonol, and hirsutenone were purified by using activity guided fractionation in the ethanolic extract of *A. japonica*. These compounds showed inhibition depending on dose concentration towards SARS-CoV PLpro by continuous fluorometric method with IC_{50} = 3 – 44.5 μM. Among all the compounds, Hirsutenone showed the most effective inhibitory effect (4.1 ± 0.3 μM) to the reference prohibitor curcumin (5.7 μM). Moreover, it was suggested that this maximum potential of inhibition was because of the manifestation of unsaturated a, b, carbonyl, and catechol groups [24].

9.5.7 NATURAL PRODUCTS MANAGING THE CHYMOTRYPSIN-LIKE PROTEASE ACTIVITY

The main viral proteinase 3 CL(pro) reins the actions of the coronavirus imitation complex, is a striking goal for chymotrypsin-like protease treatment links to nonstructural 16 proteins of the SARS Coronavirus 2. Therefore, it plays a significant part in copying the SARS Coronavirus 2, so considered a possible therapeutic mark as anti-COVID-19 drug [36]. Different natural compounds demonstrated auspicious activities against 3CL (pro) protein.

9.5.8 CHALCONES (ALKYLATED) FROM ANGELICA KEISKEI

An isolated and purified natural compound alkylated chalcones and coumarins from *A. keiskei* were examined towards SARS coronavirus 3CL(pro) inhibition by fluorescence resonance energy transfer (FRET) techniques. Alkylated chalcones showed anti SARS coronavirus chymotrypsin like protease activity in a dosage-reliance mode with a range of IC_{50} from 11.4 ± 1.4 to 129.8 ± 10.3 μM. Although kinetic studies expressed both chalcones and coumarins as good inhibitors, but xanthogelol E was the most effective inhibitor in the therapeutic line against COVID-19 [17].

9.5.9 PHLOROTANNINS IN ECKLONIA CAVA (ALGAE)

The ethanolic extract of *E. cava* consisted of nine phlorotannins. These phlorotannins were evaluated by a cell-free based method towards anti-SARS-CoV-3CL (pro) activity. Eight phlorotannins including phlorofucofuroeckol A, triphloretol A, phloroeckol-2 and 7, dioxinodehydroeckol, dieckol, eckol, and fucodiphloroethol G showed dosage-reliance prohibitory role towards SAR coronavirus chymotrypsin-like protease with IC_{50} = 2.7 ± 0.6 exhibited by dieckol and IC_{50} = 164.7 ± 10.8 μM shown by triphloretol A. Among these phlorotannins, six compounds except triphloretol, A, and eckol showed a substantial micromolar dosage-reliance inhibition of SARS-coronavirus-3CL(pro) cis-cleavage action. According to the studies of molecular docking diekcol showed resilient hydrogen bonding to the catalytic dyad comprises of Cys145 and His41 and lowermost binding energy (11.51 kcal/mol) for SARS-CoV-3-chymotrypsin like proteases, thus act as promising prohibitor of SARS-Coronavirus 3CL(pro). Structure of diekcol have two eckol groups associated by a diphenyl ether. Although differences in metabolization among phlorotannins and also their bioavailability put a question to their performances [21]. These phlorotannin have also been evidenced to effect the human gut microbiota, thus inhibiting the growth of potentially pathogenic microorganisms and proved to be beneficial to human health. Although there are limitations in their clinical usage because of the lack of analytical standards and differences in their structures and linkages with the same molecular weight (MW) [46].

9.5.10 TANSHINONES FROM SALVIA MILTIORRHIZA BUNGE

According to the findings of Park and his coworkers [16] on *S. miltiorrhiza*, the ethanolic extract at the concentration of 30 μg/ml contained six tanshinones in the plant lipophilic fraction which showed 60% prohibition towards SARS coronavirus 3CL(pro) which increases with increase in dose with an expected value of IC_{50} extending from 14.4 μM to 89.1 μM. Kinetic studies showed that the tanshinones of *S. miltiorrhiza* Bunge were non-competitive prohibitors towards SARS coronavirus 3CL(pro) with a maximum IC_{50} of 14.4 ± 0.7 μM exhibited by Dihydrotanshinone I.

9.5.11 BIFLAVONOIDS FROM TORREYA NUCIFERA SIEBOLD AND ZUCC

The ethanolic extract of leaves of *T. nucifera* were checked for their effect as anti SARS coronavirus 3CL(pro) agent by using a FRET method and reported to contain four bioflavonoids including ginkgetin, amentoflavone, bilobetin, and sciadopitysin. Although, the extract of *T. nucifera* also have eight diterpenoids exhibiting IC_{50} value ranging from 49.6 μM to 283.5 μM, but the inhibitory effect of bioflavonoids (IC_{50} = 8.3–72.3 μM) was stronger which made them competitive inhibitors towards SARS-CoV-3CL(pro). Amentoflavone was the utmost effective prohibitor exhibiting IC_{50} = 8.3 ± 1.2 μM followed by luteolin (IC_{50} = 20.0 ± 2.2 μM), quercetin (IC_{50} = 23.8 ± 1.9 μM) and apigenin (IC_{50} = 28.8 ± 21.4 μM). Molecular docking revealed that amentoflavone formed strong hydrogen bonds with SARS-CoV-3CL(pro), thus inhibiting its activity [26].

9.5.12 FLAVONOIDS

In *Pichia pastoris* GS115, seven flavonoids named ampelopsis, epigallocatechin, daidzein, puerarin, gallocatechin gallate, epigallocatechin gallate and quercetin were present which expressed their prohibitory activity towards SARS-CoV-3 chymotrypsin-like protease. Among these flavonoids gallocatechin gallate expressed 91% inhibitory activity towards SARS coronavirus 3CL(pro) followed by epigallocatechin gallate (85%), and quercetin (82%), thus, Gallocatechin gallate with IC_{50} of 47 μM was proved to be the record promising prohibitor of SARS coronavirus 3CL(pro) by establishing a hydrophobic and hydrogen bond with the dynamic site of SARS coronavirus 3Chymotrypsin like protease expressed by molecular docking studies [47]. Although, the function of this hydrogen bonds with at the active site of SARS coronavirus 3CL(pro) is difficult to predict [48].

Later in 2020, Jo, and his colleagues examined the activity of 64 flavonoids as SARS-CoV-3CL(pro) inhibitors by FRET method and reported that rhoifolin, herbacetin, and pectolinarin (20 μM) unveiled extreme prohibitory effect with IC_{50} = 27.45, 33.17, and 37.78 mM, correspondingly [49]. Furthermore, molecular docking, proved that the structure of flavonoids comprised of aromatic rings, which are hydrophobic and hydroxyl groups which are hydrophilic in nature which showed significant binding affinity to active sites of SARS-Coronavirus-3CL (pro) (Figure 9.3).

9.5.13 CRITICAL CONSIDERATIONS

This review included 15 *in vitro* studies conducted in four different countries, as 9 studies were done in Korea, 3 in Taiwan, 2 in China and 1 in Iran. These studies were published from 2011 to 2018 except 3 of which 1 was published in 2019 and 2 were published in 2020 [10, 25, 49]. On study explained the antiviral activity towards SARS coronavirus 2 [35] while the other study was on the coronavirus NL63 in humans and [25]. The methanolic, ethanolic, and water extracts of the plant were investigated in 3 studies, while 1 study was based on an herbal mixture of 11 Chinese plants. The studies were conduction on the compounds of different phytochemical classes and mostly reported compound of them were phenolics.

After analyzing all this phytopharmacological research concerned with this scenario by the practical recommendations, various factors were considered, including that most of the natural products are phenolics, quercetin, or kaempferol which belong to those phytochemical classes which have broad range biological actions under control and normal conditions. Thus, the efficiency and specificity of these active natural compounds as drugs is not very descriptive. Moreover, the methods implemented to conduct these studies did not consider the reliable sources of plant species and their standards for both plants and their products names. Among all the 15 studies, 7 studies are reported with control, but they did not justify the comparison of the positive controls, whereas, rest of the studies have not used the control, resulting in a biased result. Besides these, lack of full taxonomic statistics also considered to be a possible limitation in the methodology of these studies [51].

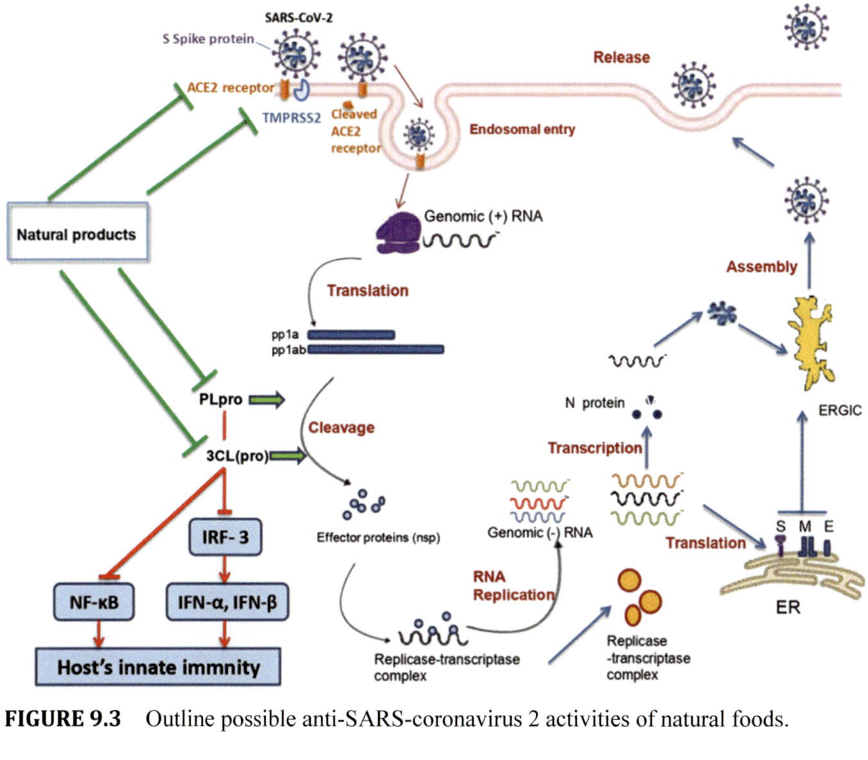

FIGURE 9.3 Outline possible anti-SARS-coronavirus 2 activities of natural foods.

In this study, a few natural compounds, including caffeic acid, dieckol, tomentin E, cryptotanshinone, hirsutenone, psoralidin, myricetin, xanthoangelol E, amentoflavone, and scutellarein, are reported to have anti SARS-Coronavirus-2 inhibition activity with an IC_{50} value ranged from 0 to 10 μM. So, these molecules were considered to be active SARS-CoV inhibitors. Among them chloroquine was reported to show inhibition activity towards both SARS-Coronavirus and coronavirus disease-19 replication with IC_{50}

8.8 μM and 1.13 to 5.47 μM, respectively, while IC_{50} of ivermectin was measured as 2 mM [52, 53]. Not surprisingly, these active molecules are phenolic in nature and their minimum bioavailability and quick eradication made them useful against COVID-9 for clinical purposes [54].

These studied plants have been used to cure reported effect in COVID-19 such as fever, infection, swellings, circulatory or heart diseases, despite the limitations, considered regarding these plants extracts and natural compounds. As a few species, showed no inhibitory effect against COVID-19, moreover, no relationship was established with their ethnopharmacological uses (Table 9.2). More research should be done to validate the safety and efficacy of these active natural compounds in the patients suffered from COVID-19. Furthermore, to enhance their clinical usefulness, the mechanisms and pathways followed by these products and some other factors including their availability, mode of action, safe doses, coverage time, pharmacokinetic profile, patients' health, stage of the disease should also be evaluated for their beneficial effects as anti-SARS-CoV-2 agent. After these studies, these active natural compounds could be a good alternative to antiviral drugs.

9.6 ROLE OF PHYTOCHEMICALS AGAINST THE COVID-19

Instead of natural products numerous imperative phytochemical compounds have capability against the CoVs [55, 56] that cause diseases in the human are discussed in details.

9.6.1 ESSENTIAL OILS

Medicinal plants such as Hyssopus officinalis, mayweeds, tea trees, Santalum, Pinus thymes, ginger, and scented plants are being used in the production of essential oil and have the antiviral activities [57–61]. Essential oil has the ability to enter the lipid double layer of viral envelops and after this it changes the fluidity of membrane [60]. Essential oil has the monoterpenes, oxygenated sesquiterpenes and phenylpropanoids and has the lipophilic natures, which is effective for disarranging the coronavirus membrane which is made up of phospholipid molecule and enter the structure of envelope proteins (E protein) of the virus during the infection [62]. Eucalyptol essential oil is obtaining from the gum trees and has the antiviral activity which effective against the COVID-19. Eucalyptus oil contain the ketone, hydroxyl, and ether molecules which are involved in the reluctance against

COVID-19 [63]. Resveratrol (terpenoids) have the ability to suppress the nucleocapsid of virus and RNA regulation and stop the replication. The cell death of Vero E6 was shown at the 125–250 μM concentration of resveratrol [64]. Jensenone compound present in essential oil of eucalyptus and showed antiviral activity to stop Mpro of SARS-Coronavirus-2 which cause the COVID-19 [65]. However, there is more research necessary to sort out the felicity of Jensenone compound can be used medicine for human.

9.6.2 ALKALOIDS

Chloroquine compound is prepared from the quinine and quinine is bitter alkaloid obtains from the cinchona tree bark. Chloroquine compound has the potential for the formulation of potent drug to cure COVID-19 because DNA of this virus has insinuated characteristics [66]. Resochin is the type of alkaloid which is being used to treat malaria and have potential against the viral diseases. Resochin medicine has the potential to stop the replication, transcription, and translation of viral nucleic acid [61]. Similarly, isoquinoline alkaloids such as palmatine and chelidonine are the intercalating alkaloid and can be used as drug candidates to the battle SARS-CoV-2 [61, 67]. Cepharanthine, fangchinoline, and tetrandrine are pharmaceutically important alkaloids purified from *Stephania tetrandra;* other species of family Menispermaceae were used against the HCoV-OC43 coronavirus which infected MRC-5 cells of lung tissue [68]. These compounds also have the anti-inflammatory and anticancer activities [68]. The use of these three compounds dramatically decreased the HCoV-OC43 cells in the human. These three alkaloids inhibited the expression of viral protein (S) and nucleocapsid (N) protein. Instead of this, mycophenolate, tylophorine, and emetine and others alkaloids had shown the significant antiviral activity [69–71].

9.6.3 PHENOLICS, FLAVONOIDS, POLYPHENOLS, AND OTHERS

Plant secondary metabolites and their derivatives like steroid, flavonoids, terpenoid, polyphenols, phenolic compounds, and important phytochemicals contain in their structure one or more hydroxyl groups. A hydrogen bond forms between the hydroxyl ion in these molecules and the positive charged amino acids residues of the virus proteins; which hinder the viral activity [61]. Wink and his coworkers [61] reported that polyphenols have the ability to bind with virus envelope and, due to this binding, stop the access of viral genome in the host cell. Viral enzyme 3C-like proteases determine the coronavirus replication complexes during the process of viral replication [72].

3C-like proteases are study during the replication of COVID-19 CoVs in the infected cells. Root extract of *Isatis indigotica* plant was used against the COVID-19 disease and it showed the effective result to this coronavirus. The root extract of this plant has the five majors' type of secondary metabolites such as sinigrin, hesperetin, indigo, β-sitosterol, β-sitosterol, and phenolic compounds, which were significantly inhibited the cleavage activity of 3C-like proteases. Plant isolated flavonoids, polyphenols, and phenolic compounds were shown very effective results against 3C-like protease coronavirus enzyme. In other studies, plant flavor compounds such as pectolinarin, gallocatechin, rhoifilin, epigallocatechin, and herbacetin are present in the seeds of *Litchi chinesis* were inhibited the replication of 3C-like proteases enzyme of CoVs [73].

All types of coronavirus such as COVID-19, NL63 Coronavirus and SARS Coronavirus attack on the human angiotensin-converting enzyme-2 receptor [74]. Therefore, phytochemicals from the plants have the ability to prevent hACE2 receptor with the interaction of COVID-19 and also increase the strengthen of this receptor to combat against the COVID-19 infection. Luteolin flavonoid, scutellarin, polyphenolic compounds such as tetra-O-galloyl-β-D-glucose extracted from *V. linariifolia* and Gallachinensis [75, 76], seeds of soybean and other plant seeds have the iron chelator like nicotianamine [77], baicalin is a flavone glycoside obtain from the extract of *S. baicalensis* [78], genus Polygonum and Rheum has an emodin [23] which has the ability to interact with ACE2 host and SARS Coronavirus S protein. In another study, cannabinoid phytochemicals were docked with viral S protein and these results indicated that these phytochemicals have the binding sites and inhibit the function of S protein [79].

In addition to, a flavonoid such as quercetin and saponin was isolated from the *T. sinensis* leaf extract and liquor ice roots, respectively [80, 81] showed strong antiviral activity against the SARS coronavirus. These compounds stop the cellular attachment and prevent the entry of virus to the human cell. More than 10,000 different compounds like drugs, natural, and synthetic are screened, and these compounds showed the effect results against the SARS coronavirus [82]. Indole alkaloids and were isolated from eucalyptus, *L. japonica* and Rauwolfia and from chestnut tree, respectively inhibited aescin the SARS coronavirus replication [82]. RNA dependent RNA polymerase is the major enzyme in the replication of SARS coronavirus, which synthesized the positive and negative strand of coronavirus RNA. A toxic steroid-like cardenolides were obtained from the plant and swine testicular cells inhibited the gastro entry of coronavirus [83]. These results showed that toxic cardenolide reduce the 50% RNA copies and suppress the viral replication [83].

Plant proteins have the antiviral activity such lectin from the *N. tabacum*, *U. dioica* and *A. porrum* was purified and pure lectin at concentration less than 1.3 μgml^{-1} showed the inhibition of viral and slow down the viral propagation [84]. These proteins in plants work as the defensive tools and can be used to cure the COVID-19 infected people. Lectin proteins have a conserved binding site and S protein of coronavirus bind in this catalytic site and inhibit the activity of virus inside the host cell. Lectin protein is a carbohydrate-binding protein in plants there are different isoforms of lectin proteins are presents that play a role in the defensive system inside the plants [84]. Moreover, several studies of flavonoids shown very effective results against the different strains of CoVs activity were listed in Table 9.2.

9.7 USE OF HERBAL MEDICINES AGAINST THE COVID-19

Different plant species have been for the synthesis of herbal medicines and these herbal medicines have the antiviral activity. Plant-based herbal medicines has a significant effect in preventing the SARS coronavirus [71]. For example, at the concentration 41.9 μgml^{-1} of *G. lucidum*, 108.4 μgml^{-1} concentration of *C. versicolor* and 198.6 μgml^{-1} concentration of *S. acutum* inhibit the replication of RNA polymerase enzyme of SARS coronavirus [95]. For cell proliferation assay, there were more than 200 Chinese plants used and assessed to find out the antiviral substances against the SARS-CoV [96]. Four herbs, i.e., *A. annua*, *P. lingua*, *L. aggregate*, and *L. radiate* were identified from this experiment which inhibited the virus activity significantly. These results showed that medicinal plants have the significant potential for the cure of SARS related diseases. However, a lycorine is a toxic alkaloid and isolated from the extract of plant and experiment results showed that it had antiviral potential and could be used for the development of antiviral medicines [96].

Chrysanthemum decoction and *Saposhnikovia divaricate* medicinal herbs and was used in China during the COVID-19 disease. These herbs are native to China and Japan. When the extract of these herbs was taken to COVID-19 infected people and people showed a better defensive system to combat against this disease. The results indicated that the use of these herb extract may change the T cell because the T cells of the host increase the defensive ability [97]. Herbal medicines were used to cure the COVID-19 disease in

TABLE 9.2 A-List of Antiviral Plants which Prohibited Various Classes of Coronavirus

Plants	Substance	Virus Type	References
C. sinensis, C longa, P. hanceana	Gallate, glucoside, and apigenin-7 catechin demethoxycurcumin	Coronavirus	[85]
H. perforatum	Hypericin	2019-nCoV NSP 14	[71]
T. indica	Tylophorine	Coronaviruses	[69]
T. indica	Tylophorine	Enteropathogenic coronavirus and transmissible gastroenteritis virus	[86]
L. radiata	Lycorine	(SARS) CoV	[70]
C. sativa	Tetrahydrocannabinol and cannabidiol	Different diseases	[87]
P. corylifolia	Bavachinin, Psoralidin, Corylifol	SARS-CoV	[20]
C. miniata	Lycorine and mycophenolate	HCoV-OC43 and MERS-CoV	[69]
A. foveolata	Silvestrol	HCoV-229E	[88]
C. sativa	Cannabidiol	Cause viral infection	[89]
B. papyrifera	Kazinol A, B, F, and J	Cysteine proteases, papain-like, and coronavirus	[90]
B. papyrifera	Polyphenols	Cysteine proteases of coronavirus	[77]
C. sinensis peel extracts, *N. sativa* and *A. hyalina*	Essential oils	Coronavirus of epithelial carcinoembryonic antigen (ECA-CoV)	[91]
E. cava	Dieckol	Porcine diarrhea	[92]
P. tomentosa	Tomentin	SARS-CoV	[22]
C. sinensis	Catechins	SARS-CoV	[93]
A. perviridis	Myricetin and Scutellarein	SARS-CoV	[18]
P. sidoides	Extract EPs® 7630	Human coronavirus (HCoV)	[94]

another study results showed that herbal medicines showed the significant and positive result to reduce the symptom and shorten the disease cycle that caused by COVID-19 infection disease [98]. However, these results showed that herbal medicines are good candidate for the development of clinical trial and *in vitro* analysis.

Crocin compound was isolated from *C. sativus* and have the remarkably antiviral activity. Crocin inhibit the replication of human coronavirus and reduced the symptoms of the disease in the infected people. *C. sativus* is medicinal herbs and is being used to treat the HIV and human coronavirus [99]. *Nerium oleander* is also herbal medicinal plants that have 11.25% digitoxigenin compound and its derivatives. These compounds and their derivatives have the anticancer and antiviral activity [100]. *Lauris nobilis* herbal plants contain the β Eudesmol compounds in low quantity, i.e., 2.39%, but this compound has a very good potential to interact with the target and showed the antibacterial antiviral activity against the different bacterial and viral diseases [101]. Docking results of these three compounds with the Coronavirus main proteases inhibited the binding site of Coronavirus main protease and controlled the replication of Coronavirus main protease [102].

9.8 USE OF FOOD PLANTS TO TREAT COVID-19 DISEASE

The immune system is very important defensive tools of human body which fight against the attack of pathogens including microorganism, viruses that cause the infection in the human body. There are 20 different types of food plants that play a role to increase the immunity and show antiviral effects against viral infections. These food plants are black pepper, turmeric, garlic, pomegranate, liquorice, ginger, tea, and many other foods plants are listed in Table 9.3. These food plants have been revealed to increase the immune system.

Food plants have the immunomodulatory function and increase the humoral and cell immunity and due to this function of food plants; some cells become activate that is non-specific to the immune system such as granulocytes, natural killer, complement systems, and macrophages. These activated cells increase the resistance against the infections. As the result of activation of these immune cells, different molecules are produced such as chemokines, interferons and cytokines and take part to increase the immune responses. During the SARS infection, immune response cells such as natural killer cells, lymphocytes, and dendritic cells (DCs) present in the spleen were decreased [103]. Results of some studies showed that during the

TABLE 9.3 Common Food Plants That have Immunomodulatory and Antiviral Potential

Plant Name	Parts	Use	References
Berberis vulgaris	Root, fruit, and stem	Boiled extract and poultice	[106–108]
Citrus aurantium	Fruit and peel	Dried peel or fruit juice	[109, 110]
Carica papaya	Fruit and leaves	Leaves are ground to prepare juice; fruit can be directly eaten	[111, 112]
Allium sativum	Bulb	Crushed and mixed with honey	[113–115]
Camellia sinensis	Leaf	Boiled and drunk	[116, 117]
Allium cepa	Bulb	Crushed and mixed with honey	[118, 119]
Glycyrrhiza glabra	Root	Dried roots extracted. The extract is vacuum dried to a dark paste, or maybe dried to a powder	[81, 120, 121]
Curcuma longa	Rhizome	Pounded, tincture, powder	[122–124]
Glycine max	Seeds	Cooked or roasted	[125–127]
Lycium barbarum	Fruit	Fresh fruit directly eaten	[128–130]
Ficus carica	Fruit, leaves	Decoction with honey	[131, 132]
Mangifera indica	Bark, leaves, roots, fruits, and flowers	Boiling or powdering of bark, leaves, root, and flowers, while fruit can be directly eaten	[133, 134]
Zingiber officinale	Root	Dried or roasted, eaten with honey	[135, 136]
Morus alba	Fruit leaf, root	Leaves and root, bark decoction or tea and fruit juice	[137, 138]
Psidium guajava	Leaves fruit, and shoots	Decoction and poultice of leaves and fruit	[139, 140]
Piper nigrum	Fruit	Dried and used as spice	[141]
Nigella sativa	Seed	Roasted an end eat	[142, 143]
Punica granatum	Bark, seeds, and fruits	Dried bark, fruit juice, decoction of seeds	[144, 145]
Piper longum	Fruit and root	Decoction	[146]
Prunus domestica	Fruit	Fresh	[147, 148]

viral infection the size of macrophages and T-lymphocytes increased at the site of viral loads [104, 105].

Liquorice is medicinal herbs that are being used to cure different types of chronic infections since ancient times. Liquorice dried and crushed roots are boiled and then prepare the root extract. The liquid crude extract can be dried to make a dark fine powder. This powder can be taken orally to cure the many types of chronic disease [149]. Glycyrrhizin is the saponin that is present in the root extract of liquorice, and this molecule show the antimicrobial, immunomodulatory, and antiviral activity [150].

Garlic is another herbal food medicine since ancient times. It was observed that fresh crushed garlic can be used with honey to enhance the immunity and also have the antimicrobial and antiviral activity. Cloves of garlic contain the several bioactive sulfur compounds, i.e., polyphenols, sulfoxide, and proteins [135, 151]. In some studies garlic show the positive significant effect on the immune cells, for example sulfur compounds such as allyl methyl sulfide, diallyl sulfide and diallyl disulfide showed the immunostimulatory reaction in mice [152]. Diallyl disulfide sulfur compound shows very good results as compared to other sulfur compounds. This compound increased the white blood cells (WBC) and antibody in mice. Sulfur containing compounds increased the quantity of spleen plaque forming cells, raised the cellularity of bone marrow and increased the positive cells of α-esterase. However, modulatory effects were observed on T lymphocyte and macrophage function by protein faction and garlic extract.

However, other food plants also show the immunostimulatory effects, like curcumin show the interaction with many immune cells such as cytokines, B, and T lymphocytes, DCs, and macrophages and also the defensive system of the host [123]. Mononuclear cells of human peripheral were enhanced the lymphoproliferative function in 72 hours with the treatment of black tea [153]. Black tea leaves contain the quercetin, negative epigallocatechin gallate, and gallic acid compounds which have the immunostimulatory effects [154]. In addition to, it was observed that fig leaves ethanolic extract boost the humoral and immune-related cell. In the past, the leaves extract of this plant was used against the cardiovascular disease, gastrointestinal (GI), respiratory, and inflammatory problems. However, mango bark methanolic extract boost immunomodulatory effects and increased the humoral antibody and slow down hypersensitivity [133]. In addition to, the *in vivo* study showed that the number of WBC, spleen, and thymus size was increased by the oral intake of mange hexane leaves extract and this result indicated that immunomodulation in WBC [155].

9.9 ETIOLOGY OF COVID-19 AND APPROACH FOR PALATABLE PLANTS

To use the natural molecules in edible plants properly against the coronavirus disease-19, it is mandatory to have an understanding of structural targets, receptors, and their mechanism of action associated with this virus. Seven human coronaviruses (HCoVs) have been identified till now and severe acute respiratory syndrome coronavirus 2 (SARS-CoV-2) also have +ssRNA along with two protein groups: structural protein and non-structural protein; structural protein included spike, envelope, matrix, and nucleocapsid while non-structural proteins comprised of nsp12-RNA-dependent RNA polymerase (RdRp), Nsp3-Papain-like proteinases, Nsp5-3C-like main protease and nsP13 SARS-CoV helicase [156, 157]. Despite of these proteins, human angiotensin-converting-enzyme-2 (ACE-2) act as a receptor of SARS-CoV-2 as essentially present in the lungs, heart, intestine, kidneys, and blood vessels can be targeted to prevent the entry of viruses into the host cells [158, 159]. The functioning of angiotensin-converting-enzyme-2 increased exponentially in diabetic patients as well as in the patients suffering from hypertension. This ACE-2 is actually a site for the replication of viruses soil the interest of developing the drugs to suppress this receptor is increasing [160]. Many plants have been reported containing phytochemicals effectively targeting viral diseases like SARS, HIV, HCV, etc. [23, 161].

The ACE-2 in human lungs serve as a binding site for S2 subunit in severe acute respiratory syndrome coronavirus 2, where virus replicate to express cellular responses like intrusion of a number of native and adaptive immune cells [162–164]. Among them, neutrophils are native, causing lungs injury while T cells are adaptive, which kill the viruses along with causing the lungs injury [165, 166]. Moreover, these T cells contain type 1 and 2 helper cells which trigger the imbalance of these cytokines thus causing a "cytokines storm" also called "cytokines surge" which increase the inflammatory actions of cytokines (TNFα, IL1, IL6, IL10) and chemokines (CXCL10 and CCL2) by apoptosis in alveoli which in turn interfere the transportation of oxygen, increase the lungs porousness and transduction of respiratory edema fluid which is concentrated with protein into the airspaces, thus reducing lungs functioning ultimately causing the death of alveoli cells in lungs resulting in ARDS (acute respiratory distress or syndrome) [74, 167] (Figure 9.4).

The main reason of deaths in coronavirus disease-19 is actually this cytokine surge along with weak immune system. Moreover, this pulmonary malfunctioning couples with the clotting of blood in which iron detach from the beta-1 chain of hemoglobin and attach to the porphyrin ring of glycoprotein, thus causing the failure of respiration [168].

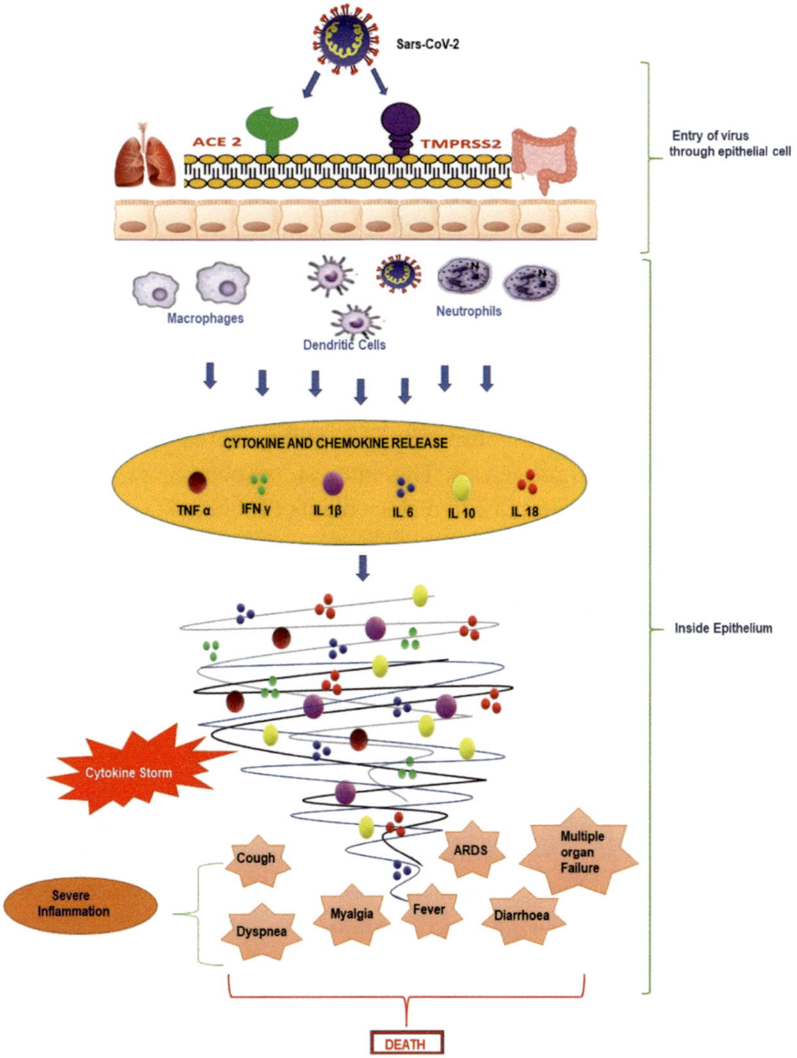

FIGURE 9.4 Etiology of coronavirus disease-19.

At the initial phase of infection of SARS-CoV-2, host immune eluding strategies lead to a prolonged incubation period consist of 2–14 days inside the human body [169]. Plants containing phytochemicals showing immunity boosting properties may serve as precautionary treatment if added in daily intake, for the prevention of COVID-19 infection and also speed up healing after infection thus, help in producing natural antiviral agents to combat this pandemic disease.

9.9.1 EDIBLE PLANTS SHOWING ANTIVIRAL PROPERTY COUNTER TO RNA VIRUSES (COVID-19)

Plants contain secondary metabolites which have been reported to be used to combat many diseases such as diabetes, atherosclerosis, cardiovascular diseases, cancer, and neurological disorders [19, 170]. From ancient times plants from Indian origin are being used to treat many diseases such as respiratory viral infections by enhancing the immunity and suppressing inflammation. Indian AYUSH system comprises of Ayurveda, Yoga Unani, Siddha, and Homeopathy medications also prevent from COVID-19 by dietary management and by improving body immunity [171] thus, increasing the interest in plants for their antiviral properties. This interest has been increasing because of phytochemicals present in these dietary plants (Table 9.4).

9.9.2 PLANTS PREVENTING ENTRY OF VIRUS IN THE HOST CELLS

Plants contain flavonoids which have the ability to bind the active site of SARS-CoV-2 protein, which is actually the site of first attachment in the host cell. The plants of family Polygonaceae contain emodin flavonoids which inhibit the contact of spike protein of SARS coronavirus and HCoV-OC43 [172]. On the other hand, lectins are the natural proteins which check the sugar groups of spike proteins of SARS-Coronavirus thus act as initial inhibitors by preventing the viral attachment to the spike protein, moreover, lectins also have potentials that viral particles bind to it and not to human cells, thus, the pathogenic cycle would not be completed [5]. Many palatable plants like *Cynara scolymus, Cassia occidentalis* and *Punica granatum* have the anti ACE agents which prevent the SARS-CoV-2 from entering the host cells [174].

9.9.3 PLANTS INHIBITING VIRAL REPLICATION

Plants have also been reported which inhibit the viral replication of severe acute respiratory syndrome coronavirus and also leads to inhibit the replication of its second strain because of similar homology; these plants include *Glycyrrhiza*

TABLE 9.4 Eatable Plants and Their Mode of Actions Against Disease-Causing Viruses

Palatable Plants	Commonly Known as	Phytochemicals	Cure Virus	Mode of Action
Abutilon indicum	Lantern	β-Sitosterol and asparagine in methanolic extract of aerial parts	Coronavirus-19	Unknown
Acalypha indica	Kuppi	Acalyphin and kaemferol in ethanolic extract of leaves	Vesicular stomatitis virus	Prohibition of protein interaction
Aegle marmelos	Bael	Marmin and marmesin in methanolic extract of all parts except flower	Human coxsackieviruses	Restricts viral replication
Agrimonia pilosa	Hairy agrimony	Catechin and quercetin in ethanolic extract of whole plant	Influenza virus	Restrict viral mRNA synthesis and replication
Allium sativum	Lehsan	Allicin, lectin, and Alliin in garlic cloves	SARS-CoV	Inhibit glycans on in spike protein to restrict the entry of virus
Aloe vera	Kwargandal	Polysaccharides and aloin in leaf extract (aqueous)	Human rhinovirus, vesicular stomatitis virus	Prevents viral attachment to host
Areca nut	Supari	Arecoline and guvacine in methanolic extract of seeds	Influenza A virus	Restriction of protease in HIV type-1
Artemisia annua	Sweet sagewort	Artemisinin ethanolic whole plant extract	Human immune disorder virus-1	Unknown
Azadirachta indica	Neem	Azadirachtin in leaf extract in methanol	Group B Coxsackieviruses	Restricts replication
Camellia sinensis	Green tea	Epigallocatechin and gallate in leaf extract (aqueous)	Bovine coronavirus, influenza virus, HIV-1	Interfere steps in virus life cycle
Cassia occidentalis	Coffee	Rhein and emodin in leaf extract (methanolic)	Human immunological disorder virus	Inhibiting HIV reverse transcriptase activity
Cicer arietinum	Gram	Dietary minerals virus in methanolic extract of aerial parts	Parainfluenza	Inhibits replication of parainfluenza-3 virus

TABLE 9.4 *(Continued)*

Palatable Plants	Commonly Known as	Phytochemicals	Cure Virus	Mode of Action
Commelina communis	Asiatic dayflower	Homonojirimycin virus in ethanolic extract of leaf and stem	Influenza (108)	Check inflammation of host sells by IFN- and IL-10 activation
Curcuma longa	Clove	Curcumin in rhizome	Pulmonary virus	Check viral replication
Cynara Scolymus	Sharifa	Cynaropicrin	Hepatitis C virus	Prevents viral entry into host cell
Embelia ribes	Vidanga	Embelin fruit extract in ethyl acetate	Influenza A virus	Interfere replication of virus
Eugenia jambolana	Jamun	Delphinidin, petunidin in leaf and bark extract (water and methanol)	Influenza virus	Affects viral envelop to restrict attachment to host cells
Gingko biloba	Ginkgo	Ginkgetin	Influenza virus (46)	Restrict sialidase enzyme activity in virus
Glycyrrhiza glabra	Mulethi	Glycyrrhizin	SARS-CoV	Prevent host cell from viral penetration and replication
Gymnema sylvestre	Gudmar	Gymnemic acid in methanolic extract of aerial parts	Coronavirus disease-19	Unknown
Hibiscus sabdariffa	Lal ambari	Hibiscus acid, citric acid in tea extract (aqueous)	H5N1 strain of influenza virus (pathogenic)	Suppress viral antigen and gene expression thus inhibiting replication
Leucas aspera	Tumba	Asperphenamate, sitosterol in methanolic extract of aerial parts	SARS-CoV	Unknown
Mangifera indica	Mango	Mangiferin in stem and bark extract (hydrochloric extract)	Influenza A virus, coxsackie B3 virus	Suppress protease enzyme activity
Momordica charantia	Karela	Momordicine, Charantin	Human immunodeficiency virus	Restrict stages of viral replication cycle

TABLE 9.4 *(Continued)*

Palatable Plants	Commonly Known as	Phytochemicals	Cure Virus	Mode of Action
Moringa oleifera	Sohanjna	Quercetin, linolenic acid in leaves extract	Human immunodeficiency virus type-1	Prohibit replication of virus
Myrica esculenta	Bayberry	Myricetin, gallic acid	SARS-CoV	Suppress helicase enzyme activity
Nigella sativa	Kalonji	Thymoquinone, thymol in dried seeds	H9N2 avian influenza virus	Restrict replication stages
Ocimum sanctum	Tulsi	Eugenol, linolenic acid in methanolic extract of aerial parts	Human immunodeficiency virus	Suppress protease activity
Olea europaea	Olive	Oleuropein in leaf extract in ethanol	Viral hemorrhagic septicemia virus	Acts on viral envelope and deactivate virus
Phaseolus vulgaris	Red bean	Phaseolin in crude been extract	Human immunodeficiency virus type-1	Suppress reverse transcriptase enzyme in HIV virus
Punica granatum	Anar	Polyphenols, ursolic acid in ethanolic peel extract	Human immunodeficiency virus	Restrict replication of virus
Solanum nigrum	Makoi	Solanine, solamargine in seed extract (methanol/chloroform)	Influenza A virus	Restrict protease (NS3) enzyme activity
Syzygium cumini	Jaman	Ellagic acid, gallic acid in leaf and bark extract	Hepatitis C virus	Mask viral envelope to inhibit entry in host cell

glabra, *Allium sativum*, etc. Some other plants as *Aloe vera*, *Gingko*, *Olea europaea*, *Cicer arietinum*, *Nigella sativa*, *Agrimonia Pilosa*, *Commelina communis*, *Mangifera indica*, *Syzygium cumini* have been reported to inhibit the replication of influenza virus. Further studies are in progress to establish a connective target between Corona and Influenza virus. Myricetin and scutellarein shows anti-SARS coronavirus helicase activity [175]. Similarly, plants have anti-HIV proteases and HIV reverse transcriptase activity and can be studied for severe acute respiratory syndrome coronavirus; these plants are *Eugenia jambolana*, *Areca nut*, *Ocimum sanctum*, *Phaseolus vulgaris*, *Phyllanthus emblica* and *Solanum nigrum*. *Azadirachta indica* (neem) and *Aegle marmelos* have anti replication effect of Coxsackie viruses may have effect against SARS-CoV-2 [176]. *Trachyspermum ammi* and *Solanum nigrum* act as inhibitory agents of protease enzymes in HCV virus and can be checked against coronavirus. Plants should be studied to inhibit the protease activity of viruses.

9.9.4 PLANTS RESTRICT THE ENTRY OF ENVELOPED VIRUSES

Lectins present in *Sambucus ebulus* have the ability to restrict the entry of enveloped viruses, although its mechanism is not known. Quertin and isorhamnetin, which are phenolic compounds in the same plant, combate Ebola virus (EBOV) while, diosgenin, and yomogenin are the flavonoids and have the ability to inhibit the entry of hepatitis C viruses (HCV) [177].

9.9.5 PLANTS INHIBIT VIRAL ACTIVITIES

Abutilon indicum, *Gymnema sylvestre*, *Leucas aspera* plants have been reported as antiviral agent of the human SARS virus. Although, *A. indicum* also have anti-influenza and anti sindbis virus activity which are agents of hepatitis B virus (HBV), *L. aspera* showed anti-MCV and anti HSV activity and *G. sylvestre* contain gymnemic acid which act against Asian influenza virus, although the mechanism of action of all these plants are unknown and have to be investigated [96, 178].

9.9.6 PLANTS EFFECTIVE IN PULMONARY DISCOMFORT

Some plants like *Zingiber officinale, Olea europaea* and *Terminalia chebula* are found to be effective in respiratory discomfort caused in SARS-CoV-2 disease. Extract from the rhizome of *Z. officinale* comprises of allicin which serves as anti-HRSV. The mechanism behind this is the secretion of IFN-β from the mucosal cells in the respiratory tract which reduced the plaque formation in mucosa. While *O. europaea* perform multiple functions like interrupting the formation of essential viral proteins, inhibit the viral assembly at the plasma membrane, viral replication in the infected cells by restricting the enzymes like transcriptase and protease [173, 179]. While, acids (chebulagic and chebulinic) in *T. chebula* did not allow the attachment and then penetration of viruses into host cells [50]. Curcumin in turmeric have anti-inflammatory and immune enhancement abilities by restricting the PHA-induced T-cell propagation, enhances NK cytotoxicity [41].

9.9.7 EATABLE ANTIVIRAL PLANTS WITH SUPPLEMENTARY ANTI-COVID-19 ACTIVITIES

In the patients of COVID-19, there is an increased response to inflammation which in turn elevate the rate of mortality. Many medicinal plants have anti-inflammatory effects due to the presence of flavonoids. Medicinal plants containing compounds including flavonoids are *Hibiscus sabdariffa, Ocimum sanctum*, *Azadirachta indica*, *Withania somnifera*, *Zingiber officinale*, *Camellia sinensis, Nigella sativa*, *Moringa oleifera*, *Agrimonia Pilosa*, *Momordica charantia* which can be added in daily diet plan of the patients to boost up their immunity as well as decreasing the inflammation caused by COVID-19, thus reducing the death rate of patients experiencing this disease. More investigative studies on these medicinal plants might prove them phytotherapeutic agents against Coronavirus Disease-19. Moreover, the active compounds in the medicinal plants act as immunoregulators thus, inhibiting the entry of virus invaders into the body [5]. As ACE2 is the site of entrance of SARS-CoV-2, so the compounds of plants block the active site for viral infection (Table 9.5). So, the anti-inflammatory, immunity-boosting and active site blockage property of the plant's derivatives should be investigated more.

9.10 CONCLUSION

For a long time, natural molecules of medicinal plants have been used as an alternative to pharmaceutical drugs to treat various diseases. With the outburst of the coronavirus disease-19 endemic in December 2019, many herbal drugs are in use which showed positive impacts on the health of coronavirus disease-19 patients, mainly in China. In this chapter, studies related to evaluating the effect of natural products of herbal plants as anti-COVID-19 agents and their use to treat COVID-19 has been discussed, but this data is still insufficient and quite emergent. Even, some natural foods exhibiting IC_{50} value below 10 μM could be deliberated as significant anti-SARS- coronavirus-2 agents. These products have the potential to hinder the proteins such as cellular receptor ACE2, papain-like or chymotrypsin-like proteinases to complete their life cycles.

TABLE 9.5 Medicinal Plants Exhibiting Anti-Inflammatory, Immunomodulatory, and/or ACE Prohibitory Activity

SL. No.	Plant Species/Family	Anti-Inflammatory	Immunomodulatory	ACE Inhibition
1.	*Abutilon indicum*	✓	✓	×
2.	*Acalypha indica*	✓	✓	×
3.	*Aegle marmelos*	✓	✓	×
4	*Agrimonia pilosa*	✓	×	×
5.	*Allium sativum*	✓	✓	✓
6.	*Aloe vera*	✓	✓	×
7.	*Areca nut*	✓	×	✓
8.	*Artemisia annua*	✓	✓	×
9.	*Azadirachta indica*	✓	✓	✓
10.	*Camellia sinensis*	✓	✓	✓
11.	*Cassia occidentalis*	✓	✓	✓
12.	*Cicer arietinum*	✓	✓	✓
13.	*Commelina communis*	✓	×	×
14.	*Curcuma longa*	✓	✓	✓
15.	*Cynara Scolymus*	✓	×	✓
16	*Embelia ribes*	✓	✓	✓
17.	*Eugenia jambolana*	✓	✓	✓
18.	*Gingko biloba*	✓	✓	✓
19.	*Glycyrrhiza glabra*	✓	✓	×
20.	*Gymnema sylvestre*	✓	✓	×
21.	*Hibiscus sabdariffa*	✓	✓	✓
22.	*Leucas aspera*	✓	✓	×
23.	*Mangifera indica*	✓	✓	✓
24.	*Momordica charantia*	✓	✓	✓
25.	*Moringa oleifera*	✓	✓	✓
26.	*Myrica esculenta*	✓	×	✓

TABLE 9.5 *(Continued)*

SL. No.	Plant Species/Family	Anti-Inflammatory	Immunomodulatory	ACE Inhibition
27.	*Nigella sativa*	✓	✓	✓
28.	*Ocimum sanctum*	✓	✓	✓
29.	*Olea europaea*	✓	✓	✓
30.	*Phaseolus vulgaris*	✓	✓	✓
31.	*Phyllanthus emblica*	✓	✓	×
32.	*Punica granatum*	✓	✓	✓
33.	*Solanum nigrum*	✓	✓	×
34.	*Syzygium cumini*	✓	✓	✓
35.	*Terminalia chebula*	✓	✓	✓
36.	*Trachyspermum ammi*	✓	✓	×
37.	*Withania somnifera*	✓	✓	✓
38.	*Zingiber officinale*	✓	✓	✓

Despite of insufficient data, this plant derived active compounds have the potential to fight against COVID-19. Moreover, further studies to investigate the therapeutic practicality of these products towards COVID-19 infection and their bioavailability as an inhibitor towards SARS-CoV-2 activity safely with their clinical validation should be considered, i.e., tannins. A series of prospective and interventional studies should be practiced to assess the potential of natural products of these herbal mixtures and medicinal plants as drugs against SARS-CoV-2 and their use as therapeutic alternative to prevent COVID-19 should be assessed.

KEYWORDS

- **ACE2**
- **antiviral plants**
- **coronaviruses**
- **COVID-19**
- **HCoV-229E**
- **lycorine**
- **SARS-CoV**

REFERENCES

1. Hong-Zhi, D., et al., (2020). Traditional Chinese medicine: An effective treatment for 2019 novel coronavirus pneumonia (NCP). *Chinese Journal of Natural Medicines, 18*(3), 206–210.
2. Khan, S., et al., (2020). Emergence of a novel coronavirus, severe acute respiratory syndrome coronavirus 2: Biology and therapeutic options. *Journal of Clinical Microbiology, 58*(5).
3. Chen, Y., et al., (2020). Structure analysis of the receptor binding of 2019-nCoV. *Biochemical and Biophysical Research Communications.*
4. Walls, A. C., et al., (2020). Structure, function, and antigenicity of the SARS-CoV-2 spike glycoprotein. *Cell.*
5. Zhou, P., et al., (2020). A pneumonia outbreak associated with a new coronavirus of probable bat origin. *Nature [Internet], 579*(7798), 270–273.
6. Jiang, S., Hillyer, C., & Du, L., (2020). Neutralizing antibodies against SARS-CoV-2 and other human coronaviruses. *Trends in Immunology*, *41*(5), 355–359.
7. Fung, T. S., & Liu, D. X., (2019). Human coronavirus: Host-pathogen interaction. *Annual Review of Microbiology, 73,* 529–557.
8. Fani, M., Teimoori, A., & Ghafari, S., (2020). Comparison of the COVID-2019 (SARS-CoV-2) pathogenesis with SARS-CoV and MERS-CoV infections. *Future Virology, 15*(5), 317–323.
9. Ceccarelli, M., et al., (2020). Editorial-differences and similarities between severe acute respiratory syndrome (SARS)-Coronavirus (CoV) and SARS-CoV-2. Would a rose by another name smell as sweet? *European Review for Medical and Pharmacological Sciences, 24*, 2781–2783.
10. Runfeng, L., et al., (2020). Lianhuaqingwen exerts anti-viral and anti-inflammatory activity against novel coronavirus (SARS-CoV-2). *Pharmacological Research, 156,* 104761.
11. Gao, D., et al., (2020). *I*dentification of a pharmacological biomarker for the bioassay-based quality control of a thirteen-component TCM formula (Lianhua Qingwen) used in treating influenza A virus (H1N1) infection. *Frontiers in Pharmacology, 11*, 746.
12. Wang, C. H., et al., (2016). A network analysis of the Chinese medicine lianhua-qingwen formula to identify its main effective components. *Molecular Biosystems, 12*(2), 606–613.
13. Lung, J., et al., (2020). The potential chemical structure of anti-SARS-CoV-2 RNA-dependent RNA polymerase. *Journal of Medical Virology, 92*(6), 693–697.
14. Pereira-Caro, G., et al., (2017). Bioavailability of black tea theaflavins: Absorption, metabolism, and colonic catabolism. *Journal of Agricultural and Food Chemistry, 65* (26), 5365–5374.
15. Luo, H., et al., (2020). Can Chinese medicine be used for prevention of coronavirus disease 2019 (COVID-19)? A review of historical classics, research evidence and current prevention programs. *Chinese Journal of Integrative Medicine,* 1–8.
16. Park, J. Y., et al., (2012). Diarylheptanoids from *Alnus japonica* inhibit papain-like protease of severe acute respiratory syndrome coronavirus. *Biological and Pharmaceutical Bulletin,* b12–00623.
17. Park, J. Y., et al., (2016). Chalcones isolated from *Angelica keiskei* inhibit cysteine proteases of SARS-CoV. *Journal of Enzyme Inhibition and Medicinal Chemistry, 31*(1), 23–30.

18. Yu, M. S., et al., (2012). Identification of myricetin and scutellarein as novel chemical inhibitors of the SARS coronavirus helicase, nsP13. *Bioorganic & Medicinal Chemistry Letters, 22*(12), 4049–4054.
19. Schwarz, S., et al., (2011). Emodin inhibits current through SARS-associated coronavirus 3a protein. *Antiviral Research, 90*(1), 64–69.
20. Kim, D. W., et al., (2014). Phenolic phytochemical displaying SARS-CoV papain-like protease inhibition from the seeds of *Psoralea corylifolia. Journal of Enzyme Inhibition and Medicinal Chemistry, 29*(1), 59–63.
21. Park, J. Y., et al., (2013). *D*ieckol, a SARS-CoV 3CLpro inhibitor, isolated from the edible brown algae *Ecklonia cava. Bioorganic & Medicinal Chemistry, 21*(13), 3730.
22. Cho, J. K., et al., (2013). Geranylated flavonoids displaying SARS-CoV papain-like protease inhibition from the fruits of *Paulownia tomentosa. Bioorganic & Medicinal Chemistry, 21*(11), 3051–3057.
23. Ho, T. Y., et al., (2007). Emodin blocks the SARS coronavirus spike protein and angiotensin-converting enzyme 2 interactio*n. Antiviral Research, 74*(2), 92–101.
24. Park, J. Y., et al., (2012). Tanshinones as selective and slow-binding inhibitors for SARS-CoV cysteine proteases. *Bioorganic & Medicinal Chemistry, 20*(19), 5928–5935.
25. Weng, J. R., et al., (2019). Antiviral activity of *Sambucus FormosanaNakai* ethanol extract and related phenolic acid constituents against human coronavirus NL63. *Virus Research, 273*, 197767.
26. Ryu, Y. B., et al., (2010). Bioflavonoids from *Torreya nucifera* displaying SARS-CoV 3CLpro inhibition. *Bioorganic & Medicinal Chemistry, 18*(22), 7940–7947.
27. Song, Y. H., et al., (2014). Papain-like protease (PLpro) inhibitory effects of cinnamic amides from *Tribulus terrestris* fruits. *Biological and Pharmaceutical Bulletin, 37*(6), 1021–1028.
28. Sigrist, C. J., Bridge, A., & Le Mercier, P., (2020*)*. A potential role for integrins in host cell entry by SARS-CoV-2. *Antiviral Research, 177*, 104759.
29. Qiu, Y., et al., (2020). Predicting the angiotensin-converting enzyme 2 (ACE2) utilizing capability as the receptor of SARS-CoV-2. *Microbes and Infection.*
30. Hoffmann, M., et al., (2020). SARS-CoV-2 cell entry depends on ACE2 and TMPRSS2 and is blocked by a clinically proven protease inhibitor. *Cell.*
31. Ortega, J. T., et al., (2020). Role of changes in SARS-CoV-2 spike protein in the interaction with the human ACE2 receptor: An in-silico analysis. *EXCLI Journal, 19*, 410.
32. Wrapp, D., et al., (2020). Cryo-EM structure of the 2019-nCoV spike in the prefusion conformation. *Science, 367*(6483), 1260–1263.
33. Adedeji, A. O., et al., (2013). Novel inhibitors of severe acute respiratory syndrome coronavirus entry that act by three distinct mechanisms. *Journal of virology, 87*(14), 8017–8028.
34. Guan, W. J., et al., (2020). Clinical characteristics of coronavirus disease 2019 in China. *New England Journal of Medicine, 382*(18), 1708–1720.
35. Yang, X., et al., (2020). Clinical course and outcomes of critically ill patients with SARS-CoV-2 pneumonia in Wuhan, China: A single-centered, retrospective, observational study. *The Lancet Respiratory Medicine*.
36. Zhang, J. J., et al., (2020). Clinical characteristics of 140 patients infected with SARS-CoV-2 in Wuhan, China. *Allergy*.
37. Fang, L., Karakiulakis, G., & Roth, M., (2020). Are patients with hypertension and diabetes mellitus at increased risk for COVID-19 infection? *The Lancet; Respiratory Medicine, 8*(4), e21.

38. Guy, J., et al., (2005). Membrane-associated zinc peptidase families: Comparing ACE and ACE2. *Biochimica et Biophysica Acta (BBA)-Proteins and Proteomics, 1751*(1), 2–8.
39. Patten, G. S., Abeywardena, M. Y., & Bennett, L. E., (2016). Inhibition of angiotensin-converting enzyme, angiotensin II receptor blocking, and blood pressure-lowering bioactivity across plant families. *Critical Reviews in Food Science and Nutrition, 56*(2), 181–214.
40. Sharifi, N., et al., (2013). Discovery of new angiotensin-converting enzyme (ACE) inhibitors from medicinal plants to treat hypertension using an in vitro assay. *DARU Journal of Pharmaceutical Sciences, 21*(1), 74.
41. Im, S. A., et al., (2010). *I*n vivo evidence of the immunomodulatory activity of orally administered Aloe vera gel. *Archives of Pharmacal Research, 33*(3), 451–456.
42. Yuan, L., et al., (2015). p53 degradation by a coronavirus papain-like protease suppresses type I interferon signaling. *Journal of Biological Chemistry, 290*(5), 3172–3182.
43. Li, S. W., et al., (2016). SARS coronavirus papain-like protease inhibits the TLR7 signaling pathway through removing Lys63-linked polyubiquitination of TRAF3 and TRAF6. *International Journal of Molecular Sciences, 17*(*5*), 678.
44. Wong, L. Y. R., Lui, P. Y., & Jin, D. Y., (2016). A molecular arms race between host innate antiviral response and emerging human coronaviruses. *Virologica Sinica, 31*(1), 12–23.
45. Lin, M. H., et al., (2018). Disulfiram can inhibit MERS and SARS coronavirus papain-like proteases via different modes. *Antiviral Research, 150*, 155–163.
46. Li, Y., et al., (2017). Extraction and identification of phlorotannins from the brown alga, *Sargassum fusiforme* (Harvey) setchell. *Marine Drugs, 15*(2), 49.
47. Nguyen, T. T. H., et al., (2012). Flavonoid-mediated inhibition of SARS coronavirus 3C-like protease expressed in *Pichia* pastoris. *Biotechnology Letters, 34*(5), 831–838.
48. Chen, D., et al., (2016). Regulation of protein-ligand binding affinity by hydrogen bond pairing. *Science Advances, 2*(3), e1501240.
49. Jo, S., et al., (2020). Inhibition of SARS-CoV 3CL protease by flavonoids. *Journal of Enzyme Inhibition and Medicinal Chemistry, 35*(1), 145–151.
50. Yadav, V., et al., (2005). Immunomodulatory effects of curcumin. *Immunopharmacology and Immunotoxicology, 27*(3), 485–497.
51. Heinrich, M., et al., (2020). Best practice in research-overcoming common challenges in phytopharmacological research. *Journal of Ethnopharmacology, 246*, 112230.
52. Keyaerts, E., et al., (2004). In vitro inhibition of severe acute respiratory syndrome coronavirus by chloroquine. *Biochemical and Biophysical Research Communications, 323*(1), 264–268.
53. Caly, L., et al., (2020). The FDA-approved drug ivermectin inhibits the replication of SARS-CoV-2 in vitro. *Antiviral Research, 178*, 104787.
54. Górniak, I., Bartoszewski, R., & Króliczewski, J., (2019). Comprehensive review of antimicrobial activities of plant flavonoids. *Phytochemistry Reviews, 18*(1), 241–272.
55. Zia-Ul-Haq, M., et al., (2021). *Alternative Medicine Interventions for COVID-19*. Springer, Cham: Springer Nature Switzerland AG 2021. XII, 284.
56. Zia-Ul-Haq, M., Dewanjee, S., & Riaz, M., (2021). *Carotenoids: Structure and Function in the Human Body*. Springer Nature Switzerland AG: Springer International Publishing. XVI, 859.
57. Li, T., & Peng, T., (2013). Traditional Chinese herbal medicine as a source of molecules with antiviral activity. *Antiviral Research, 97*(1), 1–9.

58. Akram, M., et al., (2018). Antiviral potential of medicinal plants against HIV, HSV, influenza, hepatitis, and coxsackievirus: A systematic review. *Phytotherapy Research, 32*(5), 811–822.
59. Dhama, K., et al., (2018). Medicinal and therapeutic potential of herbs and plant metabolites/extracts countering viral pathogens-current knowledge and future prospects. *Current Drug Metabolism, 19*(3), 236–263.
60. Ben-Shabat, S., et al., (2020). Antiviral effect of phytochemicals from medicinal plants: Applications and drug delivery strategies. *Drug Delivery and Translational Research, 10*(2), 354–367.
61. Wink, M., (2020). Potential of DNA intercalating alkaloids and other plant secondary metabolites against SARS-CoV-2 causing COVID-19. *Diversity, 12*(5), 175.
62. Schnitzler, P., et al., (2008). Melissa officinalis oil affects infectivity of enveloped herpesviruses. *Phytomedicine, 15*(9), 734–740.
63. Sharma, A. D., (2020). *Eucalyptol (1, 8 cineole) from Eucalyptus Essential Oil a Potential Inhibitor of COVID 19 Corona Virus Infection by Molecular Docking Studies.* Preprint.
64. Lin, S. C., et al., (2017). *Effective Inhibition of MERS-CoV Infection by Resveratrol. BMC Infectious Diseases, 17*(1), 1–10.
65. Sharma, A. D., & Kaur, I., (2020). *Molecular Docking Studies on Jensenone from Eucalyptus Essential oil as a Potential Inhibitor of COVID 19 Corona Virus Infection.* arXiv preprint arXiv:2004.00217.
66. Devaux, C. A., et al., (2020). New insights on the antiviral effects of chloroquine against coronavirus: What to expect for COVID-19? *International Journal of Antimicrobial Agents, 55*(5), 105938.
67. Ho, Y. J., et al., (2019). Palmatine inhibits Zika virus infection by disrupting virus binding, entry, and stability. *Biochemical and Biophysical Research Communications, 518*(4), 732–738.
68. Kim, D. E., et al., (2019). Natural bis-benzylisoquinoline alkaloids-tetrandrine, fangchinoline, and cepharanthine, inhibit human coronavirus OC43 infection of MRC-5 human lung cells. *Biomolecules, 9*(11), 696.
69. Shen, L., et al., (2019). High-throughput screening and identification of potent broad-spectrum inhibitors of coronaviruses. *Journal of Virology, 93*(12).
70. Suryanarayana, L., & Banavath, D., (2020). A review on identification of antiviral potential medicinal plant compounds against with COVID-19. *Int. J. Res. Eng. Sci. Manag., 3*, 675–679.
71. Yang, Y., et al., (2020). Traditional Chinese medicine in the treatment of patients infected with 2019-new coronavirus (SARS-CoV-2): A review and perspective. *International Journal of Biological Sciences, 16*(10), 1708.
72. Lin, C. W., et al., (2005). Anti-SARS coronavirus 3C-like protease effects of *Isatis indigotica* root and plant-derived phenolic compounds. *Antiviral Research, 68*(1), 36–42.
73. Gong, S., et al., (2008). A study on anti-SARS-CoV 3CL protein of flavonoids from *Litchi chinensis* sonn core. *Chinese Pharmacological Bulletin, 24*, 699–700.
74. Letko, M., Marzi, A., & Munster, V., (2020). Functional assessment of cell entry and receptor usage for SARS-CoV-2 and other lineage B betacoronaviruses. *Nature Microbiology, 5*(4), 562–569.
75. Yi, L., et al., (2004). Small molecules blocking the entry of severe acute respiratory syndrome coronavirus into host cells. *Journal of Virology, 78*(20), 11334–11339.

76. Wang, W., et al., (2016). Neuroprotective effect of scutellarin on ischemic cerebral injury by down-regulating the expression of angiotensin-converting enzyme and AT1 receptor. *PloS One, 11*(1), e0146197.
77. Takahashi, S., et al., (2015). Nicotianamine is a novel angiotensin-converting enzyme 2 inhibitor in soybean. *Biomedical Research, 36*(3), 219–224.
78. Deng, Y., et al., (2012). Inhibitory activities of baicalin against renin and angiotensin-converting enzyme. *Pharmaceutical Biology, 50*(4), 401–406.
79. Tallei, T. E., et al., (2020). Potential of plant bioactive compounds as SARS-CoV-2 main protease (Mpro) and spike (S) glycoprotein inhibitors: A molecular docking study. *Scientifica.*
80. Chen, C. J., et al., (2008). Toona sinensis roem tender leaf extract inhibits SARS coronavirus replication. *Journal of Ethnopharmacology, 120*(1), 108–111.
81. Cinatl, J., et al., (2003). Glycyrrhizin, an active component of liquorice roots, and replication of SARS-associated coronavirus. *The Lancet, 361*(9374), 2045, 2046.
82. Wu, C. Y., et al., (2004). Small molecules targeting severe acute respiratory syndrome human coronavirus. *Proceedings of the National Academy of Sciences, 101*(27), 10012–10017.
83. Yang, C. W., et al., (2018). The cardenolide ouabain suppresses coronaviral replication via augmenting a Na+/K+-ATPase-dependent PI3K_PDK1 axis signaling. *Toxicology and Applied Pharmacology, 356,* 90–97.
84. Yonesi, M., & Rezazadeh, A., (2020). *Plants as a Prospective Source of Natural Anti-viral Compounds and Oral Vaccines Against COVID-19 Coronavirus.* Preprint.
85. Khaerunnisa, S., et al., (2020). *Potential Inhibitor of COVID-19 Main Protease (Mpro) from Several Medicinal Plant Compounds by Molecular Docking Study.* Preprints 202003022684.
86. Yang, C. W., et al., (2010). Identification of phenanthroindolizines and phenanthroquino-lizidines as novel potent anti-coronaviral agents for porcine enteropathogenic corona-virus transmissible gastroenteritis virus and human severe acute respiratory syndrome coronavirus. *Antiviral Research, 88*(2), 160–168.
87. Hill, K. P., (2020). Cannabinoids and the coronavirus. *Cannabis and Cannabinoid Research, 5*(2), 118–120.
88. Müller, C., et al., (2018). Broad-spectrum antiviral activity of the eIF4A inhibitor silvestrol against corona-and picornaviruses. *Antiviral Research, 150*, 123–129.
89. Orzalli, M. H., & Kagan, J. C., (2017). Apoptosis and necroptosis as host defense strategies to prevent viral infection. *Trends in Cell Biology, 27*(11), 800–809.
90. Park, J. Y., et al., (2017). Evaluation of polyphenols from *Broussonetia papyrifera* as coronavirus protease inhibitors. *Journal of Enzyme Inhibition and Medicinal Chemistry, 32*(1), 504–512.
91. Ulasli, M., et al., (2014). The effects of *Nigella sativa* (Ns), *Anthemis hyalina* (Ah) and *Citrus sinensis* (Cs) extracts on the replication of coronavirus and the expression of TRP genes family. *Molecular Biology Reports, 41*(3), 1703–1711.
92. Kwon, H. J., et al., (2013). In vitro antiviral activity of phlorotannins isolated from *Ecklonia cava* against porcine epidemic diarrhea coronavirus infection and hemagglutination. *Bioorganic & Medicinal Chemistry, 21*(15), 4706–4713.
93. Roh, C., (2012). A facile inhibitor screening of SARS coronavirus N protein using nanoparticle-based RNA oligonucleotide. *International Journal of Nanomedicine, 7,* 2173.

94. Michaelis, M., Doerr, H. W., & Cinatl, Jr. J., (2011). Investigation of the influence of EPs® 7630 a herbal drug preparation from *Pelargonium sidoides*, on replication of a broad panel of respiratory viruses. *Phytomedicine, 18*(5), 384–386.
95. Fung, K. P., et al., (2011). Immunomodulatory activities of the herbal formula Kwan du Bu Fei dang in healthy subjects: A randomized, double-blind, placebo-controlled study. *Hong Kong Medical Journal= Xianggang yi xue za zhi, 17*, 41–43.
96. Li, S. Y., et al., (2005). Identification of natural compounds with antiviral activities against SARS-associated coronavirus. *Antiviral Research, 67*(1), 18–23.
97. Poon, P., et al., (2006). Immunomodulatory effects of a traditional Chinese medicine with potential antiviral activity: A self-control study. *The American Journal of Chinese Medicine, 34*(01), 13–21.
98. Hsu, C. H., et al., (2006). Can herbal medicine assist against avian flu? Learning from the experience of using supplementary treatment with Chinese medicine on SARS or SARS-like infectious disease in 2003. *Journal of Alternative & Complementary Medicine, 12*(6), 505–506.
99. Soleymani, S., et al., (2018). Antiviral effects of saffron and its major ingredients. *Current Drug Delivery, 15*(5), 698–704.
100. Boff, L., et al., (2019). Potential anti-herpes and cytotoxic action of novel semisynthetic digitoxigenin-derivatives. *European Journal of Medicinal Chemistry, 167*, 546–561.
101. Astani, A., Reichling, J., & Schnitzler, P., (2011). Screening for antiviral activities of isolated compounds from essential oils. *Evidence-Based Complementary and Alternative Medicine*.
102. Aanouz, I., et al., (2020). Moroccan medicinal plants as inhibitors against SARS-CoV-2 main protease: Computational investigations. *Journal of Biomolecular Structure and Dynamics*, 1–9.
103. Zhan, J., et al., (2006). The spleen as a target in severe acute respiratory syndrome. *The FASEB Journal, 20*(13), 2321–2328.
104. Farcas, G. A., et al., (2005). Fatal severe acute respiratory syndrome is associated with multiorgan involvement by coronavirus. *Journal of Infectious Diseases, 191*(2), 193–197.
105. Gu, J., et al., (2005). Multiple organ infection and the pathogenesis of SARS. *Journal of Experimental Medicine, 202*(3), 415–424.
106. Wu, Y., et al., (2011). In vivo and in vitro antiviral effects of berberine on influenza virus. *Chinese Journal of Integrative Medicine, 17*(6), 444–452.
107. Shin, H. B., et al., (2015). Inhibition of respiratory syncytial virus replication and virus-induced p38 kinase activity by berberine. *International Immunopharmacology, 27*(1), 65–68.
108. Kalmarzi, R. N., et al., (2019). Anti-inflammatory and immunomodulatory effects of barberry (Berberis vulgaris) and its main compounds. *Oxidative Medicine and Cellular Longevity*.
109. Shen, C. Y., et al., (2017). Structural characterization and immunomodulatory activity of novel polysaccharides from *Citrus aurantium* Linn. variant Amara Engl. *Journal of Functional Foods, 35*, 352–362.
110. Mannucci, C., et al., (2018). Clinical pharmacology of citrus aurantium and *Citrus* sinensis for the treatment of anxiety. *Evidence-based Complementary and Alternative Medicine*.
111. Kala, C. P., (2012). Leaf juice of *Carica papaya L.* a remedy of dengue fever. *Med. Aromat. Plants, 1,* 109.

112. Pandey, S., et al., (2016). Anti-inflammatory and immunomodulatory properties of *Carica* papaya. *Journal of Immunotoxicology, 13*(4), 590–602.
113. Ishikawa, H., et al., (2006). Aged garlic extract prevents a decline of NK cell number and activity in patients with advanced cancer. *The Journal of Nutrition, 136*(3), 816S–820S.
114. Clement, F., Pramod, S. N., & Venkatesh, Y. P., (2010). Identity of the immunomodulatory proteins from garlic (Allium sativum) with the major garlic lectins or agglutinins. *International Immunopharmacology, 10*(3), 316–324.
115. Liu, C. T., et al., (2009). Effect of supplementation with garlic oil on activity of Th1 and Th2 lymphocytes from rats. *Planta Medica, 75*(03), 205–210.
116. Zvetkova, E., et al., (2001). *Aqueous extracts of Crinum latifolium* (L.) and *Camellia* sinensis show immunomodulatory properties in human peripheral blood mononuclear cells. *International Immunopharmacology, 1*(12), 2143–2150.
117. Chen, C. N., et al., (2005). Inhibition of SARS-CoV 3C-like protease activity by theaflavin-3, 3'-digallate (TF3). *Evidence-Based Complementary and Alternative Medicine, 2*(2), 209–215.
118. Mirabeau, T. Y., & Samson, E. S., (2012). Effect of *Allium cepa* and *Allium sativum* on some immunological cells in rats. *African Journal of Traditional, Complementary and Alternative Medicines, 9*(3), 374–379.
119. Gansukh, E., et al., (2017). Nature nominee quercetin's anti-influenza combat strategy—Demonstrations and remonstrations. *Reviews in Medical Virology, 27*(3), e1930.
120. Jeong, H. G., & Kim, J. Y., (2002). Induction of inducible nitric oxide synthase expression by 18β-glycyrrhetinic acid in macrophages. *FEBS Letters, 513*(2, 3), 208–212.
121. Raphael, T., & Kuttan, G., (2003). Effect of naturally occurring triterpenoids glycyrrhizic acid, ursolic acid, oleanolic acid and nomilin on the immune system. *Phytomedicine, 10*(6, 7), 483–489.
122. Srivastava, R. M., et al., (2011). Immunomodulatory and therapeutic activity of curcumin. *International Immunopharmacology, 11*(3), 331–341.
123. Catanzaro, M., et al., (2018). Immunomodulators inspired by nature: A review on curcumin and echinacea. *Molecules, 23*(11), 2778.
124. Momtazi-Borojeni, A. A., et al., (2018). Curcumin: A natural modulator of immune cells in systemic lupus erythematosus. *Autoimmunity Reviews, 17*(2), 125–135.
125. Hayashi, K., et al., (1997). Inhibitory activity of soy saponin II on virus replication in vitro. *Planta Medica, 63*(02), 102–105.
126. Kinjo, J., et al., (1999). Hepatoprotective effects of oleanane glucuronides in several edible beans. *Natural Medicines* [= 生薬學雜誌], *53*(3), 141–144.
127. Anitha, T., et al., (2015). Evaluation of in vitro immunomodulatory effects of soybean (glycine max. l) extracts on mouse immune system. *International Journal of Pharmaceutical Sciences and Research, 6*(5), 2112.
128. Tang, W. M., et al., (2012). A review of the anticancer and immunomodulatory effects of *Lycium barbarum* fruit. *Inflammopharmacology, 20*(6), 307–314.
129. Cheng, J., et al., (2015). An evidence-based update on the pharsmacological activities and possible molecular targets of *Lycium barbarum* polysaccharides. *Drug Design, Development and Therapy, 9*, 33.
130. Byambasuren, S. E., Wang, J., & Gaudel, G., (2019). Medicinal value of wolfberry (Lycium barbarum L.). *J. Med. Plants Stud., 7*(4), 90–97.
131. Idolo, M., Motti, R., & Mazzoleni, S., (2010). Ethnobotanical and phytomedicinal knowledge in a long-history protected area, the Abruzzo, Lazio and Molise National Park (Italian Apennines). *Journal of Ethnopharmacology, 127*(2), 379–395.

132. Patil, V. V., Bhangale, S. C., & Patil, V. R., (2010). Studies on immunomodulatory activity of *Ficus carica. Int. J. Pharm. Pharm. Sci., 2*(4), 97–99.
133. Makare, N., Bodhankar, S., & Rangari, V., (2001). Immunomodulatory activity of alcoholic extract of *Mangifera indica* L. in mice. *Journal of Ethnopharmacology, 78*(2, 3), 133–137.
134. Garrido, G., et al., (2004). In vivo and in vitro anti-inflammatory activity of *Mangifera indica* L. extract (VIMANG®). *Pharmacological Research, 50*(2), 143–149.
135. Sahoo, B., & Banik, B., (2018). Medicinal plants: Source for immunosuppressive agents. *Immunology: Current Research, 2*, 106.
136. Mahboubi, M., (2019). *Zingiber officinale Rosc.* essential oil, a review on its composition and bioactivity. *Clinical Phytoscience, 5*(1), 1–12.
137. Bagachi, A., Semwal, A., & Bharadwaj, A., (2013). Traditional uses, phytochemistry and pharmacology of *Morus alba* Linn.: A review. *Journal of Medicinal Plants Research, 7*(9), 461–469.
138. Grienke, U., et al., (2016). Discovery of prenylated flavonoids with dual activity against influenza virus and *Streptococcus pneumoniae. Scientific Reports, 6*(1), 1–11.
139. Gutiérrez, R. M. P., Mitchell, S., & Solis, R. V., (2008). Psidium guajava: A review of its traditional uses, phytochemistry and pharmacology. *Journal of Ethnopharmacology, 117*(1), 1–27.
140. Ravi, K., & Divyashree, P., (2014). *Psidium guajava*: A review on its potential as an adjunct in treating periodontal disease. *Pharmacognosy Reviews, 8*(16), 96.
141. Chaudhry, N., & Tariq, P., (2006). Bactericidal activity of black pepper, bay leaf, aniseed and coriander against oral isolates. *Pakistan Journal of Pharmaceutical Sciences, 19*(3), 214–218.
142. Ahmad, A., et al., (2013). A review on therapeutic potential of *Nigella sativa*: A miracle herb. 2013. *Asian Pacific Journal of Tropical Biomedicine, 3*(5), 337–352.
143. Koshak, A. E., et al., (2018). Comparative immunomodulatory activity of *Nigella sativa* L. preparations on proinflammatory mediators: A focus on asthma. *Frontiers in Pharmacology, 9*, 1075.
144. Bhowmik, D., et al., (2013). Medicinal uses of *Punica* granatum and its health benefits. *Journal of Pharmacognosy and Phytochemistry, 1*(5).
145. Howell, A. B., & D'Souza, D. H., (2013). The pomegranate: Effects on bacteria and viruses that influence human health. *Evidence-Based Complementary and Alternative Medicine*.
146. Koul, I. B., & Kapil, A., (1993). Evaluation of the liver protective potential of piperine, an active principle of black and long peppers. *Planta Medica, 59*(05), 413–417.
147. Kayano, S. I., et al., (2002). Antioxidant activity of prune (Prunus domestica L.) constituents and a new synergist. *Journal of Agricultural and Food Chemistry, 50*(13), 3708–3712.
148. Walle, T., et al., (2003). Effect of dietary flavonoids on oral cancer cell proliferation: Bioactivation by saliva and antiproliferative mechanisms. In: *Cancer Epidemiology Biomarkers & Prevention*. Amer Assoc. cancer research 615 chestnut St., 17th Floor, Philadelphia, PA.
149. Asl, M. N., & Hosseinzadeh, H., (2008). Review of pharmacological effects of *Glycyrrhiza* sp. and its bioactive compounds. *Phytotherapy Research: An International Journal Devoted to Pharmacological and Toxicological Evaluation of Natural Product Derivatives, 22*(6), 709–724.

150. Seki, H., et al., (2008). Licorice β-amyrin 11-oxidase, a cytochrome P450 with a key role in the biosynthesis of the triterpene sweetener glycyrrhizin. *Proceedings of the National Academy of Sciences, 105*(37), 14204–14209.
151. Anywar, G., et al., (2020). Medicinal plants used by traditional medicine practitioners to boost the immune system in people living with HIV/AIDS in Uganda. *European Journal of Integrative Medicine, 35*, 101011.
152. Kuttan, G., (2000). Immunomodulatory effect of some naturally occurring sulphur-containing compounds. *Journal of Ethnopharmacology, 72*(1, 2), 93–99.
153. Chattopadhyay, C., et al., (2012). Black tea (Camellia sinensis) decoction shows immunomodulatory properties on an experimental animal model and in human peripheral mononuclear cells. *Pharmacognosy Research, 4*(1), 15.
154. Kumar, D., et al., (2012). A review of immunomodulators in the Indian traditional health care system. *Journal of Microbiology, Immunology and Infection, 45*(3), 165–184.
155. Shailajan, S., et al., (2016). Standardized extract of *Mangifera indica* L. leaves as an antimycobacterial and immunomodulatory agent. *Pharmacognosy Communications, 6*(3).
156. Barnard, D. L., & Kumaki, Y., (2011). *Recent developments in anti-severe acute respiratory syndrome coronavirus chemotherapy. Future Virology, 6*(5), 615–631.
157. Belouzard, S., et al., (2012). Mechanisms of coronavirus cell entry mediated by the viral spike protein. *Viruses, 4*(6), 1011–1033.
158. Wan, Y., et al., (2020). Receptor recognition by the novel coronavirus from Wuhan: An analysis based on decade-long structural studies of SARS coronavirus. *Journal of Virology, 94*(7).
159. Majeed, J., Ajmera, P., & Goyal, R. K., (2020). Delineating clinical characteristics and comorbidities among 206 COVID-19 deceased patients in India: Emerging significance of renin-angiotensin system derangement. *Diabetes Research and Clinical Practice, 167*, 108349.
160. Scotti, N., et al., (2010). Plant-based anti-HIV-1 strategies: Vaccine molecules and antiviral approaches. *Expert Review of Vaccines, 9*(8), 925–936.
161. Cascella, M., et al., (2021). *Features, Evaluation, and Treatment of Coronavirus (COVID-19).* Statpearls [internet].
162. Xu, Z., et al., (2020). Pathological findings of COVID-19 associated with acute respiratory distress syndrome. *The Lancet Respiratory Medicine, 8*(4), 420–422.
163. Tian, S., et al., (2020). Pulmonary pathology of early-phase 2019 novel coronavirus (COVID-19) pneumonia in two patients with lung cancer. *Journal of Thoracic Oncology, 15*(5), 700–704.
164. Tomar, B., et al., (2020). Neutrophils and neutrophil extracellular traps drive necroinflammation in COVID-19. *Cells, 9*(6), 1383.
165. Small, B. A., et al., (2001). CD8+ T cell-mediated injury in vivo progresses in the absence of effector T cells. *The Journal of Experimental Medicine, 194*(12), 1835–1846.
166. Channappanavar, R., & Perlman, S., (2017). Pathogenic human coronavirus infections: Causes and consequences of cytokine storm and immunopathology. In: *Seminars in Immunopathology*. Springer.
167. Rizzo, P., et al., (2020). *COVID-19 in the Heart and the Lungs: Could we "Notch" the Inflammatory Storm?* Springer.
168. Prompetchara, E., Ketloy, C., & Palaga, T., (2020). Immune responses in COVID-19 and potential vaccines: Lessons learned from SARS and MERS epidemic. *Asian Pac. J. Allergy Immunol., 38*(1), 1–9.

169. Heinrich, M., & Gibbons, S., (2001). Ethnopharmacology in drug discovery: An analysis of its role and potential contribution. *Journal of Pharmacy and Pharmacology, 53*(4), 425–432.
170. Patra, J. K., et al., (2019). *Ethnopharmacology and Biodiversity of Medicinal Plants.*: CRC Press.
171. Ye, Q., Wang, B., & Mao, J., (2020). *T*he pathogenesis and treatment of the cytokine storm' in COVID-19. *Journal of Infection, 80*(6), 607–613.
172. Keyaerts, E., et al., (2007). Plant lectins are potent inhibitors of coronaviruses by interfering with two targets in the viral replication cycle. *Antiviral Research, 75*(3), 179–187.
173. Kan, A., Özçelik, B., & Kartal, M., (2009). In vitro antiviral activities under cytotoxic doses against herpes simples type-1 and parainfluenza-3 viruses of *Cicer arietinum L. African Journal of Pharmacy and Pharmacology, 3*(12), 627–631.
174. Elsebai, M. F., Mocan, A., & Atanasov, A. G., (2016). Cynaropicrin: A comprehensive research review and therapeutic potential as an anti-hepatitis C virus agent. *Frontiers in Pharmacology, 7*, 472.
175. Musarra-Pizzo, M., et al., (2019). *T*he antimicrobial and antiviral activity of polyphenols from almond (Prunus dulcis L.) skin. *Nutrients, 11*(10), 2355.
176. Kilianski, A., et al., (2013). Assessing activity and inhibition of middle east respiratory syndrome coronavirus papain-like and 3C-like proteases using luciferase-based biosensors. *Journal of Virology, 87*(21), 11955–11962.
177. Badam, L., et al., (2002). In vitro antiviral activity of Bael (Aegle marmelos Corr) upon. *Journal of Communicable Diseases, 34*(2), 88–99.
178. San, C. J., et al., (2013). Fresh ginger (Zingiber officinale) has anti-viral activity against human respiratory syncytial virus in human respiratory tract cell lines. *Journal of Ethnopharmacology, 145*(1), 146–151.
179. Xie, F., (2016). Broad-spectrum antiviral effect of chebulagic acid and punicalagin on respiratory syncytial virus infection in a BALB/c model. *Int. J. Clin. Exp. Pathol., 9*(2), 611–619.

CHAPTER 10

COVID-19 Pandemic and Traditional Chinese Medicines

ROHEENA ABDULLAH,[1] AYESHA TOOR,[1] HINA QAISER,[2] AFSHAN KALEEM,[1] MEHWISH IQTEDAR,[1] TEHREEMA IFTIKHAR,[3] MUHAMMAD RIAZ,[4] and DOU DEQIANG[5]

[1]*Department of Biotechnology, Lahore College for Women University, Lahore, Pakistan, E-mail: roheena_abdullah@yahoo.com (R. Abdullah)*

[2]*Department of Biology, Lahore Garrison University DHA Phase VI Sector C, Lahore, Pakistan*

[3]*Department of Botany, Government College University Lahore, Pakistan*

[4]*Department of Pharmacy, Shaheed Benazir Bhutto University, Sheringal, Pakistan*

[5]*College of Pharmacy, Liaoning University of Traditional Chinese Medicine, Dalian Campus, China*

ABSTRACT

Coronavirus disease 2019 (COVID-19) pandemic has hit almost every part of the earth due to its highly infectious nature. Various therapeutic strategies aiming at prevention and treatment are being explored to combat this disease within the domains of traditional Chinese medicine (TCM). TCM offers many advantages when it comes to effective treatment plan. It has proved very fruitful in alleviating the symptoms at every stage of the disease and holds great potential to improve the cure rate, reduce death incidence and enhance rehabilitation. The integration of western medicine along with TCM has enabled China to attain good clinical efficacy with respect to disease deterrence and management. Treatment guidelines publicized by The National Health Commission of the People's Republic of China for diseased individuals based upon the severity level of the disease. This chapter evaluates the potential of TCM as medicaments for COVID-19. For in COVID-19 prevention and treatment it will be helpful in exploring current standing of TCM.

10.1 INTRODUCTION

In 2019 at the end of December numerous cases with unknown cause concerning viral pneumonia, were found in Wuhan, which is a city situated in the Hubei province of China. This unknown viral pathogen was named On February 11th, 2020 by the World Health Organization (WHO) as the Coronavirus Disease (COVID-19) [1]. It was suggested that the responsible pathogen for causing the disease belongs to coronavirus family *Coronaviridae* by The International Committee on Taxonomy of viruses (ICTV) and named it as Severe Acute Respiratory Syndrome Coronavirus 2 (SARS-CoV-2) [2]. Amongst recurrent symptoms are fever, fatigue, and dry cough. In more severe cases, they include acute respiratory distress syndrome and dyspnea meaning shortness of breath, speech, and/or movement loss, chest pain or pressure. Some rare cases also appear to be asymptomatic but still highly contagious. The virus is highly contagious and the outbreaks of COVID-19 occur at mass scale due to its risk of airborne transmission. Around 14% of corona patients require hospitalization along with oxygen support. Out of these 14% of the severe cases, approximately 5% of patients are transferred to intensive care unit (ICU) due to severity of disease [3, 4].

China has proposed a blending of therapeutic treatment for corona patients of traditional Chinese medicine (TCM) and conventional Western medicine. Recovery of the first COVID-19-patient by using the symptomatic treatment by TCM was announced on January 27th, 2020 by The State Administration of TCM. By March 23rd, 2020 the rate of affectivity of treatment of COVID-19 patient reached above 90% in 91.5% confirmed patients. The use of TCM can alleviate mild symptoms in the patients and prevent the patients from developing severe cases and reduce fatality rate. "Diagnosis and Treatment of Pneumonia Caused by Novel Coronavirus Infection" (Trial Ver. 4) was announced on January 27, 2020 by the Office of the State Administration of TCM and General Office of National Health and Health Commission of China. This issued version outlined the TCM herbal medicine treatment program along with implementation of TCM and Western Medicine [4, 5].

The therapy that TCM imparts is a treatment with concoction of Chinese herbs depending on different symptoms in different patients using Chinese diagnostic patterns. Several studies reported various Chinese herbal mixtures like Qingfei Paidu Decoction, Lianhua Qingen Capsule, Shufeng, Jeidu Capsule. All of these possess the ability of blocking the replication and proliferation of viral particles [5].

10.2 HISTORY

The history of Chinese Medicine goes back to Second Century B.C. The oldest written scriptures contain description of diseases from Shang Dynasty era (1600–1046 BBC) but no defined medical techniques are explained in the manuscripts. The manipulation of Yin and Yang using moxibustion and acupuncture is explained in similar manner to that of modern era in the book Yellow Emperor's Inner Canon (the first clear evidence of medical practice in TCM found in history) [6].

The history of TCM can be summarized by listing important scriptures and doctors (Figure 10.1).

10.2.1 SHAMANISTIC SHANG DYNASTY (1766–1122 BC)

The people from Shang era were religious. They believed that illness was equal to being cursed by the ancestors or the possession of demonic entity, as a result of upsetting them. So, majority of the healing practices involved appeasing ancestors with different rituals or expulsion of demons from bodies. For these purposes, people turned to arbitrators versed in talking to ancestors called Shamans, who then asked for assistance from their deity "Shang Ti." Most of scriptures from this era contained philosophical ideas [7, 8].

The first non-philosophical scripture, written by Huang Di Nei Jing (Yellow Emperor), contained the usage of herbs. Huang Di's "Yellow Emperor's Internal Classics" consisted of two parts; The Spiritual Pivot and The Book of Plain Questions. The book contained usage of TCM involved in various cases. The anatomy and physiology of body was also included [9].

10.2.2 ZHOU DYNASTY (1045–221 BC)

In Zhou Dynasty, the Imperial doctors included four different fields of research such as dietetic, diseases, sores, and veterinary. Their approved remedies are based on herbal, animal, and mineral materials in their arsenals. Zhang Zhongjing, Hua Tou, and Wang Shuhe are the famous doctors of Zhou Dynasty. Zhang Zhongjing produced complete set of treatment principles in his work on external heat disorders, epidemics, jaundice, and gynecology. Hua Tou invented an anesthetic using powdered cannabis called "Mafei San." This anesthetic, when taken orally, caused the loss of consciousness in patients. Therefore, aiding doctors in performing elaborate surgeries. Wang Shuhe explained the relationship between pulse, pathology, and physiology by introducing a pulse reading theory, and divided the pulse into 24 types [7, 8].

10.2.3 EASTERN HAN DYNASTY (206 BC–220 AD)

The first Chinese pharmacopeia was compiled by Shen-Nong of Han dynasty titled as "Shen-Nong's Classic of Herbal Medicine." The scripture contained medical herbs categorized by their properties along with their dosage and usage in combination with different herbs.

Zhong Zhahjing wrote "Treaties on Cold-Induced Miscellaneous Diseases," laying down the foundation of diagnosis using the interpretation of signs and symptoms along with the overall indication of health. The book focused on different types of fevers and various forms of influenzae [7, 9].

10.2.4 JIN DYNASTY (265 BC –420 AD)

Huangfu Mi wrote the first book entitled "Systematic Classic of Acupuncture and Moxibustion" on how physical ailments can be treated by acupuncture, acupressure, and moxibustion. Huangfu Mi discovered approximately 350 different pressure points and meridians of Qi in human body that can be manipulated to prevent and cure diseases [7, 9].

10.2.5 TANG DYNASTY (618 BC –907 AD)

Sun Simiao of Tang dynasty was the most knowledgeable medical scientist who understood all the aspects of Chinese Medicine including acupuncture, internal medicine, gynecology, pediatrics, physiology, anatomy, pathology, herbs, diagnosis, prescription, treatment, and other various theories of TCM. He wrote a separate book on children and women's remedies [7, 8].

10.2.6 SONG DYNASTY (960 BC –1297 AD)

In 1247, Song Ci of Song dynasty published a book called "Collected Cases of Injustice Rectified." It comprised of information on human anatomy, detoxification, coronary method, and emergency method. This text is the one of the first scriptures, which uses forensic medicine and methodology to explain cause of death using medical evidence [7, 8].

10.2.7 YUAN DYNASTY (1279 BC –1368 AD)

Hwa Shou of Yuan dynasty published the results of his thorough research related to acupuncture points and meridians in "Shisi Jing Fahui (An Explosion of 14 Meridians) which then became the basis of the present theory on meridians and their Collaterals [7, 10].

10.2.8 MING DYNASTY (1368 BC –1644 AD)

In Ming dynasty, Acupuncture became the principle treatment throughout the China. Countless texts and scriptures written during Ming dynasty are still consulted even to this day. Zhenjiu Dauan by Xu Feng, Zhenjiu Juying Fahui by Gao Wu, Zhenfeng Liuji by Wu Ku are some of the famous books that are still consulted in this era. In 1530, Wang Ji wrote Zhengjiu Wendui, a comparative study on technical differences in Acupuncture and Moxibustion. It led to discovery of new acupuncture points [7, 10].

10.2.9 QING DYNASTY (1644 BC –1912 AD)

Upon the arrival of Qing dynasty, the use of acupuncture became scarce to the point of it entering into the period of prohibition. The principle treatment in China shifted towards "Young" Western Medicine and TCM [10]. Accounts of TCM along with Western Medicine written by Zhang Xichun drew the ire of Chinese government and their attempt to abolish this integrated practice in medical schools [7, 9].

With discovery of penicillin in 1928 and its miraculous work, TCM was tossed aside for a long period of time. The TCM drought came to end in the era of Chairman Mao who was a Chinese communist revolutionary in 1970. His work resulted in modernization of Traditional Chinese techniques and aligned them to western beliefs. This evolution became the basis for the incorporation of TCM in medical schools and hospitals of present era [9].

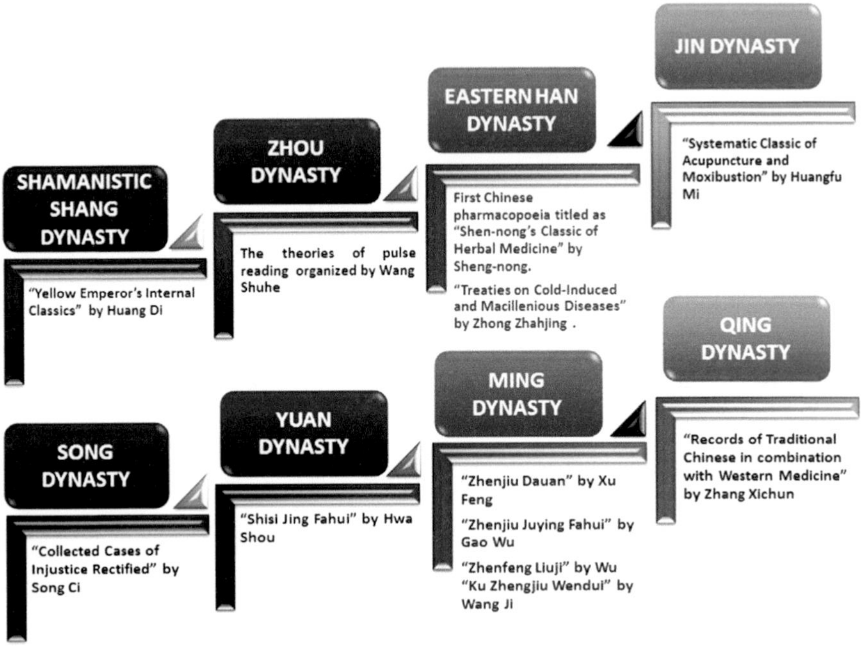

FIGURE 10.1 Development of TCM in four major sovereignties.

10.3 TRADITIONAL CHINESE MEDICINE (TCM): A HOLISTIC APPROACH

Holistic therapies are seen in ancient times of some healing traditions like those from Western societies in which Holistic medicine was used in 300 BC, during the era of Hippocrates in Ancient Greece. Holistic medicine is a hypernym used to describe various therapies of treating a patient as a whole person. Holism is philosophy that believes in the treatment of all three elements of human being; the mind, body, and spirit in order to achieve a complete healing of any nature. Holistic medicine includes analysis of all the elements affecting the health of an individual like physical, environmental, nutritional, emotional, and spiritual life style. A Holistic medicine practitioner takes into consideration the overall health of an individual including physical, emotional, and mental health before prescribing any kind of treatment [11].

Ancient Chinese philosophical thoughts are the basis of holism in TCM. According to these philosophical thoughts, TCM uses comprehensive analysis of time-space-human theory in order to explain illnesses and stresses upon the integration of human's social background, mental psychology, living conditions and quality of life. All fields of TCM including pathology, psychology, physiology, diagnoses, treatment, etc., pervade holism. The concept of holism in TCM has a deeper meaning than simple holism. For example, "Wuzang" (five different organs) in TCM does not mean five physical organs but five functional systems of human body [11].

Holism in TCM has two meanings. One, TCM marks human body to be a single complete entity in which all tissues and organs interact both physiologically and pathologically influencing each other. So, changes in the conditions of Yin and yang, viscera, qi, and blood of body are responsible of pathological changes, whereas the human body, as a whole entity, interacts with eternal environment. The human body is in constant contact with eternal environment and factors like climate, geographical location, working, and family environment. All of these factors affect the human health. TCM not only marks human body as a single unified entity, but also explains its interaction with environmental factors [11].

10.4 TRADITIONAL CHINESE MEDICINE (TCM) TECHNIQUES

Traditional Chinese medicine relies upon two principle theories which are discussed in subsections.

10.4.1 WU XING THEORY

The first theory is the five-element theory called "Wu Xing theory," which divides universe into five elements including Huo (fire), Jin (metal), Mu (wood), Shui (water) and Tu (earth). It was further proposed that the human body also comprises of these elements. So, these five elements are used for the treatment of different illnesses as each element corresponds to specific organ. For example, the element of fire corresponds to heart, the element of earth to digestive system, the element of metal to lungs, water element corresponds to kidneys and wood element to liver. Figure 10.2 represents the different techniques that are used for treatment in Chinese medicine [12].

10.4.2 MERIDIAN THEORY

Meridian theory is the core component of TCM elaborating how life and diseases work. It also explains how different therapies affect the illnesses. According to this theory, a hierarchal network of channels called 'meridians' exist in the human body. Around 14 main meridians are distributed throughout the body longitudinally from which smaller branched channels "collateral' and "sub collateral' arise. These run throughout the whole body to distribute the vital life (energy) force called qi. Qi is a vital substance and the energy sustaining the body. It mainly runs through the body in the interspaces of muscles or interstices between different tissues like vessels and bones found along the longitudinal axis in our body. The points from which 'I' leaves or enter the meridians are called acupoints. There are 365 acupoints present along the 14 main meridian channels that allows the qi to leave meridians and enter sub collateral channels. These acupoints are used to maintain balance of qi in human body. So, any imbalance in qi results in illness [13]. Figure 10.2 summarizes the techniques used in TCMs.

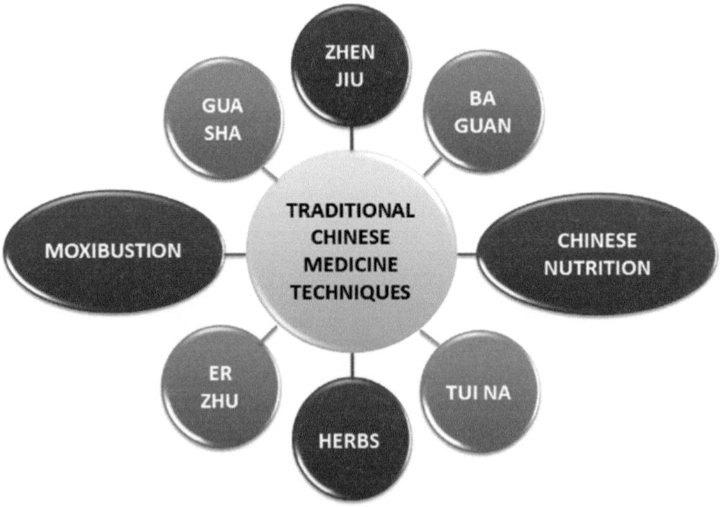
ZHEN JIU
GUA SHA
BA GUAN
MOXIBUSTION
TRADITIONAL CHINESE MEDICINE TECHNIQUES
CHINESE NUTRITION
ER ZHU
TUI NA
HERBS

FIGURE 10.2 Traditional Chinese medicine techniques.

10.4.3 ZHEN JIU (ACUPUNCTURE)

Acupuncture is the act of inserting thin needles in human body at different acupoints at superficial skin, subcutaneous tissue, and muscle level. Any imbalance or blockage in qi results in valetudinarianism. As soon as the flow is restored to its balanced state, the health of mind and body is restored. The acupuncture needles are inserted in specific acupoints to manipulate the qi flowing through the body. It aims to restoring the balance. In China, Acupuncture is mainly used for pain relief [12, 14].

10.4.4 BA GUAN (CUPPING)

Cupping is the technique that uses small glass cups to produce suction on the skin. These cups are strategically placed on specific points on fleshy parts of the body like stomach and back to restore the balance of qi in body. In this technique, cotton soaked in inflammable substance like alcohol is burned inside the small cups removing all the oxygen present is the cups. Then these heated cups are placed on the surface of the body. As the air in the cups cools down, it creates a vacuum in the cups which helps them to stick to the skin. When these cups are removed from the body, they produce suction action which bruises the skin of the body. The bruising experience is rather relaxing instead of being painful and stimulates blood flow and Qi. Respiratory problems are usually treated by Ba Guan [12, 14].

10.4.5 GUA SHA (SCRAPING)

Scrapping is a folk treatment which uses smooth flat surfaced objects like ceramic spoons, coins, animal bones or shaped rocks to scrape the moist surfaced skin in order to release toxins from the body and remove any obstructions present in the qi. Scrapping is rather a painful process as the skin is scraped till red welts form on the treating area. Despite the painful procedure, Gua Sha is believed to use for blood stagnation elevation and muscle relaxation by increasing the blood flow. Scrapping technique is usually used to treat chronic pain and fevers [12, 14].

10.4.6 TUI NA MASSAGE

The literal meaning of Tui Na is 'push and grasp.' This specific form of massage uses motions like kneading, rolling, pressing, and rubbing using acupressure on specific points on the body through fingers and hands. Sometimes herbs, ointments, and heat are used to enhance the effects of massage.

Tui Na regulates the flow of qi in the meridians and focuses on providing treatment for specific musculoskeletal problems instead of just providing relaxation [12, 14].

10.4.7 CHINESE HERBS

In herbology treatment of TCM, herbs are combined into formulas that are dispensed in the form of traditional tea, capsules, liquid extracts, granules, or powdered extracts. Most of the herbs used in TCM are extracted from seeds, roots, leaves, and bark of the plants like ginseng, ginger, licorice, cinnamon, etc. [14].

10.4.8 CHINESE NUTRITION

Nutrition is considered as first line of defense in TCM regarding health. Nutrition is a mode of dieting in TCM. It involves using the 5 tastes; spicy, sour, bitter, sweet, and salty in daily diet. These five tastes are considered to have different effects on human body. For example, spicy food has a warm effect on body while salty, sour, and bitter food has cooling effect [14].

10.4.9 ER ZHU (EAR CANDLING)

Ear candling is the technique in which a hollow candle is placed over the ear and is burned at the opposite end. This technique a believed to remove wax and debris from the ear and relieves headache. It also treats allergies. But scientifically this technique is proved to be harmful to the body, in case the wax of the melting candle falls in the ear. This technique is also proved to be ineffective to treat any headache, allergies or removal of ax and debris from ear. So, in the light of scientific evidences, this practice has mostly been abandoned in China [12].

10.4.10 MOXIBUSTION

Moxibustion technique is the activity of burning moxa, mugwort root made from a dried spongy herb '*Artemesia vulgaris*' near the skin. Moxa, on burning, produces large amount of smoke and pungent odor along with heat that warms and invigorate blood. Resultantly, it increases qi flow in meridians.

There are two types of moxibustion techniques. In direct moxibustion, cone shaped moa is placed in direct contact with acupoint on skin and burned. The heating sensation produces a pleasant feeling on the skin. On the other hand, in indirect moxibustion stick, moxa is burned at one end and held close to the area being treated until the area turns red. Historically, moxibustion therapy is used to relieve menstrual pain in women [15].

10.5 DIAGNOSTIC METHODS OF TRADITIONAL CHINESE MEDICINE (TCM)

The description of disease diagnostic principles in TCM is first found in Yellow Emperor's Classic of Internal Medicine. Later on, the principles for disease diagnosis were proposed by famous scholar Zhang Zhongjing in his book 'Treaties on Cold-Induced and Miscellaneous Diseases.' In the modern era, TCM physicians still use these principles as guidelines to determine the nature and location of pathological changes in body. The eight principles of diagnosis act as guiding rules for the purpose of diseases diagnosis and differentiating syndromes. Each of the eight principles generalizes a unique characteristic of clinical manifestation. The complete picture of patient can only be analyzed by applying eight principles of diagnosis together. These principles are "Yin, yang, heat, cold, excess (shi), deficiency (xu), interior, and exterior (Figure 10.3). These principles make four pairs of opposing terminologies in which Yin and yang serve as the root of remaining six principles and group them into two categories under them. In this grouping the yin category includes the interior, cold, and deficiency and the yang include the exterior, heat, and excess [16].

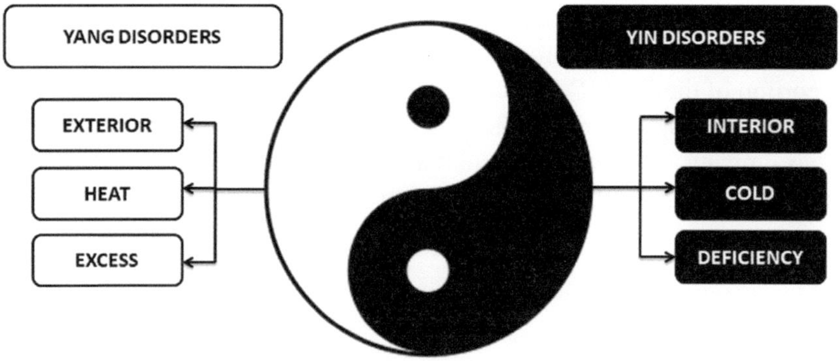

FIGURE 10.3 Classification of Yin/Yang disorders.

10.5.1 YIN/YANG

Opposite interrelated aspects of the Yin and yang theory is found in nature, clinical features, and disease. As all the clinical features of disease can be categorized under either yin or yang terminologies, so these two principles become the foundation of other six principles. In clinical diagnosis, physician first determine whether the symptom can be categorized as Yin or yang. Yin type symptoms are associated with inhibition, quietude, deterioration, and gloominess. For example, low spiritedness, slow, week, and deep pulse, pale complexion, coldness in limbs, white coating on pale tongue, and loose bowels, clear profuse urine. On the other hand, yang type symptoms are associated with excitation, restlessness, and hyperactivity. For example, irritability, rolling, and rapid pulse or surging and floating, hot sensations in body, reddening of face, loud voice, coarse breathing, thirst, abdominal pain, sparse yellow urine, constipation, and yellow coating on deep red colored tongue [16].

10.5.2 EXTERIOR AND INTERIOR

Exterior and interior diagnosing principle is significant for exogenous disease diagnosis as their causative factor is stemmed from outside of the body. The development of such diseases occurs from outer to inner part of body and their severity increases with their progression. Exterior type diseases are the diseases that occur in meridians, muscles, and body surface. On the other hand, interior type diseases are the diseases that occur in internal organs, blood, and qi [16].

10.5.2.1 EXTERIOR TYPE SYNDROME

Exterior type syndrome is the condition that results from the invasion of exogenous pathogens in body through mouth, nose or skin and affect the superficial portion of the body. Fever, chills, disinclination to wind, headache, body aches, thin coating on tongue and floating pulse are general clinical features that accompany exterior type conditions. Other generalized signs comprise of coughing and sneezing, runny nose, sore throat, and nasal congestion [16].

10.5.2.2 INTERIOR TYPE SYNDROME

The conditions that are caused by pathological changes deep inside the body involving internal organs, Qi, blood, and bone marrow are referred to as interior type syndrome. Mental stress, physical strain, and improper diet along with exogenous pathogens are the factors that cause interior type syndromes. Interior types of syndromes are considerably severe and run longer course of disease accompanied with organ dysfunction. Clinical symptoms of interior type syndrome differ from person to person [16].

10.5.3 HEAT AND COLD

Heat and cold are indications of the body reflecting the balanced Yin and yang state of body that represents two different aspects of disease. Heat and cold, despite being opposite in nature have the tendency to coexist and develop a complex syndrome of cold and heat [16].

10.5.3.1 COLD TYPE SYNDROMES

Recessive conditions occurring due to imbalance in yin and yang state, with increase in yin energy and deficiency of yang energy in the body are cold syndromes. Cold syndromes can also occur due to exposure to exogenous cold. Sensitivity to low temperature, preference for warmth, pale complexion, bland taste, pale tongue with white glossy coating, coldness in limbs, weariness, loose bowels, clear copious urine, clear, and thin body discharges and slow or tense pulse are the clinical features that accompany cold type syndromes [16].

10.5.3.2 HEAT TYPE SYNDROMES

Excitatory conditions due to excess yang and decreased yin energy in the body or invasion of exogenous heat in the body are heat syndromes. Reddening of face, disinclination to heat, thirst, predilection for cold, irritability, constipation, thick, and yellow body discharges, sparse yellow urine, yellow, and dry coating on red tongue and rapid pulse are the clinical features of heat syndromes [16].

Under certain circumstances cold and heat syndromes have the ability to transform into each other. For instance, the invasion of pathogenic cold causes diseases that are cold in nature but turn to heat if it stays long enough in the body [16].

10.5.4 EXCESS (SHI) AND DEFICIENCY (XU)

During the course of disease, the conflicting forces between pathological factors and body's resistance are analyzed and generalized with the help of two principles of *xu* and *shi* [16].

10.5.4.1 DEFICIENT (XU) TYPE SYNDROME

The conditions that arise in the body due to body's weak defense against the disease, instead of overabundance of pathogens are referred to deficient syndromes. The motifs of this syndrome include deficiency in Qi, Yin, and yang, body fluids, blood, and nutrient levels along with bone marrow depletion. Common clinical features of *xu* syndromes include drowsiness, low-spiritedness, pallor skin color, shortness of breath, coldness in limbs, palpitation, diarrhea, frequent or incontinence urination pale tongue and weak thready pulse. Most patients having chronic diseases, weak health and inherent defects suffer from *xu* syndrome [16].

10.5.4.2 EXCESS (SHI) TYPE SYNDROME

The conditions that result because of abundance of pathogenic factors while the body is in prime health with strong disease preventing forces, resulting in strong confrontation between the opposite forces are referred to deficient syndromes. Qi sluggishness, sluggishness of fluid flow, phlegm impediment or blood stasis can also be the cause of excess syndromes along with the invasion of pathogenic factors. Common clinical features of excess syndrome include fever, distension pain that worsens on pressing, difficulty in urination, constipation, unconsciousness, irritability, chest stuffiness, coarse breathing, unwarranted throat discharges, thick greasy tongue coating and excessive forceful pulse. *Shi* syndromes usually manifest as sudden attacks accompanied with strong clinical symptoms in people with strong physique [16].

10.5.5 PILLARS OF DIAGNOSTICS IN TCM

Chinese Traditional Medicine has a quite different approach in diagnosing diseases in patients as compared to Western Medicine. TCM use four methods of diagnostics which are commonly referred to four pillars of diagnostics in

TCM. Each pillar provides information that is combined for the diagnosis and adds up to the holistic view of examination [17, 18].

10.5.5.1 INSPECTION

Inspection or looking is the visual part of diagnosis that is used to analyze color and luster of skin and face along with observation of different body features like eyes, ears, and tongue. In TCM, tongue examination takes quite precedence as its condition like color, shape, texture, coating, and moisture level corresponds to different conditions of "zang fu" organs that can reveal the particulars of a disease and its progression. Five organs that fall in the category of zang are heart, lungs, spleen, liver, and kidney. On the other hand, the six organs in the body that fall in fu category are stomach, gall, and urinary bladder, small, and large intestine and sanjiao (triple energizer) [17, 18].

10.5.5.2 AUSCULTATION

Auscultation refers to examination of peculiar sounds as the sound of someone's voice is indicator of health. TCM particularly classifies sounds into five different types: laughing, singing, groaning, weeping, and shouting. Auscultation also outstretches to olfaction which is examination of body odor despite it being considered separate from sound in Western Medicine [17, 18].

10.5.5.3 PALPATION

Palpation is examination of body by feeling specifically the wrist pulse, abdomen, and meridian points in body. Different type of pulses like choppy, rapid, strong, slow, weak, shallow, etc., after examination of wrist pulse at various points provide insight to physical and mental condition of the patient. During abdominal examination, TCM practitioner looks for tender or painful areas along with hot or cold, sweaty, swollen, and discolored areas to gain insight into the condition of body [17, 18].

10.5.5.4 INQUIRY

Inquiry refers to part of examination which includes gaining insight to patient's past health and habits by asking different questions. Traditionally,

TCM diagnosis includes 10 questions that range from diet patterns to sleeping patterns. After diagnosing of a specific pattern of disharmony in the body, TCM practitioner prescribes specific treatment to the patient [17, 18].

All of the external symptoms of the body reflect condition of the health of internal organs and systems of a patient. The information, provided by whole examination by employing four pillars of examination, paints a clear picture of a patient's condition that allows the professional to develop complete understanding of patient and recommend relevant treatment plan that addresses the disparities in the qi of body (Figure 10.4) [17, 18].

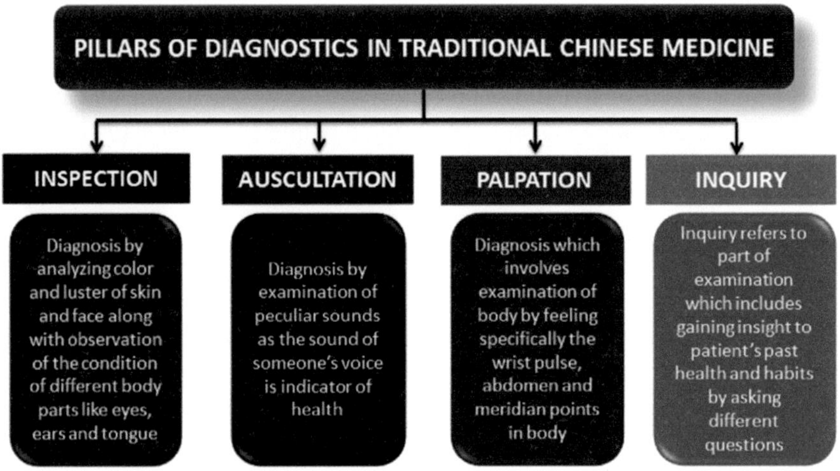

FIGURE 10.4 Pillars of diagnostics in TCM.

10.6 CORONA AND TCM

TCM's concept of diseases place Corona (COVID-19) in the category as it is an infectious disease of virulent nature with epidemic factors [19]. COVID-19 has been listed by China as a Class B infectious disease but the containment plan and preventive measures for COVID-19 have been taken according to the outlines of Class A infectious diseases. Main source of COVID-19 infection spread, presently, are novel Coronavirus infected patients, as well as the infected patients who are asymptomatic. So, contagious capacity of COVID-19 is ranged from medium to slightly high. The SARS-CoV-2 virus which incubate the body for almost one week. The longest incubation period observed in COVID-19 patients is

14 days but in some rare cases an incubation period of as long as 24 days is also observed [20].

In Chinese history, hundreds of epidemic and pandemic events have been dealt with the help of TCM which has amassed a huge amount of effective therapeutic experiences and treatments. For example, Chinese dealt with Small pox epidemic in Song Dynasty with the help of variolation and in 2003 Chinese doctors used TCM integrated with Western Medicine to fight against SARS. TCM have also shown high cure rate along with low mortality rate in the patients of Corona in China [19].

On January 22, 2020 treatment priority of COVID-19 was shifted towards TCM by National Health Commission (NHC) of People's Republic of China. In trial Ver. 3 of treatment, four syndromes and their corresponding formulas were included in COVID-19 diagnosis and treatment. In the later trial ver., including 4 and 5 the pestilent toxin treatment that blocks the lungs with the help of Xuanfei Baidu formula was adopted. Later on, the formula was further developed during trial version 6 and 7 for simultaneous treatment of lungs syndromes with dampness and toxin retention. In trial version 7 of treatment, Qingfei Paidu Decoction was recommended by NHC for treatment of mild to critical COVID-19 patients. Additionally, Linhua Qingwen Capsule and Jinhua Qinggan Granule were recommended by NHC for treatment of fever during COVID-19. During moderate and critical period of disease Xuebijing injection was also used for treatment plan during clinical observation. Eventually, TCM doctors recommended an effective therapeutic treatment against COVID-19 comprising of Lianhua Qingwen Capsule, Qingfei Paidu Decoction, Jinhua Qinggan Granule, Xuanfei Baidu Formula, Xuebijing Injection, and Huashi Baidu Formula, cumulatively named "Three TCM Prescriptions and Three Medicines" [19].

10.6.1 STAGE DIFFERENTIATION OF COVID-19 IN TCM

TCM has differentiated and categorized disease progression in case of COVID-19 into four main categories so treatment plan of COVID-19 is also based on the stages (Figure 10.5). The four stages include the initial mild, the progressive severe, the extremely severe and the final recovery convalescent stage [20]. Following are symptoms associated with these four stages of disease progression in case of COVID-19:

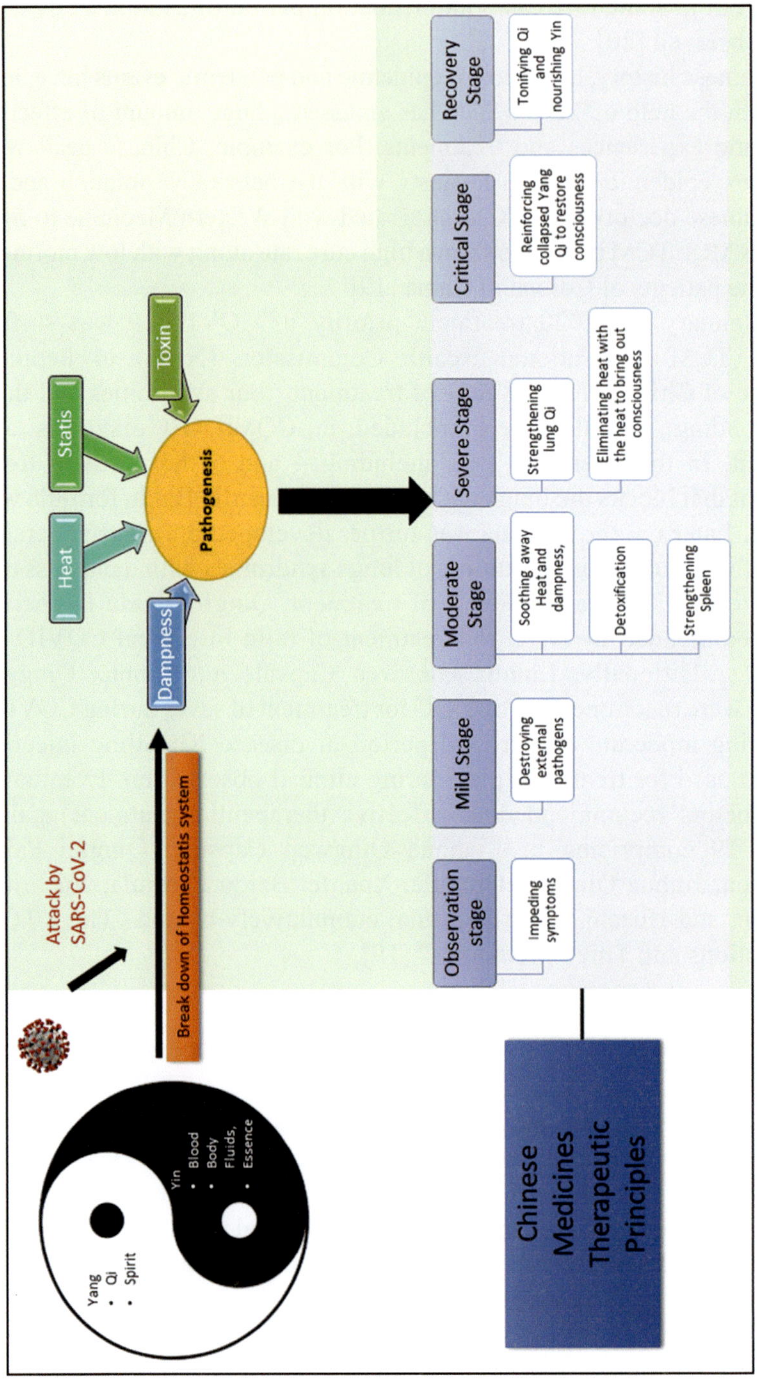

FIGURE 10.5 Chinese medicine therapeutic principles applied to the COVID-19 treatment.

10.6.1.1 INITIAL STAGE

In the initial stage of COVID-19, 'fever without cold' is considered to be the main symptom. Additional symptoms that accompany fever include insomnia and distress, dry cough, polydipsia, angina pectoris, occasional myalgia, loose stool, runny nose, nasal congestion, absence of perspiration, absence of excessive heat or irritability caused by heat sensation, no sore throat, dark red tongue, or tongue with redness around the edges, thin white coating on tongue and varying pulse without fixed point [20].

10.6.1.2 PROGRESSIVE STAGE

High fever, asthma, breathlessness, laborious movements, exacerbation of fatigue, exacerbation of cough, incessant dry cough with reduced phlegm, polydipsia, blueness of lips and nails, increased palpitation, lightheadedness, delirium, dyspepsia, dark red tongue, smooth pulse, constipation or loose stools, difficulty in urination, bloating, and abdominal distension, are main clinical features associated with progressive stage of COVID-19[20].

10.6.1.3 EXTREME STAGE

Without proper treatment at progressive stage, the symptoms of disease can further aggravate that would lead to the severe stage of disease categorized as Extreme stage. High fever, dyspnea, blue colored lips, darkening of skin tone, extreme fatigue, distress, fainting spells, difficulty in urination, warm or cold limbs, dark red tongue and rapid thinning pulse are the main clinical features of extreme stage of COVID-19. Some patients during this stage developed low grade fever or no fever at all during clinical observation period [20].

10.6.1.4 RECOVERY STAGE

Only mild symptoms are found among patients during recovery stage of disease, high fever subsides with improvement in mental state, mild fever, exhaustion, sticky stool, and mild loss in appetite. Fibrosis is observed among patients during recovery stage in computerized tomography (CT). Dampness in lungs is completely eliminated in recovery stage but residual evil is observed in the body with deficiency in spleen and lung Qi during demonstration of disease pathogenesis [20].

10.7 TCM APPLICATION FOR COVID-19 TREATMENT WITH STAGE PROGRESSION IN DISEASE

Syndrome differentiation and COVID-19 treatments with stage progression in disease is required in case of TCM treatment (Table 10.1). Removal of dampness, prompting blood circulation and resolving pooling of blood are priorities of treatment plan.

Heat, dampness, and turbidity are very difficult to separate even if epidemic toxin consists of them. Dampness is usually categorized as Yin and is treated with warm tonic herbs which contradict the removal of heat, requiring the use of cold and cool drugs. Dampness is drained along with removal of heat and turbidity from body using combinations of herbs at different stages of disease. Usually, warm herbs are used at early stages and cold herbs are used at later stage of disease so as to deal with dampness, heat, and turbidity [20].

As soon as lungs shadow appears, treatment of affected persons ought to be initiated with therapeutics that evoke blood circulation and resolve blood pooling problems. During different stages of treatment, products that promote blood circulation, eliminate blood pooling, dredge blood vessels, reduce damage in alveoli, prevent fibrosis in pulmonary interstitials and reduce aftermaths of disease are used. The basis of using these is those pathological reports which indicate increased blood volume and hemorrhage in vessels and organs, edema, inflammation in pulmonary interstices and diffused alveolar in body which are indications of blood stasis [20].

10.7.1 TREATMENT AT INITIAL STAGE

In the initial stage treatment, plan follows the clearance of damp heat by treating shangjiao membrane to cure lungs. The treatment plan also includes separation and dissipation of dampness, heat, and smooth release of lung Qi. Sanren Decoction and Huopu Xialing. Decoction principle is followed to screen the toxin potential to enter inside the body and pacify dampness, remove dirt, enhance Qi flow, resolve, and relieve blood pooling and vessels. The combination prescription constitutes of peilan, doukou, xingren, fuling, zexei, guanghuoxiang, banxia, huashi, danzhuye, yiyiren, chishao, mudanpi, and tongco [20].

TABLE 10.1 Stage Differentiation and Treatment of COVID-19

Stage	Clinical Manifestation	Treatment Plan	Prescribed TCM
Initial	Fever without cold, insomnia, fatigue, dry cough, polydipsia, angina pectoris, occasional myalgia, loose stool, runny nose, nasal congestion, absence of perspiration, absence of excessive heat or irritability caused by heat sensation, dark red tongue with thin white coating and varying pulse without fixed point	Clearance of damp heat by treating shangjiao membrane to cure lungs, separation, and dissipation of dampness, smoothen release of lung Qi	Sanren Decoction and Huopu Xialing Decoction comprising of peilan, banxia, guanghuoxiang, doukou, fuling, zexie, yiyiren, chishao, xingren, huashi, tongcao, danzhuye, and mudanpi
Progressive	High fever, asthma, breathlessness, laborious movements, exacerbation of fatigue, exacerbation of cough, incessant dry cough with reduced phlegm, polydipsia, blueness of lips and nails, increased palpitation, lightheadedness, delirium, dyspepsia, dark red tongue, smooth pulse, constipation or loose stools, difficulty in urination, bloating, and abdominal distension	removal of dampness, removal of toxins, and transferring of aromatics to the lung, removal of yin heat ensuing cooling of blood	Shengjiang Powder comprising of guanghuoxiang, peilan, banxia, chenpi, dafupi, houpo, heye, jiangcan, and chantui. Jiedu Huoxue Decoction, chaihu, taoren, honghua, chishao, shengdihuang, danggui, lianqiao, gegen, gancao, jianghuang, and dahuang
Extreme	High fever, dyspnea, blue colored lips, darkening of skin tone, extreme fatigue, distress, fainting spells, difficulty in urination, warm or cold limbs, dark red tongue, and rapid thinning pulse	Disseminating lung Qi, rectifying body's essence Qi, enhancing blood flow, removal of toxins and rescuing inverse	Shenfu Sini Decoction comprising of fuzi, gancao, ganjiang, suhexiang, longnao, anxixiang, xiangfu, muxiang, tanxiang, chenxiang, ruxiang, dingxiang, bibo, baizhu, hezi, and zhusha
Convalescent	High fever subsides with improvement in mental state, mild fever, exhaustion, sticky stool, and mild loss in appetite	Dispose of remaining evil in body, enhancing lung circulation, reinvigorate spleen and build up healthy Qi	Xue's Wuye Lugen Decoction comprising of bohe, fresh lotus leaf, huoxiang leaf, dongguazi leaf, lugen, and peilan

Doukou, banxia, peilan, and guanghuoxiang are used for regulation of Qi, drying, and aromatization; lung Qi is promoted by xingren; for removal of dampness yiyiren, huashi, tongcao, danzhuye, and fuling are used Fuling, Zexie, Huashi, Tongcao, Danzhuye, and Yiyiren are used; and chishao and mudanpi resolve blood pooling in body. Sanjiao Qi mechanism can be smoothening, dampness can be dissipated and dissolved, blood stasis can be resolved, and collaterals can be dredged using the combination of these herbs [20].

10.7.2 TREATMENT AT PROGRESSIVE STAGE

Heat of the body can be increased due to the toxins causing dampness in lungs leading to lungs infection and deterioration in functioning of lungs. So, treatment plan at progressive stage includes removal of dampness, detoxification, and aromatizing the lungs, elimination of yin heat ensuing blood cooling. In this treatment the combination of Jiedu Huoxue Decoction with Shengjiang Powder, and including Lei's aromatic turbid-resolving method, are employed. Shengjiang Powder constitutes of guanghuoxiang, peilan, banxia, chenpi, dafupi, houpo, heye, jiangcan, and chantui while Jeidu Huoxue Decoction constitutes of taoren, chaihu, honghua, chishao, shengdihuang, danggui, lianqiao, gegen, gancao, jianghuang, and dahuang herbs [20].

Peilan, banxia, and guanghoxiang are efficient in dampness removal and revitalize spleen and stomach; chempai improves Qi circulation in the body; huopo and dafupi are used together to eliminate dampness and promote circulation in body; heye is used for reducing the heat in body and murkiness in lungs, jiangcan, and chantui are used to for reduction of the dampness in the body along with removal of gas produced, detoxification, and bringing down heat in body. Chaihu of Jiedu Huoxue Decoctiom can sift liver and Qi of the body; taoren and honghua are used for sorting out blood pooling and enhancing blood flow; danggui, shengdihuang, and chishao are used for reduction of body heat, hence cooling blood and improving its nutrient constitution; gegen and lianqiao are used for reduction of body heat and removal of toxins from body; gancao is used to restore Qi and to invigorate the spleen; jianghuang is used for Qi dispersion and lessen blood stasis; and dahuang is used for subsiding body heat [20].

10.7.3 TREATMENT AT EXTREME STAGE

Lungs can be closed due to presence of dampness and heat if disease is not properly treated at progressive stage. Qi and Yin treatment at extreme stage of

COVID-19 include disseminating lung Qi, rectifying Qi, enhancing blood flow, removal of toxins and rescuing inverse. Based upon the treatment plan following can be used: Three Treasures (zixue and zhibao dan, angong niuhuang pill) and Shenfu Sini, Decoction or Suhe Xiang Pill. Shenfu Sini Decoction constitutes of fuzi, gancao, ganjiang, suhexiang, longnao, anxixiang, xiangfu, muxiang, tanxiang, chenxiang, ruxiang, dingxiang, bibo, Baizhu, hezi, and zhusha [20].

Fuzi of Shenfu Sini Decoction is used to warm and strengthen kidney. Gancao is lucrative for Qi; to warm stomach and spleen, cold elimination, and ganjiang assist in Yang dredge blood vessels; suhexiang help Qi flow, eliminate phlegm and open orifices to awaken mind; to rouse mind longnao is used; anxixiang has the capability to circulate blood and Qi and remove dirt; xiangfu pacifies liver, synchronize Qi and alleviate depression; muxiang is capable of soothing Sanjiao; Qi is relieved by tanxiang and sluggishness in stomach; descending of Qi by chenxiang, warming middle energizer of Sanjiao and controlling Qi by warming kidney; ruxiang improves blood circulation; bibo and dingxiang warms stomach and spleen, assist Qi circulation and bring down cold symptoms; baizhu reinvigorate spleen and transfer dampness and helps remove turbidity and dampness in Sanjiao with the help of aromatic herbs; hezi prevents Qi consumption by heat and alleviate pain; zhusha is capable of removing toxins from heart and soothe mind; and shuiniujiao clear out fire and. Zixue dan or angong niuhuang pill can be employed while removing heat and suhe xiang pill and be consumed in case of closed Yin [20].

10.7.4 TREATMENT AT CONVALESCENT STAGE

Weakness dominates the body at recovery stage of disease. Xue's Wuye Lugen Decoction can be utilized to dispose of remaining evil in body, enhancing lung motion, reinvigorate spleen and build up healthy Qi in body as bohe, fresh lotus leaf, huoxiang leaf, dongguazi leaf, lugen, and peilan in decoction hover and expose remaining evil in body [20].

Peilan leaf, bohe, fresh lotus and huoxiang leaf are aromatic and rejuvenate spleen while dongguazi and lugen are used to infiltrate the body. Lugen decoction is capable of disseminating, purifying, and infiltration [20].

10.8 ORAL TCM FOR COVID-19 TREATMENT

Therapy has proven to be beneficial using TCM for multi target and -linked treatment. Multiple TCM herbal formulations are being employed to treat recent havoc of COVID-19. Many Chinese formulas constituting of variety of herbs have shown remedial effects on COVID-19 (Figure 10.6 and Table 10.2).

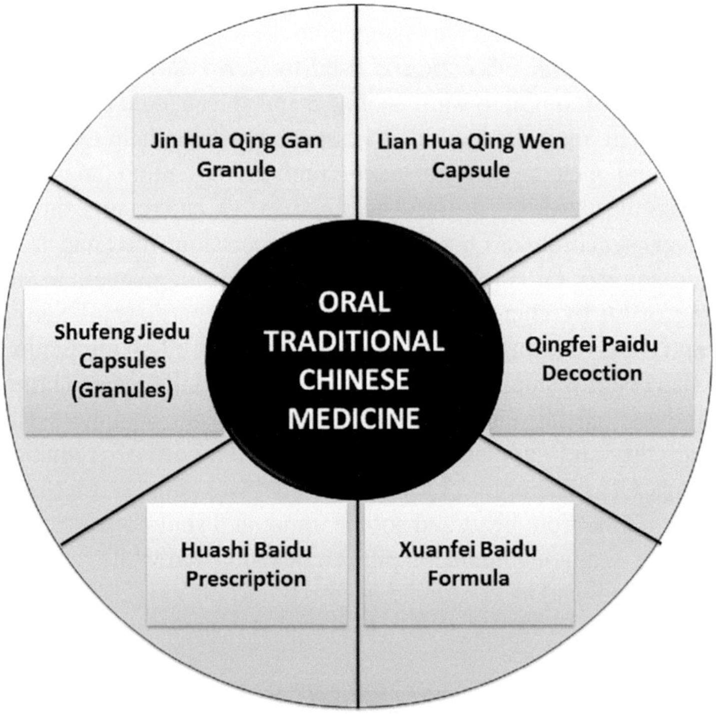

FIGURE 10.6 Oral TCM for COVID-19 treatments.

10.8.1 JIN HUA GINGGAN GRANULE

Jin Hua Qinggan granules are antiviral, effectively regulate immune system and used to treat plague diseases [21]. It mainly constitutes of Semen *Armeniacae amarum* (kuxingren), Forsythiae Fructus (lianqiao), Arctii Fructus (niubangzi), *Menthae haplocalycis* Herba (bohe), Glycyrrhizae Radix et Rhizoma (gancao), Lonicerae Japonicae Flos (jinyinhua), Scutellariae Rdix (huangqin), Anemarrhena Rhizoma (zhimu), Gypsum Fibrosum (shigao), Ephedrae Herba (mahuang), Artemisiae Annuae (qinghao) and Fritillariae Thunbergii Bulbus (zhebeimu) herbs [19]. In clinical practice, Jin Hua Qing Gan has been recommended in the guidelines of NHC for treating

TABLE 10.2 Composition and Mode of Action of Oral TCM

SL. No.	Decoction	Composition	Mode of Action
1.	Jin Hua Qing Gan Granule	Semen Armeniacae Amarum (kuxingren), Forsythiae Fructus (lianqiao), Arctii Fructus (niubangzi), Menthae Haplocalycis Herba (bohe), Glycyrrhizae Radix et Rhizoma (gancao), Lonicerae Japonicae Flos (jinyinhua), Scutellariae Rdix (huangqin), Anemarrhena Rhizoma (zhimu), Gypsum Fibrosum (shigao), Ephedrae Herba (mahuang), Artemisiae Annuae (qinghao) and Fritillariae Thunbergii Bulbus (zhebeimu)	Control several signaling pathways by binding to SARS-CoV-2 3CL hydrolase by interacting with ACE 2, BCL 2, HSP90AA1, CASP3, HSP90AB1, PTGS 1, PTGS 2 and NCOA 2 molecules, modulates cytokine storm, inhibit arachidonic Acid pathway (AA metabolic pathway and promote pneumonia inflammatory exudate absorption
2.	Lian Hua Qing wen capsule	Gypsum Fibrosum (shigao), Menthol (bohenao), Glycyrrhizae Radi et Rhizoma (gancao), Houttuyniae Herba (yuxingcao), Rhei Radi et Rhizoma (dahuang), Forsythiae Fructus (lianqiao), processed Semen Armeniacae Amarum (chao kuxingren), processed Ephedrae Herba (zhi mahuang), Dryopteridis Crassirhizomatis Rhizoma (mianmaguanzhong), Rhodiolae Crenulatae Radix et Rhizoma (hongjingtian), Pogostemonis Herba (guanghuoxiang), Lonicerae Japonicae Flos (jinyinhua) and Isatis Radix (ban lan gen)	Reduce IL-6, CCL2/MCP-1, CXCL-10/IP-10 and TNF-α that act as proinflammatory cytokines, inhibit SARS-CoV-2 replication in Vero E6 cells
3.	Shufeng Jeidu capsules	Ban Lan Gen (radix isatidis), Bupleurum, Forsythia, Verbena, *Rhizoma Phragmitis* Communis (reed root), *Glycyrrhiza glabra* (licorice), *Polygonum cuspidatum* (Japanese knotweed) and *Bupleurum falcatum* (Chinese thoroughwax)	Inhibitory activity against NF-kB/MAPK signaling, prevent regulation of NF-kB mRNA, inhibit expression of inflammatory cytokines, reduce levels of lactic acid, increase in partial pressure in lungs tissue alleviating symptoms related to lungs infection by prompt absorption of lung inflammation
4.	Qingfei Paidu decoction	Asari Radix et Rhizoma (xixin), Atractylodis Macrocephalae Rhizoma (baizhu), Belamcandae Rhizoma (shegan), Asteris Radix (ziwan), Armeniacea Semen (xingren), Aurantii Fructus Immaturus (zhishi), Ephedrae Herba (mahuang), processed Glycyrrhizae Radix et Rhizoma (zhigacao), Dioscoreae Rhizoma (shanyao), Pinelliae	anti-viral and anti-inflammatory characteristics, regulate STAT1, MAPKs, JUN, IL-6, RELA, and AKT1 inhibiting inflammatory reactions in body, reduce lung injury, regulate immune functions, and preserve nerve function

TABLE 10.2 *(Continued)*

SL. No.	Decoction	Composition	Mode of Action
		Rhizoma Praeparatum Cum Zingibere et Alumine (jiang banxia), Citri reticulatae Pericarpium (chenpi), Gypsum Fibrosum (sheng shigao), Alismatis Rhizoma (zexie), Pogostemonis Herba (huoxiang), Polyporus (zhuling), Bupleuri Radix (chaihu), Poria (fuling), Farfarae Flos (donghua), Cinnamomi Ramulus (guizhi), Zingiberis Rhizoma Recens (shengjiang) and Scutellariae Radix (huanqing)	
5.	Huashi Baidu prescription	Poria (fuling), Gypsum Fibrosum (sheng shigao), Armeniacae Semen (xingren), Tsaoko Fructus (caoguo), Astragali Radix (sheng huangqi), Magnoliae officinalis Cortex (houpo), Peoniae Radix Rubra (chishao), Pinellinae Rhizoma Praeparatum (fa banxia), Rhei Radix et Rhizoma (sheng dahuang), Glycyrrhizae Radix (gancao), Lepidii/Descurianiae (tinglizi), Atracytlodis Rhizoma (cangzhu), Pogostemonis Herba (huoxiang) and Ephedrae Herba (sheng mahuang)	Regulate inflammatory response and inhibit cytokine storm
6.	Xuanfei Baidu formula	Phragmitis Rhizoma (lugen), Atractylodis Rhizoma (maocangzhu), Ephedrae Herba (sheng mahuang), Lepidii/Descurainiae Semen (tinglizi), Glycyrrhizae Radix et Rhizoma (gancao), Citri Grandis Exocarpium rubrum (huajuhong), Verbenae Herba (mabiancao), Artemisiae Annuae Herba (qinghao), Pogostemonis Herba (guanghuoxiang) Coicis Semen (sheng yiyiren), Armeniacae Semen Amarum (kuxingren), Gypsum Fibrosum (sheng shigao) and Polygoni Rhizoma et Radix (huazhang)	Suppress excessive immune response and regulates inflammatory factors including chemokines and related T cells Th17, Th1, Th2, IL-6, CXCL8, etc.

patients of COVID-19 during medical observation. The use of Jin Hua Qing Gan as adjuvant therapy alleviated fever, cough, fatigue, sputum, and anxiety in COVID-19 patients along with reduction in hospitalization time period [21, 22].

The mechanism of action of Jin hua ginggan has been revealed by molecular docking and network pharmacology techniques to be its ability to modulate numerous cellular routes by interacting with SARS-CoV-2 3CL hydrolase and ACE 2, BCL 2 (B-cell lymphoma 2), HSP90AA1, CASP3, HSP90AB1, PTGS 1, PTGS 2 and NCOA 2 molecules because of the presence of Oxylin A, baicalein, and kaempferol which serve as active compounds of formula [19]. The hydrolase SARS-CoV-2 3CL is an important enzyme involved in SARS-CoV-2 replication. In Forsythiae Fructus Forsythiaside A, in Ephedrae Herba Ephedrine, Chlorogenic acid in Lonicerae Japonicae Flos were identified to have high affinity for SARS-CoV-2 3CL hydrolase and ACE 2 and can act as potential inhibitors to stop ACE 2 and SARS-CoV-2 S binding successfully prohibiting viral invasion in host cells [23]. Moreover, Jin hua qinggan acts directly on the virus and modulates cytokine storm associated with COVID-19 mortality. The inhibition of arachidonic acid pathway (AA metabolic pathway) reduces cytokine storm as AA metabolic pathway is involved in synthesis of inflammatory cytokines. So, Jin hua qinggan is an anti-COVID-19 force because it deals with cytokines storm. Jin hua qinggan promotes pneumonia inflammatory exudate absorption without any unfavorable effects on patients [24]. Dysregulated cytokines produced in body is considered to be the hallmark of Corona patients. In severe cases of Corona elevated levels of IL-2, -4, -6 and -10 and TNFα have been observed. Particularly incessant increase in IL-6 levels due to SARS-CoV-2 infection led to deregulation of immune system which correlated with severity and mortality of patients. Additionally significant decrease in CD4+ and CD8+ T-cells and reduction in Natural killer cells (NK) to produce IFN-γ has been observed in patients. Decreased IFN-γ led to improper immune response as IFN-γ acts as central mediator of anti-viral immunity by enhancing MHC class 1 pathway, IFN-α/β activity and Th1 dependent immune response. Jinhua qinggan granule upregulated IFN-γ levels and down regulated IL-6 levels and played immunomodulatory role to regulate immune system response [25]. The average time for nucleic acid detection test to become negative in patients treated with Jin hua qinggan granules is 7± 4 days. Around 7 days positive to negative nucleic acid conversion rate was significantly higher among patients given adjuvant treatment of Jin hua qinggan granules as compared to patients treated with only Western medicine. After 7-day treatment using Jinhua qinggan granules significant decrease in pulmonary inflammation promoting pneumonia inflammatory exudate absorption and significant increase in blood cell count (especially leukocytes and lymphocyte) was observed which indicated improvement in immune system recovery in patients with COVID-19 [26] In hua, qinggan is usually used 3 times for 5 to 7 days by dissolving one to two bags of it in boiling water [24].

10.8.2 LIAN HUA QING WEN CAPSULE

Yinqiao Powder and Fang Ma Xing Shi Gan Tang are used for the development of Lian hua qingwen capsule [22]. Lianhua Qingwen constitutes of Gypsum Fibrosum (shigao), Menthol (bohenao), Glycyrrhizae Radi et Rhizoma (gancao), Houttuyniae Herba (yuxingcao), Rhei Radi et Rhizoma (dahuang), Forsythiae Fructus (lianqiao), processed Semen Armeniacae Amarum (chao kuxingren), processed Ephedrae Herba (zhi mahuang), Dryopteridis Crassirhizomatis Rhizoma (mianmaguanzhong), Rhodiolae Crenulatae Radix et Rhizoma (hongjingtian), Pogostemonis Herba (guanghuoxiang), Lonicerae Japonicae Flos (jinyinhua) and Isatis Radix (ban lan gen) [19]. Using rapid ultraperformance liquid chromatography together with quadrupole time of flight mass spectrometry and diode array detector 12 chemical markers were quantified in majority of constituents of lianhua qingwen capsules. These representative compounds include chlorogenic acid, cryptochlorogenic acid, salidroside, forsythoside E, hperin, glycyrrhizic acid, phillyrin, rutin, sweroside, forsythoside A, rhein, and amygdalin. While high performance liquid chromatography revealed caffeic acid, chlorogenic acid, phillyrin, rutin, forsythoside A, isochlorogenic acid B and isochlorogenic acid C to be the main components of Lianhua qingen capsules [27]. Kaempferol, luteolin, oxalin, and quarcetin are the active components of Lianhua qingwen and are involved in the reduction of phlegm, cough, and fever, immune control, and broad-spectrum anti-bacterial and antiviral effects by targeting and regulating MAPK and Hepatitis B cellular mechanisms [24].

Lianhua qingwen reduces IL-6, CCL2/MCP-1, CXCL-10/IP-10 and TNF-α that act as proinflammatory cytokines and *In vitro* analysis has shown its ability to prevent SARS-CoV-2 replication in Vero E6 cells affecting virus on morphological level and increased cure rate in COVID-19 patients [21]. Lianhua qingwen capsules plays protective role by blocking early stages of viral infection (0–2 hours) and regulate immune response by reducing IL-6,

IL-8 gene expression, TNF-α levels, nuclear factor kappa B (NF-kB) activation, Monocyte chemoattractant protein 1 (MCP-1) and interferon inducible protein 10 (IP-10) [27]. Lianhua qingwen therapeutic effect increases significantly by combining it with drugs like azithromycin injection, potassium dehydroandograpolide succinate injection and tanreqing injection while treating influenza H1N1 patients. Moreover, ribavirin, and vitamin C are also used in combination with Lianhua Qingwen to combat viral upper respiratory infections. So, Lianhua qingwen alleviates clinical symptoms of patients suffering from COVID-19 and also attenuate SARS-CoV-2 virus [19]. Usually, four capsules of Lianhua qingwen are prescribed three times a day for 14 days duration to patients [24]. Documented adverse drug reaction (ADR) relevant to Lianhua qingwen capsules included incidence of gastrointestinal (GI) reactions including diarrhea, GI discomfort, and abdominal distention; skin and its accessory injuries; itching and rash. The complex composition of Lianhua qingwen capsules stand for multiple targets and pleiotropic effects but it may also lead to adverse Ning of Acute respiratory distress syndrome [27, 28].

10.8.3 SHUFENG JIEDU GRANULES (CAPSULES)

These granules are utilized in treatment of severe and short term upper respiratory tract infections because they possess characteristic broad spectrum anti-viral affect. The inhibiting activity of Shufeng jiedu capsules has proved to be effective against para-influenza virus, H1N1, respiratory syncytial virus (RSV), herpes simplex virus (HSV) type 1 and 2, adenivirus, coxsackievirus B4 and B5. The capsules constitute of Ban Lan Gen (radix isatidis), Bupleurum, Forsythia, Verbena, Rhizoma Phragmitis Communis (reed root), Glycyrrhiza glabra (licorice), Polygonum cuspidatum (Japanese knotweed) and Bupleurum falcatum (Chinese thoroughwax) that are effective for alleviation of inflammatory effects [21, 29].

Physovenine, luteolin, quercetin, beta-setosterol, wogonin, kaempferol, bbicuculline, acacetin, stgmasterol, isorhamnetin, medicarpin, formononetin, and 7-Methoxy-2-methyl isoflavone are active compounds found in shufeng jiedu capsules [29, 30]. Shufeng jiedu possesses inhibitory activity against the cellular mechanism of NF-kB and MAPK, down regulates expression of NF-kB mRNA and inhibit inflammatory cytokines. Reduction in levels of lactic acid produces the inhibitory effect on signaling pathways and the increase in partial pressure in lungs tissue alleviates symptoms related to lungs infection by prompt absorption of lung inflammation. For treatment of mild cases of Corona NHC guidelines recommend the use of Shufeng jiedu capsules under clinical observation [21].

10.8.4 QINGFEI PAIDU DECOCTION

The treaties on exogenous febrile and miscellaneous diseases contain Shegan mahuang decoction, Maxiang shigan decoction, Xiao cai hu decoction and Wuling powder as classic prescriptions that are combined to make Qingfei paidu decoction. Qingfei paidu decoction constitutes a total of 21 herbs that are Asari Radix et Rhizoma (xixin), Atractylodis Macrocephalae Rhizoma (baizhu), Belamcandae Rhizoma (shegan), Asteris Radix (ziwan), Armeniacea Semen (xingren), Aurantii Fructus Immaturus (zhishi), Ephedrae Herba (mahuang), processed Glycyrrhizae Radix et Rhizoma (zhigacao), Dioscoreae Rhizoma (shanyao), Pinelliae Rhizoma Praeparatum Cum Zingibere et Alumine (jiang banxia), Citri reticulatae Pericarpium (chenpi), Gypsum Fibrosum (sheng shigao), Alismatis Rhizoma (zexie), Pogostemonis Herba (huoxiang), Polyporus (zhuling), Bupleuri Radix (chaihu), Poria (fuling), Farfarae Flos (donghua), Cinnamomi Ramulus (guizhi), Zingiberis Rhizoma Recens (shengjiang) and Scutellariae Radix (huanqing) [19, 31].

Ten significantly effective compounds including luteolin, quercetin, kaempferol, beta-sitosterol, naringenin, baicalein, nobiletin, wogonin, stigmasterol, and isorhamnetin in Qingfei paidu decoction possesses anti-viral and anti-inflammatory characteristics. Network pharmacology has revealed active compounds quercetin, luteolin, and kaempferol to regulate STAT1, MAPKs, JUN, IL-6, RELA, and AKT1 inhibiting inflammatory reaction in body, reduce lung injury, regulate immune functions, and preserve nerve function in COVID-19 patients. Molecular docking examination of some core compounds of Qingfei paidu decoction like tussilagone, shionone, ergosterol, etc., revealed their binding activity to SARS-CoV-2 3CL hydrolase and ACE 2 effectively inhibiting SARS-CoV-2 S protein and ACE 2 interaction [19, 32]. Western medicines sodium chloride injection, interferon α2b injection, methylprednisolone sodium succinate injection, moxifloxacin hydrochloride, lopinavir, and ritonavir tablets used in combination with Qingfei paidu decoction provide better treatment in severe COVID-19 cases, while improve pulmonary conditions in patients when used in combination with Kaletra [19]. Nausea, vomiting, dizziness, rash, mild diarrhea, and dermatitis were some common adverse reactions of Qingfei paidu decoction. But all adverse reactions were mild in nature and were resolved without any separate treatment [32].

10.8.5 HUASHI BAIDU PRESCRIPTION

Diagnosis and treatment Trail Ver. 6 and 7 protocol of COVID-19 Huashi baidu prescription revealed its ability to deal with epidemic toxins that block lungs from causing lungs syndromes. This prescription constitutes of total of 14 herbs including Poria (fuling), Gypsum Fibrosum (sheng shigao), Armeniacae Semen (xingren), Tsaoko Fructus (caoguo), Astragali Radix (sheng huangqi), Magnoliae officinalis Cortex (houpo), Paeoniae Radix Rubra (chishao), Pinellinae Rhizoma Praeparatum (fa banxia), Rhei Radix et Rhizoma (sheng dahuang), Glycyrrhizae Radix (gancao), Lepidii/Descurianiae (tinglizi), Atracytlodis Rhizoma (cangzhu), Pogostemonis Herba (huoxiang) and Ephedrae Herba (sheng mahuang) [19]. Network pharmacology and molecular docking studies revealed quercetin, kaempferol, beta-sitosterol, stigmasterol, lopinavir, ritonavir, naringenin, baicalein, isorhamnetin, formononetin, and remdesivir as active compounds of Huashi baidu prescription. Quercetin and Baicalein are flavonoids and quercetin showed high binding affinity to ACE 2 3CL and baicalein shoed high binding affinity to SARS-CoV-2 3CL hydrolase inhibiting SARS-CoV-2 and ACE 2 interaction. Additionally, quercetin reduced angiogenesis, capillary brittleness, and apoptosis. Huashi baidu prescription targeted TNF, HIF-1, MAPK, P13-Akt and NOD like receptor signaling routes and control cytokines like IL-1β, -6 and TNF-α. The latter two are commonly involved in cytokine inflammatory response. By targeting MAPK signaling pathway quercetin regulated inflammatory response of immune system [33]. Huashi baidu prescription provided multi linked extensive management of Corona by inhibiting cytokine and inflammatory response and improved clinical signs proved by physical and chemical examination, and lung CT scan thereby preventing long-term hospital stay. Examination of kidney and liver functions of patients treated with Huashi baidu prescription proved that prescription had no adverse effects on the body [19].

10.8.6 XUANFEI BAIDU FORMULA

Professor Qingquan Liu and CAS academician Boli Zhang recommended Xuanfei Baidu Formula for treatment of damp toxin retention in the patients of lung syndromes. The formula constitutes of total 13 herbs that are Phragmitis Rhizoma (lugen), Atractylodis Rhizoma (maocangzhu), Ephedrae Herba (sheng mahuang), Lepidii/Descurainiae Semen (tinglizi), Glycyrrhizae Radix et Rhizoma (gancao), Citri Grandis Exocarpium rubrum (huajuhong), Verbenae Herba (mabiancao), Artemisiae Annuae Herba (qinghao), Pogostemonis Herba (guanghuoxiang) Coicis Semen (sheng yiyiren), Armeniacae Semen Amarum (kuxingren), Gypsum Fibrosum (sheng shigao) and Polygoni Rhizoma et Radix (huazhang). Xuanfei baidu formula took part in suppression of inflammatory storm and excessive activation of immune response in patients of COVID-19 [19].

Xuanfei baidu formula regulates inflammatory factors including chemokines and related T cells Th17, Th1, Th2, IL-6, CXCL8 (C-X-C motif chemokine ligand 8), etc. This duplex regulatory effect resulted in improvement of COVID-19 related symptoms. The regulation of inflammatory response, in the early stages of disease, and enhancement of immune response in the late stages of diseases resulted in efficient and accelerated recovery in moderate cases of disease and prevented the transformation of these moderate cases into severe cases [19].

10.9 TCM INJECTIONS FOR COVID-19 TREATMENT

Herbal formulas that are injected intravenously for treatment of COVID-19 is summarized in Figure 10.7 and Table 10.3.

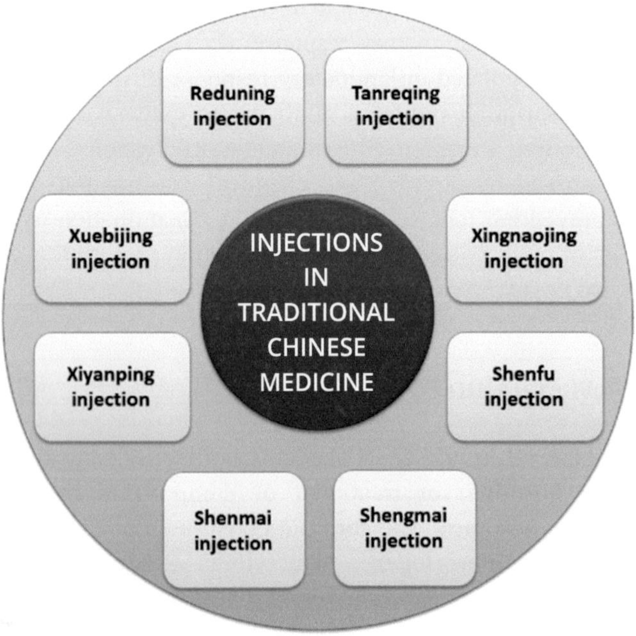

FIGURE 10.7 Traditional Chinese medicine injections for COVID-19 treatment.

TABLE 10.3 Composition and Mode of Action of TCM Injection for COVID-19 Treatment

SL. No.	Injection	Composition	Mode of Action	Pharmacological Action
1.	Xiyanping injection	Andrographis Herba	Regulates inflammatory factors (TNFα and IL-6) levels	Reduces inflammation, inhibit replication of virus, reduce infection, inhibit concurrent bacterial infections, and reduce cardiovascular damage.
2.	Xuebinjing injection	Red peony (Radix Paeoniae Rubra), chuanxiong (Ligusticumchuanxiong Hort), salvia miltiorrhiza, safflower (*Carthamus tinctorius*) and angelica (*Angelica sinensis*)	Reduces plasma IL-6 and TNFα levels	Regulates systemic inflammatory response syndrome, sepsis
3.	Reduning injection	Artemisia annua, Flos Lonicerae and Gardeniae Fructus	Regulate IL-6, CASP3, MAPK1, CCL2, HIF1, IL-17 and C-type lectin receptor	Antiviral, anti-inflammatory, immunomodulatory effects
4.	Tanreqing injection	Bear bile powder, goat horn, *Scutellaria baicalensis*, honeysuckle, and forsythia	Reduces TGF-β1, TNF-α and α-SMA expression levels	Decrease inflammation and fibrotic destruction of lung tissues, inhibit alveolar wall cells apoptosis
5.	Xingnaojing injection	Musk, turmeric, borneol, gardenia, curcumenone, curcumenol, curzerenone, and germacrone	Reduces CRP and TNF-α indexes in serum, increase CD3+, CD4+ levels and reduce CD8+ levels	Inhibit inflammatory response
6.	Shenfu injection	Red ginseng and black monkshood	Reduce IL-6 levels, increase peripheral blood cells (CD3+, CD4+, CD8+, T-cells) content reduces the value of serum procalcitonin and increases levels of IgA, IgM, and IgG	Increase immunity, maintains pro inflammatory and anti-inflammatory response balance
7.	Shenmai injection	Ophiopogon japonicas and red ginseng	Elevate anti-inflammatory factor levels, reduce inflammatory factors levels, reduce WBC content, reduce C-reactive protein, and reduce procalcitonin levels	Regulate inflammatory response and inhibit cytokine storm.
8.	Shengmai injection	Ginseng Radix et Rhizoma, Ophiopogonis Radix and Schisandrachinensis	Reduce ANP levels, reduce ET levels, increase PG12 and PG12//TXA2 levels	Inhibit inflammatory response, improve breathing and vascular microcirculation

10.9.1 XIYANPING INJECTION

Xiyanping injection is involved in curing cough, detoxification, soothing away fever and dysentery. Clinically Xiyanping injection is used in TCM for treating bacterial diseases, bronchitis, and tonsillitis [21]. Xiyanping injection contains Andrographis Herba [34]. Andrographolide compound is the active compound of the herb in xiyanping injection that acts as antipyretic and anti-inflammatory. A diterpene bicycle ring and a γ lactone ring together form andrographolide and the structural double bonds determine the anti-inflammatory activity of the injection. An experiment involving treatment of various influenza viruses by administering andrographolide compound proved that its activity could reduce inflammatory cytokine expression, reduce viral load, lessen viral load, lessen pathological changes in lungs, inhibit apoptosis and increase survival rate of infected [21].

In case of COVID-19 patients Xiyanping injection aids in reducing inflammation and improving symptoms like fever, cough, rattling sounds in lungs and strengthen immunologic responses along with liver functions. Despite the absence of clinical studies of Xiyanping injection against COVID-19, NHC guidelines recommend its use in the progressive stage of the disease [21].

10.9.2 XUEBIJING INJECTION

Xuebijing injection constitutes red peony (Radix Paeoniae Rubra), chuanxiong (Ligusticumchuanxiong Hort), salvia miltiorrhiza, safflower (Carthamus tinctorius) and angelica (Angelica sinensis) [21, 33] and is involved in treating septicemia, acute respiratory distress syndrome (ARDS), pneumonia, chronic obstructive pulmonary disease, and other censorious illnesses in China. Safflower yellow A, danshensu, protocatechualdehyde, ligustrazine, ferulic acid and paeoniflorin are active compounds of xuebijing injection and reduce levels of inflammatory cytokines like TNF-α and IL-6 in plasma when administered to patients of severe pneumonia along with traditional treatment. Activated T-cells and mononucleae cells produces multifunctional cytokine IL-6 that regulate acute immune response and hematopoiesis in response to infection while various mononuclear macrophages produce transmitter TNF-α that is involved in inflammatory response to infections. But overexpression of IL-6 and TNF-α leads to lungs damage, severe inflammatory response, cytokine storm and multiple organ damage. Seven-day treatment ith xuebijing injection significantly reduced IL-6 levels, body temperature was observed and nucleic acid test became negative much faster in patients treated with xuebijing injection as compared to other patients. Flow cytometry revealed significant increase in CRP levels of peripheral blood count and decrease in lymphocyte count in COVID-19 patients. Lymphocytopenia is considered to be one of the hallmarks of disease and degree of decrease determines severity of SARS-CoV-2 infection. Lymphocytopenia, severe inflammatory response and monocyte infiltration in lungs due to infection serves as major cause of death in COVID-19 patients [21, 35, 36].

The clinical trials of Xuebijing injection, involving 44 COVID-19 positive individuals, revealed that lung CT after treatment showed increased rete of lesion absorption compared to patients that were not administered the injection. Despite the smaller sample size, NHC recommend the use of Xuebijing injection in severe stage of COVID-19 [21].

10.9.3 REDUNING INJECTION

This injection constitutes of Artemisia annua, Flos Lonicerae and Gardeniae Fructus and has anti-pyretic, -viral, and -inflammatory pharmacological properties. In treatment of upper respiratory tract infection and acute Bronchitis has shown to be effective [21, 34]. Reduning injection in combination with biapenem has a better curative effect to treat critical pneumonia and improves patients' symptoms such as: improved lung function and blood gas indexes and reduced serum inflammatory factor levels [21].

The antiviral, anti-inflammatory, and immunomodulatory effects of Reduning injection is due to the presence of compounds such as luteolin, rutin, quercetin, and isorhamnetin that act through various signaling pathways on CASP3, MAPK1, IL-6, IL-17, CCL2, H1F1 (histone H1) and C-type lectin receptor. Active compounds in Reduning injection have the ability to bind to PLP, ACE 2 and Mpro and inhibit SASR-CoV-2 invasion in host cells. Despite no current clinical studies regarding the use of Reduning injection in COVID-19 patients NHC guidelines recommend its use in the advanced stages of disease [21, 37, 38].

10.9.4 TANREQING INJECTION

Tanreqing injection, composed of Bear Bile powder, *Scuttelaria baicalensis* (baikal skullcap), Horny Goat weed, Forsythia, and Lonicera (honeysuckle), is involved in detoxification, reducing cough and phlegm and soothing away fever in the body. Clinically it is used for treating acute bronchitis, acute aggravation of chronic bronchitis, lower respiratory tract infections and early pneumonia. *In vitro* studies show that active compound in Tanreqing injection quercetin and luteolin have anti-viral activity against anti-influenza A and have the ability to reduce α-SMA, TNF-α and TGF-β1, reduce inflammation, reduce fibrotic destruction of rat lungs tissue and hinder alveolar wall cells apoptosis [21–34].

Molecular docking and network pharmacology studies theorize treatment of COVID-19 using synergistic approaches. Despite the absence of clinical studies, NHC recommend use of injection in the progressive stages of disease [21].

10.9.5 XINGNAOJING INJECTION

Xingnaojing injection constitutes of Curcuma longa (turmeric), musk, Gardenia, Borneol, Curcumenone, Germacrone, Curzerenone, and Curcumenol and is clinically used for the treatment of pneumonia, respiratory failure, acute cerebrovascular disease, pulmonary encephalopathy, acute poisoning, viral encephalitis, cranio cerebral injury, sepsis, and acute viral infectious fevers [21, 39].

In elderly, while treating mycoplasmal pneumonia, Xingnaojing injection in combination with zithromycin reduces serum inflammation index levels of CRP and TNFα, increases CD3+ and CD4+ levels and reduces CD8+ levels. During adjuvant treatment, in case of ventilator-associated pneumonia, Xingnaojing injection inhibit serum IL-6 overexpression and probability of inflammatory response is further reduced by CRP and TNFα, hence reducing damage to multiple organs. Under NHC guidelines, Xingnaojing injection is recommended for treating extremely severe cases of COVID-19 [21].

10.9.6 SHENFU INJECTION

Shenfu injection, composed of Panax ginseng and *Aconitum napellus* (black monkshood), is used for treating cardiovascular diseases, cerebrospinal diseases, septicemia, severe pneumonia, multiple organ dysfunction and treatment of tremors. In case of sepsis, Shenfu injection maintains balanced anti-inflammatory and pro-inflammatory response by increasing number of peripheral blood cells expressing CD3+, CD4+ and CD8+ receptors, T-cells, and reducing IL-6 levels. Shenfu injection also reduces the value of serum procalcitonin and upsurges IgM, IgA, and IgG in body fluids of elderly patients having chronic lung infection [21].

Shenfu injection in combination with antibiotics reduce the sol. E-selection content and von Willebrand factor (vWF), which enhance vascular endothelial cells function and diminishing myocardial damage, cough, shortens fever duration, lung damage in severe pneumonia, and enhance blood oxygen levels. Shenfu injection reduces TNF-α and IL-1β hence reducing the expression of pro-inflammatory by preventing HMGB1/NF-κB signaling routes and prevents cytokine storms. NHC recommends the use of Shenfu injection for the treatment of critical COVID-19 patients [21].

10.9.7 SHENMAI INJECTION

This injection constitutes of Panax ginseng and Ophiopogon japonicas (mondo grass) and treat neutropenia, coronary heart disease, chronic pulmonary heart disease, viral myocarditis. It reduces side effects of chemotherapy and improve immune functions of tumor patients [21, 34]. The recovery rate increases in the patients of severe pneumonia when administered Shenmai injection as adjuvant treatment as it elevates levels of anti-inflammatory factors, lessen levels of inflammatory factors, reduce white blood cells (WBC) count, C-reactive protein (CRP) and procalcitonin levels [21].

In a clinical study involving pneumonia patients on ventilators, two different dosages of shenmai injections (high and low) were administered. The results indicated reduction in CRP, WBC, and procalcitonin levels and elevation in peripheral blood cells exhibiting CD4+/CD8+. These results were more pronounced when high dosage was used. In case of sepsis treatment, shenmai injection improves immune function in the patients by enhancing NK, IgM, CD3+, CD4+ and complement C3 levels. These clinical studies prove that shenmai injection can improve critical symptoms like viral infection, lung inflammation and drug induced lung injury in critical cases of COVID-19 and NHC guidelines also recommend the use of shenmai injection for treating extremely severe cases of COVID-19 [21].

10.9.8 SHENGMAI INJECTION

Shengmai injection constitutes *Radix ophiopogonis*, *Schisandra chinesis* (five flavor berry) and Ginseng Radix et Rhizoma and is clinically prescribed for cerebrovascular and cardiovascular disease treatments. It plays protective role in many organs. Shengmai injection in combination with traditional treatment of systemic inflammatory response syndrome improve breathing and vascular microcirculation by reducing the levels of endothelin (ET) and atrial natriuretic peptides (ANP) and upregulate the levels of PG12/TXA2 and plasma prostacyclin (PG12). The results of a clinical study showed that Shengmai injection improved cure rate in elderly patients suffering from pulmonary infections and multiple organs dysfunction. Schisandra chinensis in Shengmai enhance body's immune function and increase splenic white nucleus pulposus lymph node cortex volume. Clinical trial proved that Schisandra chinensis in Shengmai when administered in immunosuppressed mice increases their splenic and lymph node weight [21].

The clinical features of Shengmai can improve symptoms like lung inflammation, drug-induced disease lung injury and virus infection in COVID-19 patients so NHC recommend its use in treatment of critical cases [21].

10.10 NOVEL COMPOUNDS TARGETING SARS-COV-2

In such a short time, developing new agents against SARS-CoV-2 is both costly and time consuming. Therefore, many scientists screened various substances used in Chinese medicine that target viruses and found many naturally occurring compounds possessing abilities to combat SARS-CoV-2. Most compounds discovered seemed to be working against SARS-CoV-2 are of flavonoid category. Flavonoids are the compounds produced by plants as part as secondary metabolites and play defensive role by exhibiting abundant of biological activities like antiviral, anti-oxidation, anti-tumor, anti-inflammatory effects, and prevention of cardiovascular and cerebrovascular diseases, etc.

The structure of flavonoid compound comprises of two aromatic rings joined together by a 3-carbon chain forming structure C6-C3-C6. The inhibitory effect produced by flavonoid compounds on macrophages and mast cell upon cytokine release is increased by different patterns of hydroxylation in B ring of compound. Flavonoid compounds inhibit the synthesis of pro inflammatory compounds like cytokines and eicosanoids and inhibit transcription factor (NF-Kb) activation and initiate anti-inflammatory activity by activating protein-1. Moreover, flavonoid compounds have the affinity to bind to S protein, helicase, and ACE 2 protease site leading to conformational changes and prohibiting the interaction of SARS-CoV-2 and ACE 2 protein. These actions lead to inhibit cellular entry of SARS-CoV-2 and also alleviate clinical symptoms and increase cure rate in COVID-19 patients (Table 10.3) [24].

10.10.1 HESPERETIN

Hesperetin is flavonoid compound obtained from citrus fruits' pericarp and is characteristic anti-inflammatory and anti-oxidant compound. *In vitro* cell lysis assay of Hesperetin showed the ability to inhibit SARS-CoV 3C like protease cleavage activity depending on the dose. Hesperetin has affinity for binding to 3C like protease along with its affinity for main protein in RBD domain of virus protein prohibiting interaction between SARS-CoV-2 protein and ACE 2 protein [24].

10.10.2 BAICALIN

Biaclin is a flavonoid compound displaying neuro-protective effect along with anti-oxidant and anti-inflammatory activities. Biaclin is mainly found in *Scutellaria baicalensis* extract which is a flowering plant in family Lamiaceae. *In vitro* study using cell line of fetal Rhesus kidney-4 cells (fRhK-4) proved that biaclin has anti-SARS-CoV activity. Molecular docking study proved the affinity of biaclin for ACE 2 receptor, prohibiting the interaction of SARS-CoV S protein and ACE 2 protein [24].

10.10.3 CURCUMIN

Curcumin is phenolic compound that is present in extract of Turmeric rhizome and has anti-viral, -oxidant, -inflammatory, and -cancerous actions. With its dose from 3.3 to 10 μmol/L, it plays inhibitory role on replication of SARS-CoV particles and at IC_{50} of 40 μmol/L, it has an inhibitory effect on 3C like protease. Curcumin is also responsible for blocking cytokine storm by blocking the release of cytokines such as IL-1 and -6 and TNF-α, during patient treatment. Molecular docking using virtual screening showed the affinity of curcumin for PLpro, protease domain of ACE 2 receptor (PD-ACE 2) and RBD of spike glycoprotein (RBD-S) that can prohibit the interaction between viral and ACE 2 domains [24].

10.10.4 GLYCYRRHIZIC ACID

Glycyrrhizic acid, also known as glycyrrhizin, is an active compound of Glycyrrhiza glabra L (licorice) possessing anti-viral, anti-oxidant, and immunomodulatory activities and stabilize the cell membranes. Glycyrrhizic acid is responsible for inhibiting replication of SARS-CoV-2 particles and hinders penetration of virus into host cell. When 600 mg/l is used as $EC_{50,}$ glycyrrhizin is considerably less effectual during and after period of viral penetration but 2,400 mg/l as EC_{50} is the most effective dose in this regard. A combination of curcumin, glycyrrhizin, and vitamin C has been identified by System biology tools to be effective to regulate body's immune response produced against SARS-CoV-2 infection. This combination targets Toll like signaling pathways and NOD like signaling pathways and inhibit P13K/AKT, NF-kB, and MAPK signaling pathway preventing cytokine storm thereby inhibiting excessive inflammatory response. Glycyrrhizin also regulate ACE 2 activity by binding to ACE2, 3C like protease, Spike, P like protease, and RdRp [24].

10.10.5 LUTEOLIN

Luteolin is a natural flavonoid that inhibits proliferation of tumor cells and is also anti-inflammatory and anti-oxidant in nature. With EC_{50} of 10.6 µmol/l, luteolin proved to be effective for inhibition of cleavage activity of SARS-CoV and at EC_{50} of 20.2 µmol/l, it can inhibit SARS-CoV 3C like protease activity. Molecular docking has shown strong interaction of Luteolin with SARS-CoV-2 via 3C like protease, RdRp, P like protease, and Spro [24].

10.10.6 RUTIN

Rutin is a flavonoid having biological activities like anti-viral, anti-oxidant, neuroprotective, and anti-inflammatory effects. It is an active compound of Lianhua Qingwen and inhibits replication of different RNA viruses like enterovirus A71 and influenza A virus. Molecular dynamics simulation has shown that Rutin has the ability to bind SARS-CoV-2 Mpro' pocket preventing interaction of viral and cell substrate complex (Table 10.4) [24].

10.11 INTEGRATED TCM AND WESTERN MEDICINE FOR COVID-19

Western medicine and TCM are based on different theoretical systems with their unique characteristics, advantages, and disadvantages. TCM basically

TABLE 10.4 Source, Pharmacological Action, and Mode of Action of Flavonoid Compounds Against COVID-19

SL. No.	Flavonoid	Source	Pharmacological Action	Mode of Action
1.	Hesperetin	Pericarp of citrus	Anti-oxidant and anti-inflammatory activities	Inhibit SARS-CoV 3C-like protease cleavage activity by bind to 3C like-protease and have affinity for main protein in SARS-CoV-2 RBD domain prohibiting interaction of SARS-CoV-2 protein and ACE 2 protein
2.	Baicalin	*Scutellaria baicalensis* Georgi extract	Neuro-protective effect, anti-oxidant, and anti-inflammatory activities	Affinity for ACE 2 receptor prohibiting the interaction of SARS-CoV S protein and ACE 2 protein
3.	Curcumin	Rhizome of turmeric	Inhibit anti-cancerous, anti-viral, anti-inflammatory, antioxidant activities, block cytokine storm and inhibit interaction of viral RBD and ACE 2 protein	Block inflammatory cytokine (TNF-α, IL-1 and IL-6) release, inhibitory effect on SARS-CoV replication, inhibitory effect on PLpro, 3C like protease, affinity for PD-ACE 2 and RBD-S of virus
4.	Glycyrrhizic acid	*Glycyrrhiza glabra* L	Immunomodulatory activity, anti-viral activity, and membrane stabilizing activity, inhibit excessive inflammatory response and regulate ACE 2 activity	Inhibit SARS-CoV replication and penetration of in host cell, acts on Toll like signaling pathway, NOD like signaling pathway, PI3K/AKT, NF-Kb and has affinity to bind to ACE2, 3C like protease, Spike, P like protease, and RdRp.
5.	Luteolin	Reseda luteola	Inhibits proliferation of tumor cells, inhibit virus entry and proliferation, has anti-inflammatory and anti-oxidant activity.	Inhibit cleavage activity of SARS-CoV, inhibit SARS-CoV 3C like protease, interaction affinity for SARS-CoV-2, 3C like protease, RdRp, P like protease, and Spro
6.	RUTIN	Citrus plants	Anti-oxidant, anti-inflammatory, antiviral activities, and neuroprotective effects	Inhibits RNA viruses like Enterovirus A71 and Infuenza A virus influenza A virus and enterovirus A71 and bind to SARS-CoV-2 Mpro' pockets

use holistic approach in diagnosing and treating diseases while Western based medical practice uses common law of disease and focus on treatment through disease analysis. In case of COVID-19 treatment, integrated TCM and Western medicine has proven to be most effective in China. Clinical studies have proved that integrated medicine has effectively decreased mortality rate along with alleviating symptoms in COVID-19 patients as compared to sole use of Western medicine.

Nelfinavir in combination with spilanthol enhance control of viral replication and reduce risk of disease transmission and progression in case of COVID-19 patients. Around 11 studies from 6 different databases on meta-analysis and systematic review of efficiency and safety of Western TCM integrated approach for Corona treatment have shown positive findings. The cure rate, severity of illness, hospital stay duration and development of symptoms were effectively controlled in case of integrated medicine as compared to treatment provided by sole use of Western medicine. A different systematic review suggested improvement in total efficacy, rate of sputum production and cough severity among patients when given integrated medicine [24].

10.12 *SANYINZHIYI* AND COVID-19

The outbreak started in late December (temperature 2–4°C) under wet and cold conditions. Low temperature and humidity could facilitate the transmission and acquiring of the pathogen. Upon infection, the virus could deteriorate lungs and spleen and lessens the Qi production. TCM builds treatment plan according to *Sanyinzhiyi. Sanyinzhiyi* principle belongs to Chinese medicine that modifies treatment plan of a disease based on external factors like climate, geographical site, epidemic conditions, and individual characteristics. Under holistic perspective of TCM pertaining to *Sanyinzhiyi,* the entire human, his nature and his society is taken into consideration when forming a treatment plan. For example, Central, East, South, and Southwest areas of China have warm and humid climatic conditions therefore TCM usually employ *Attractylodes lancea* (thnub), *Agastache rugosa* (wrinkled giant hyssop/Korean mint) and some other Chinese herb-based medicines for heat clearance, detoxification, reinforcing spleen and clearing out dampness. On the other hand, in regions like North, Northeast, and Northwest China where climatic conditions are cold, wet, and toxic, *Scrophularia ningpoensis* (ningpo figwory/Chinese figwort) and other TCM medicines are employed for clearing out cold and wind, detoxification, removing dampness, nourishing Yin and moistening dryness [40].

10.13 TCM-BASED COVID-19 PREVENTION

TCM recommends early prevention and treatment to avoid worsening patient's condition and preventing relapse of infection for better control of transmittable pathogenic diseases. TCM helps in prevention of viral respiratory infections in general population by keeping away from evil Qi while retaining vital Qi. This is achieved by using active TCM therapy for patients especially belonging to high-risk category. It also strongly advocates preventive measures for both the uninfected and recovered individuals restoring vital Qi. TCM also prevent viral respiratory infections by promoting immune regulatory functions, strengthening body resistance, harmonizing Yin Yang, and removing pathogenic elements [40].

Clinical manifestation and pathogenesis of Corona suggests that this disease occur and developed by causing overwhelming Yin fire in lungs and deterioration of splenic and stomach functions. This suggests that COVID-19 can be prevented by clearing Yin fire and strengthening stomach and spleen by providing effective nutrients [40].

10.13.1 EPIDEMIC PREDICTION BASED ON FIVE MOVEMENTS AND SIX QI

Effect of natural climate change on human organ function can be predicted using theory of "five movements and six qi." Moreover "three-year epidemic formation" theory proposes that an epidemic might occur in next three years if abnormalities are observed in climatic operations and migrations. TCM has the ability to accurately predict the time of occurring of outbreak of disease allowing doctors and paramedics to prepare beforehand [41].

10.13.2 PREVENTION USING TCM DECOCTION

TCM decoctions are recommended to people that are isolated at home to prevent COVID-19. Usually, TCM decoctions consists of aromatic compounds that provide autoimmunity and help avoiding sickness. Vital Qi is maintained by TCM prescriptions that are based on "Natural Factor theory." Pharmacological studies in this modern era have proved ability of TCM prescriptions to inhibit virus by relieving surface humidity, clearing away heat and detoxification. TCM inhibits viruses in two ways. Firstly, by heat clearing and detoxifying, it leads to the direct inhibition of viruses with the use of compounds like Lonicera, Folium Isatidis, and Scutellaria. Secondly TCM inhibit viral attack by inhibiting inflammatory response mediated by viral attack with the help of Acanthopanax senticosus, Salvia, and Gentiana. As TCM uses holistic approach it regulates body's systems by targeting multiple organs [41].

10.13.3 PREVENTION OF DISEASE USING HERBAL INCENSE

TCM employs traditional aromatherapy as preventive measures for people who are uninfected but exposed to virus. Herb sachets containing herbs like *Atractylodes lancea*, *Artemisia argyi* (silver wormwood) and *Phellodendron amurense* (amur cork tree) are used for aromatherapy and have proved to impart significant protection against viral diseases [41].

10.13.4 PREVENTION AND TREATMENT USING ACUPUNCTURE AND MOXIBUSTION

Acupuncture and moxibuxtion are the treatments that have been employed by Chinese people since ancient times and have made a vital contribution in anti-epidemic action in China. In the face of terrific disaster of COVID-19, both acupuncture and moxibustion have been employed by Chinese doctors for purpose of preventing and treating COVID-19. Acupuncture and Moxibustion Intervention for COVID-19 (second edition) have demonstrated the use of acupuncture and moxibustion treatment by dividing it into three phases, i.e., medical observation which includes suspected cases, clinical treatment which is confirmed cases and the convalescence or recovering cases [41].

Suspected cases were inserted acupuncture needles in CV6 (qihai), LI4 (hegu), LI11 (quchi), BL12 (fengmen), BL13 (feishu), BL20 (pishu), LU5 (chize), LU10 (yuji), SP6 (sanyinjiao) and ST36 (zusanli) acupoints for the purpose of stimulating vital Qi, enhancing the viscera's defense, and stimulating functions of the lungs and spleen. In confirmed cases, needles were administered in CV4 (guanyuan), CV6 (qihai), CV12 (zhongwan), CV17 (danzhong), CV22 (tiantu), BL11 (dazhu), BL12 (fengmen), BL13 (feishu), BL15 (xinshu), BL17 (geshu), L14 (hegu), LU1 (zhongfu), LU5 (chize), LU6 (kongzui), LR3 (taichong), SP6 (sanyinjiao) and ST36 (zusanli) Hegu acupoints to protect viscera, dispel pathogens and stimulate spleen and lung vital function. During convalescence phase, Qi CV6 (qihai), CV12 (zhongwan), PC6 (neiguan), ST36 (zusanli) and ST25 (tianshu) acupoints were targeted to eliminate remaining virus, reinstate vitality, and restore the function of lungs and spleen [41].

Chinese Scientists suggested that the use of moxibustion is not only for prevention and treatment of COVID-19 but also helps to improve quality of life. DU14 (dazhui) and LI11 (quchi) points can be used to treat fever by moxibustion technique. Similarly, moxibustion on BL13 (feishu), DU14 (dazhui) and EX-B1 (dingchuan) for cough treatment; moxibustion on CV12 (zhongwan), ST36 (zusanli) and ST25 (tianshu) for upper digestive system discomfort and moxibustion on CV4 (guanyuan), CV6 (qihai) and ST36 (zusanli) for fatigue can be fruitful in this regard [41].

10.14 NETWORK PHARMACOLOGICAL STUDIES FOR TREATMENT AND PREVENTION OF COVID-19

Anti-inflammatory, anti-viral, immunoregulation activities and transcriptional control by various components targeting multiple signaling pathways and chemokines can be the possible mechanisms of treating COVID-19 by TCM as proved by various network pharmacological studies (Figure 10.8).

10.14.1 ANTI-VIRUS PATHWAYS

3CL hydrolase (Mpro) is vital component for SARS-CoV-2 replication. 3CL hydrolase (Mpro) possesses ability of proteolytic processing of viral polyproteins (proteins vital for replication and functioning of virus). On the other hand, ACE 2 acts as a receptor required by the virus to enter host cell. Hence, with the help of molecular docking and network pharmacological studies, scientist determined that binding energy of Mpro and ACE 2 with Jin hua qinggan granule, Lian hua qingwan capsule, Xuebijing injection and Tanreqing Injection is upright and can be used for inhibition of viral entry and replication in the cell. Moreover, QingfeiPaidu Decoction and

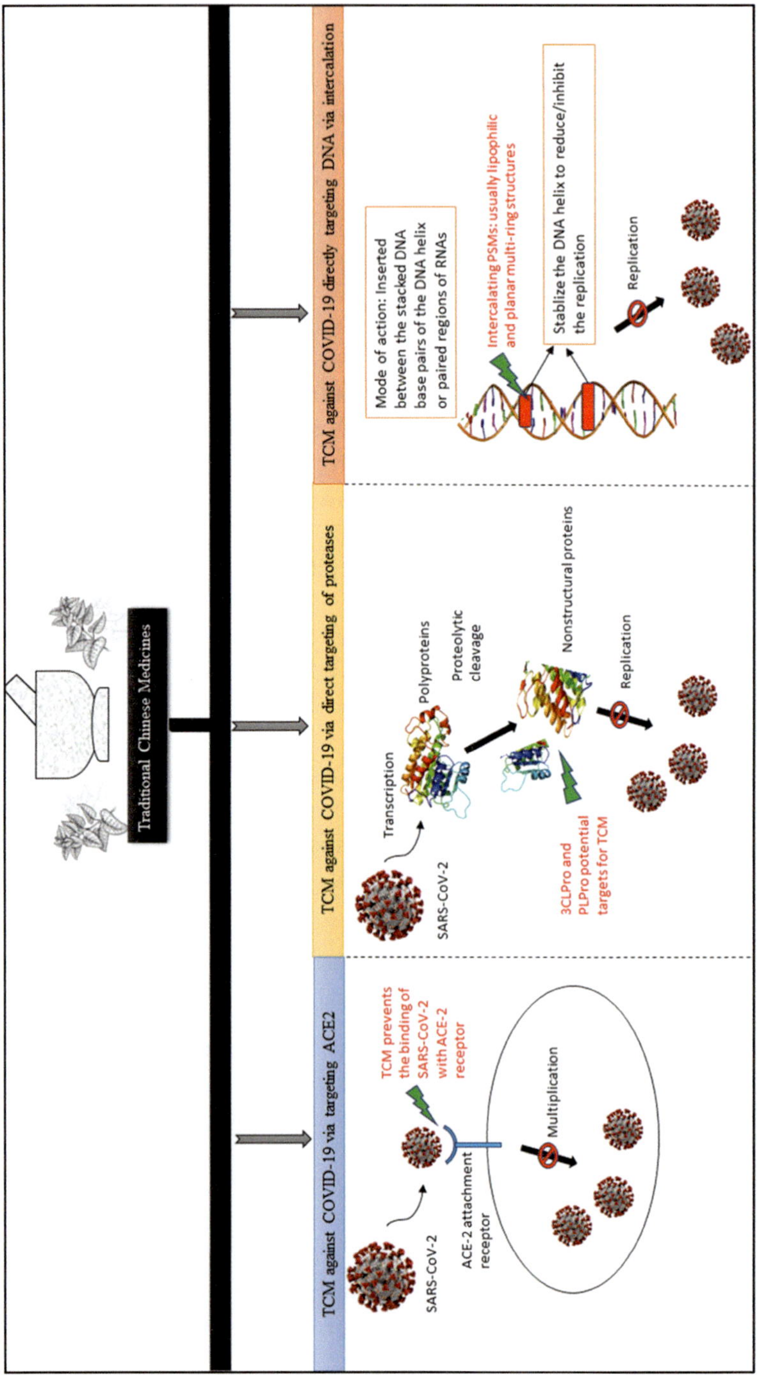

FIGURE 10.8 Potential target mechanisms of TCM against COVID-19.

Xuebijing injection can regulate phosphatidylinositol-3kinase/total protein kinase (PI3K-Akt) which is necessary for regulation of cell proliferation, angiogenesis, viral replication, viral assembly, and pathogenicity. Some naturally occurring flavonoids like baicalin, hesperetin, glycyrrhizin, and nicotinamide have antiviral activities and can play an important role to neutralize COVID-19 through ACE 2 receptor [34].

10.14.2 ANTI-INFLAMMATION PATHWAYS

One of many pathogenic mechanisms that COVID-19 triggers in the body is cytokine storm in which various inflammatory factors like IFNα, IFNβ, IL-1, IL-6, IL-12 and TNFα are produced by the body. Cytokines are produced as a result of inflammatory factors production which cause damage to cells and organs. Therefore, severity of disease and mortality rate can be reduced in the patients by reducing body's cytokine storm. TCM concoctions that contain *Agastache rugosa* (Korean mint), Moslae herba, *Flos Chrsanthemi* indici and *Artemisia annua* (sweet wormwood) have the ability to act on TNF, MAPK, NF-κB signaling pathways and suppress cytokine levels in the body. TCM concoctions containing above components are Jin Hua Qing Gan Granule, Shengjiang powder, Huashi Baidu Prescription, QingfeiPaidu Decoction, Maxing Shigan Decoction, Xuebijing injection, Reduning injection and Xiyanping Injection. The arachidonic acid (AA) metabolic pathway is also involved in the production of various inflammatory factors like TNF, IFN, interleukins, and monocyte chemo attractant protein 1 (MCP-1), etc. So, by mediating AA metabolic pathway with TCM decoctions, cytokine storm can be prevented. TCM medicines like Jin Hua Qing Gan Granule, Xuebijing injection, Reduning injection, QingfeiPaidu Decoction and Tanreqing injection have inhibitory effect on arachidonic acid (AA) metabolic pathway and are crucial for alleviating cytokine storms. Other than these medicines some naturally occurring flavonoids like vitamin C, curcumin, and glycyrrhizin also have the ability to prevent cytokine storm [34].

10.14.3 IMMUNOREGULATION PATHWAYS

Immune cells are activated and recruited by the signaling of virus infected cells and produce various chemokines and inflammatory cytokines further recruiting additional immune cells to the lesion area leading to excessive immune response and body damage [19]. Cytokine storm occurs after increase in cytokines during a short time. Upon SARS-CoV-2 invasion CD4+ T-cells are activated into helper T-cells-1 (Th-1 cells) which secretes granulocyte macrophage colony stimulating factor (GM-CSF). GM-CSF increases IL-6 levels and further induces CD14+ CD16+ monocytes. An immense increase in CD14+IL-1β+ promote upsurge in IL-1β levels in COVID-19 patients. Furthermore, Th-17 also recruits neutrophils, macrophages/monocytes and activate cytokine cascades like IL-1β, -6, etc., on the site of infection and IL-6 acts as a mediator of cytokine storm [42]. TCM can restore normal physiological functions of the body by controlling and alleviating excessive immune response. Network pharmacology has shown that Lianhua qingwen capsule and SARS-CoV-2 have total of 55 common target sites which are enriched in the innate immune pathways that are regulated by Toll like receptors INF-1 and inflammatory factors like TNF and IL-17. Therefore, Lianhua qinqwen capsule can be used to neutralize SARS-Co-V-2. Moreover, Tanreqing injection has the ability to overcome TNF, MAPK, and EGFR (epidermal growth factor receptor) signaling pathways helping in inhibition of activated cytokines and elimination of inflammatory factors leading to alleviation of cytokine storm [23]. Bitter almonds contain Vitamin B17 also known as Amygdalin which is toxic glycoside compound and plays immunoregulatory role. For example, Vitamin B17 inhibits the expression of inflammatory factors like sICAM-1 and TNF-α [19].

10.14.4 OTHER SIGNALING PATHWAYS

Network pharmacology has also predicted some other signaling pathways that are targeted by TCM prescriptions and control COVID-19. For example, Huoxiang Zhengqi oral liquid can reduce the levels of cytokines and lactate dehydrogenase protecting lung cells from damage alongside improving oxygenation index and alleviating systemic symptoms. Shufeng Jiedu Capsule can target signaling pathways like Toll like receptors, HIF-1, IL-17 and may also act on PTGS (prostaglandin endoperoxide synthase), IL-6, IL-10, and transcription activator-1 (STAT-1) thereby helps in treating and preventing COVID-19. Huashi Baidu Prescription is also used for treatment of Corona and network pharmacological studies demonstrated to have 49 potential common targeting sites specific for SARS-CoV-2 including TNF, IL-6, -1β, MAPK1 and -8. Similarly, Shengmai injection targets signaling pathways like caspase (CASP), PTGS, and NOS and is used for treating COVID-19 [34].

Network pharmacological studies have also demonstrated that many naturally occurring herbs can also be used for treatment of COVID-19 because of their ability to target multiple signaling pathways and multiple targets. Agastache rugosa have 16 active components that act on Toll, MAPK, and other signaling pathways and 10 related targets to deal with SARS-CoV-2. Rhubarb can treat COVID-19 by targeting 31 signaling pathways and 49 corresponding targets. Similarly, Quercetin and Epigallocatechin gallate are also used for the treatment of COVID-19 because of their potential affinity for IL-6, ACE2 and SARS-CoV-2 [34].

10.15 TCM EMOTIONAL THERAPY

TCM uses holistic approach so mental health is an important factor along with physical health during treatment plan and adopt methods related to emotional conditioning to manage patient's health and banish negative emotion while enforcing immune system. In response of COVID-19, psychological state of public has been plunged, so various strategies of TCM emotional therapy have been employed to maintain mental health. Calm emotion method, music delight method, diversion of attention method, suggestive indication method and auricular pressing method are employed to make emotional adjustments in public which enables them to survive stressful situations and maintain sanity. Additionally, TCM promotes use of nutrients, healthy diet, appropriate exercise, and healthy living conditions to improve physical, mental, and emotional health of people [40].

10.16 CONCLUSION

COVID-19 has become a global crisis and a great many untiring efforts are being carried out to fight this disease. At the present, there is no specific antiviral drug and supportive treatment is choice of action. TCM holds an ancient history of fighting epidemics of the past. In China, TCM is being generally and profoundly engaged in therapeutics concerning COVID-19 and has assumed a positive part in this crisis. COVID-19 therapeutic approaches focusing on the combined use of TCM and western medicine can be fruitful as it is shown to effective in alleviating the symptoms and increasing the overall cure rate of COVID-19. However, TCM based diagnosis and treatment actually need target assessment rules and elaborate scientific studies have to be conducted if its viability has to be established. The modernization of the TCM must be based upon proof-based medicines validated through advanced scientific methods. We trust that, by the commitment of TCM, joined with current scientific advances and the coordination of global partners, COVID-19 could be viably controlled and treated.

KEYWORDS

- **acute respiratory distress syndrome**
- **COVID-19**
- **endothelin**
- **prevention**
- **traditional Chinese medicine**
- **treatment**
- **western medicine**

REFERENCES

1. Li, J. L., Chen, X., Yang, W. N., Xu, X. M., Lu, L. Y., Wang, J., Kong, Y. X., & Zheng, J. H., (2020). Traditional Chinese medicine for the treatment of pulmonary fibrosis a protocol for systematic review and meta-analysis of overview. *Medicine, 99*, e21310. Baltimore.
2. Wu, Y., Ho, W., Huang, Y., Jin, D. Y., Li, S., Liu, S. L., Liu, X., et al., (2020). SARS-CoV-2 is an appropriate name for the new coronavirus. *The Lancet, 395*, 949, 950.
3. Larsen, J. R., Martin, M. R., Martin, J. D., Kuhn, P., & Hicks, J. B., (2020). Modeling the onset of symptoms of COVID-19. *Frontiers in Public Health.* doi: 10.3389/fpubh.2020.00473.
4. Liu, D., Yu, Y., Chen, Y., & Tang, S., (2020). Efficacy of integrative traditional Chinese and Western medicine for the treatment of patients infected with 2019 novel coronavirus (COVID-19). *Medicine, 99*, e20781. Baltimore.
5. Li, Y., Liu, X., Guo, L., Li, J., Zhong, D., Zhang, Y., Clarke, M., & Jin, R., (2020)., (2020). Traditional Chinese herbal medicine for treating novel coronavirus (COVID-19) pneumonia: Protocol for a systematic review and meta-analysis. *Systematic Reviews, 9*, 6.
6. Hua, G., & Jing, S., (2000). Yin Yang is the great principle of heaven and earth-the influence of guanzi on the theory of yin-yang in the yellow emperor's inner canon. *Chinese Journal of Basic Medicine in Traditional Chinese Medicine, 6*, 11–13.
7. Michael, T., (2015). Shamanism theory and the early Chinese Wu. *Journal of the American Academy of Religion, 83*, 649–696.
8. Zhang, Q., (2015). *An Introduction to Chinese History and Culture* (pp. 385–408). Reflection on ancient Chinese science and technology China Academic Library, Berlin, Heidelberg, Springer.

9. Zhu, Y. P., & Woerdenbag, H. J., (1995). Traditional Chinese herbal medicine. *Pharmacy World and Science, 17*, 103–112.
10. Zhuang, Y., Xing, J. J., Li, J., Zeng, B. Y., & Liang, F. R., (2013). History of acupuncture research. *International Review of Neurobiology, 111*, 1–23.
11. Ke, H., (2019). Modern holistic medicine from the perspective of traditional Chinese medicine. *International Journal of Complementary and Alternative Medicine, 12*, 1–6.
12. Jiang, W. Y., (2005). Therapeutic wisdom in traditional Chinese medicine: A perspective from modern science. *Trends in Pharmacological Sciences, 26*, 558–563.
13. Zhang, W. B., Wang, G. J., & Fuxe, K., (2015). Classic and modern meridian studies: A review of low hydraulic resistance channels along meridians and their relevance for therapeutic effects in traditional Chinese medicine. *Evidence-Based Complementary and Alternative Medicine, 2015*, 1–14.
14. Gao, H., Wang, Z., Li, Y., & Qian, Z., (2011). Overview of the quality standard research of traditional Chinese medicine. *Frontiers of Medicine, 5*, 195–202.
15. Chan, K., (1995). Progress in traditional Chinese medicine. *Trends in Pharmacological Sciences, 16*, 182–187.
16. Wang, X., Zhang, A., Sun, H., & Wang, P., (2012). Systems biology technologies enable personalized traditional Chinese medicine: A systematic review. *The American Journal of Chinese Medicine, 40*, 1109–1122.
17. Xu, J., & Yang, Y., (2009). Traditional Chinese medicine in the Chinese health care system. *Health Policy, 90*, 133–139.
18. Xutian, S., Zhang, J., & Louise, W., (2009). New exploration and understanding of traditional Chinese medicine. *The American Journal of Chinese Medicine, 37*, 411–426.
19. Luo, H., Gao, Y., Zhang, S., Chen, H., Liu, Q., Tan, D., Han, Y., et al., (2020). Reflections on treatment of COVID-19 with traditional Chinese medicine. *Chinese Medicine, 15*, 1–14.
20. Wang, S. X., Wang, Y., Lu, Y. B., Li, J. Y., Nyamgerelt, M., & Wang, W. W., (2020). Diagnosis and treatment of novel coronavirus pneumonia based on the theory of traditional Chinese medicine. *Journal of Integrated Medicine, 18*, 275–283.
21. Wang, C., Sun, S., & Ding, X., (2021). The therapeutic effects of traditional Chinese medicine on COVID-19: A narrative review. *International Journal of Clinical Pharmacy, 43*, 35–45.
22. Chen, H., Song, Y. P., Gao, K., Zhao, L. T., & Ma, L., (2020). Efficacy and safety of Jinhua qinggan granules for coronavirus disease 2019 (COVID-19). *Medicine, 99*, e20612. Baltimore.
23. Ren, Y., Yin, Z. H., Dai, J. X., Yang, Z., Ye, B. B., Ma, Y. S., Zhang, T., & Shi, Y. Y., (2020). Evidence-based complementary and alternative medicine exploring active components and mechanism of Jinhua qinggan granules in treatment of COVID-19 based on virus-host interaction. *Natural Product Communications, 15,* 1–11.
24. Qiu, Q., Huang, Y., Liu, X., Huang, F., Li, X., Cui, L., Luo, H., & Luo, L., (2020). Potential Therapeutic effect of traditional Chinese medicine on coronavirus disease 2019: A review. *Frontiers in Pharmacology, 11*, 570893.
25. Kageyama, Y., Aida, K., Kawauchi, K., Morimoto, M., Ebisui, T., Akiyama, T., & Nakamura, T., (2020). *Jinhua Qinggan Granule, a Chinese Herbal Medicine Against COVID-19, Induces Rapid Changes in the Plasma Levels of IL-6 and IFN-γ. medRxiv*, 2020.06.08.20124453.
26. Zengli, L., Xiuhui, L., Chunyan, G., Li, L., Xiaolan, L., Chun, Z., Yin, Z., et al., (2020). Effect of Jinhua qinggan granules on novel coronavirus pneumonia in patients. *Journal of Traditional Chinese Medicine, 40*, 467–472.

27. Li, L. C., Zhang, Z. H., Zhou, W. Z., Chen, J., Jin, H. Q., Fang, H. M., Chen, Q., etal., (2020). Lianhua qingwen prescription for Coronavirus disease 2019 (COVID-19) treatment: Advances and prospects. *Biomedicine and Pharmacotherapy*, *130*, 110641.
28. Hu, C., Liang, M., Gong, F., He, B., Zhao, D., & Zhang, G., (2020). Efficacy of Lianhua Qingwen compared with conventional drugs in the treatment of common pneumonia and COVID-19 Pneumonia: A meta-analysis. *Evidence-Based Complementary and Alternative Medicine*, *2020,* 15.
29. Chen, X., Yin, Y. H., Zhang, M. Y., Liu, J. Y., Li, R., & Qu, Y. Q., (2020). Investigating the mechanism of Shufeng Jiedu capsule for the treatment of novel Coronavirus pneumonia (COVID-19) based on network pharmacology. *International Journal of Medical Sciences*, *17*, 2511–2530.
30. Zhao, Y., Hu, J., Song, J., Zhao, X., Shi, Y., & Jiang, Y., (2020). Exploration on shufeng jiedu capsule for treatment of COVID-19 based on network pharmacology and molecular docking. *Chinese Medicine*, *11*, 9–18.
31. Yuan, Z., Hongyan, X., Yan, L., Tianhao, L., Haipo, Y., Xiaoxu, F., & Chungyuang, X., (2020). Qingfei paidu decoction for treating COVID-19: A protocol for a meta-analysis and systematic review of randomized controlled trials. *Medicine*, *99*.
32. Ren, W., Ma, Y., Wang, R., Liang, P., Sun, Q., Pu, Q., Dong, L., Mazhar, M., Luo, G., & Yang, S., (2021). Research advance on Qingfei Paidu decoction in prescription principle, mechanism analysis and clinical application. *Frontiers in Pharmacology*, *11*, 589714.
33. Tao, Q., Du, J., Li, X., Zeng, J., Tan, B., Xu, J., Lin, W., & Chen, X. L., (2020). Network pharmacology and molecular docking analysis on molecular targets and mechanisms of Huashi Baidu formula in the treatment of COVID-19. *Drug Development and Industrial Pharmacy*, *46*, 1345–1353.
34. Dai, Y. J., Wan, S. Y., Gong, S. S., Liu, J. C., Li, F., & Kou, J. P., (2020). Recent advances of traditional Chinese medicine on the prevention and treatment of COVID-19. *Chinese Journal of Natural Medicines*, *18*, 881–889.
35. Guo, H., Zheng, J., Huang, G., Xiang, Y., Lang, C., Li, B., Huang, D., et al., (2020). Xuebijing injection in the treatment of COVID-19: A retrospective case-control study. *Annals of Palliative Medicine*, *9*.
36. Luo, Z., Chen, W., Xiang, M., Wang, H., Xiao, W., Xu, C., Li, Y., Min, J., & Tu, Q., (2021). The preventive effect of xuebijing injection against cytokine storm for severe patients with COVID-19: A prospective randomized controlled trial. *European Journal of Integrative Medicine*, *42*. doi: 10.1016/j.eujim.2021.101305.
37. Chenggang, C., Zelong, Z., Shengnan, K., & Tao, X., (2020). Reducing injection combined with western medicine for pneumonia: A protocol for systematic review and meta-analysis. *Medicine, 99*. doi: 10.1097/MD.0000000000022757.
38. Jia, S., Luo, H., Liu, X., Fan, X., Huang, Z., Lu, S., Shen, L., et al., (2021). Dissecting the novel mechanism of reduning injection in treating Coronavirus Disease 2019 (COVID-19) based on network pharmacology and experimental verification. *Journal of Ethnopharmacology*, *273*. doi: 10.1016/j.jep.2021.113871.
39. Pan, W., Yang, L., Fang, W., Lin, L., Li, C., Liu, W., Gan, G., Fan, J., Zou, J., Wang, Z., & Pan, H., (2015). Determination of five sesquiterpenoids in xingnaojing injection by quantitative analysis of multiple components with a single marker. *Journal of Separation Science, 38,* 3313–3323.

40. Wu, X. V., Dong, Y., Chi, Y., Yu, M., & Wang, W., (2020). Traditional Chinese medicine as a complementary therapy in combat with covid-19—A review of evidence-based research and clinical practice. *Journal of Advanced Nursing, 77,* 1635–1644.
41. Zhao, Z., Li, Y., Zhou, L., Zhou, X., Xei, B., Zhang, W., & Sun, J., (2020). Prevention and treatment of COVID-19 using traditional Chinese medicine: A review. *Phytomedicine.* doi: 10.1016/j.phymed.2020.153308.
42. Yang, L., Liu, S., Liu, J., Zhang, Z., Wan, X., Huang, B., Chen, Y., & Zhnag, Y., (2020). COVID-19: Immunopathogenesis and immunotherapeutics. *Signal Transduction and Targeted Therapy, 5*, 1–8.

CHAPTER 11

The Role of Natural Products in COVID-19

IQRA AKHTAR,[1] SUMERA JAVAD,[1] TEHREEMA IFTIKHAR,[2] AMINA TARIQ,[1] HAMMAD MAJEED,[3] ASMA AHMAD,[1] MUHAMMAD ARFAN,[4] and M. ZIA-UL-HAQ[5]

[1]*Department of Botany, Lahore College for Women University, Lahore, Pakistan, E-mail: zif_4@yahoo.com (S. Javad)*

[2]*Department of Botany, Government College University Lahore, Pakistan*

[3]*Knowledge Unit of Science, University of Management and Technology, Iqbal Campus, Sialkot, Pakistan*

[4]*Department of Botany, Division of Science and Technology, University of Education Lahore, Punjab, Pakistan*

[5]*Office of Research, Innovation and Commercialization, Lahore College for Women University, Lahore–54000, Pakistan*

ABSTRACT

Antiviral treatment for COVID-19 is need of the hour along with development of vaccine. A lot of work is being carried out since December 2019, to treat this infectious disease but still with no results. Nature is full of such marvelous treasure of chemicals, which has a number of hidden characteristics, and we need to explore those for their biological activities. A lot of work was done on natural products and their effects on SARS CoV when the world came across the infection in 2003. Coronavirus causing SARS CoV-2 (also known as SARS COVID-19) has pretty much genomic resemblance with the SARS CoV. Therefore, it is believed that herbal treatments which were valid for SARS CoV may be equally effective against SARS CoV-2. Therefore, a thorough study has been done to review the antiviral activities of plants and their phytochemicals, particularly against coronaviruses (CoVs).

11.1 INTRODUCTION

The chemical compounds acquired from living organisms like plants, animals, bacteria, fungi, or algae are called natural compounds. Natural compounds have gained a factual importance as traditional medicines with the passage of time. They themselves and their derivatives occupy an essential space in pharmaceutical and related industries. They exhibit a multi-dimensional chemical structure with an array of biological functions [1]. Natural products have always been a back bone for drug discovery due to their chemical diversity, structural variability, and biochemical specificity because nature has always solutions, what our job is? To search them [2].

They have been used as antibacterial, antifungal, anti-inflammatory, anti-cancerous, antihypertension, and a lot more. Lovastatin, Artemisinin, Vinblastine, Micafungin are a few examples of natural products being used as medicines [3]. A number of them are also FDA approved and in clinical use in the USA and other parts of the world as well. These natural compound-based drugs are also preferred by a number of people due to their lesser side effects and lesser prices.

Natural compounds also have a long history to be used as antivirals. Viral diseases have always caused a distressing health situation for mankind. World is facing a constant threat of novel viruses causing infections with every passing day [4]. Vaccinations have proven their effectiveness against a number of viral diseases like mumps, measles, small pox, polio, and chickenpox, etc. But still, vaccination is a failure for a number of viral infections like AIDS, hepatitis C, etc. Furthermore, development of a vaccine takes time, and a costly treatment for developing countries [5]. Therefore, a vital role may be played by natural products as antivirals.

Story of infections goes to December 2019, when a strange type of pneumonia was reported from Wuhan city of China, which spread throughout the world and transformed into the first pandemic of the century, causing an alarming number of deaths per day worldwide [6]. There are a lot of efforts being made since December 2019, to treat this acute sickness, also known as severe acute respiratory syndrome (SARS) COVID-19 caused by coronavirus. As it is a new virus, therefore, efforts are being made tirelessly for its treatment. A lot of research and funds are devoted to the vaccine development worldwide. But due to the highly mutable nature of this RNA virus, vaccination would not be a long-term solution to this virus. It is the reality associated with RNA viruses as they do not have a proofreading mechanism of RNA replicating enzymes, which increases the chances of genetic errors or mutations [7–9].

In such a situation, natural compounds can cure the sickness or at least can relieve the symptoms to relieve the patients and can boost one's immunity to enable them to fight the illness. There are a lot of complexities associated with COVID-19 infections and the severity of conditions depend upon the body reactions of the symptoms. That is why COVID-19 infection may be carried without symptoms, with mild symptoms or with severe life-threatening sickness. In this regard lifestyle and eating habits of the patient play a significant role, both pre and post infection [10, 11]. Herbal products, carrying a mixture of precious natural compounds really worked for SARS (caused by coronaviruses) in 2003. Healthy life style does not mean or it does not ensure that coronavirus is not going to infect someone. Rather it implies to reduce the severity of the clinical symptoms and their complexities produced due to COVID-19 infection [12]. It is really important to concentrate on plant based or other natural compounds for possible COVID-19 treatment in future due to a number of reasons. Therefore, in this chapter, different aspects of COVID-19, its causative agent and proposed natural metabolites to treat the COVID sickness, are discussed in detail.

11.2 CORONAVIRUSES (COVS) AND COVID-19

Coronavirus causing COVID-19 is a member of genus beta-coronavirus and subgenus sarbecovirus. It is an enveloped forward sense ssRNA virus with spikes on its surface. Its total diameter is reported to be 125 nm [13]. The helical genomic nuclear material (RNA) is covered by a protein coat and an outer enfolded protein shell. Then outermost is lipid bilayer envelope with various structural proteins like spikes (Figure 11.1) [6, 14, 15]. Another type is also discovered, known as COV-2 which is quite similar to SARS-CoV and MERs-CoV, i.e., 72–79% and 51.8% respectively, but more infectious [16, 17].

Coronavirus is very active to spread among the human race, it may be by direct contact, or respiratory microdroplets which can stay in the air for much longer. They also have a great capacity to survive over various surfaces tolerating a range of temperatures and pH values, ultimately, once again infecting a new host without direct contact [18, 19].

11.3 COVID-19 INFECTION AND NATURAL PRODUCTS

It involves the binding of the SARS-CoV Spike protein to its cellular receptor angiotensin-converting enzyme 2 (hACE2) which is present on the cell membrane of outer cells of human lungs and its life cycle begins [20].

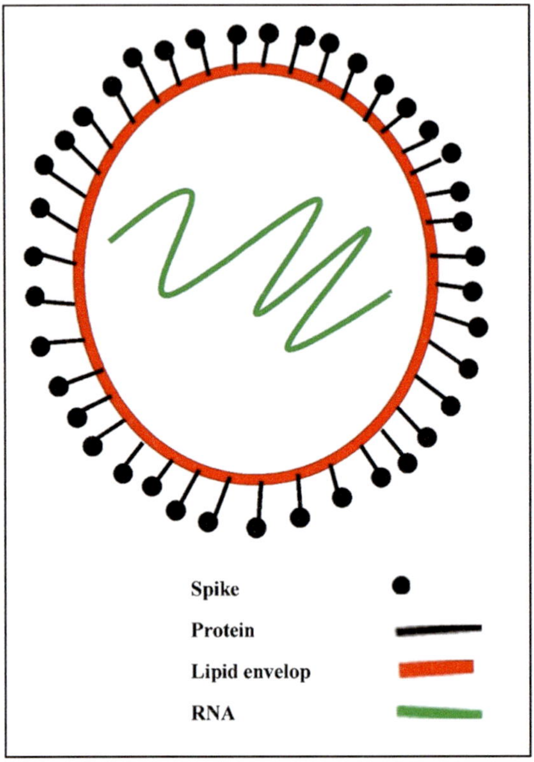

FIGURE 11.1 Coronavirus.
Source: Adapted from: Jahan and Onay (2020) [6].

Viruses of zoonotic origin (viruses which can mutate themselves to change their host from some animal to another like human) like CoVs are not easy to study, and extensive research budgets are being deployed to find an effective treatment for patients affected by coronavirus. For this purpose, at first structure elucidation of virus, its source, genome, and infection mechanism are necessary to be known. Another difficulty, while treating viruses, particularly, RNA viruses is their ability to mutate, which make it difficult to prepare any broad-spectrum antiviral agent. This mutating ability of viruses also make them resistant to antiviral drugs as well. If synthetically developed medications for viruses are discussed, there are also related a number of unwanted side effects causing a lot of health problems other than viral sickness. Therefore, a natural drug, particularly a plant-based drug can open new horizons to face the complexities, sickness, and side effects produced by coronavirus and synthetic antiviral agents [6, 21–23].

Natural products have a long history of use, as readily available treatments, for the ailments either caused by viruses or other microbes. They are being preferred due to their low cost, lesser side effects and easy availability. There is a dire need of extensive research for a metabolic profile of such reported active plants from different regions of the world to exploit this green treasure to compete with pandemics like COVID-19. A Swiss philosopher and botanist, Philippus Aureolus Theophrastus Bombastus von Hohenheim, once said "All that man needs for health and healing has been provided by God in nature, the challenge of science is to find it." [24]. Plants contain an array of natural compounds with different structures and different biological activities. These bioactive compounds may have very strong antiviral activities like essential oils, alkaloids, phenolics, glycosides, and saponins (Figure 11.2).

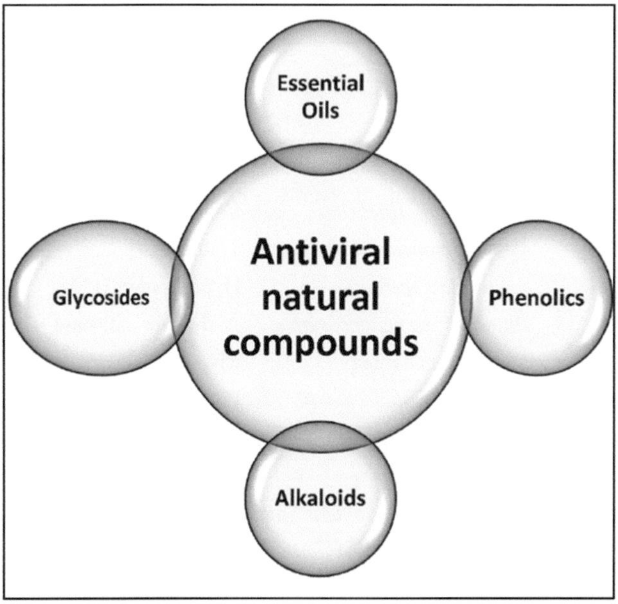

FIGURE 11.2 Plant metabolites mainly working as antivirals.

11.4 NATURAL PRODUCTS AND DRUG DISCOVERY

Natural products are known to possess a broader diversity in chemical space and, as a result, have produced a profound impact on chemical biology and drug development (Table 11.1). Drug discovery and formulation using plant metabolites as raw material has always been a challenging task. This process of drug discovery usually consists of following steps:

- Extraction of bioactive compounds;
- Isolation of these compounds;
- Characterization;
- Structure elucidation;
- Pharmacological investigation;
- Preclinical, and clinical trials;
- Final approval.

TABLE 11.1 List of Some FDA Approved Drugs Developed from Natural Compounds Extracted from Plants

Natural Compound	Source Plant	Used for Treating	References
Artemisinin	*Artemisia annua*	Malaria	[24, 27]
Colchicine	*Colchicum autumnale*	Gout	[27]
Crofelemer	*Croton lechleri*	AIDs	[24]
curcumin	*Curcuma longa*	Alzheimer's disease	[28]
Deserpeidine	*Rauwolfia canescens*	Hypertension	[24]
Docetaxel	*Taxus brevifolia*	Cancer	[24, 29]
Ematine	*Cephaelis ipecacuanha*	Vomiting	[24]
Lovastatin	*Aspergillus terreus*	Hyperlipidemia	[24]
Rivastigmine	*Physostigma venensosum*	Alzheimer's disease	[28]
Silymarin	*Silybum marianum*	Liver diseases	[30]
Taxol	*Taxus brevifolia*	Cancer	[31]
Ternatolide	*Ranunculus ternatus*	Tuberculosis	[24]
Thymol	*Thymus vulgaris*	Fungal infections	[32]
Tubocurarine	*Chondodendron tomentosum*	Muscle soreness	[24]
Veregen	*Camellia sinensis*	Perianal warts	[24, 33]
Yohimbine	*Pausinystalia yohimbe*	Aphrodisiac	[24]

These all stages are time consuming and a little bit expensive but once developed, an herbal drug is a true reward. Far-reaching research is one of the basic requirements with the involvement of modern technology and instrumentation to speed up the process of discovering the natural drug molecules. Stepping forward techniques are gas chromatography-mass spectrometry, nuclear magnetic resonance (NMR), high performance liquid chromatography, liquid chromatography, infrared spectroscopy, etc. These techniques have really helped in all above said procedures of drug discovery. Furthermore, targeted extraction techniques including microwave assisted extraction, ultrasonic extraction, supercritical fluid extraction, etc., has made the process faster and cheaper. Nowadays, using of software and information technology to screen new molecules and interconnect globally has paved the way to new horizons to rely more on natural compounds for treatments. Simply Powerful new technologies are revolutionizing natural herbal drug discovery [25, 26].

Options for treatment of COVID-19 can be divided into two main groups, firstly the development of vaccine, secondly reproducing and relying on the already approved drugs or chemical compounds [34].

11.5 HISTORY OF NATURAL DRUGS

In 2600 BC, Mesoamerica, used plant based pharmaceutical products for the first time. They used clay tablets. There are indications that they had an extensive pharmaceutical system consisting of around 1,000 herbal medicines including described oils from different plant species like *Cypresses sempervirens* (Cypress), *Eucalyptus*, and *Commiphora*. There use is even continuous at present age for the treatment of inflammation, cold, flu, and coughing fits [36]. The knowledge of drug and medication in Egypt was estimated around 2000 BC, contain about 700 plant derived drugs. In Ebers Papyrus, plant-based medicines have been reported around 1550 BC [37, 38] ranges from infusions, tablets, balms, and gargles. For thousands of years, Traditional Chinese Medicines (TCM) have been thoroughly recorded [39] and Chinese Materia Media is the main source of this information:

- Wu She Er Bing Fang (1100 BC) had an assemblage of 52 medications;
- Shannong Herbal (100 BC) had a record of 365 medicines;
- A record of 850 medicines from Tang Herb (659 AC) [36];
- The Ayurveda framework has been recorded since the first millennium BC [40].

The Western world's awareness of plant-derived therapeutics is largely based on Roman and Greek cultures. In fact, a compendium was published by Theophrastus (a Greek philosopher and a scientist) in 100 BC. It contained a lot of knowledge about medicinal herbs and their uses. There are also research reports that in 1st century AC Roman Pliny the Elder and Greek physician Dioscorides published material on preparation, handling, and usage of medicinal plants. Then in second century AC, Greek (Rome) Galen published data about medicinal plants [41, 42].

German, Irish, English, and French monasteries also retained western plant-based medicinal expertise throughout the dark and Middle Ages (5th to 12th centuries). Arabs have enshrined Greek-Roman information, complemented it with their own tools and herbs from ancient Chinese and Indian medication, uncommon in the Greco-Roman community [37]. Furthermore, the Arabs made significant contributions to the study of pharmacy and medicine in the eighth century, establishing independent pharmacies through the Persian pharmacist, surgeon, scholar, and philosopher Avicenna and works like the *Canon Medicinae*. About the 10th century, in the south of Italy, the Arab medicinal culture stumbled upon the Greco-Roman herbal and pharmaceutical philosophy in about 10th century. It was in the south of Italy when a great contribution was made by establishing the famous Salerno school, which was a primary and preliminary stage at first and then took the shape of modern university. This whole scenario was maintained and encouraged by Emperor Federico II and regarded.

Then Greek physician Dioscorides invented the paper press, which revived the Greco-Roman knowledge of plants once again in the 15th and 16th centuries. This made it possible to print the herbal books like "The Mainz Herbal" by Herbarius Moguntinus and "The German Herbal" in 1484. These printed books were then distributed among all over the Europe. Later on, both books were edited by Gutenberg's partner Peter Schoffer, in 1530 [41].

In 1804, an analgesic and sleep-inducing agent morphium was isolated from opium. This was named Morhine. Its name was derived from Greek myth, which describes "Morpheus as a god of dreams." It was a real milestone in the logical development of drugs from plants [43]. Friedrich Serturner, a German herbalist's assistant, discovered a new class of medicines called alkaloids. Following the discovery of morphine, researchers turned their attention to other medicinal plants, and throughout the 19th century, a huge range of plant substances, mainly alkaloids such as nicotine, caffeine, quinine, capsaicin, atropine, cocaine, colchicine, and codeine were extracted and isolated from their natural origins [44, 45].

Herbalists, the founding fathers of the modern pharmaceutical industry, extracted, and purified compounds like alkaloids, and the first example was H. E. Merck in Darmstadt (Germany), who began extracting morphine as well as other alkaloids in 1826. Salicylic acid was the first chemical substance formed by chemical synthesis in 1853 [45]. Alexander Fleming, who discovered penicillin in 1928. Penicillin is a compound which had antibacterial properties. This compound is basically produced by a fungal strain known as *Penicillium chrysogenum*. And this was the true beginning of modern drugs which had anti-lactam action. It was considered as the most influential discovery in the area of natural substances at the beginning of the 20th century. As a result of this development, several basic research activities were centered on separating substances from bacterial species. Scientific and economic establishments supported such developers afore and through World War II. After this scenario of World War II, this became the trend of the drug industry to develop and establish a modern drug company/companies which have the capability to produce antibacterial components from microbes [46]. During all this time period, drug industries were focused to discover antibiotics like gentamicin, streptomycin, and tetracycline. They were expanding their research programs just to target natural compounds related to fermentation technology to work as antibiotics. Each pharmaceutical company has created a discovery program for the treatment of various diseases like bacterial, fungal, and infectious diseases during the second half of the 20th century. In the 70's a new significant area of study was started with the finding of 2 new molecules, namely, mevinolin, and compactin. These molecules belonged to the class Statins and they opened new horizons for plant-based drug researchers. These compounds were efficient to inhibit the synthesis of cholesterol, so they were named "everyday medication" [47].

11.6 MODE OF ACTION OF NATURAL PRODUCTS

Influenza virus, rhinoviruses, enteroviruses, along with CoVs cause the majority of lower respiratory tract infections, and these pathogens can help in boosting the bacterial pneumonia infections, thus deteriorating the situation for patients [30].

Natural products have complex chemical structures but yet simpler mechanisms to work against viruses and other microbes. Plant based drugs or active molecules can act at any level, like they can interrupt the entry of viral particles into the host cells. They can also stop the viral replication and signal transduction. Plant products are also reported to inhibit the action of viral enzymes like neuraminidase in influenza virus infection [48]. Plant products also enhance the phagocytic capability of macrophages, thus boosting the immune response of host cell [49]. Flavonoids from plants are known to reduce the inflammatory reactions of host cells in response to viral infections by reducing the productions of interleukins and other cytokines [50]. But these are very few examples, and they need an elaborative evaluation to get more promising results.

Natural compounds derived from plants have a number of mechanisms by which they can act as antiviral compounds. TCM has a lot of related home-grown knowledge which can be used to fight against COVID by following up on various sub-atomic targets. The sub-atomic targets for natural products against COVID include:

- S glycoprotein;
- COVID primary 3CL(pro);
- RdRp;
- PLpro;
- Kinase; and
- Other N proteins, for example, viral helicase [51, 52].

11.6.1 TARGETING S GLYCOPROTEIN

The principal antigen present at the viral surface is the COVID spike (S) glycoprotein which has the objective of killing antibodies during disease, therefore considered as the main focal point of immunization plan of virus. Two main functions are performed by the COVID-19 S protein, which are the key roles. These include to establish the virus-cell connection and for intervention of viral layer fusion with host cell during disease. Mode of action of natural products may be related to the hindering of the S protein/ spike protein/or surface binding protein. This S protein of coronavirus is usually glycosylated, and plant based letins can adhere with them easily as they have a tendency to react with glycosylated compounds [53].

Different antiviral natural compounds attack and target antiviral S glycoprotein. For example, emodin, is a plant secondary metabolite (extracted and isolated from Rhei). It hinders the S protein from binding with ACE2. Its hindering effect on S protein is dose dependent. Thus, it has strong antiviral activity against SARS-CoV. This antiviral potential depends upon it focusing on the S protein. As SARS COVID-2, also known as SARS COVID-19, has much genomic resemblance with SAES CoV, so it is assumed that the same mechanism will work for both for most of the time with a very few exceptions. Concentrates of *Lonicera Japonica* Flos and *Eucalyptus globulus* have been accounted for having antiviral potential against SARS-CoV because of their capacity to disturb the preparation/synthesis of envelope, made up of glycoprotein for virus assembly. Saikosaponins secluded from *Bupleuri radix* applied as an antiviral agent against HCoV-22E9. Saikosaponin B2 are found to be disturbing the viral glycoproteins (S-proteins). Due to which, the viral entrance by blocking viral connection and infiltration. *Stephaniae tetrandrae* Radix has reported to have an alkaloid, i.e., Bis-benzylisoquinoline alkaloids-tetrandrine which has strong antiviral effect on HCoV-OC43 [46]. This antiviral potential of this particular alkaloid is maintained by hindering the function of S-protein [54]. S proteins can also be blocked by blocking their amino acids at active sites [55].

11.6.2 TARGETING ON PROTEASES

The life cycle of the COVID virus depends upon two types of proteases, i.e., 3CLpro (3 chymotrypsin like cysteine protease) and PLpro (Papain like proteases). These proteases are responsible for the translation of genomic RNA into viral proteins (structural as well as non-structural) which are required for the life cycle continuation of the virus. 3CLpro is a monomer in native form, but when attached to substrate, it forms a dimer. Each monomer of 3CLpro consists of 2 domain. As this enzyme is required for viral replication, so this enzyme can be a possible important target of antiviral natural compounds.

Both of these above said proteases may be good targets of antiviral drugs. They should be considered as two viable drug targets when working on anti SARS COV medication because these are playing vital roles in viral replication and ultimately dispersal. There are a number of reports about the discovery of antiviral drugs attacking on 3CLpro and PLpro and ultimately killing the virus. Coumarins, chalcones, and flavanones from *Angelicae sinensis* Radix are reported, in one research work, having a dose dependent inhibitory effect on 3CLpro [56]. It is also reported that 3CLpro of SARS-CoV and SARS COVID-19 differ in just 12 amino acids. Therefore, leading compounds as anti 3CLpro are already present in literature, therefore an antiviral targeting this enzyme may be a possible future for COVID-19 treatment [57]. History of treatment of HCV and HIV has also shown the success of protease inhibitory compounds. There is a lot of literature available on plants like *Camellia sinensis, Angelica keiskei, Cullen corylifolium, Isatis tinctoria,* whose extracts have potential antiviral activities because they inhibited the activity of viral proteases as described in Figure 11.3 [58].

11.6.3 TARGETING ON RDRP

RNA replicases of coronavirus, also known as RdRp boost up and catalyzes the RNA replication from viral RNA template. This is a common and essential protein which is a part of all RNA viruses. These are vital parts of the viral life cycle with no DNA so a part of replication, outside the central dogma. RdRps are working with RNA replication, RNA recombination and mRNA synthesis for protein synthesis. RdRps are also considered as an interesting and vital target of antiviral agents working against coronavirus. Many natural compounds have been discovered which initially target RdRp. Theaflavin, antioxidant polyphenols of tea leaves, have a marked role in suppressing the viral RNA replication by blocking RdRp [59].

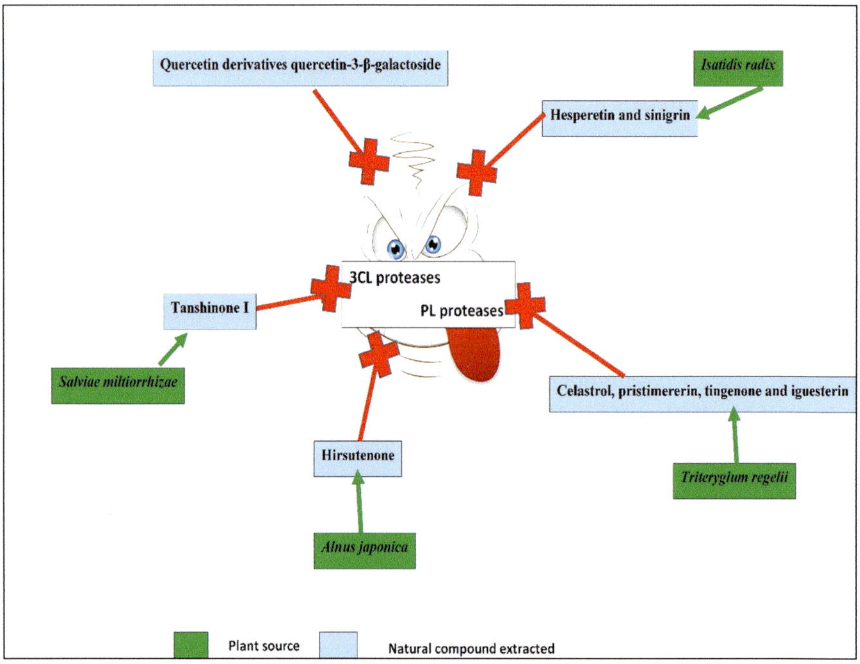

FIGURE 11.3 Natural compounds targeting 3CLpro and PLpro enzymes as antiviral strategy.
Source: Adapted from Mandal et al. [58].

11.6.4 TARGETING ON N PROTEINS

The solitary and primary protein of coronavirus which is related with RTC (replication Transcription complexes), is known as N protein. It basically joins with the gRNA or guide RNA which is a fundamental step for joining of infectious material to host DNA. It is also a part of ribonucleoprotein complex of the virus, thus playing a role in the structural organization of the virus. For this purpose, this protein has a network of action with other N proteins, M proteins and gRNAs. In CoVs, particularly, N protein is primarily responsible for the encapsidation of viral genome to expose it and to start the viral life cycle. It is considered as a very vital step of coronavirus infection cycle in the host. Therefore, targeting N proteins can get rid of corona infection. Resveratrol is known to target N proteins to get rid of coronavirus infect and it is a natural compound being extracted from a number of plants like can berries, chocolate, *Polygonum cuspidatum, Vitis vinifera*, etc. [60].

11.6.5 REDUCING THE EXPRESSION OF ACE2

Various alkaloids and other natural products have been reported to reduce the expression of ACE2, which in turn has inhibitory effects on viral entry. Natural compounds reported are piperine, berberine, thebaine, curcumin, etc., which have a strong inhibiting effect on ACE2 [61]. Naringine and naringenin from citrus peels can bind to ACE 2 with lesser binding energy as compared to other competitors, making them a strong candidate for anti-COVID-19 treatment [62].

11.6.6 TARGETING ION CHANNELS

Ion channel in the host cell membrane support the release of viruses from infected cells and the dispersal of infection to other cells. Inhibition of 3A proteins also inhibit the viral release from cell. This step can also be target of natural drugs to weaken the symptoms and to decrease the viral load [63].

11.6.7 TARGETING HELICASES

This group of enzymes is involved in unwinding of genome. Therefore, if these are blocked, viral replication can be stopped. Bananins are reported in this regard to have anti-helicase activity against SARS CoV without being hazardous to the host cell activity. There are iodobananins eubananins and vanillin bananins which can be a hope for the future of COVID-19 treatment [64].

11.6.8 INHIBITING TMPRSS 2

Transmembrane protein serine 2 is usually required for virus entry into the cell. Therefore, a choice of antiviral can be made by making TMPRSS 2 a target for the natural compound. There are reports that compounds like Myricitin, quercetin, naringin neospheridin have anti TMPRSS 2 activity [65, 66].

11.6.9 OTHER TARGETS

Some natural compounds like glycyrrhizin, extracted from *Glycerhiza glabra*, can target other proteins other than 3CLpro, S protein, RdRp, PLpro, or N proteins. They can act against protein kinase C. This protein is responsible for the upregulation of nitrous synthase and production.

Some natural products like scutellarein and myricetin can target SARS-COV helicase enzyme, which in turn is responsible for viral replication and proliferation in host cells [67].

11.7 MOLECULAR DOCKING

There are a number of computational tools available now which accelerate the drug discovery and decrease the budget of discovery. These tools help us to understand the fact that a chemical compound can be used in a drug or not. We can also make an estimation of the mechanism of drug action and its possible safe dose. These computational techniques involve Chemoinformatics, Network Pharmacology, Molecular Similarity, Pharmacogenomics De Novo Design, Quantitative Structure-Activity Relation and Molecular Docking, etc. [68–70].

Molecular docking is a common and modern technique which is used now a day to discover new drug formulas. A number of software are in use for this purpose. This procedure can analyze small molecules for their interaction with the binding sites of target enzymes or proteins. The capacity of a molecule to bind with minimum energy is searched out. This binding of natural products and target proteins depend upon the shape of the molecule and electrostatic forces between them. Its' such a successful method that it can be used for such target proteins whose structure is still undiscovered but can be done with some homologous structures as in the case of various proteins involved in SARS CoV and COVID-19 infections [61].

11.8 HEALING PERSPECTIVE OF VARIOUS MEDICINAL PLANTS AGAINST SARS-COVID

11.8.1 ALCEA DIGITATA (BOISS.) ALEF

This is a medicinal plant of family Malvaceae with predominant antioxidant, antimicrobial, anti-inflammatory, antitussive, and expectorant properties. Its flowers have a history of being used for the treatment of neck and head cancer along with lung related infections. This plant has a number of phenolics, vitamin C, carotenoids, and flavones, etc., which are in use for lung diseases. An *in vitro* study has also shown that it has inhibition activity or blocking activity against ACE-2 receptor. It is also a promising candidate for therapeutic solution of corona [71].

11.8.2 ALLIUM SATIVUM L.

Garlic or *Allium sativum* belongs to *Amaryllidaceae*. It has a long history where humans used it as a spice. It is famous worldwide and is a part of different daily food dishes. It is also used for a number of home remedies for various ailments. It is an aromatic herb. Extracts of *A. sativum* exhibit antifungal, antibacterial, antioxidant, anticarcinogenic, antidiabetic, antihypertensive, reno-protective, and anti-atherosclerotic. Its cloves possess several potent components, i.e., allicin, alliin, vinyldithiins, ajoenes (Figure 11.4), and flavonoid, which are the secret of its biological activities. These components or natural drugs also inhibit the ACE 2 site, thus blocking viruses to enter in the host cell [72].

11.8.3 AMMI VISNAGA

Ammi visnanga is a member of the Apiaceae family and rich in ϒ-pyrones and coumarins. One of the active components is Cromolyn which is used as a drug as its sodium salt. In COVID-19, some of the death are reported due to cardiac failure. It has already been reported that during viral myocarditis, inflamed heart can be treated with cromolyn. It is very effective for controlling inflammation and cytokine storms. It is used as an anti-asthmatic. It is basically a stabilizer of mast cells by interfering with the calcium transport across the cell membrane of mast cells under the effect of an antigen.

Therefore, it then inhibits the release of leukotrienes and histamines from mast cells.

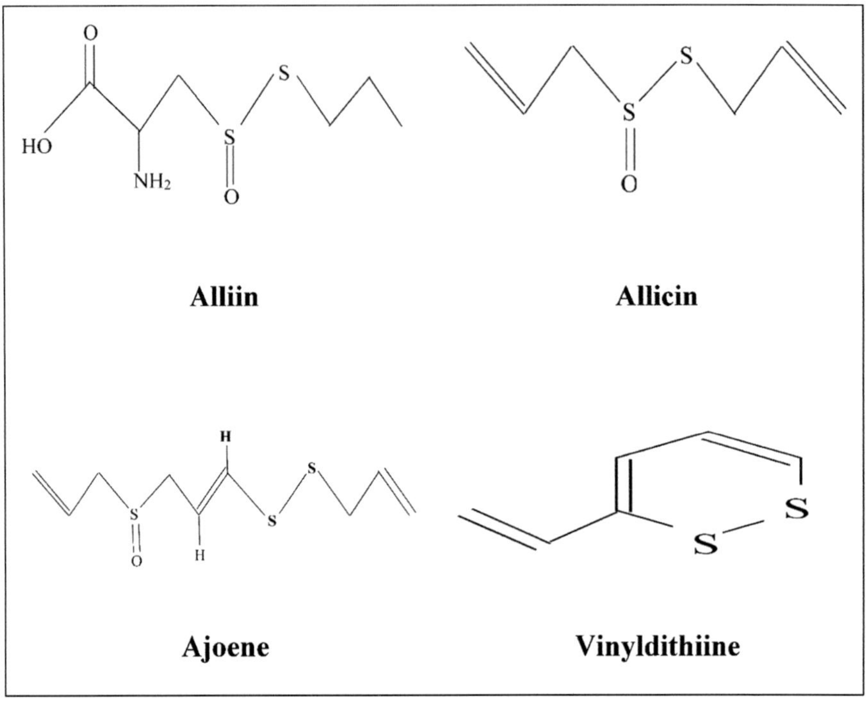

FIGURE 11.4 Structures of active antiviral components of *Allium sativum*.
Source: Adapted from Dethier et al. [73].

It is also involved in reducing the viral cell replication. It may be given to patients in the form of nasal spray or nebulizer, making it more effective for patients with worsened condition (Figure 11.5) [74, 75].

11.8.4 BUPLEURUM SPECIES

These are the member of family Apiaceae and very much dispersed in northern hemisphere. It is a very old and famous medicine from TCMs. These plants are reported to be possessing antiviral activity, particularly against HCoV-22E9. Dried root extract of these bupleurum species is considered as very effective for viral infections. Its active ingredient is saikosaponins which are in fact triterpene saponin glycosides with potent antiviral activity.

There are four main kinds of saikosaponins namely SSa, SSb, SSc, and SSd. SSa, SSb, and SSd types are particularly very active against SARS COV infections and influenza viruses. These glycosides hinder the early stages of replication of the virus. These are also investigated to be helpful in initiating the immune response against coronavirus by involving monocytes and lung neutrophils [77].

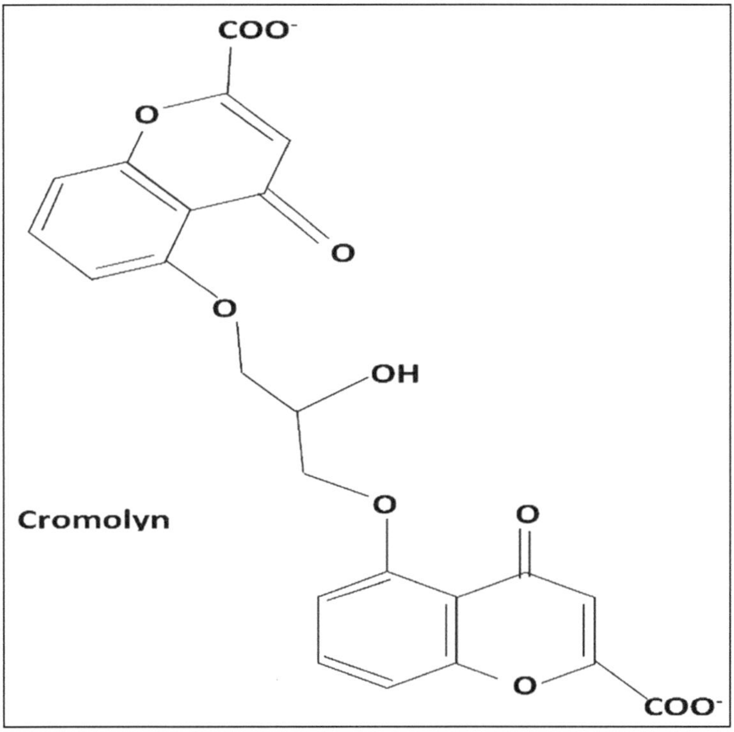

FIGURE 11.5 Structure of cromolyn.

Source: Adapted from: Cheng et al. [76].

11.8.5 *CAMELLIA SINENSIS*

Tea plant or *C. sinensis* is one of the most famous evergreen shrub of family Theacea. Tea is one of the leading beverage, common in every culture and climate. Its extract contains theaflavins which is a group of compounds varying with R and R' as shown in Figure 11.6. It is reported to show anti-herpes simplex virus (HSV) activity as it blocks the entry of virus into host cell and stops the spread of disease [78]. Five reported polyphenols have also shown the predominant antiviral action against influenza A and B viruses [79]. There are also researches carried out on the effects of tea polyphenols on SARS CoV-2, due to their previously reported antiviral activities. It was then successfully reported that tea polyphenols have strong inhibitory action on 3CLpro of this virus [80]. Due to this activity of tea polyphenols, the virus loses its ability to process its polyprotein and its infectious cycle slows down and finally stops. This also has positive effects on the health of other vital signs of the body.

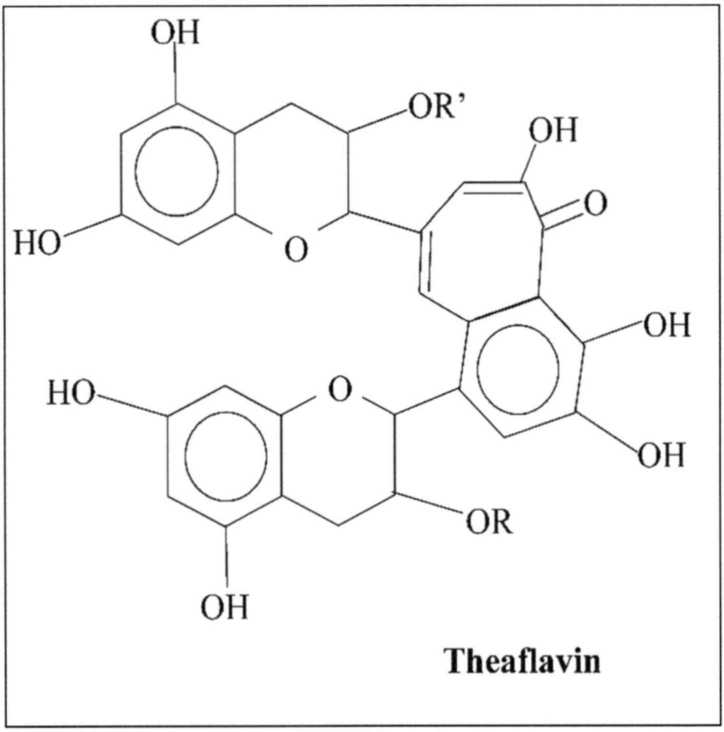

FIGURE 11.6 Structure of theaflavin.
Source: Adapted from: Maiti and Banerjee [82].

Mhatre et al. [81] reported a molecular level docking experiment for epigallocatechin and theaflavins of tea to search for their antiviral targets inside SARS-CoV-2 infectious cycle. They successfully reported that tea extracts with epigallocatechin (predominantly in green tea) and theaflavins (predominantly in black tea) had a higher affinity for viral proteins to stop their active sites as compared to approve and already in use antiviral drugs. Epigallocatechin are found to be more effective in treating the COVID-19. Molecular visualization also approves that these natural compounds have higher affinity to bind and block the active sites of viral proteins [81, 82].

11.8.6 CERASUS AVIUM (L.) MOENCH

Cerasus avium (L.) Moench, otherwise known as sweet cherry, is a member of rosacea family. It is well known plant for antibacterial, antifungal, antioxidant, and antiviral activities of its extracts. This plant is also well known to act on ACE 2 receptors. A couple of experiments have shown the hidden potential of this plant to act against coronavirus, which should be explored more for some practical solution of the global problem of COVID-19 [71, 72].

11.8.7 CITRUS AURANTIUM L.

Bitter orange, a member of family rutaceae, has many essential natural components (hesperidin, naringin) with well-known antimicrobial and antiviral activities. This plant is well known for treatment of lung diseases, anxiety, and prostate cancer, etc. [83]. It is also reported to be blocking the entry of CoVs into the host cell by interacting with ACE-2 site.

11.8.8 CITRUS LIMON

C. limon is a member of the citrus family or Rutaceae and is considered as a remedy for flu, common cold, and other allergies by local Chinese and other Asian countries. Its juice is rich in vitamin C and a number of flavonoids like quercetin, rutin, naringenin, and hesperidin along with functional terpenes like limonene.

Quercetin is a common flavonoid that is found in a number of medicinal plants. Lemon (*C. limon*) is also rich in quercetin. It has shown strong anti-influenza virus activity previously [84]. Quercetin is known to impair the expression of influenza virus protein [85]. It was particularly found very active against initial stages of viral attack. It has also been in common use since a long for treating common cold [86]. Quercetin also showed predominant detrimental effects on hepatitis C virus (HCV) by hindering the replication of virus inside the host cells quercetin can control the viral load directly itself or by host mediated interference to the viral life cycle [87]. It can suppress the activities of various viral enzymes like proteases, reverse transcriptases, DNA gyrases and polymerases [88–91]. The half-life of quercetin in human body is 25 hours, so its higher levels in blood plasma can be easily maintained for longer to treat viral infections without multiple doses [92].

Although quercetin is found in a number of plant sources, but here it is suggested with lemon. Synergism of quercetin with vitamin C is suggested and stressed by a number of researchers [93–95] for treatment of COVID-19 particularly. A paradox associated with quercetin, also known as quercetin paradox is, it is soon oxidized to O-quinone and O semiquinone in the body where these metabolites can interact with thiol groups of proteins, forming toxic compounds [96]. But these metabolites can be recycled again in the presence of vitamin C, therefore, vitamin C in fact increases absorbance of quercetin in the body [93].

Vitamin C is also important for boosting and maintaining the immune response. Vitamin C has direct as well as indirect antiviral activity. Indirect antiviral activities include increase in interferons, supporting lymphocytes, reducing inflammation, modulating cytokines, and even during the acute respiratory distress syndrome caused due to sepsis [97–101]. One human study, carried out on Russian soldiers, helped them to protect themselves from pneumonia by taking a dose of 300 mg/person of vitamin C [102]. Therefore, a multidrug tactic may be proposed for the treatment of COVID-19. Molecular docking has also supported rutin as a strong drug against main protease of COVID-19, with optimal solubility, non-cancerous, and non-toxic side effects [103, 104].

Other flavonoids found are hesperidin and naringenin, both have strong antiviral activities as well. Saha et al. [105] reported after analyzing 248 plant compounds through molecular docking software that hesperidin and (-)-epigallocatechin gallate had the most prominent binding energies for catalytic part of RNA dependent RNA polymerase of SARS Coronavirus 2 [105]. Synergistic doses of hesperidin with naringenin have also been suggested which can be a great remedy for COVID-19 [106]. Therefore, overall lemon juice and fruit and even its peels can pave the way to strong antiviral drug against the present pandemic (Figure 11.7).

11.8.9 *COLCHICUM AUTUMNALE*

C. autumnale is a member of the family Colchaceae, also commonly known as crocus roots. This plant is famous for its alkaloid production, known as colchicine. Colchicine interrupts the production of tubulin in the cells which otherwise are responsible for collagen secretion. So, colchicine can be considered as anti-fibrotic compound. Its overdose is fatal.

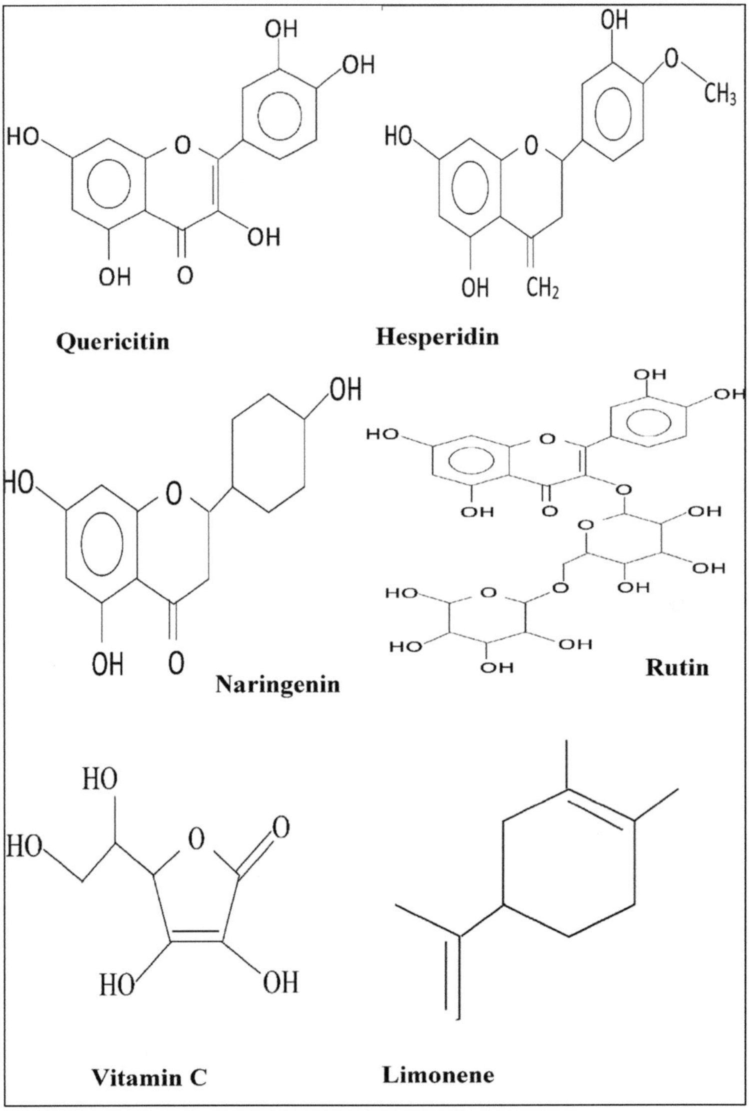

FIGURE 11.7 Bioactive natural components of *Citrus limon.*
Source: Adapted from: Choi et al. [84]; Kim et al. [107]; Salehi et al. [108]; Ganeshpurkar and Saluja [109]; National Center for Biotechnology Information [110, 111].

Colchicine has been recommended by a number of researchers for the treatment of COVID-19 treatment. COVID-19 infection has three main phases:

- Early phase in which virus invades the lung parenchyma;
- Second or pulmonary phase which is characterized by the lung tissue injury and onset of host immune response; and
- Formation of inflammatory cascade in which inflammasomes are produced.

In fact, these inflammasomes are responsible for deteriorated condition of COVID-19 patients and their multiple organ failure, leading to death. Inflammasomes are consisting of a number of immune protein with activated neutrophils and macrophages. Neutrophils are directly or indirectly involved in the formation of thrombus and an increase in the serum α thrombin level. This condition has been reported in COVID-19 patients [112, 113]. Cytokine reactive protein is produced and can cause cardiogenic shocks [114, 115].

Colchicine is reported to inhibit neutrophil activity and it can also stop the activity of inflammasomes and can prevent cytokine movements. Colchicine is also considered as a good option alkaloid for future research in search of medication for Patients of COVID-19; as it is not immune response trigger, not suppressor, but it just stops the movement of signaling proteins by altering the tubulins [116–119].

11.8.10 CURCUMA LONGA

C. longa, a commercially and medicinally important member of family Zingiberaceae with a lot more secondary metabolites being stored in its rhizome. Main component of its rhizome extraction is curcumin, which is a hydrophobic polyphenol beta di-ketone (Figure 11.8). It is a famous Chinese, Siddha, and Ayurveda medicine [120]. It has proven antioxidant, analgesic, antiviral, and antimicrobial activities. It has been proved to be safe for human use at a dose of 12 g per day dose [121, 122]. Although there are some researches showing negative effects of higher or overdoses of curcumin but positive impacts of antiviral treatments by curcumin outweigh its minor negative impacts.

It has a number of benefits which indicate that it can play its stronger rule in controlling COVID-19 infection. Curcumin has the ability to modulate molecular targets. It can regulate transcription or can activate the signaling pathway at the cellular level [123]. Curcumin has a real versatility to act on viruses (Figure 11.9). It can attack on viruses by opting various targets. Curcumin abrogates the viral envelop proteins. They attack on viral envelop to destroy it. Curcumin hinders the viral replication by modulating the signaling pathways of cells. Curcumin associates with lipid membrane of virus and causes a non-linear thinning and weakening of membrane, finally causing destruction of viral membrane [124]. Curcumin is also reported to affect the fluidity of viral envelopes, which ultimately affects the entry of virus into the host cell [125]. Recent studies have shown that curcumin loaded on silver nanoparticles is more effective against enveloped viruses.

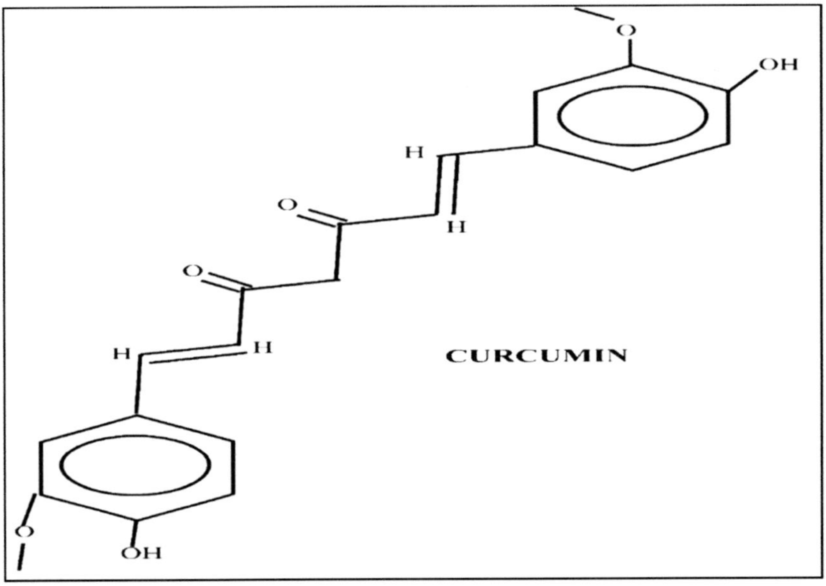

FIGURE 11.8 Structure of curcumin.
Source: Adapted from: Gupta et al. [121].

Curcumin is efficiently involved in suppressing intercellular signaling cascades of human cells, which is required for viral replication. As viruses use these signaling pathways and ubiquitin protease system for their own replication by hijacking the host signaling system, curcumin can stop them here [92]. Curcumin controls infections caused by HCV and HBV by suppressing the signaling pathway of AKT/PBK or NF-kB pathway [126, 127]. Curcumin can target cellular transcription system, where it controls peroxisome activated receptor ϒ co-activator, by which it can minimize the infections caused by hepatitis B virus (HBV) [128].

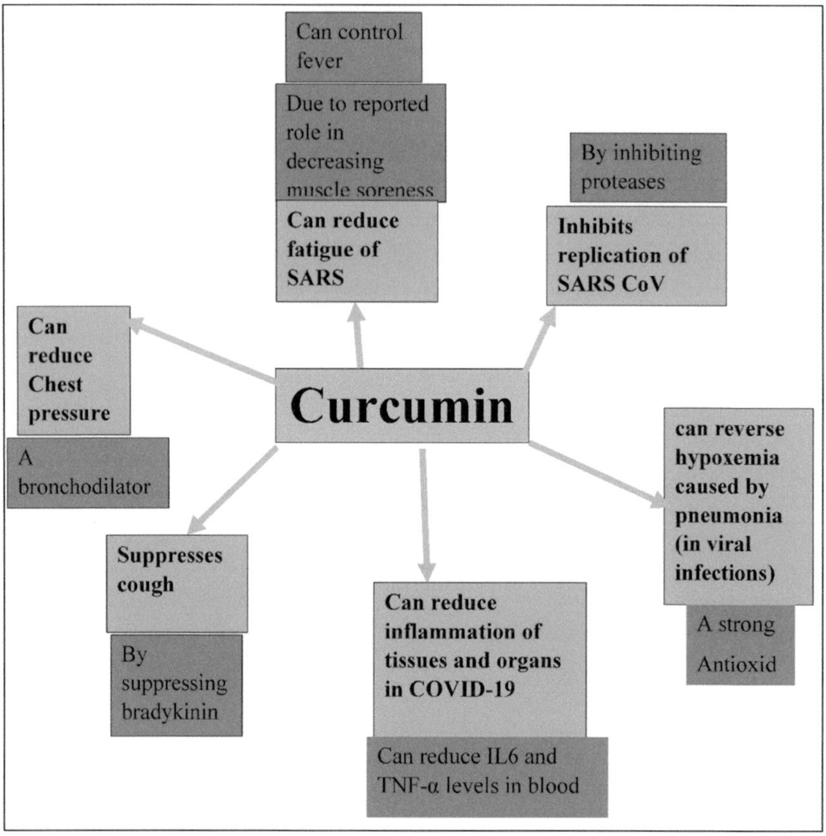

FIGURE 11.9 Proposed actions of curcumin against COVID-19.
Source: Adapted from: Ingolfsson et al. [124]; Anggakusuma et al. [125]; Xu et al. [126]; Kim et al. [127].

Curcumin also takes action on post transcriptional and post translational modifications. Curcumin can improve Dicer expression, thus inhibiting viral expression [129]. For dengue virus treatment, curcumin has been found to work on viral protein degradation [130].

11.8.11 GLYCERHIZAE GLABRA

G. glabra is a famous plant for its anti-inflammatory and cough depressant activity. Glycyrrhizin, a triterpene saponin derived from its bark, has predominant antiviral activity. It is reported to be most effective during viral adsorption period. It can also hinder the replication of a number of respiratory viruses [131, 132]. ACE2, the only receptor of COVID-19 has shown a strong affinity for glycyrrhizin [133]. It has also been suggested that slight modification of glycyrrhizin can produce a possible antiviral against COVID-19 [134].

Glycyrrhizin (Figure 11.10) can modulate the cytokine activity but not acting as an immunosuppressant. It also helps the cells to get rid of reactive oxygen species (ROS) being produced during viral infection, thus reducing the activity of signaling proteins. As a consequence, the intensity of cytokine storm is reduced [135]. Glycyrrhizin plays its role in following ways, i.e.,

- By blocking the entry points of viruses;
- ACE2 independent anti-inflammatory mechanism;
- ACE2 dependent anti-inflammatory mechanism.

Molecular docking method also gave good results for glycyrrhizin [136].

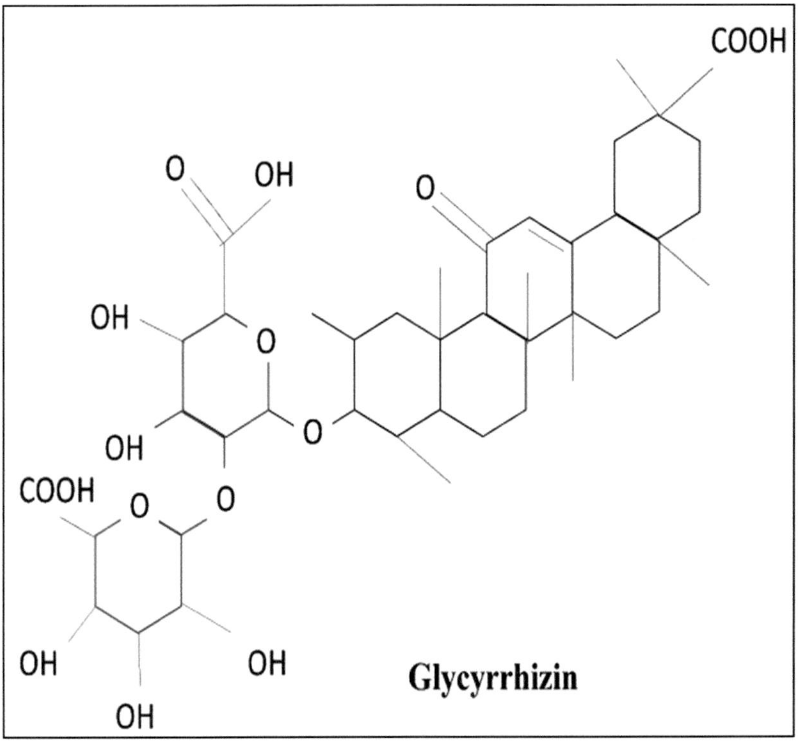

FIGURE 11.10 Structure of glycyrrhizin.

Source: Adapted from: Bailly and Vergoten [136].

Glycyrrhizin causes a halt in the action of 11-beta-hydroxysteroid dehydrogenase, which causes cortisol to interact with mineral corticoid receptor, causing a high level of aldosterone in blood. This in turn causes downregulation of ACE2 enzyme.

11.8.12 LYCORIS RADIATE

This plant belongs to the family Amaryllidaceae and found commonly in Korea, China, and Nepal. It contains a toxic, crystalline alkaloid known as lycorine. It shows broad-spectrum antiviral activities [137]. Lycorine has the ability to inhibit RNA synthesis and protein synthesis. It has been found very active against zika virus [138], poliovirus [139], HSV [140] and SARS-CoV [141]. There are different mechanisms of this single potent alkaloid molecule to inhibit the infectious activities of different viruses. Lycorine has also been tested against SARS COV-2 infection *in vitro* with very promising results. It, along with oxysophoridine and gemcitabine, stopped the viral replication. It was further explained that doses of these compounds were safe for human cell lines as well (Figure 11.11) [142].

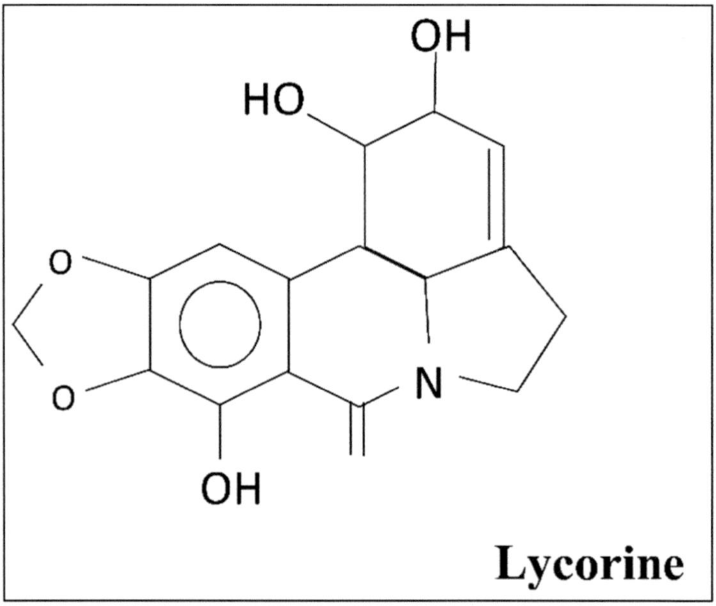

FIGURE 11.11 Structure of lycorine.
Source: Adapted from: Wang et al. [137].

11.8.13 *NIGELLA SATIVA*

It belongs to the family Ranunculaceae and also known as black cumin/black seed. It is known to have antiviral, antibacterial, antifungal, antioxidant, and anti-cancerous activities. It has also been suggested as probable herbal care and treatment for SARS COVID-19 sickness [143]. In COVID-19 immune system is over-activated, also called "cytokine storm." During this process a huge number of cytokines and chemokines are produced, which causes an increased production of micro-thrombus. This leads to multiple organ failure. This hyper activated immune cell response during COVID-19 infection is considered as the main reason for the complexity of patients and ultimately their death. It has been, therefore, suggested by the number of researchers and medical experts that aggressive immunomodulatory treatment at the start of COVID-19 infection an increase the survival percentage and probability of the patient [144, 145].

Essential oils of *N. sativa* are reported to have immunomodulatory effects (IME). Its IME is believed to be mediated by natural killer cells and T-lymphocytes in the host cell [146]. *N. sativa* essential oils also act as bronchodilator. They have the potential to increase the Peak and Maximal Expiratory Flow of patients' lungs. Therefore, they can cause a soothing effect on the lungs and respiratory tract stress and congestion caused by COVID-19 infection [147].

Seed powder and essential oils of *N. sativa* have anti-asthmatic potential as well [148]. It shows antihistamine potential, thus controlling the allergic reactions of the lungs and bronchoconstriction. It reduces the production of histamines and leukotrienes in the body and is also known to block the receptors of histamines, thus having a great control over allergic reactions [149].

Thymoquinone (Figure 11.12), which is an active ingredient of the *N. sativa* extract, has been reported to enhance the activity and survival of CD8+ve cells, thus boosting the immune system against viral antigens [150]. It has also the capability of reducing the formation of microthrombus in the body, thus reducing the chances of COVID-19 induced multiple organ failure [145].

Thymoquinone, when combined with other bioactive constituents, like artemisinin, curcumin, hesperidin, has also shown synergistic anti-viral and antimalarial activities. Development of hydrophobic nano-carriers for thymoquinone has also enhanced the antiviral activity of compound. Hydrophobic carriers help to release the herbal medicine to the targeted lung cells, but also help it to stick to lipophilic envelop of SARS COVID-19 [150]. It has also been reported to be SARS COVID-19 protease inhibitor, thus affecting the viral replication, and hindering the COVID infection from severity [151].

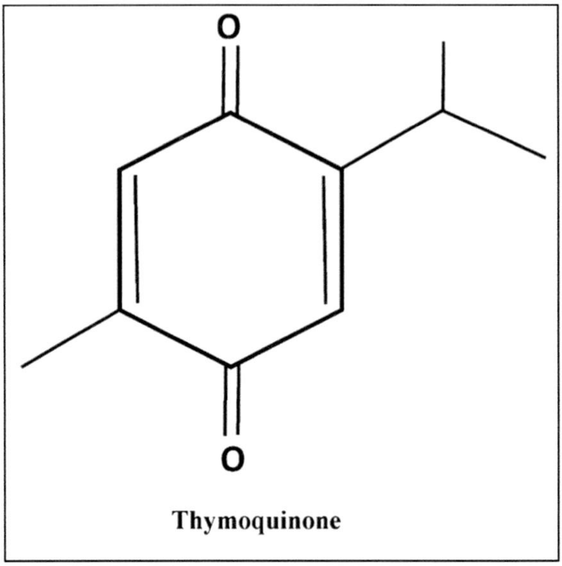

FIGURE 11.12 Structure of thymoquinone.
Source: Adapted from: National Center of Biotechnology [152].

11.8.14 ORIGANUM DICTAMNUS

Pirintsos et al. [153] reported that a combo of essential oils from *O. dictamnus, Thymbra capitate,* and *Salvia fruiticosa* was very effective against viral infections in human beings like influenza virus infections, upper respiratory tract infections and rhinoviruses. Their mode of action included impaired transcription of viral proteins by translocation of viral nuclear proteins [153–156].

11.8.15 POLYGONUM MULTIFLORUM THUNB

This plant is also a member of the family Polygonaceae and mostly found in China, Japan, and Korea. Its root tubers are extracted for biologically active extract. This exudate is used to treat a number of ailments like joint pains, scrofula, rubella, paralysis, malaria, hypercholesterolemia, inflammation, and viral sickness. This plant also acts on ACE-2 receptor site. Ho et al. [157] reported that the bioactive component in this plant is also emodin working in the same way as in Chinese rhubarb. They also suggested that it would be highly appreciable to focus on emodin as anti-corona treatment, source plant may vary, but emodin may be the solution to the problem [157].

11.8.16 *RHEUM PALMATUM L.*

Chinese rhubarb or *Rheum palmatum* L. is a member of Polygonaceae. Its habitat is usually high altitude, and it is very common in the mountains of Gansu, Sichuan, and Shaanxi (China). It is a well-known medicinal herb acting as astringent and laxative. It is used as a treatment for liver bile disease, hemorrhoids, stomachache, etc. It has a series of natural bioactive metabolites, and a few of them are rhein, aloe-emodin, emodin, physcion, and chrysophanol with very eminent biological activities including antibacterial, antipyretic, antiviral, antispamolytic, laxative as well as antiviral.

Emodin is an active ingredient of extract from *R. palmatum.* It is an anthraquinone and has strong antiviral potential as it can reduce the mRNA expression [158]. Emodin is also active against influenza virus. It reduces the virus replication in a dose dependent manner. It is also known to upregulate the antiviral genes like IFN β and ϒ, etc., and finally controlling the influenza virus infection [159]. Emodin has also been reported to be treating HBV and HSV in time and dose dependent manner [159–161].

It is tested against SARS COV-1 as it has the potential to bind with the ACE-2 site. It is a strong competitor of SARS coronavirus for ACE-2 site. In this way it stops and restricts the entry of coronavirus into the host cell. Extracts of root tubers of this plant are rich in emodin and are reported to be very active in blocking the viral entry into host cells in an *in vitro* studies [157]. Emodin plays its role against SARS COV 1 as it stops its entry into the host cell. It is accomplished by obstructing the attachment of S-protein and host cell membrane enzyme ACE2. This emodin (Figure 11.13) can be a possible therapeutic manager of COVID infections [163].

Genome of SARS COVID-19 is divided into 14 open reading frames. 5' end has only one open reading frame encodes a polyprotein which produces 16 non-structural proteins for virus after processing. 3' end has 13 open reading frames translating 4 structural proteins, namely M (matrix protein), E (small envelop proteins), S (spike proteins) and N (nucleocapsid phosphoproteins). As discussed earlier, antiviral drugs can target any of the above structural proteins, but spike proteins can mutate easily, thus avoiding drug attack. Antivirals attacking on viral proteases also interfere with host cell enzymes, thus creating problem for the host cell. So, N protein can be a good target for the antiviral drugs. Many natural compounds like emodin have the capability to attack and block the N protein of coronavirus, thus inhibiting the packaging of viral entities and blocking the spread of infection. Emodin can also block the RNA binding N-terminus of N proteins of coronavirus [164–166].

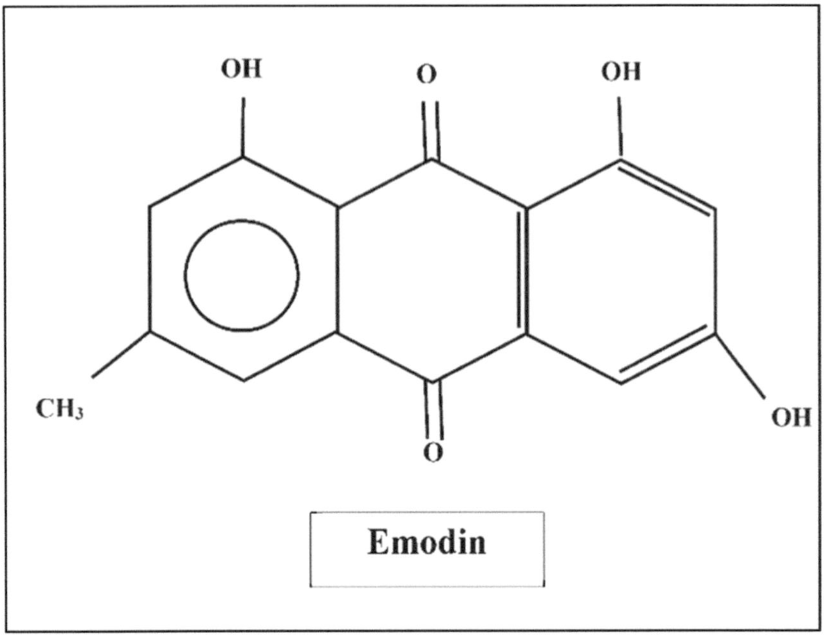

FIGURE 11.13 Structure of emodin, a strong candidate natural metabolite as anti-COVID-19. *Source:* Adapted from: Ho et al. [157].

Rhein is also an anthraquinone, extracted from *R. palmatum, Aloe vera*, etc., derivatized to form Diacerin. Diacerin is obtained by deacetylation of rhein (Figure 11.14) and is a FDA approved medicinal natural compound used for the treatment of osteoarthritis. This natural compound has also profound antiviral potential. It is documented earlier that that Diacerin (active component rhein) inhibits a number of inflammation doorways caused by viral infection. It stops the replication of hepatitis B-virus. Diacerin also stops the entry of flu virus into human lung cells. Most important is that it, like emodin, interferes with the attachment between ACE2 and SARS COVID-19 S-proteins. Thus, Diacerin can act against SARS COVID-19 by reducing viral entry into cells and by reducing host cell overactive immune response [167, 168].

11.8.17 *TARAXACUM OFFICINALE*

This plant belongs to the family Asteraceae and is very well known for its anti-inflammatory, antibacterial, and antifungal activities. This herbaceous plant is rich in phytochemical composition including a number of phenolics, flavonoids, and glycosides. One of the glycosidic compounds is cichorrin which is basically a coumarin glycoside. This plant has been reported to be hindering the chronic pro-inflammatory cytokine storm produced due to SARS CoV [169, 170]. The main reason is found to be cichorin. Molecular docking experiment also suggested the best fit for cichorin out of 100 compounds isolated from Mexican medicinal plants. It blocks the RTP site of RdRP enzyme, Nsp, and papain like proteases of CoVs [171].

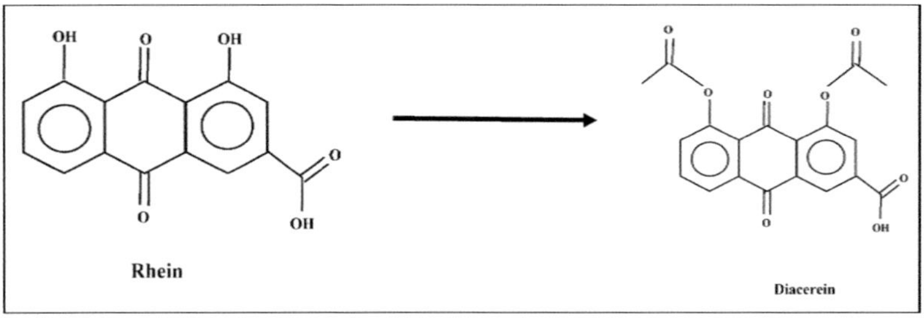

FIGURE 11.14 Acetylation of rhein to form diacerein.
Source: Adapted from: Kaur et al. [167].

Luteolin is another reported antiviral component of *T. officinale* extract. Luteolin is an antioxidant and ant cancerous compound along with recognized antiviral properties. Chemically it is a flavonoid. It has been reported to be active against the Japanese encephalitis virus both *in vivo* and *in vitro* [172]. There are also earlier reports showing that luteolin interferes with the entry of the SARS CoV virus of the 2003 epidemic [173, 174]. Flavonoids like luteolin has very less or no toxicity at all, so they can be made a part of daily diet easily and can be suggested to patients of old age even for the treatment of COVID-19 or to build the immunity wall against this infection. These flavonoids have the reported ability to interfere with the functions of three major proteins of COVID-19 infection [175, 176]. It can also be used as a part of daily diet as functional food.

Luteolin is also known for its vaso-relaxation process [177], therefore it can also be used to treat the hypertension complexities in worsen conditions of COVID-19. Furthermore, molecular docking experiments also provided data for least binding energy of luteolin for binding sites of three major infectious proteins of COVID-19, i.e., 3CLpro, PLpro, and ACE2 (Figure 11.15) [178].

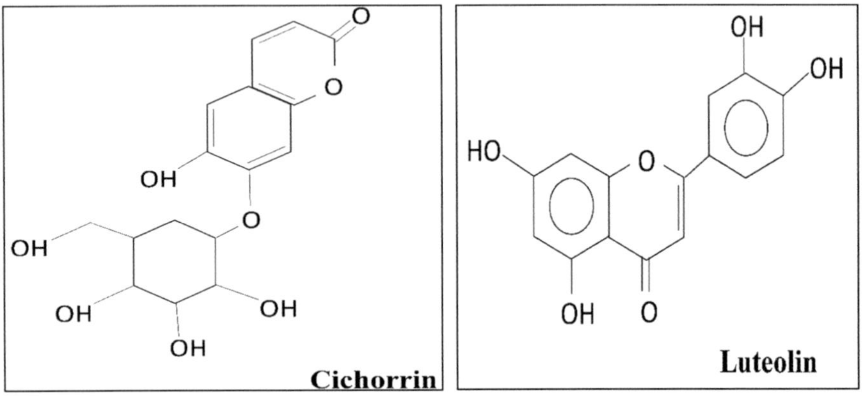

FIGURE 11.15 Structure of cichorrin and luteolin.
Source: Adapted from: Rivero-Segura and Gomez-Verjan [171].

11.8.18 THYMUS VULGARIS

T. vulgaris is a member of the family Lamiaceae and is well known for its essential oils. Extracts and essential oils of this plant have proven antiviral activity. Its active ingredients are carvacrol and thymol (Figure 11.16) [179]. They have a long history of being used for treatment of cough, upper respiratory tract, and bronchitis, etc. [180]. Thyme herb is active against human influenza virus, HSV and human rhinoviruses [179]. Its essential oils can inhibit the entry of virus into the cell or can interfere with the replicating viral entities. These have also proved to relieve the symptoms and complexities associated with viral infection like muscle pain, etc. This is done by reducing the amounts of interleukins 8 and interleukins 1β [181] and hindering the viral proliferation [182]. Antioxidants present in thyme extracts boosts and strengthens the immune system to cope with attacking viruses. Thyme extract is also used as a muscle relaxant, therefore, its use as a symptom reliever of COVID-29 seems to be effective [183, 184]. Their mode of action and time of maximum advantage should be determined.

Protein-ligand docking design has been used to predict the role of thymol against COVID-19. Thymol and carvacrol have shown a high docking score for inhibiting receptor-binding domain (RBD) of S protein of COVID-19. This S protein is the main protein which is responsible for viral entry into the human cell. On the basis of such findings, USA Canada have already approved disinfectants for surfaces using thymol extract [185–187].

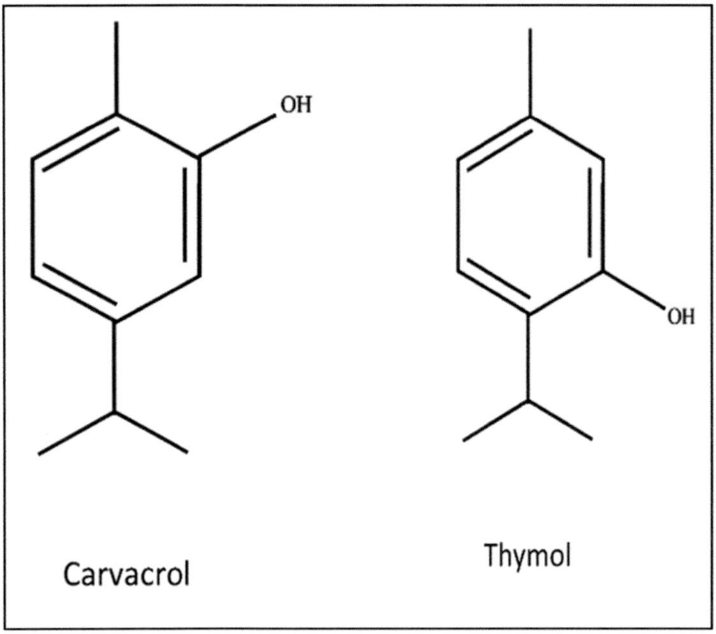

FIGURE 11.16 Two antiviral isomers-carvacrol and thymol from *T. vulgaris*.
Source: Adapted from: Kulkarni et al. [186].

Sardari et al. [184] reported reduction in chest pain, fever, anorexia, cough, headache, fatigue, and other COVID-19 related problems in patients when treated with 5 mL extract of Thyme (in form of syrup) twice a day for one week [184].

11.8.20 HONEY

Honey has been recommended for respiratory tract infections since long. It has immunomodulatory as well as anti-inflammatory functions. It has already been in record that consumption of honey on a daily basis reduces the severity of acute respiratory distress syndrome. There are recommendations that 1,200 mg/g of honey should be used on a daily basis as it can increase the immunity of the body against a number of common ailments [188, 189]. The chemical composition of honey is shown in Figure 11.17 [190, 191]. It shows that honey is rich in phenolic acids and flavonoids, which poses a strong antioxidant capacity to honey [192, 193].

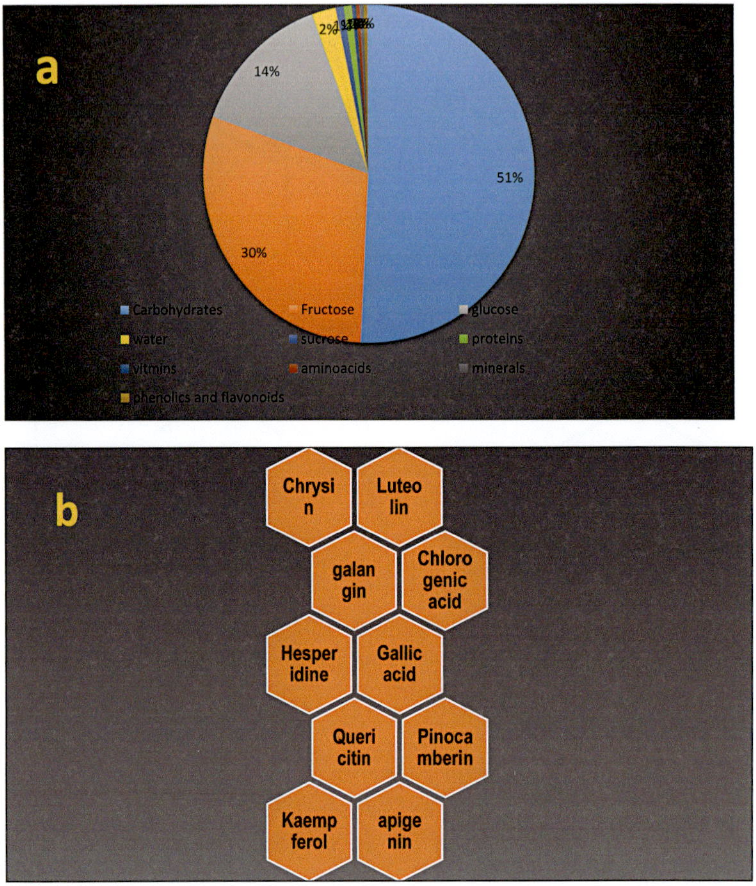

FIGURE 11.17 (a) General composition of honey; (b) flavonoids and phenolics of honey.
Source: Adapted from: Cianciosi et al. [190]; Al-Hatamleh et al. [191].

Honey is a proven biological suppressor of mitogen-activated protein kinase (MAPK) and nuclear factor-kappa B. These two moieties are responsible for the inflammation in the body. This can be controlled by using honey. It has been also reported that symptoms of COVID-19 may take 14 days to appear, and consumption of honey with other plant products during these initial days can reduce the severity of the COVID-19 attack. Honey is also known to increase the bacterial sensitivity for different drugs. Therefore, honey may also be suggested to reduce the post-COVID infection complexities [194].

Clinical trial of honey against COVID-19 is already in progress [195]. Furthermore, honey can increase the level of T and B lymphocytes (B cells) to fight the infection. It can reduce the blood cholesterol. Propolis, which is bee wax, which they form to protect their hives, is also rich in antioxidants and its liposomes have been prepared for targeted delivery inside the organism. Solid lipid nanoparticles have been also on the way to increase the efficiency of propolis, and it is suggested that these liposomes and nanoparticles will be helpful in treating the COVID-19 (Table 11.2) [196, 197].

11.9 COVID-19 AND LIFESTYLE

Common symptoms of COVID-19 are depicted in Figure 11.18. Whereas complexities include lymphopenia, pneumonia, acute lung injury, acute heart injury, RNAemia, and cytokine storm [162]. If this disease is controlled at the initial level, serious circumstances can be avoided.

It is worthwhile to mention here that the severity of this alarming disease can be reduced by improving the eating habits and life styles. A number of bioactive natural compounds discussed earlier may be a part of our regular diet. Therefore, plants containing these natural compounds can act as functional food for us.

These plants, when used as food, will not only increase our immunity but will also purify our internal system from products of infection and stress, like ROSs. So, prevention is always better than cure. This can be continued in treatment related to COVID-19 with the help of natural products. Research is needed in this part to formulate the daily recommended doses of these natural local foods as a therapy for COVID.

11.10 CONCLUSION

It is concluded here that plants and natural plant-based drugs have a proven and tested antiviral activities; therefore, having a great potential to work against COVID-19. There are a number of natural products which are already under clinical trials to check their efficacy to treat this contagious and fatal infection. Although production of a plant based natural drug is a time-consuming process, but it has a long-term effectiveness. They can also be considered as functional food parts and can be added to the daily food, thus treating the immune system of the body before and after the infection. Intense research is needed in this field to contribute towards the treatment of COVID-19 in this pandemic situation.

TABLE 11.2 Some Other Possible Antiviral Medicinal Plants Against COVID-19

SL. No.	Plant and Family	Active Component	Biological Activity/Active Against	Mechanism of Action of Extractor Natural Metabolite Isolated	References
1.	*Artemisia annua* L. Asteraceae	Flavonoid, quercetine, triterpenes, polyphenols, sterols, polysaccharides, saponins, dicaffeoylquinic acid	Dengue virus, hepatitis C, HIV, HSV1, human cytomegalovirus and poliovirus, RSV	Hinders the enzymatic activity of 3CLPro; to inhibit the enzymatic activity of 3CLPro	[198]
2.	*Aglaia odorata Meliaceae*	Flavaglines like aglain	Herpes simplex	Hinders proteases	[199]
3.	*Lycoris radiate* (L) Amaryllidaceae	Lycorine	Antiviral effects on Coxsackievirus Herpes simplex virus, Human immunodeficiency virus (HIV) and measles virus, Poliovirus, SARS-CoV	Inhibiting virus replication, preventing autophagy. Reduces the JNK phosphorylation, causes reduction in signaling and finally autophagy is stopped.	[198]
4.	*Sambucus nigra* L. *Caprifoliaceae*	Flavonoids, lectins, anthocyanin	Common cold, urinary tract edema, influenza, HSV-1, HIV, and other rheumatic diseases.	Block virus entry, controls the symptoms	[200, 201]
5.	*Salvia miltiorrhiza* Bunge *Lamiaceae*	Flavonoids, triterpenoids, lipophilic diterpenoids and hydrophilic phenolics	Thrombosis, removing blood stasis, other cardiovascular diseases, atherosclerosis, improving blood circulation, angina pectoris and antiviral activity of HIV-1	Can stop enzyme "RdRp" from doing its function and playing its role in viral replication	[202]
6.	*Eleutherococcus senticosus* (Rupr. and Maxim.) Maxim *Araliaceae*	Phenols, lignans, coumarins, phenylpropanoids, afzelin, anthocyanin, flavonoids, hyperin, kaempferol, phenolic acids, quercetin, rutin, triterpenic acids,	Altitude sickness, chronic coughing, diabetes, ischemic heart disease, neurodegenerative disorders, cancer, chronic fatigue	Inhibit replication of influenza virus	[203]

TABLE 11.2 *(Continued)*

SL. No.	Plant and Family	Active Component	Biological Activity/Active Against	Mechanism of Action of Extractor Natural Metabolite Isolated	References
7.	*Acacia arabica* (Lam.) Willd. *Fabaceae*	Steroidal sapogenin aglycone ascorbic acid, epicatechin-3-gallate, ferulic acid, flavonoids, CH_3-3,4,5-$(OH)_3C_6H_5$, isoferulic, myristic, oleic and palmitic acid, *para*-coumaroyl glucoside, *p*-coumaroylquinic acid, quercetin 3-O-(4′-O-acetyl)-rhamnopyranoside	H9N2 influenza disease, Newcastle disease, bursal disease virus, skin diseases	Extract of this plant inhibits the replication of viruses and their multiplication inside the host cells	[204]
8.	*Ocimum sanctum* L. *Lamiaceae*	Alkanoids, anthocyanins, tannins, flavonoids, saponins, phenols, and triterpenoids	Anxiety, arthritis, asthma, back pain, cardiac, cough, diarrhea, dysentery, eye disorders, fever, genitourinary disorders, H9N2 influenza disease, insect, and scorpion bites, malaria, otalgia	Extracts of this plant deter the Immunodeficiency Virus infection. And sometimes, they are also responsible for blocking/masking/hindering the non-definite interaction of host and viral parasite. They do so by preventing the action of glycoproteins like S proteins	[205]
9.	*Pelargonium sidoides* DC. *Geraniaceae*	Proanthocyanidins, methoxycoumarin, and prodelphinidins.	Membranous virus-like coronaviruses is specifically considered as very sensitive to extracts	Very effective and efficient in impeding the influenza virus to enter into host cell	[206]
10.	*Echinacea purpurea* *Asteraceae*	Alkylamides, caffeic acids and chicoric acids	Common colds and respiratory problems	Stimulate the release of numerous cytokines by macrophages. Macrophages are the cells which do not have the SARS COVID-19 receptors on their surface.	[207]

TABLE 11.2 *(Continued)*

SL. No.	Plant and Family	Active Component	Biological Activity/Active Against	Mechanism of Action of Extractor Natural Metabolite Isolated	References
11.	*Curcuma longa* Zingiberaceae	Curcumin	Antiviral, antimicrobial, anti-inflammatory, COVID related hypertension illness.	During hypertension, amount of angiotensin-converting enzyme (ACE) is increased in the blood. Curcumin acts as ACE inhibitor and also activates the homeostasis mechanism to control the enzyme amount (42, 44 45 of 3). But use of curcumin may also increase ACE 2.	[208–211]
12.	*Zingiber officinales* Zingiberaceae	Essential oils, zingiberene	Can treat dry cough, fever, wooziness (all phase 1 symptoms) and GI as well as lymphocytopenia, thrombocytopenia, and CRP-C reactive protein	Reduce viral load	[212, 213]
13.	*Isatis indigotica* Fortune *Cruciferae*	Aloe-emodin, Hesperetin, Indican, Indigo, Indirubin, Sinigrin, Beta-Sitosterol	Treatment of SARS-CoV-1-infected patients	It has inhibitory effects on 3CLpro, thereby inhibiting the entry and replication of the virus.	[214]

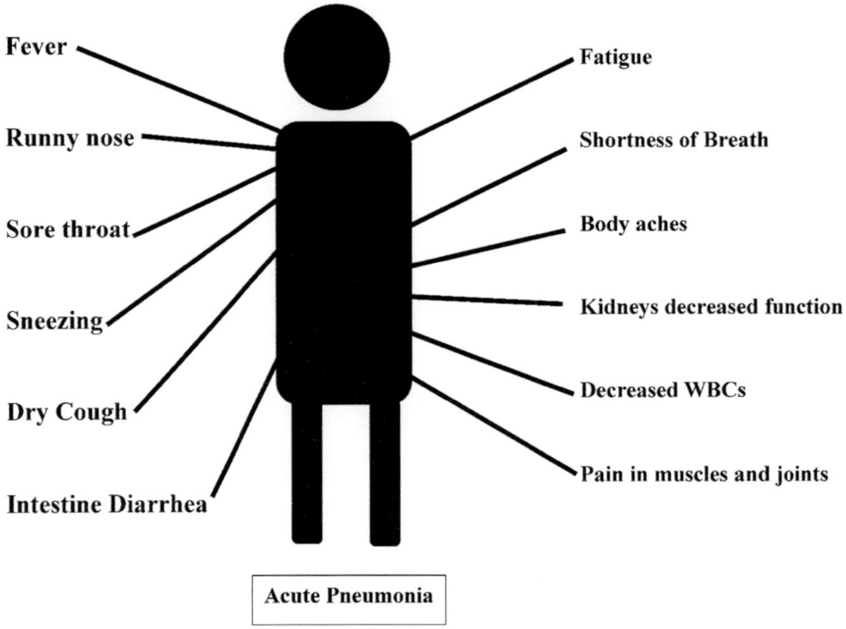

FIGURE 11.18 Symptoms of coronavirus infection.
Source: Adapted from: Huang et al. [162].

KEYWORDS

- **COVID-19**
- **curcumin**
- **mitogen-activated protein kinase**
- **natural products**
- **replication transcription complexes**
- **severe acute respiratory syndrome**

REFERENCES

1. Parul, S., Mangal, M., Singh, H., Gajendra, P., Raghava, S., Subhash, S., & Agarwal, M., (2020). Naturally occurring plant-based anticancer compound-activity-target database. *Nucleic Acids Research, 41*(1), 1124–1129.

2. Feher, M., & Schmidt, J. M., (2003). Property distributions: Differences between drugs, natural products, and molecules from combinatorial chemistry. *Journal of Chemical Information and Computer Scientists, 43*, 218–227.
3. Koehn, F. E., & Carter, G. T., (2005). The evolving role of natural products in drug discovery. *Nature Reviews Drug Discovery*, 206–220.
4. Zhang, Q., Wang, Y., Qi, C., Shen, L., & Li, J., (2020). Clinical trial analysis of 2019-nCoV therapy registered in China. *Journal of Medical Virology, 92*, 540.
5. Kitazato, K., Wang, Y., & Kobayashi, N., (2007). Viral infectious disease and natural products with antiviral activity. *Drug Discovery and Therapeutics, 1*(1), 14–22.
6. Jahan, I., & Onay, A., (2020). Potentials of plant-based substance to inhabit and probable cure for the COVID-19. *Turkish Journal of Biology, 44*(3), 228.
7. Richman, D. D., (2006). The impact of drug resistance on the effectiveness of chemotherapy for chronic hepatitis B. *Hepatology, 32*, 866–867.
8. Yin, C., De-Clercq, E., & Neyts, J., (2006). Lamivudine, adefovir and tenofovir exhibit long-lasting anti-hepatitis B virus activity in cell culture. *Journal of Viral Hepatitis, 7*, 79–83.
9. Shafer, R. W., Haas, D. W., & Smeaton, L. M., (2009). Pharmacogenetics of long-term responses to antiretroviral regimens containing efavirenz and/or nelfinavir: An adult aids clinical trials group study. *Journal of Infectious Diseases, 192*, 1931–1942.
10. Stoian, A. P., Toth, P. P., Kempler, P., & Rizzo, M., (2020). Gender differences in the battle against COVID-19: Impact of genetics, comorbidities, inflammation and life style on differences in outcomes. *International Journal of Clinical Practice*. doi.org/10.1111/ijcp.13666.
11. Almeida, B. P. G., (2020). the key role of zinc in elderly immunity: A possible approach in COVID-19? *Brazilian Journal of Nutrition, 38*, 65–66.
12. Gasmi, A., Chirumbolo, S., Peana, M., Noor, S., Menzel, A., Dadar, M., & Bjorklund, G., (2021). The role of diet and supplementation of natural products in COVID-19 prevention. *Biological Tree Element Research*. doi.org/10.1007/s12011-021-02623-3.
13. Boopathi, S., Poma, A. B., & Kolandaivel, P., (2020). Novel 2019 coronavirus structure, mechanism of action, antiviral drug promises and rule out against its treatment. *Journal of Biomolecular Structure and Dynamics*. doi: 10.1080/07391102.2020.1758788.
14. Lu, W., Zheng, B. J., Xu, K., Schwarz, W., Du, L., Wong, C. K., Chen, J., et al., (2020). Severe acute respiratory syndrome-associated coronavirus 3a protein forms an ion channel and modulates virus release. *Proceedings of Natural Academy of Sciences USA, 103*, 12540–12545.
15. Zhou, H. Q., Song, H. D., Tu, C. C., Zhang, G. W., Wang, S. Y., Zheng, K., Lei, L. C., et al., (2020). Cross-host evolution of severe acute respiratory syndrome coronavirus in palm civet and human. *Proceedings of National Academy of Sciences, USA, 102*, 2430–2435.
16. Coutard, B., Valle, C., De- Lamballerie, X., Canard, B., Seidah, N., & Decroly, E., (2020). The spike glycoprotein of the new coronavirus 2019-nCoV contains a furin-like cleavage site absent in CoV of the same clade. *Antiviral Research, 176*, 104742.
17. Ren, W. W., Wang, Y. M., Wu, Z. Q., Xiang, Z. C., Guo, L., Xu, T., et al., (2020). Identification of a novel coronavirus causing severe pneumonia in human: A descriptive study. *Chinese Medical Journal, 133*(9), 1015–1024.
18. Moriyana, M., Hugentobler, W. J., & IwasakI, A., (2010). Seasonality of respiratory viral infections. *Annual Reviews of Virology, 7*, 83–101.

19. Lai, S. T., Peiris, J. S., Poon, L. L., Guan, Y., & Yam, L. Y., (2007). Coronavirus as a possible cause of severe acute respiratory syndrome. *Lancet, 361*, 1319–1325.
20. Letko, M., Marzi, A., & Munster, V., (2020). Functional assessment of cell entry and receptor usage for SARS-CoV-2 and other lineage B beta coronaviruses. *Natural Microbiology, 5*, 562–569.
21. Oyston, P., & Robinson, K., (2012). The current challenges for vaccine development. *Journal of Medical Microbiology, 61*, 889.
22. Ghildiyal, R., Prakash, V., Chaudhary, V. K., Gupta, V., & Gabrani, R., (2020). Phytochemicals as antiviral agents: Recent updates. *Plant-Derived Bioactives, 12*, 279.
23. Qamar, M. T., Alqahtani, S. M., Alamri, M. A., & Chen, L. L., (2020). Structural basis of SARS-CoV-2 3CLpro and anti-COVID-19 drug discovery from medicinal plants. *Journal of Pharmaceutical Analysis, 26*.
24. Akindele, A. J., Agunbiade, F. O., Sofidiya, M. O., Awodele, O., Sowemimo, A., Ade-Ademilua, O., et al., (2020). COVID-19 pandemic: A case for phytomedicines. *Natural Product Communications, 15*(8), 1–9.
25. Akhtar, I., Javad, S., Yousaf, Z., Iqbal, S., & Jabeen, K., (2019). Review: Microwave assisted extraction of phytochemicals is an efficient and modern approach for botanicals and pharmaceuticals. *Pakistan Journal Pharmaceutical Science, 32*(1), 223–230.
26. Siddiqui, M. H., Al-Whaibi, M. H., Faisal, M., & Al- Sahli, A. A., (2014). Nano-silicon dioxide mitigates the adverse effects of salt stress on *Cucurbita pepo* L. *Environmental Toxicology and Chemistry, 33*(11), 2429–2437.
27. Klayman, D. L., (1985). Qinghaosu (Artemisinin): An antimalarial drug from China. *Science, 228*, 1049–1055.
28. Kumar, A., Singh, A., & Aggarwal, A., (2017). Therapeutic potential of herbal drugs for Alzheimer's disease: An overview. *Indian Journal of Experimental Biology, 55*, 63–73.
29. Zhao, P., & Astruc, D., (2012). Docetaxel nanotechnology in anticancer therapy. *ChemMedChem*, *7*(6), 952–972.
30. Safa, O., Hassaniazad, M., Farashahinejad, M., Davoodian, P., Dadvand, H., Hassanipour, S., & Fatalipour, M., (2020). Effects of ginger on clinical manifestations and paraclinical features of patients with severe acute respiratory syndrome due to COVID-19: A structured summary of a study protocol for a randomized controlled trial. *Trials, 21*, 841.
31. Kingston, D. G. I., Samranayake, G., & Ivey, C. A., (1990). The chemistry of taxol, a clinically useful anticancer agent. *Journal of Natural Product, 53*(1), 1–12.
32. Kubinec, R., Blasko, J., Galbava, P., Jurdakova, H., Sadecka, J., Pngallo, D., Buckova, M., & Puskarova, A., (2020). The antifungal activity of vapor phase of odorless thymol derivative. *Peer Journal, 8*. doi.org/10.7717/peerj.9601.
33. Ogle, N., (2009). Green tea *Camellia sinensis. Australian Journal of Medical Herbalism, 21*(2), 44–48.
34. Twomey, J. D., Luo, S., Dean, A. Q., Bozza, W. P., Nalli, A., & Zhang, B., (2020). COVID-19 update: The race to therapeutic development. *Drug Resistance, 53*, 100733.
35. Chilamakuri, R., & Agarwal, S., (2021). COVID-19: Characteristics and therapeutics. *Cells, 10*, 206.
36. Cragg, G. M., & Newman, D. J., (2005). Plants as a source of anticancer agents. *Journal of Ethnopharmacology, 100*(1, 2), 72–79.
37. Cragg, G. M., & Newman, D. J., (2013). Natural Products: A continuing source of novel drug leads. *Biochimica Biophysica Acta, 1830*(6), 3670–3695.

38. Borchardt, J. K., (2002). The beginnings of drug therapy: Ancient Mesopotamian medicine. *Drug News Perspectives, 15*, 187–192.
39. Unschuld, P. U., (1986). *Medicine in China: A History of Pharmaceutics*. University of California Press.
40. Patwardhan, B., (2005). Ethnopharmacology and drug discovery. *Journal Ethnopharmacology, 100,* 50–52.
41. Sneader, W., (2005). Drugs originating from the screening of dyes. *Drug Discovery*. 10.1002/0470015535.ch27.
42. Atanasov, A. G., Wang, J. N., Gu, S. P., Bu, J., Kramer, M. P., & Baumgartner, L., (2015). Honokiol: A non-adipogenic PPARgamma agonist from nature. *Biochimica Biophysica Acta, 1830,* 4813–4819.
43. Dias, A., Uzuner, H., Bauer, R., Fan, T. P., & El-Nezami, H., (2012). Traditional Chinese medicine research in the post-genomic era: Good practice, priorities, challenges and opportunities. *Journal of Ethnopharmacology, 140*, 458–468.
44. Felter, W. H., & Lloyd, J. U., (1898). *King's American Dispensatory*. Ohio Valley Co, Cincinnati.
45. Kaiser, H., (2008). Von der Pflanze zur Chemie Die Frühgeschichte der "Rheumamittel" *Z. Rheumatology*, 67: 252–262.
46. Baker, D. W., Chu, M., Oza, U., & Rajgarhia, V., (2007). The value of natural products to future pharmaceutical discovery. *Natural Product Research*, 24, 1225–1244.
47. Verpoorte, R., Choi, Y. H., & Kim, H. K., (2005). Ethnopharmacology and systems biology: A perfect holistic match. *Journal of Ethnopharmacology, 100*, 53–56.
48. Sahoo, M., Jena, L., Rath, S. N., & Kumar, S., (2016). Identification of suitable natural inhibitor against influenza A (H_1N_1) neuraminidase protein by molecular docking. *Genomics & Informatics, 14*(3), 96–103.
49. Muraoka, K., Yoshida, S., Hasegawa, K., Nakanishi, N., Fukuzawa, I., Tomita, A., & Cyong, J. C., (2004). A pharmacologic study on the mechanism of action of *Kakkon-to*: Body temperature elevation and phagocytic activation of macrophages in dogs. *The Journal of Alternative and Complementary Medicine, 10*(5).
50. Eng, Y. E., Lee, C. H., Lee, W. C., Huang, C. C., & Chang, J. S., (2019). Unraveling the molecular mechanism of traditional Chinese medicine: Formulas against acute airway viral infections as examples. *Molecules, 24*(19), 10.3390/molecules24193505.
51. Biancardi, E., Fennell, M., Rawlinson, W., & Thomas, P. S., (2016). Viruses are frequently present as the infecting agent in acute exacerbations of chronic obstructive pulmonary disease in patients presenting to hospital. *International Medicinal Journal, 46*(10), 1160–1165.
52. Xian, Y., Zhang, J., Bian, Z., Zhou, H., Zhang, Z., lin, Z., & Xu, H., (2020). Bioactive natural compounds against human coronaviruses: A review and perspective. *Acta Pharmaceutica Sinica B, 10*(7), 1163–1174.
53. Maurya, V. K., Kumar, S., Prasad, A. K., Bhatt, M. L. B., & Saxena, S. K., (2020). Structure-based drug designing for potential antiviral activity of selected natural products from Ayurveda against SARS-CoV-2 spike glycoprotein and its cellular receptor. *Virus disease, 31*, 179–193.
54. Kim, H. E., Kim, H. J., & Chang, J., (2019). Superior immune responses induced by intranasal immunization with recombinant adenovirus-based vaccine expressing full-length SPIKE protein of Middle East respiratory syndrome coronavirus. *PLoS One, 14*(7).

55. Liang, X., & Li, Z. Y., (2010). Ion channels as antivirus targets. *Virologica Sinica, 25*, 267–280.
56. Park, H. R., Yoon, H., Kim, M. K., et al., (2012). Synthesis and antiviral evaluation of 7-O-arylmethylquercetin derivatives against SARS-associated coronavirus (SCV) and hepatitis C virus (HCV). *Archives of Pharmacological Research, 35*, 77–85. https://doi.org/10.1007/s1227 2-012-0108-9.
57. Macchiagodena, M., Pagliai, M., & Procacci, P., (2020). *Inhibition of the Main Protease 3CLPro of the Corona Virus Disease 19 via Structure-Based Design and Molecular Modeling*. Available at https://arxiv.org/pdf/2002.09937.pdf (accessed on 6 August 2021).
58. Mandal, A., Jha, A. K., & Hazra, B., (2021). Plant products as inhibitors of coronavirus 3CL protease. *Frontiers in Pharmacology*. doi: 10.3389/fphar.2021.583387.
59. Ding, Z. Y., Wang, Y. H., Huang, Y. C., Lee, M. C., Tseng, M. J., Chi, Y. H., & Huang, M. L., (2017). Outer nuclear membrane protein kuduk modulates the LINC complex and nuclear envelope architecture. *Journal of Cell Biology*, (9), 2827–2841.
60. Tian, B., & Liu, J., (2020). Resveratrol: A review of plant sources, synthesis, stability, modification and food application. *Journal of Science of Food and Agriculture, 100*(4), 1392–1404.
61. Habib, P. T., Ayad, M. S., & Hassanein, S. E., (2020). *In Silico Analysis of 716 Natural Bioactive Molecules from Atlantic Ocean Reveals Candidate Molecule to Inhibit Spike Protein*. Research Square Preprint. doi.org/10.21203/rs.3.rs-156623/v1.
62. White, K. M., Rosales, R., Yildiz, S., Kehrer, T., Miorin, L., Moreno, E., Jangra, S., Uccellini, M. B., Rathnasinghe, R., Coughlan, L., et al., (2021). Plitidepsin has a potent preclinical efficacy against SARS-CoV-2 by targeting the host protein eEF1A. *Science*. In press.
63. Parthasarathy, K., Ng, L., Lin, X., Liu, D. X., Pervushin, K., Gong, X., et al., (2008). Structural flexibility of the pentameric SARS coronavirus envelope protein ion channel. *Biophysics Journal*, *95*(6), L39–L41.
64. Tanner, J. A., Zheng, B. J., Zhou, J., Watt, R. M., Wong, K. L., et al., (2005). The admantane derived bananins are potent inhibitors of the helicase activities and replication of SARS coronavirus. *Chemical Biology, 12*, 303–311.
65. Hoffmann, M., Kleine-Weber, H., Schroeder, S., Kruger, N., Herrler, T., Erichsen, S., et al., (2020). SARS-CoV-2 cell entry depends on ACE2 and TMPRSS2 and is blocked by a clinically proven protease inhibitor. *Cell, 181*, 271–280.
66. Rahman, N., Basharat, Z., Yousuf, M., Castaldo, G., Rastrelli, L., & Khan, H., (2020). Virtual screening of natural products against type II transmembrane serine protease (TMPRSS@), the priming agent of coronavirus 2 (SARS-CoV-2). *Molecules, 25*(10), 2271.
67. Yu, M. Y., Lee, J., Lee, J. M., Kim, Y., Chin, Y. W., Jee, J. G., Keum, Y. S., & Jeong, Y. J., (2015). Identification of myricetin and scutellarein as novel chemical inhibitors of the SARS coronavirus helicase, nsP13. *Bioorganic and Medical Chemistry Letters, 22*(12), 4049–4054.
68. Ou-Yang, S. S., Lu, J. Y., Kong, X. Q., Liang, Z. J., Luo, C., & Jiang, H., (2012). Computational drug discovery. *Acta Pharmacologica Sinica, 33*, 1131–1140.
69. Pech-Puch, D., Perez, P. M., Lenis, R. O. A., Rodriguez, J., & Jimenez, C., (2020). Marine natural products from the Yucatan peninsula. *Marine Drugs, 18*, 59.

70. Si, Y., Xu, X., Hu, Y., Si, H., & Zhai, H., (2021). Novel quantitative structure-activity relationship model to predict activities of natural products against COVID-19. *Chemical Biology and Drug Design, 97*, 978–983.
71. Heidary, F., Varnaseri, M., & Gharebaghi, R., (2020). The potential use of Persian herbal medicines against COVID-19 through angiotensin-converting enzyme. *Archives of Clinical Infections and Diseases, 15*.
72. Ziai, S. A., Heidari, M. R., Amin, G. H., Koochemeshki, A., & Heidari, M., (2009). Inhibitory effects of germinal angiotensin-converting enzyme by medicinal plants used in Iranian traditional medicine as antihypertensive. *Journal of Kerman University of Medical Sciences, 16*, 134.
73. Dethier, B., Hanon, E., Maayoufi, S., et al., (2013). Optimization of the formation of vinyl dithiins, therapeutic compounds from garlic. *European Food Research and Technology, 237*, 83–88.
74. Yousefi, H., Mashouri, L., Okpechi, S. C., Alahari, N., & Alahari, S. K., (2021). Repurposing existing drugs for the treatment of COVID-19/SARS-CoV-2 infection: A review describing drug mechanisms of action. *Biochemistry and Pharmacology, 183*, 114296.
75. National Center for Biotechnology Information, (2021). *PubChem Compound Summary for CID 27503, Cromolyn Sodium*. Retrieved from: https://pubchem.ncbi.nlm.nih.gov/compound/Cromolyn-sodium (accessed on 6 August 2021).
76. Cheng, P. W., Ng, L. T., Chiang, L. C., & Lin, C. C., (2006). Antiviral effects of saikosaponins on human coronavirus 229E *in vitro*. *Clinical and Experimental Pharmacology & Physiology, 33* (7), 612–616. doi: 10.1111/j.1440-1681.2006.04415.
77. National Center for Biotechnology Information, (2021). *PubChem Compound Summary for CID 27503, Cromolyn Sodium*. Retrieved from: https://pubchem.ncbi.nlm.nih.gov/compound/Cromolyn-sodium (accessed on 6 August 2021).
78. Oliveira, A., Prince, D., Lo, C. Y., Lee, L. H., & Chu, T. C., (2015). Antiviral activity of theaflavin digallate against herpes simplex virus type 1. *Antiviral Research, 118*, 56–67.
79. Yang, Z. F., Bai, L. P., Huang, W., Li, X. Z., Zhao, S. S., Zhong, N. S., & Jiang, Z. H., (2014). Comparison of in vitro antiviral activity of tea phenols against influenza A and B viruses and structure-activity relationship analysis. *Fitoterapia*, *93*, 47–53.
80. Jang, M., Park, Y. I., Cha, Y. E., Namkoong, S., Lee, J. I., & Park, J., (2020). Tea polyphenols EGCC and theaflavin inhibit the activity of SARS-CoV-2 3CLprotaese *in vitro. Evidence-Based Complimentary and Alternative Medicine*, 5620838.
81. Mhatre, S., Naik, S., & Patravale, V., (2021). A molecular docking study of EGCG and theaflavin digallate targets of SARS-CoV-2. *Computers in Biology and Medicine, 129*, 104137.
82. Maiti, S., & Banerjee, A., (2020). SARS-CoV-2 spike protein central channel with reference to the hydroxychloroquinone interaction: Bioinformatics and molecular docking study. *Drug Development Research, 82*(1), 86–95.
83. Sun, Y., Zhang, H., Sun, Y., Zhang, Y., Liu, H., Cheng, J., Bi, S., & Zhang, H., (2009). Study of interaction between protein and main active components in *Citrus auritium* L. by optical spectroscopy. *Journal of Luminescence*, *130*, 270–279.
84. Choi, H. J., Song, J. H., Park, K. S., & Kwon, D. H., (2009). Inhibitory effects of quercetin 3-rhamnoside on influenza A virus. *European Journal of Pharmaceutical Sciences, 37*, 329–333.
85. Wu, C., Liu, Y., Yang, Y., Zhang, P., Wang, Y., et al., (2020). Analysis of therapeutic targets from SARS-CoV-2 and discovery of potential drugs by computational methods. *Acta Pharm. Sinica B, 10*, 766–788.

86. Ansari, W. A., Ahamad, T., Khan, M. A., Khan, Z. A., & Khan, M. F., (2021). *Luteolin: A Dietary Molecule as Potential anti COVID-19 Agent.* Research Square Preprint, doi.org/10.21203/rs.3.rs-35368/v1.
87. Rojas, A., Del, C. J., Clement, S., et al., (2016). Effect of quercetin on hepatitis C virus life cycle: From viral to host targets. *Scientific Reports*, *6*, 31777.
88. Shinozuka, K., Kikuchi, Y., Nishino, C., Mori, A., & Tawata, S., (1988). Inhibitory effect of flavonoids on DNA dependent DNA and RNA polymerases. *Experientia*, *44*, 882–885.
89. Bachmetov, L., Gal, T. M., Shapira, A., Vorobeychik, M., Galam, G. T., Sathiyamoorthy, P., et al., (2012). suppression of hepatitis C virus by the flavonoid quercetin is mediated by inhibition of NS3 protease activity. *Journal of Viral Hepatitis, 19*, e81–88.
90. Spedding, G., Ratty, A., & Middleton, E. J., (1989). Inhibition of reverse transcriptase by flavonoids. *Antiviral Research*, *12*, 99–110.
91. Cushnie, T. P., & Lamb, A. J., (2005). Antimicrobial activity of flavonoids. *International Journal of Antimicrobial Agents, 26*, 343–356.
92. Castillo, M. H., Perkins, J. H., Doerr, R., Hassett, J. M., et al., (1989). the effects of the bioflavonoid quercetin on squamous cell carcinoma of head and neck region. *American Journal of Surgery, 158*, 351–355.
93. Biancatelli, R. M. L. C., Berrill, M., Catravas, J. D., & Marik, P. E., (2020). Quercetin and vitamin C: An experimental, synergistic therapy for the prevention and treatment of SARS-CoV-2 related disease (COVID-19). *Frontiers in Immunology*. doi: 10.3389/fimmu.2020.01451.
94. Boots, A. W., Kubben, N., Haenen, G. R., & Bast, A., (2003). Oxidized quercetin reacts with thiols rather than with ascorbate: Implication for quercetin supplementation. *Biochemical and Biophysical Research Communications, 308*, 560–565.
95. Bors, W., Michel, C., & Schikora, S., (2005). Interaction of flavonoids with ascorbate and determination of their univalent redox potentials: A pulse radiolysis study. *Free Radical Biology and Medicine, 19*, 45–52.
96. Awad, H. M., Boersma, M. G., Boeren, S., Van, D. W. H., Van, Z. J., Van, B. P. J., et al., (2002). Identification of o-quinone/quinone methide metabolites of quercetin in a cellular in vitro system. *FEBS Letters, 520*, 30–34.
97. Carr, A. C., & Maggini, S., (2017). Vitamin C and immune functions. *Nutrients, 9*, 1211.
98. Leibovitz, B., & Siegel, B. V., (1981). Ascorbic acid and immune response. *Advances in Experimental and Medicinal Biology, 135*, 1–25.
99. Dey, S., & Bishayi, B., (2018). Killing of *S. aureus* in murine peritoneal macrophages by ascorbic acid along with antibiotics chloramphenicol or ofloxacin: Correlation with inflammation. *Microbiology of Pathogens, 115*, 239–250.
100. Furuya, A., Uozaki, M., Yamasaki, H., Arakawa, T., & Arita, K. M. A. H., (2008). Antiviral effects of ascorbic and dehydroascorbic acids in vitro. *International Journal of Molecular Medicines, 8*, 167.
101. Fowler, A. A., Truwit, J. D., Hite, R. D., Morris, P. E., Dewilde, C., Priday, A., et al., (2019). Effect of vitamin C infusion on organ failure and biomarkers of inflammation and vascular injury in patients with sepsis and sever acute respiratory failure: The CITRIS-ALI randomized clinical trial. *JAMA, 322*, 1261–1270.
102. Kimbarowski, J. A., & Mokrow, N. J., (1967). Colored precipitation reaction of the urine according to kimbaroeski (FARK) as an index of ascorbic acid during treatment of viral influenza. *Das Deutsche Gesundheitswesen, 22*, 2413–2418.

103. Al-Zahrani, A. A., (2020). Rutin as a promising inhibitor of main protease and other protein targets of COVID-19: In silico study. *Natural Product Communications*. doi.org/10.1177/1934578X20953951.
104. Rahman, F., Tabrez, S., Ali, R., Alqahtani, A. S., Ahmed, M. Z., & Rub, A., (2021). Molecular docking analysis of rutin reveals possible inhibition of SARS-CoV-2 vital proteins. *Journal of Traditional and Complementary Medicines, 11*(2), 173–179.
105. Saha, S., Rajat, N., Poonam, V., Amresh, P., & Diwakar, K., (2021). Discovering potential RNA dependent RNA polymerase inhibitors as protective drug against COVID-19: As in silico approach. *Journal of Pharmacology*, 12. doi.org/10.3389/fphar.2021.634047.
106. Meneguzzo, F., Ciriminna, R., Zabini, F., & Pagliaro, M., (2020). Review of evidence available on hesperidin rich products as potential tools against COVID-19 and hydrodynamic based extraction as a method of increasing their production. *Processes, 8*, 549.
107. Kim, J., Wie, M. B., Ahn, M., Tanaka, A., Matsuda, H., & Shin, T., (2019). Benefits of hesperidin in central nervous system disorders: A review. *Anatomy and Cell Biology, 52*(4), 369–377.
108. Salehi, B., Fokou, P. V. T., Sharifi-Rad, M., et al., (2019). Therapeutic potential of naringenin: A review of clinical trials. *Pharmaceuticals, 12*(1), 11. Basel.
109. Ganeshpurkar, A., & Saluja, A. K., (2017). The pharmacological potential of rutin. *Saudi Pharmaceutical Journal, 25*(2), 149–164.
110. National Center for Biotechnology Information, (2021). PubChem Compound Summary for CID 54670067. *Ascorbic Acid*. Retrieved from: https://pubchem.ncbi.nlm.nih.gov/compound/Ascorbic-acid (accessed on 6 August 2021).
111. National Center for Biotechnology Information, (2021). PubChem Compound Summary for CID 440917. *D-Limonene*. Retrieved from: https://pubchem.ncbi.nlm.nih.gov/compound/D-Limonene (accessed on 6 August 2021).
112. Vordenbaumen, S., Sander, O., Bleck, E., et al., (2012). Cardiovascular disease and serum defensin levels in systemic lupus erythematosus. *Clinical and Experimental Rheumatology, 30*, 364–370.
113. Biswas, S., Thakur, V., Kaur, P., Khan, A., Kulshrestha, S., & Kumar, P., (2021). Blood clots in COVID-19 patients: Simplifying the curious mystery. *Medicinal Hypotheses, 146*. doi: 10.1016/j.mehy.2020.110371.
114. Qin, C., Zhou, L., Hu, Z., et al., (2020). Dysregulation of immune response in patients with coronavirus 2019 (COVID-19) in Wuhan, China. *Clinical Infections and Diseases, 71*, 762–768.
115. Belkaid, Y., & Rouse, B. T., (2005). Natural regulatory T cells in infectious disease. *Natural Immunology, 6*, 353–360.
116. Cronstein, B. N., Molad, Y., Reibman, J., et al., (1995). Colchicine alters the quantitative and qualitative display of selectins on endothelial cells and neutrophils. *Journal of Clinical Investigation, 96*, 994–1002.
117. Martinon, F., Pétrilli, V., Mayor, A., et al., (2006). Gout-associated uric acid crystals activate the NALP3 inflammasome. *Nature, 440*, 237–241.
118. Martinez, G. J., Celermajer, D. S., & Patel, S., (2018). The NLRP3 inflammasome and the emerging role of colchicine to inhibit atherosclerosis-associated inflammation. *Atherosclerosis, 269*, 262–271.
119. Reyes, A. Z., Hu, K. A., Teperman, J., Muskardin, T. L. W., Taradif, J. C., Shah, B., & Pillinger, M. H., (2020). Anti-inflammatory therapy for COVID-19 infection: The case for colchicine. *Annals of the Rheumatic Diseases*. doi: 10.1136/annrheumdis-2020-219174.

120. Zhou, Y., Xie, M., Song, Y., Wang, W., Zhao, H., Tian, Y., & She, G., (2016). Two traditional Chinese medicines *Curcumae radix* and *Curcumae Rhizoma*: An ethnopharmacology, phytochemistry, and pharmacology review. *Evidence-Based Complementary and Alternative Medicine*, 4973128. http://dx.doi.org/10.1155/2016/4973128.
121. Gupta, S. C., Patchva, S., & Aggarwal, B. B., (2013). Therapeutic roles of curcumin: Lessons learned from clinical trials. *AAPS Journal, 15*(1), 195–218. http://dx.doi.org/10.1208/s12248-012-9432-8.
122. Mathew, D., & Hsu, W. L., (2018). Antiviral potential of curcumin. *Journal of Functional Foods*, 40, 692–699.
123. Ravindran, J., Prasad, S., & Aggarwal, B. B., (2009). Curcumin and cancer cells: How many ways can curry kill tumor cells selectively? *AAPS Journal, 11*(3), 495–510. http://dx.doi.org/10.1208/s12248-009-9128-x.
124. Ingolfsson, H. I., Thakur, P., Herold, K. F., Hobart, E. A., Ramsey, N. B., Periole, X., & Andersen, O. S., (2014). Phytochemicals perturb membranes and promiscuously alter protein function. *ACS Chemical Biology, 9*(8), 1788–1798. http://dx.doi.org/10.1021/cb500086e.
125. Anggakusuma, C. C. C., Schang, L. M., Rachmawati, H., Frentzen, A., Pfaender, S., & Steinmann, E., (2014). Turmeric curcumin inhibits entry of all hepatitis C virus genotypes into human liver cells. *Gut., 63*(7), 1137–1149. http://dx.doi.org/10.1136/gutjnl-2012-304299.
126. Xu, F., Mu, X. L., & Zhao, J., (2009). Effects of curcumin on invasion and metastasis in the human cervical cancer cells caski. *Chinese Journal of Cancer Research, 21*(2), 159–162. http://dx.doi.org/10.1007/s11670-009-0159-8.
127. Kim, K., Kim, K. H., Kim, H. Y., Cho, H. K., Sakamoto, N., & Cheong, J., (2010). Curcumin inhibits hepatitis C virus replication via suppressing the Akt-SREBP-1 pathway. *FEBS Letters, 584*(4), 707–712. http://dx.doi.org/10.1016/j.febslet.2009.12.019.
128. Rechtman, M. M., HarNoy, O., BarYishay, I., Fishman, S., Adamovich, Y., Shaul, Y., & Shlomai, A., (2010). Curcumin inhibits hepatitis B virus via down-regulation of the metabolic coactivator PGC-1alpha. *FEBS Letters, 584*(11), 2485–2490. http://dx.doi.org/10.1016/j.febslet.2010.04.067.
129. Ahmed, J., Tan, Y., & Ambegaokar, S., (2017). Effects of curcumin on vesicular stomatitis virus (VSV) infection and dicer-1 expression. *The FASEB Journal, 31*(1), 622.11–622.11. Available at: https://faseb.onlinelibrary.wiley.com/doi/abs/10.1096/fasebj.31.1_supplement.622.11 (accessed on 24 August 2021).
130. Padilla, S. L., Rodriguez, A., Gonzales, M. M., Gallego, G. J., & Castano, O. J., (2014). Inhibitory effects of curcumin on dengue virus type 2-infected cells *in vitro*. *Archives of Virology, 159*(3), 573–579. http://dx.doi.org/10.1007/s00705-013-1849-6.
131. Cinatl, J., Morgenstern, B., Bauer, G., Chandra, P., Rabenau, H., & Doerr, H. W., (2003). Glycyrrhizin, an active component of liquorice roots, and replication of SARS-associated coronavirus. *Lancet, 361*, 2045, 2046. doi: 10.1016/S0140-6736(03)13615-X.
132. Hoever, G., Baltina, L., Michaelis, M., Kondratenko, R., Baltina, L., Tolstikov, G. A., et al., (2005). Antiviral activity of glycyrrhizic acid derivatives against SARS coronavirus. *Journal of Medicinal Chemistry, 48*, 1256–1259. doi: 10.1021/jm0493008.
133. Chen, H., & Du, Q., (2020). *Potential Natural Compounds for Preventing 2019-nCoV Infection*. Preprints, 2020-2020010358.
134. Luo, P., Liu, D., & Li, J., (2020). Pharmacological perspective: Glycyrrhizin may be as efficacious therapeutic agent for COVID-19. *International Journal of Antimicrobial Agents, 55*, 105995.

135. Tong, T., Hu, H., Zhou, J., Deng, S., Zhang, X., Tang, W., et al., (2020). Glycyrrhizic-acid-based carbon dots with high antiviral activity by multisite inhibition mechanisms. *Small, 16*(13), e1906206.
136. Bailly, C., & Vergoten, C., (2020). Glycyrrhizin: An alternative drug for the treatment of COVID-19 infection and the associated respiratory syndrome? *Pharmacology and Therapeutics, 214*, 107618.
137. Wang, P., Li, L. F., Wang, Q. Y., Shang, L. Q., Shi, P. Y., & Yin, Z., (2014). Anti dengue virus activity and structure –activity relationship studies of licorine derivatives. *ChemMedChem, 9*(7), 1522–1533.
138. Chen, H., Zizhao, L., Xu, J., Li, Z., Long, H., Li, D., Lin, L., et al., (2020). Antiviral activity of lycorine against zika virus in vivo and in vitro. *Virology, 546*, 88–97.
139. Hwang, Y. C., Chu, J. J., Yang, P. L., Chen, W., & Yates, M. V., (2008). Rapid identification of inhibitors that interfere with poliovirus replication using a cell based assay. *Antiviral Research, 77*, 232–236.
140. Renard, J. N., Kim, T., Imakura, Y., Kihara, M., & Kobayashi, S., (1989). Effect of alkaloids isolated from *Amaryllidaceae* on herpes simples virus. *Research in Virology, 140*, 115–128.
141. Li, S. Y., Chen, C., Zhang, H. Q., Guo, H. Y., Wanng, H., Wang, L., Zhang, X., et al., (2005). Identification of natural compounds with antiviral activities against SARS-associated coronavirus. *Antiviral Research, 67*, 18–23.
142. Zhang, Y. N., Zhang, Q. Y., Li, X. D., Xiong, J., Xiao, S. Q., Wang, Z., Zhang, Z. R., et al., (2020). Gemcitabine, lycorine and oxysophoridine inhibit novel coronavirus (SARS-CoV-2) in cell culture, *Emerging Microbes and Infections, 9*(1), 1170–1173.
143. Maiden, N. M. P., Prophetic medicine- *Nigella sativa* (black cumin seeds)- potential herb for COVID-19? *Journal of Pharmacopuncture, 23*(2), 62–70.
144. Ingraham, N. E., Lotfi-Emran, S., Thielen, B. K., Techar, K., Morris, R. S., Holtan, S. G., et al., (2020). Immunomodulation in COVID-19. *Lancet Respiratory Medicines*. S2213-2600(20)30226-5.
145. Khan, M. A., & Younas, H., (2020). Potential implications of black seed and its principal constituent thymoquinone in the treatment of COVID-19 patients. *Current Pharmaceutical Biotechnology*. https://doi.org/10.2174/1389201021999201110205048.
146. Salem, M. L., (2005). Immunomodulatory and therapeutic properties of the *Nigella sativa* L. seed. *International Immunopharmacology*, 5(13, 14), 1749–1770.
147. Boskabady, M. H., Mohsenpoor, N., & Takaloo, L., (2010). Antiasthmatic effect of *Nigella sativa* in airways of asthmatic patients. *Phytomedicine, 17*(10), 707–713.
148. Salem, A. M., Bamosa, A. O., Qutub, H. O., Gupta, R. K., Badar, A., Elnour, A., et al., (2017). Effect of *Nigella sativa* supplementation on lung function and inflammatory mediators in partly controlled asthma: A randomized controlled trial. *Annals of Saudi Medicine, 37*(1), 64–71.
149. Ansari, M. A., Ahmed, S. P., Haider, S. A., & Ansari, N. L., (2006). *Nigella sativa*: A non-conventional herbal option for the management of seasonal allergic rhinitis. *Pakistan Journal of Pharmacy, 23*(2), 31–35.
150. Salem, M. L., Alenzi, F. Q., & Attia, W. Y., (2011). Thymoquinone, the active ingredient of *Nigella sativa* seeds, enhances the survival and activity of antigen specific CD8-positive T cells *in vitro. Brazillian Journal of Biomedical Sciences, 68*(3), 131–137.
151. Kadil, Y., Mouhcine, M., & Filali, H., (2020). In silico investigation of the SARS CoV2 protease with thymoquinone, the major constituent of *Nigella Sativa. Current Drug Discovery Technologies, 17*, 1. https://doi.org/10.2174/1570163817666200712164406.

152. National Center for Biotechnology Information, (2021). PubChem Compound Summary for CID 10281, Thymoquinone. Retrieved from: https://pubchem.ncbi.nlm.nih.gov/compound/Thymoquinone (accessed on 6 August 2021).
153. Pirintsos, S. A., Bariotakis, M., Kampa, M., Sourvinos, G., Lionis, C., & Castanas, E., (2020). The therapeutic potential of the essential oil of *Thymbra capitata* (L.) cav., *Origanum dictamnus* L. and *Salvia fruticosa* mill. and a case of plant-based pharmaceutical development. *Frontiers in Pharmacology, 400*(11), 522213.
154. Duijker, G., Bertsias, A., Symvoulakis, E. K., Moschandreas, J., Malliaraki, N., Derdas, S. P., Tsikalas, G. K., et al., (2015). Reporting effectiveness of an extract of three traditional Cretan herbs on upper respiratory tract infection results from a double-blind randomized controlled trial. *Journal of Ethnopharmacology, 163*, 157–166.
155. Anastasaki, M., Bertsias, A., Pirintsos, S. A., Castanas, E., & Lionis, C., (2017). Post-market outcome of an 340 extract of traditional Cretan herbs on upper respiratory tract infections: A pragmatic, prospective 341 observational study. *BMC Complement Alternative Medicines, 17*, 466.
156. Tseliou, M., Pirintsos, S. A., Lionis, C., Castanas, E., & Sourvinos, G., (2019). Antiviral effect of an essential oil combination derived from three aromatic plants (*Coridothymus capitatus* (L.) Rchb. f., *Origanum dictamnus* L. and *Salvia fruticosa* Mill.) against viruses causing infections of the upper respiratory tract. *Journal of Herbal Medicine*, 17–18.
157. Ho, T. Y., Wu, S. L., Chen, J. C., Li, C. C., & Hsiang, C. Y., (2007). Emodin blocks the SARS coronavirus spike protein and angiotensin-converting enzyme 2 interaction. *Antiviral Research, 74*(2), 92–101.
158. Liu, Z., Ma, N., Zhong, Y., & Yang, Z. Q., (2015). Antiviral effect of emodin from *Rheum palmatum* against coxsackievirus B_5 and human respiratory syncytial virus *in vitro. Journal of Huazhong University of Science, Technology and Medical Sciences, 35*(6), 916–922.
159. Li, S. W., Yang, T. C., Lai, C. C., Huang, S. H., Liao, J. M., Wan, L., Lin, Y. J., & Lin, C. W., (2014). Antiviral activity of aloe-emodin against influenza A virus via galectin-3 up-regulation. *European Journal of Pharmacology, 5*, 125–132. doi: 10.1016/j.ejphar.2014.05.028.
160. Shuangsuo, D., Zhengguo, Z., Yunro, C., Xin, Z., Baofeng, W., Lichao, Y., & Yanan, C., (2006). Inhibition of the replication of hepatitis B virus *in vitro* by emodin. *Medical Science Monitor, 12*(9), BR302–306.
161. Xiong, H. R., Luo, J., Hou, W., Xiao, H., & Yang, Z. Q., (2011). The effect of emodin, an anthraquinone derivative extracted from the roots of *Rheum tanguticum,* against *Herpes simplex* virus *in vitro* and *in vivo. Journal of Ethnopharmacology, 133*(2), 718–723.
162. Huang, C., Wang, Y., Li, X., Ren, L., Zhao, J., Zhang, L., Zhang, L., Fan, G., Xu, J., Gu, X., Cheng, Z., Yu, T., Xia, J., et al., (2020). Clinical features of patients infected with 2019 novel coronavirus in Wuhan, China. *Lancet, 395*, 497–506.
163. Dabaghian, F., Khanavi, M., & Zarshenas, M. M., (2020). Bioactive compounds with possible inhibitory activity of angiotensin-converting enzyme-II; a gate to manage and prevent COVID-19. *Medical Hypotheses, 143*, 109841. doi: 10.1016/j.mehy.2020.109841.
164. Cong, Y., Ulasli, M., Schepers, H., Mauthe, M., V'kovski, P., Kriegenburg, F., Thiel, V., et al, (2020). Nucleocapsid protein recruitment to replication-transcription complexes plays a crucial role in coronaviral life cycle. *Journal of Virology, 94*, e-01919.
165. Gordon, D. E., Jang, G. M., Bouhaddou, M., Xu, J., Obernier, K., O'meara, M. J., Guo, J. Z., et al., (2020). *A SARS-CoV-2-Human Protein-Protein Interaction Map Reveals Drug Targets and Potential Drug-Repurposing*. BioRxiv. https://doi.org/10.1101/2020.03.22.002386.

166. Rolta, R., Yadav, R., Salaria, D., Trivedi, S., Imran, M., Sourirajan, A., Baumler, D. J., & Dev, K., (2020). *In silico* screening of hundred phytocompounds of ten medicinal plants as potential inhibitors of nucleocapsid phosphoproteins of COVID-19: An approach to prevent virus assembly. *Journal of Biomolecular Structure and Dynamics*. doi: 10.1080/07391102.2020.1804457.
167. Kaur, D., Kaur, J., & Kamal, S. S., (2019). Diacerein, its beneficial impact on chondrocytes and notable new clinical applications. *Brazilian Journal of Pharmaceutical Sciences, 54*(4), doi.org/10.1590/s2175-97902018000417534.
168. Oliveira, P. G., Termini, L., Durigon, E. L., Lepique, A. P., Sposito, A. C., & Boccardo, E., (2020). Diacerein: A potential multi-target therapeutic drug for COVID-19. *Medical Hypotheses, 144*, 109920.
169. Froese, N. T., & Van, A. R. C., (2003). Distribution and interference of dandelion (*Taraxacum* officinale) in spring canola. *Weed Science, 51*, 435–442.
170. DelValle, D. M., Kim-Schulze, S., Huang, H. H., Beckmann, N. D., Nirenberg, S., Wang, B., Lavin, Y., Swartz, T. H., Maddueri, D., & Stock, A., (2020). An inflammatory cytokine signature predicts COVID-19 severity and survival. *Nature Medicines, 26*, 1636–1643.
171. Rivero-Segura, N. A., & Gomez-Verjan, J. C., (2021). In silico screening of natural products isolated from Mexican herbal medicines against COVID-19. *Biomolecules 11*, 216–228.
172. Fan, W., Qian, S., Qian, P., & Li, X., (2016). Antiviral activity of luteolin against Japanese encephalitis virus. *Journal of Viruses Research, 220*, 112–116.
173. Yi, L., Yuan, K., Qu, X., Chen, J., Wang, G., Zhang, H., Luo, H., et al., (2004). Small molecules blocking the entry of severe acute respiratory syndrome coronavirus into host cells. *Journal of Virology, 78*(20), 11334–11339.
174. Chen, F., Chan, K. H., Jiang, Y., Kao, R. Y., Lu, H. T., Fan, K. W., Chang, V. C., et al, (2004). In vitro susceptibility of 10 clinical isolates of SARS coronavirus to selected antiviral compounds. *Journal of Clinical Virology, 31*, 69–75.
175. Wong, S. S. Y., & Yuen, K. Y., (2008). the management of coronavirus infections with particular reference to SARS. *Journal of Antimicrobial Chemotherapy, 61*, 437–441.
176. Lopez, L. M., (2009). Distribution and biological activities of the flavonoid luteolin. *Mini-Reviews in Medicinal Chemistry, 9*(1), 31–59.
177. Si, H., Wyeth, R. P., & Liu, D., (2014). The flavonoid luteolin induces nitric oxide production and arterial relaxation. *European Journal of Nutrition, 53*(1), 269–275.
178. Shawan, M. M. A. K., Halder, S. K., & Hasan, M. A., (2021). Luteolin and abyssinone II as potential inhibitors of SARS-CoV-2: An in silico molecular modeling approach in batteling the COVID-19 outbreak. *Bulletin of National Research Center, 45*(1), 27.
179. Kowalczyk, A., Przychodna, M., Sopata, S., Bodalska, A., & Fecka, I., (2020). Thymol and thyme essential oil-new insights into selected therapeutic applications. *Molecules, 25*, 4125. doi: 10.3390/molecules25184125.
180. Nilima, T., Silpi, B., Rakesh, N. B., & Monali, R., (2013). Antimicrobial efficacy of five essential oils against oral pathogens: An *in vitro* study. *European Journal of Dentistry, 7*, 71–77.
181. Nabissi, M., Marinelli, O., Morelli, M. B., et al., (2018). Thyme extract increases mucociliary-beating frequency in primary cell lines from chronic obstructive pulmonary disease patients. *Biomedicine Pharmacotherapy, 105*, 1248–1253. doi: 10.1016/j.biopha.2018.06.004.

182. Kordali, S. K. R., Mavi, A., Cakir, A., Ala, A., & Yildirim, A., (2005). Determination of the chemical composition and antioxidant activity of the essential oil of *Artemisia dracunculus* and of the antifungal and antibacterial activities of Turkish *Artemisia absinthium*. *Journal of Agriculture and Food Chemistry, 53*(24), 9452–9458. doi: 10.1021/jf0516538.
183. Buechi, S., Vögelin, R., VonEiff, M. M., Ramos, M., & Melzer, J. J. C. M. R., (2005). Open trial to assess aspects of safety and efficacy of a combined herbal cough syrup with ivy and thyme. *Complementary Medicine Research, 12*(6), 328–332.doi: 10.1159/ 000088934.
184. Sardari, S., Mobaien, A., Ghassemifard, L., Kamali, K., & Khavasi, N., (2021). Therapeutic effect of thyme (*Thymus vulgaris*) essential oil on patients with COVID-19: A randomized clinical trial. *Journal of Advances in Medical and Biomedical Research, 29*(133), 83–91.
185. Walls, A. C., Park, Y. J., Tortorici, M. A., Wall, A., McGuire, A. T., & Veesler, D., (2020). Structure-function and antigenicity of the SARS-CoV-2 spike glycoprotein. *Cell, 181*, 281–292.
186. Kulkarni, S. A., Nagarajan, S. K., Ramesh, V., Palaniyandi, V., Selvam, S. P., & Madhavan, T., (2020). Computational evaluation of major components from plant essential oils as potent inhibitors of SARS-CoV-2 spike protein. *Journal of Molecular Structure, 1221*, 128823.
187. Zhang, Y., & Kutateladze, T. G., (2020). Molecular structure analyses suggest strategies to therapeutically target SARS-CoV-2. *Nature Communications, 11*, 2920.
188. Sulaiman, S. A., Hasan, H., Deris, Z. Z., Wahad, M. S. A., Yusof, R. C., Naing, N. N., et al., (2011). The benefit of Tualang honey in reducing acute respiratory symptoms among Malaysian hajj pilgrims: A preliminary study. *Journal of ApiProduct ApiMedicinal Science, 3*(1), 38–44.
189. Al-Waili, N. S., (2003). Effects of daily consumption of honey solution on hematological indices and blood levels of minerals and enzymes in normal individuals. *Journal of Medicinal Food, 6*(2), 135–140.
190. Cianciosi, D., Forbes-Hernandez, T. Y., Afrin, S., Gasparrini, M., Reboredo-Rodriguez, P., Manna, P. P., & Zhang, J., Bravo, L. L., Martinez, F. S., Agudo, T. P., et al., (2018). Phenolic compounds in honey and their associated health benefits: A review. *Molecules, 23*, 2322.
191. Al-Hatamleh, M. A. I., Boer, J. C., Wilson, K. L., Plebanski, M., Mohamud, R., & Mustafa, M. Z., (2020). Antioxidant-based medicinal properties of stingless bee products: Recent progress and future directions. *Biomolecules, 10*, 923.
192. Ahmed, S., Sulaiman, S. A., Baig, A. A., Ibrahim, M., Liaqat, S., Fatima, S., et al., (2018). Honey as a potential natural antioxidant medicine: An insight into its molecular mechanisms of action. *Oxidative Medicine and Cellular Longevity*, 8367846.
193. Kek, S. P., Chin, N. L., Yusof, Y. A., Tan, S. W., & Chua, L. S., (2014). Total phenolic contents and color intensity of Malaysian honeys from the *Apis* spp. and *Trigona* spp. bees. *Agriculture and Agricultural Science Procedia, 2*, 150–155.
194. Zandi, K., Teoh, B. T., Sam, S. S., Wong, P. F., & Mustafa, M. R., (2011). In vitro antiviral activity of fisetin, rutin and naringenin against dengue virus type 2. *Journal of Medicinal Plant Research, 5*(23), 5534–5539.
195. Tantaway, M. A., (2020). *Efficacy of Honey Treatments in Patients with Novel Coronavirus*. Clinical Trial. Gov. Identifier NCT04323345.
196. Mani, R., & Natesan, V., (2018). Chrysin: Sources, beneficial pharmacological activities and molecular mechanism of action. *Phytochemistry, 145*, 187–196.

197. Refaat, H., Mady, F. M., Sarhan, A., Rateb, H. S., & Alaaeldin, E., (2021). Optimization and evaluation of propolis liposomes as a promising therapeutic approach for COVID-19. *International Journal of Pharmaceutics, 592*, 120028.
198. Prasad, A., Muthamilarasan, M., & Prasad, M., (2020). Synergistic antiviral effects against SARS-CoV-2 by plant-based molecules. *Plant Cell Reports, 39*, 1109–1114.
199. Schulz, G., Victoria, C., Kirschning, A., & Steinmann, E., (2021). Rocaglamide and silvestrol: A long story from antitumor to anticorona virus compounds. *Natural Products Reports, 38*, 18–23.
200. Mlynarczyk, K., Dorota, W., & Lysiak, G. P., (2018). Bioactive properties of *Sambus nigra* L. as a functional ingredient for food and pharmaceutical industry. *Journal of Functional Foods, 40*, 377–390.
201. Harnett, J., Oakes, K., Care, J., Leach, M., Brown, D., Cramer, H., Pinder, T. A., et al., (2020). The effects of *Sambucus nigra* berry on acute respiratory viral infections: A rapid review of clinical studies. *Advances in Integrative Medicine, 7*, 240–246.
202. Benarba, B., & Pandiella, A., (2020). Medicinal plants as sources of active molecules against COVID-19. *Frontiers in Pharmacology*. doi: 1 0.3389/fphar.2020.01189.
203. Ponossian, A., & Brendler, T., (2020). The role of adaptogens in prophylaxis treatment of viral respiratory infections. *Pharmaceuticals, 13*, 236. doi: 10.3390/ph13090236.
204. Deogade, M. S., (2020). Agnihotra [Homa]- an Ayurveda therapy in the prevention and control of Covid-19. *International Journal of Research in Pharmaceutical Sciences, 1*, 304–309.
205. Ghoke, S. S., Sood, R., Kumar, N., Pateriya, A. K., Bhatia, S., Mishra, A., Dixit, R., Singh, V. K., Desai, D., Kulkarni, D. D., et al., (2018). Evaluation of antiviral activity of *Ocimum sanctum* and *Acacia arabica* leaves extracts against H9N2 virus using embryonated chicken egg model. *BMC Complementary and Alternative Medicine, 18*, 174.
206. Theisen, L. L., & Muller, C. P., (2012). EPs ®7630 (Umckaloabo), an extract from *Pelargonium sidoides* roots, exerts anti-influenza virus activity *in vitro* and *in vivo*. *Antiviral Research, 94*(2), 147–156.
207. Singer, J., Jonsdottir, H. R., Albrich, W. C., Strasser, M., Zust, R., Ryter, S., Rahel, A. G., et al., (2020). *In vitro* virucidal activity of echinoforce, an *Echinaceae purpurea* preparation, against coronaviruses, including common cold coronavirus 229E and SARS-CoV-2. *Virology Journal, 17*, 136. doi.org/10.1186/s12985-020-01401-2.
208. Akinyemi, A. J., Adedara, I. A., Pome, G. R., et al., (2015). Dietary supplementation of ginger and turmeric improves reproductive function in hypertensive male rats. *Toxicology Reports, 2*, 1357–1366.
209. Morsch, Y., Wang, W., Li, M., et al., (2016). Curcumin exerts its antihypertensive effect by down-regulating the AT1 receptor in vascular smooth muscle cells. *Scientific Reports, 6*, 1–8.
210. Leong, X. F., (2018). Positive spice for hypertension: Protective role of *Curcuma longa*. *Biomedical and Pharmacology Journal, 11*(4), 1829–1840.
211. Fang, L., Karakiulakis, G., & Roth, M., (2020). Are patients with hypertension and diabetes mellitus at increased risk for COVID-19 infection? *e Lancet Respiratory Medicine, 8*(4), 21.
212. Haridas, M., Sasidhar, V., Nath, P., Abhithaj, J., Sabu, A., & Rammanohar, P., (2021). Compounds of *Citrus medica* and *Zingiber officinale* for COVID-19 inhibition: In silico evidences from cues from Ayurveda. *Future Journal of Pharmaceutical Sciences, 7*, 13.

213. Wibowo, D. P., Mariani, R., Hasanah, S. U., & Aulifa, D. L., (2020). Chemical constituents, antibacterial activity and mode of action of elephant ginger (*Zingiber officinale var* officinale) and emprit ginger rhizome *Zingiber officinale* var. amarum*)* essential oils. *Pharmacognosy Journal, 12*(2), 404–409.
214. Lin, C. W., Tsai, F. J., Tsai, C. H., Lai, C. C., Wan, L., Ho, T. Y., et al., (2005). Anti-SARS coronavirus 3C-like protease effects of *Isatis indigotica* root and plant derived phenolic compounds. *Antiviral Research, 68*, 36–42.

CHAPTER 12

Nanomedicine Against COVID-19

SAIMA ZULFIQAR,[1] ZUNAIRA NAEEM,[1] SHAHZAD SHARIF,[1] AYOUB RASHID CH.,[1] M. ZIA-UL-HAQ,[2] and MARIUS MOGA[3]

[1]Materials Chemistry Laboratory, Department of Chemistry, GC University Lahore, Lahore–54000, Pakistan, E-mail: mssharif@gcu.edu.pk (S. Sharif)

[2]Office of Research, Innovation and Commercialization, Lahore College for Women University, Lahore–54000, Pakistan

[3]Faculty of Medicine, Transilvania University of Brasov, Brasov–500036, Romania

ABSTRACT

Almost the whole world is in crisis due to novel COVID-19 pandemic, which has surpassed territorial, political, ideological, religious, cultural, and academic boundaries, due to severe acute respiratory syndrome coronavirus-2. It is an open challenge for the chemists and engineers to develop the effective drug and vaccine for its prevention as well as treatment. Even though much work has started but still there is no effective procedure. Even though the widespread clinical study of patients is introduced multiple drug targets, but there is no successful therapy till date. In such miserable situation, nanomaterials could be used to prevent the infection before and after getting into the host body. The nanomaterials can be used in the form of nanoparticles, engineered drugs, Nano vaccines or nanomedicines. This chapter covers the use of nanotechnology for the development of therapeutic nanoparticles, nanocarriers, engineered drugs, vaccines, vaccine adjuvants as well as quantum dots to be used for the treatment and prevention of this infection.

12.1 INTRODUCTION

Molecular mechanisms followed by viruses evolved with millions of years for entering into cells with chances of survival for a long period of time followed by turning on the defense system, its inhibition and modification mechanisms [1]. When it was realized in 1990 that viruses have the ability to transfer genes with great efficacy, then non-harmful ones were employed for developing "Recombinant Viral vectors" to be used in applications of gene therapy [2–4]. For the improved performance in drug delivery, efforts were made in order to make the viral vectors safer and development of a method following the intrinsic mechanism by viruses according to their capabilities. These efforts resulted in the establishment of nanomedicine in which various nanosystems have the capacity to transfer the genes in the same way as carried out by viruses. Many delivery systems following the molecular mechanism of viruses have been developed in nanomedicine and biomedical fields for the applications of cancer therapy and regenerative medicines [5, 6]. But it is also the fact that nanotechnology does not only focus on "VIROLOGY" for development of the medical field but is also on the front-line for destroying the infectious viruses.

Viral diseases are not only involved in increasing the mortality rate but also effect the economy worldwide significantly [7]. Treatment of these diseases relies on infecting the gradual processes of viral biological clock by using vaccines and therapeutics. But with the passage of time, many viruses also develop a shield against these treatments; therefore need remains for developing more effective drugs (Table 12.1).

Some common viral diseases have been described in Figure 12.1.

12.1.1 CORONAVIRUS

This viral disease was first reported in 1931 which is not only harmful for humans but also for birds and various species of animals like mammals. The first virus, isolated from the body of humans in 1965 was HCoV-229E and prototype murine coronavirus strain was isolated in 1949. Researches made since 1970 revealed its replication and pathogenic mechanism. Its identification in humans for the first time showed that it could cause acute lungs infections and hence affect the respiration. Other central nervous system (CNS) related diseases, gastrointestinal (GI) as well as hepatic processes were also observed in humans, birds, and animals [9].

TABLE 12.1 Symptoms Shown in Patients by Different Types of HCoVs

HCoVs	Symptoms	Incubation period
HKU1	Fever, Cough, Respiratory Tract Illnes (RTI), Sneezing, Dyspnea, and Pneumonia	2-4 days
229E	Fever, Chills, Cough, Acute Rhinorrhea, Measles, Nasal Congestion and Discharge, Headache, Throat Sore	2-5 days
OC43	Fever, Cold, Cough, Sputum, Dyspnea, Headache, Nasal Congestion and Discharge, Sneazing, Throat Sore	2-5 days
NL63	Fever, Cough, Cold, Respiratory Distress, Wheeze, Rales, Rhinorrhea Tachypnea, Hypoxia	2-4 days
MERS-CoV	Fever, Cough, Cold, Shortness of Breath, Gastrointestinal symptoms, Sore Throat, Arthralgia, Diarrhea, Vomiting, Pneumonia, Acute Renal Impairment, Multiple Organ Failure, Rapid Kidney FAilure.	2-13 days
SARS-CoV	Fever, Cough, Cold, Rigor, Shortness of Breath, Gastrointestinal Symptoms, myalgias, Headache, Malaise, Dyspnea, Respiratory Distress, Diarrhea, Pneumonia	2-11 days
SARS-CoV-2 (COVID-19)	Fever, Cough, Cold, Sore Throat, Nasal Congestion and Rhinorrhea, Diarrhea, Asymptomatic, Damage of Organ functions, Acute kindney and Cardiac Infection, Liver Dysfunction, Pneumothorax	2-14 days (may be 24 days)

Source: Adapted from: Ref. [9]; Open access source.

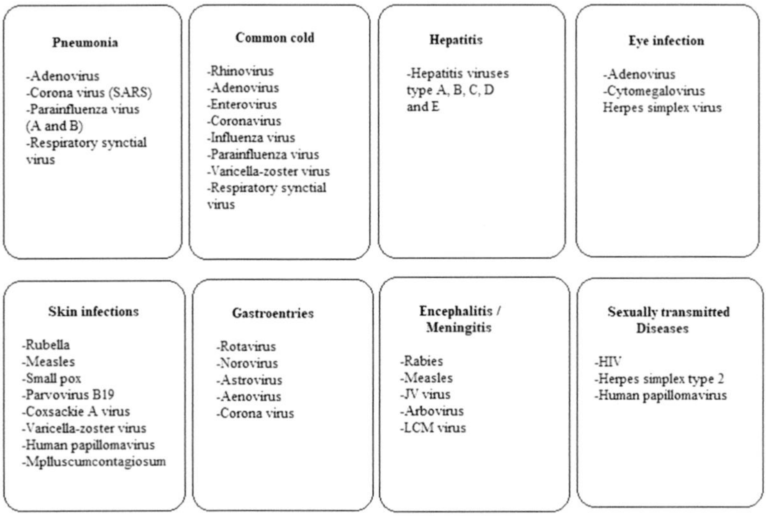

FIGURE 12.1 Common infections caused by viruses.

Source: Adapted from: Ref. [8]; Open access source.

Belonging to "Coronaviridae family," coronaviruses (CoVs) comprised variety of viruses with wide spectrum of activity which are divided in four sub-sections; Alpha, Beta, Gamma, and Delta. These are referred to as corona because spikes on their surfaces resemble the shape of crown. CoVs are in the envelop of positive-sense RNA genome (single-stranded) with nucleocapsid having helical symmetry with 125 nm diameter and range from 27–34 kilobases (Figure 12.2). First outbreak of coronavirus was happened in China, which lead to acute "Respiratory Syndrome" epidemic in 2003. While in 2012, it was emerged for the second time in Saudi Arabia which resulted in Middle-East Respiratory Syndrome [10].

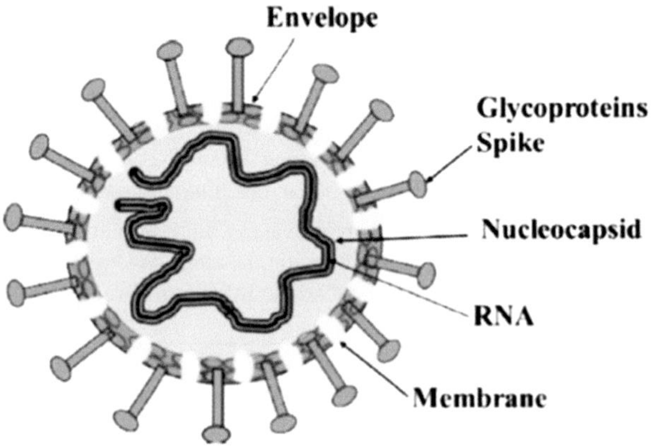

FIGURE 12.2 Structure of CoVirus.
Source: Reprinted from Ref. [9]. © 2020 Wiley□VCH Verlag GmbH & Co. KGaA, Weinheim. Open access.

During December 2019, a novel strain of CoVs was identified that caused severe infections to the people of Wuhan (China) and was labeled as SARS-COV-2. On January 30, 2020 an emergency on global health was announced by WHO committee as many cases reported and confirmed and the disease was given a name COVID-19 officially in February, 2020. Its sites for Coronavirus Infectious Disease. The virus became the headline due to its fast spread which caused mortality. A number of cases is increasing day by day due to its high mobility, which can be tracked on the official website of the World Health Organization (WHO). The transmission of disease from one to other person is mainly due to sneezing, talking, and coughing, which produce small respiratory drops and the disease is very similar to the Influenza [11].

The complete symptoms are not present in-patient suffering from COVID-19 so a detail diagnosis cannot be done. Guan et al. studied percentages of symptoms in 1,099 patients and reported that in China 44% people had fever before going to hospital and 89% patients got fever when they were in hospital. Some had cough, others have fever or shortness of breath. The virus infects the other person when an already infected one comes in close contact to a healthy person, touching the infectious surface or touching the eyes, nose, and mouth. It takes 12–14 days for developing of infection and beginning of symptoms. At the start of this pandemic, it was believed that coronavirus droplets could not travel beyond two meters and even do not stand in the air. But reports revealed the virus remain viable for 4 hrs. On copper, 3 hrs; on aerosols, 2–3 days on stainless steel/plastic and 1 day on cardboard [12].

This virus has four structural proteins, multiple nonstructural proteins as well as accessory pigments. Nonstructural proteins synthesize coronavirus viral RNA, as described in Table 12.2.

Researchers also revealed that persons with weak immunity or suffering from illnesses like lung diseases, cardiovascular disease, and hypertension have high chances of mortality than the healthy ones. The main factors cooperating to the developing of ARDS (acute respiratory distress syndrome) are the organ failure, age, dysfunction of coagulation and neutrophilia, which even lead to death. However, there is still a need to study the disease more with more number of patients under observation. Researches on SARS-COV-2 genome sequence showed that it highly resembles with other strains of coronavirus causing respiratory infections like SARS-COV. Moreover, it has also been revealed that the virus requires a 'Surface-receptor' in the cells of humans and 'angiotensin-converting Enzyme-2' (ACE2) for effective up-take in hosts' cells. The domain of SARS-COV-2 which shows affinity for ACE2 is C-terminal domain. As for causing the infection, binding of viral S-protein to ACE2 is highly crucial, so most of the studies involve developing treatment by focusing on this critical step.

Three strategies have been proposed to block ACE2 binding in the following ways:

- Use of antibodies in the vaccines which specifically interacts with the S-protein of virus, interfering in its interaction with ACE2.
- A recombinant ACE2 protein which is soluble and shows activity like "Decoy Receptor" should be administrated in order to scavenge the virus, preventing its uptake to the cells of the host.
- Virus S protein binding with ACE2 can also be prevented by inhibiting the essential proteases of the host followed by fusion of cell membrane, which is involved in enabling the virus intracellular delivery [28].

TABLE 12.2 Functions of Nonstructural Proteins

Type of non structural proteins	Functions
nsp1	Promotes degradrtion of cellular mRAN and blocks translation of host cell, obstructive immunity, inhibitsintereferon signal
nsp2	Unknown functions
nsp3	Multi domain large transmenmbrane protein;its functions include: 1. N-protein interacts with Ac and Ub 11 domains 2. Cytokine expression promotes due to ADRP activity 3. Viral polyprotein cleaved by PLPro/Deubiquitinase domain, which blocks host innate immunity 4. unknown functions of NAB, SUD, Ubl2, G2M, andY domain
nsp4	Potential transmembrane scaffold protein, plays a role in DMVs formation
nsp5	Chymotripsin like protease,m main protease cleaves viral polypeptides, inhibits interefron signal
nsp6	Restricts expression of autophagosome, potential transmembrane scaffold protein inhibits double membrane vesicle formation
nsp7	Foramtion ofhexadecameric complex(cofactor) with nsp8 & nsp12, plays a role as processivity clamp and primase for RNA polymerase
nsp8	Forms hexadecameric comlex with nsp7 & nsp11, may act as processing activity clamp and primase for RNA polymerase
nsp9	RNA binding protein, Dimerization
nsp10	Stimulates 2-0-MT and ExoN activities, scaffold protein for nspl4&nsp16
nsp11	Unknown functions
nsp12	Primer and RNA dependant, RNA polymerase
nsp13	RNA helicase, 5'-triphosphatase
nsp14	Exoribonuclease activity for viral genome proffreading, N7-Mtase activity adds 5'-cap to viral RNAs, 3',5'-triphosphatase
nsp15	nsp 15 endonuclease, envasion of dsRNA sensors
nsp16	2'-0Mtase, avoiding MDA5 recognition negative regulation of innate immunity

Source: Reprinted from Ref. [9]. © 2020 Wiley□VCH Verlag GmbH & Co. KGaA, Weinheim. Open access.

The first key event involved in binding of S protein of virus with ACE2 at molecular level is depicted in Figure 12.3.

Symptoms related to COVID-19 develop after a week or several days with already load of virus in the lungs so, there is a need to develop an

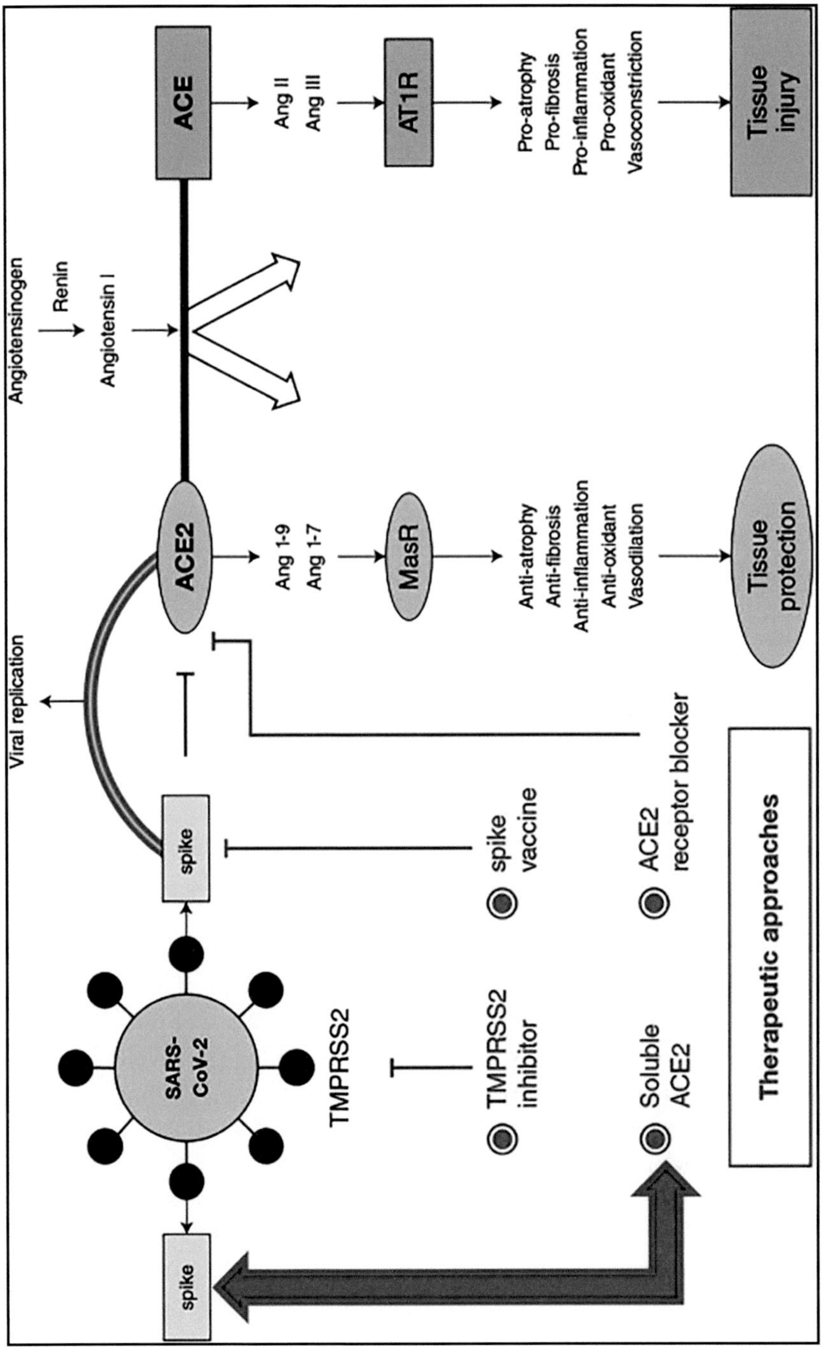

FIGURE 12.3 Binding of ACE 2 with S protein of virus.
Source: Reprinted with permission from Ref. [243]. © 2020 Springer Nature.

approach which not only can avoid the infections but is also at the forefront to attack the pre-existing viruses in the host cells. It will prevent the processes of multi-pleorgan failure and hyper inflammation in the lungs, which can threaten the life. Food and Drug Administration (FDA) is following a "drug repurposing" process in order to develop COVID-19 novel drugs with a focus on the interaction mechanism of viral proteins and host proteomes.

In order to improve conditions, early diagnosis is necessary so that if a person is not infected with a virus, he should not be quarantined in hospital. Otherwise, there is a chance that the person with negative result will become positive due to positive patients in hospital. The drugs and vaccines are in progress for patients suffering from this virus, but they are not completed, so the best way to avoid it is to take preventive measures such as isolation and identifying people who came in direct contact with patients having COVID-19 positive.

12.1.2 NANOMATERIALS

Nanoscience focuses on applications and advancement of 1 to 100 nm (nanoscale) structures of atoms and molecules which are employed with variable morphology, surface chemistry, and composition (Figure 12.4). Nanocarriers are widely known for the drug delivery to the specified target without affecting the healthy cells, detection of viral infections during early stages, delivery of combined therapeutics by crossing cellular barriers and nano-vaccines interacting with tissues of infected organs [12].

Nanoscience is basically based on approaches to attack the viruses by nanomaterials like acid-functionalized carbon nanotubes (multi-walled) and blocking the interaction of virus protein to the ACE2 receptor in case of COVID-19 (Figure 12.5). Nanocarriers are effectively involved in the delivery of antigens and antigen-adjuvant combinations with the ease of functionalization at surface level but however, the forefront demand is the development of a nano-agent in the medical field which can deliver the most suitable concentration at the right target within an appropriate period of time. Figure 12.5 explains how nanomaterials are effective in the treatment of COVID-19.

Some efforts are also required for efficient management by RNA-mediated interface technology to handle multiple virus-related illnesses at the same time. However, the limitations are associated to validity of therapeutics with interfering RNA in clinical activity, poisoning due to some reactions by immune system and RNA not able to transverse the membrane due to high molecular weight (MW) and negative charge density. These all limitations can be avoided with the use of nano-carriers/particles to develop the novel approaches which can efficiently inhibit replication by virus. For example, silver nanoparticles modified with curcumin were prepared using a green approach and showed high activity against infection caused by syncytial virus [9]. Table 12.3 summarizes the nanotechnology-based therapeutics which are efficient against viral infection and inhibition.

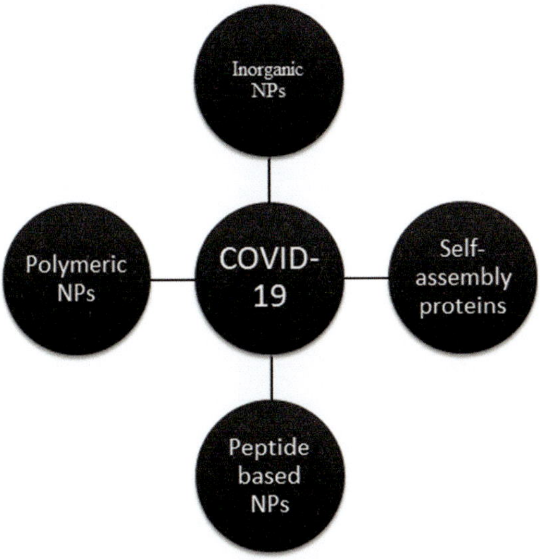

FIGURE 12.4 Role of nanoscience against COVID-19.

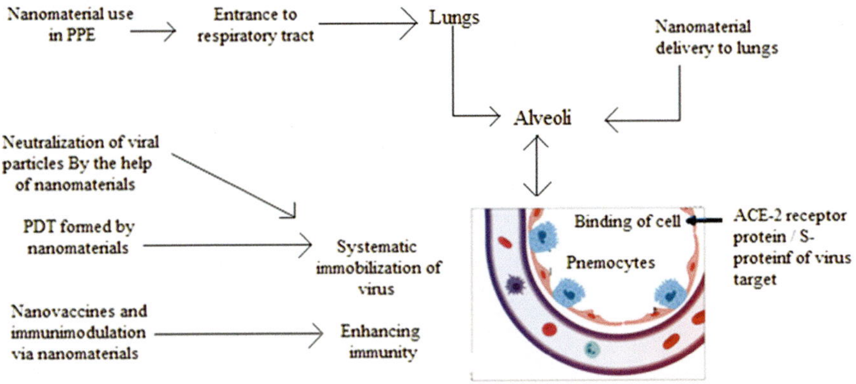

FIGURE 12.5 General representation of role of different nanomaterials in treatment of COVID-19.

Source: Adapted from Ref. [28]; Open access source. © 2020 American Chemical Society.

TABLE 12.3 Nanotechnology-based Viral Therapeutics

Nanoplatform	Properties	Drug	Virus
Silver (Ag)	Monodisperse and uniformerly spherical highly stable (>28 days), Ag NPs loaded with Am on their surface less cytotoxic than free AgNPs or AM	Adamantine (AM)	H1N1
Selenium (Se)	1) Uniformerly spherical, more stable, superior antiviral effect on kidney cells treated with H1N1 and less cytotoxicity of AM loaded Se NPs than free Se NPs	Adamantine (AM)	H1N1
	2) Uniformerly spherical, superior antiviral effect on kidney cells treated with H1N1 and less cytotoxicity of OTV loaded Se NPs than free Se NPs	Oseltamivir (OTV)	H1N1
PEG-PLGA	Uniformerly spherical, NPs loaded with Diphyllin and bafilomycin, high biocom-patibility and antiviral activity towards NP drugs than free drugs	Diphyllin & Bafilomycin	H1N1
PLGA	Uniform spherical/smooth surface NPs three GCV prodrugs can be seperately loaded on PLGA NPs: non-toxic NPs	Gangiclovir (GCV)	HSV-1
HPAC	Non-loading efficiency: HPAC, non-toxic towards human epithelial cells (vaginal, corneal), foreskin fibroblasts, HeLa cells, cell viability >75%	Acyclovir (ACV)	HSV
PLGA	Polydisperse particles loaded with LAM, slow NPs degradation in simulated intestinal fluid PBS; molecular interaction between polymer and LAM confirmed by FTIR & DSC	Lamivudine (LAM)	HIV
PLGA	Spherical/smooth surface NFVNPs; almost narrow distribution	Efavirenz (EFV)	HIV
PEO-PCL	Spherical PEO-PCL NPs with smooth surface: SQV is encapsulated into PEO-PCL NPs	Squinavir (SQV)	HIV
PLGA-PEG	Spherical shape for those loaded with SAHA ans NFV: size of nanoparicles varies depending upon SAHA or NFV	Suberoylanilide hydroxamic acid (SAHA) & NFV	HIV
Hybrid NPs (PLGA, PLA, MMA-SPM, & PMMA)	Almost spherical NPs: nontoxic NPs	LAM+AZT (Zidovudine)	HIV

TABLE 12.3 *(Continued)*

Nanoplatform	Properties	Drug	Virus
PM Acoated MNP	Uniformly spherical NPs conjugated with ENF: nontoxic in vivo & in vitro NPs conjugated with ENF	Enfuvirtude (ENF)	HIV
Chitosan nanospheres	Spherical nanospheres with smooth surface polydisperse;86% Vero cell viability; ACV encapsulation efficiency	(ACV)	HSV
PG dendrimer	Antiviral effect in vitro: nontoxic peptide-PG conjugates in vitro	Peptides	IAV
DSPC+MPEG + DSPE (LNPs)	In-vitro anti-HIV; Do not show any local reaction, whilewithin normal limit, animal platelets were observed	LPV+TFV+RTV	HIV
PEG & phospholipids (LNPs)	LNPs loaded with drugs:upto 96 % incorporation efficiency	ATV+TFV+RTV	HIV
Micelles (NiPam)	Copolymers self-assembled in multicellar aggregates by hydrodynamic: high muco-adhesion & cytocompatibility properties	EFV	HIV

HSV → Herpes Simplex Virus: PG → Polyglycerol: IAV → Influenza A virus: LPV → Lopinavir TFV → Tenofovir: RTV → Ritonavir: ATV → Atazanavir: RSPC → 1,2-Distrearoyl-sn-glycero-3-phosphocholine

Source: Adapted from: Ref. [8]. Open access source.

On the other hand, Table 12.4 enlists the nanomaterials especially engineered for CoVs inhibition.

TABLE 12.4 Engineered Nanomaterials for Inhibition of Coronavirus Infection

NPs	Virus	Mode of Action
Chiral Au-NPs-Quantum dots composites	CoVs	Chiral plasmon-exciton symptoms
Graphene oxide (Go) sheets	Felin CoVs	Organism model: fcwf-4 cells, DF-1 cells: Association with Viral lipid tails leading to aggregation and rupture of the envelop
Go sheets Ag-NPs	Feline CoVs	Association with viral lipid tails leading to aggragation with attachment of Ag-NPs with -SH group of protein and rupture of the envelop
Carbon electrode modified with Au-NPs	MERS-CoVs	Recombinant spike protein S1 has been employed as a biomarker: sensor is based on indirect competition between free virus in the sample and immobilized MERS-CoV protein for a fixed concentration of added antibody to the sample
Au-NPs-Adjuvanted S protein	SARS-CoVs	Stimulates significant antigen-specific IgG response against SARS-related CoV infection
Cationic carbon dots based on curcumin	CoVs: porcine epidemic diarrhea virus (PEDV)	Inhibition of viral proliferation: structure of surface protein in viruses has been changed, prohibiting viral entry, cationic carbon dots based on curcumin can supress synthesis of -ve stranded RNA and budding of virus, and and accumulation of reactive oxygen species by virus.Furhtermore, it suppress viral replication by stimulating formation of interferon stimulating genes and pro-inflammatory cytokines
Glutathione-cappedAg$_2$S nanoclusters	(PEDV)/ CoV	Ag$_2$S nanoclusters treatment prohibits fotmation of viral -ve stranded RNA and budding. It +vely regulates production of Interferon stimulating genes and expression of pro-inflammation cytokines, which may inhibit CoV proliferation and infection
Chiral Zirconium Quantum Dots	CoVs	Fluorescence properties of immuno-conjugated quantum dots-magneto-plasmonic NPs

Source: Adapted from: [31]; Open access source.

12.2 HOW CORONAVIRUS INFECTS A PERSON?

Viral-spike glycoproteins are the reasons behind the entrance of coronavirus into the cells of the victim [32, 33]. The viral spike basically consists of two subunits which are named as; S1 and S2. Receptor linking site in the S1 subunit of virus allows its binding with cells of host. Host range can be determined for coronavirus by a critical step, i.e., "receptor binding." Coronavirus for which host is the human contains receptors such as:

- Aminopeptidase N (APN) for the HCOV-229E;
- Dipeptidyl peptidase 4 for MERS-CoV;
- 9-O-acetylated Sialic acid for HCoV-HKU1; and
- Angiotensin-converting enzyme-ACE2 for the SARS-COV and HCOV-OC43 [34].

The recently discovered COVID-19 shows strong coordination with the ACE2 of human and bat cells through its receptor-binding domain (RBD) [34]. In the case of the S2 subunit, there is a specialized "Fusion Machinery" which induces strong affinity between the host cells and coronavirus. Afterwards, protease activities in the coronavirus by the host cells cleave the S at S2 fusion peptide [35]. When the virus has entered in the host, it gets un-coated followed by translation of a viral genomic RNA-ORF1 which encodes a polyprotein (pp1a). As the translation of ORF1 proceeds further, a longer polyprotein (pp1ab) is produced [36].

These produced polyproteins generate 15 to 16 non-structural proteins via autoproteolytic cleavage. These nonstructural proteins are responsible for some significant activities like:

- nsp12 can encode the RNA-polymerase activity which is RNA-dependent [23];
- nsp3, nsp4, and nsp6 through spherules or DMV (double-membrane vesicle) can mediate the rearrangement of cell-membrane;
- nsp3 and nsp5 can encode the protease-PLpro just like papain [37] and major activities of protease-Mpro sequentially [38, 39].

Moreover, the transcription complex of coronavirus is held and further assembled at the DMVs. The whole biological clock, multiplication process and pathogenicity of COVID-19 virus is the same as that of SARS-COV-2 [40, 41].

12.3 INACTIVATION OF CORONAVIRUS

Being highly stable, it is necessary to inactivate SARS-CoV; for this purpose, bleach, povidone-iodine, ethanol, benzalkonium chloride, chloroxylenol, and chlorhexidine, are commonly used disinfectants depending upon the configuration of the material infected with it [42]. Nowadays, nanotechnology is widely used in almost every field of life. It is preferably used, because it does not affect the healthcare and housekeeping staff; even though, chemical-based, nanoparticle-based, and bio-based disinfectants are used. Nanomaterial and nanoparticles exhibit the characteristic of inactivation of bacteria, fungi, yeasts, and viruses via different pathways.

12.3.1 INACTIVATION BY NANO-ROOTED DEVICES

Medically, nanoparticles of copper, zinc, and silver have inherent characteristics against different microbes. These are used because these do not contain bulk material and metal ions; on the other hand, the release of metal ions is a slow process, which kills the microbes at their location. There is no efflux pump for expel of nanoparticles accumulated with the cells [43]. The most commonly used silver nanoparticles are employed in medical treatments, like dressing of lacerations, in urinary and intravascular catheters, in paints as zeolites, in food trays as biocides [44, 45]. It is also used against monkeypox virus, HIV-1, MS2, UZ1 and bacteriophages, as well as murine noroviruses MNV1 [46–49].

Silver nanoparticles are used for antiviral properties. We can use it through different mechanisms such as by dissolving nanoparticles of silver (0) forming Ag^+ ions which show antiviral properties. Silver also has strong interaction with sulfur groups and interacts at functional domains of various enzymes. It can also interconnect with viruses' proteins present at the surface or get into the host cell by making interaction with enzymes that contain thiols by blocking their function of virus multiplication. These nanoparticles use was hypothesized by Zodrow et al.; and Gusseme et al. for bacteriophage MS2 and MNV-1, respectively [48, 50]. Silver based nanoclusters are used for the blockage of porcine epidemic diarrhea virus (PEDV) by hampering the formation of viral RNA strand, and these nanoclusters show antiviral ability without formation of Ag+ ions [51].

Silver ions and nanoclusters show different behavior in their action and target viruses or cells that are infected. Silver nanoclusters are clustered within the cell where viruses are performing their activities such as nucleocapsids assembly, but these are not released outside the cell but Ag (I) are accumulated at other areas and they are removed steadily, and they interact with viruses by inhibiting their activity. This was studied by Elechiguerra et al. and Orlowski for HIV-1 and HSV-2 when displayed to silver nanoparticles having a layer of tannic acid. Elechiguerra et al. studied and examine the diameter of nanoparticles as 10 nm, and these nanoparticles are weakly interacted with virus and Orlowski studied that size matters a lot and larger size of NP inhibits blocking in a good way. Gusseme used 11.2 nm nanoparticles, and they showed very good activity by inhibiting virus in an effective way [48]. Ag NPs' coating on virus surface results in breakdown of membrane or virus envelope. Ag NPs present in filters have the property to show antiviral activity against bacteriophage MS2 [52].

Copper also exhibits antimicrobial properties and have also antiviral properties [53]. In 1979 copper was studied for poliovirus and it showed good efficiency as studied by Murray [54]. Copper was also taken into consideration for HuCoV-229E coronavirus and also some other forms most specifically against SARS-CoV-2. Its residence time is of six days on smooth surfaces such as Teflon, glass, stainless steel, but on surfaces which contain copper, its residence time is less than 60 minutes [55]. On copper-based materials virus is broken down. This occurs due to the release of copper ions onto the surface followed by viral attack after production of reactive oxygen species (ROS) [53]. The residence time span of SARS-CoV-1 and SARS-CoV-2 is less than four hours as compared to plastic and steel where they remain for 2–3 days. The mechanism is used for inactivation of envelope proteins (E protein) by using ions of copper [56]. For healthcare purposes, copper-based alloys are brasses can be used for doorknobs and bed rails.

Catalysts are made by using a small percentage of copper or silver along with aluminum oxide, such as 10% of copper with aluminum oxide and 5% of silver with Al_2O_3 which will inhibit SARS-CoV virus in 20 and 5 minutes, respectively and use for air disinfection [57]. When copper and copper oxide nanoparticles are brought into contact with living cells, these are converted to ions [58, 59]. Nanoparticles small size enables them to cover huge surface area as well as enhance the speed of dispersion of copper ions. Antimicrobial activity is increased by using nanostructured copper.

Nanoparticles have efficient ability to stop the activity of viruses by spraying them at areas that are dirty and masks, blouses, etc. Masks containing copper oxide are used, and they showed great anti-viral activity of influenza virus [60] and these copper oxide-based particles should also be checked for SARS-CoV-2.

The antiviral characteristics of copper and silver nanoparticles is increased using iron along with them [61]. The derivatives of graphene are also studied, and they showed great inactivation properties. Graphene oxide sheets and derivatives of graphene having sulfur group are used for herpes simplex virus (HSV) type-1 [62]. Graphene oxide folios reduction by heating and hyper branching with polyglycerol and sulfation are also produced as graphene-originated biomimetics [63–65]. Heparin sulfate and heparin sulfate both have antiviral properties [66, 67], but they are not used due to the reason of anticoagulation. Sulfated graphene oxide hyperbranched glycerol (rGo-hPG) is found good in hampering the strains of orthopox and herpes virus but unable to stop its spread from cell to cell. Since virus particles are positively charged and graphene oxides have negative charge so there is great interaction between the two in terms of electrostatics. The presence of negative charge on graphene oxide and rGO capable of recessing the infection of PEDV, EV71 (enterovirus 71), H9N2 and pseudorabies viruses [68, 69]. It is due to the negative charge we can use other nanomaterial having two dimensions which have the property to suppress the infections caused by both gram-negative as well as gram-positive strains of bacteria such as $Ti_3C_2T_x$ MXene [70].

The derivatives of graphene can also bind to virus antibody which are specific and have shown antiviral properties in grotavirus, in subtypes of avian influenza virus (AIV), which are H-5 (AIV H-5) and H-7 (AIV H-7), and influenza virus H1N1 [71, 72].

12.3.2 PHOTOTHERMAL INACTIVATION

Photothermal treatment is also called plasmonic photothermal treatment because heating is produced by noble metals in the presence of light; this condition is analogous to Plasmon resonance [73]. This characteristic is exhibited by nanomedical researchers to destroy the cancer cells preferable via gold nanoparticles that have less toxicity than silver nanoparticles. Loeb et al. reported that intense heat, to kill viral protein, from gold nanoparticles can be produced by irradiation of sunlight; this experiment was performed onto the surfaces of bacteriophages MS2 and PR772 coated with gold nanorods as well as nanocubes [74]. Here killing of virus by this technique requires close contact with heat. On the other hand, femtosecond pulsed laser was poured onto gold nanorods to halt the metabolism of murine leukemia virus (MLV) by Nazari et al. who put forward this mechanism as plasmon-enhanced shockwave generation which requires no close contact of nanoparticles and virus, but lowers the interconnection of various proteins of virus with the receptors of the host cell [75].

12.3.2.1 INACTIVATION BY PHOTOCATALYTIC NANOPARTICLES

The most common nanoparticles of titanium oxide exhibit the property of photocatalysis, as they have no toxicity, are inert as well as show no corrosion on irradiation of light [76]. Titanium oxide is being used in paint and lacquer industry, self-cleaning windows as well as to purify water [44, 77]. These also purify the air from volatile organic compounds on exposure of UV light. Some researchers have found discharge of toxic compounds when photocatalytic titanium oxide is used to purify air; this has marked question on its use in above mentioned applications. When UV light is irradiated onto the surface of the photocatalytic material, an electron is activated from the outermost orbital and moves to the uppermost conduction orbital leaving behind an empty space having a positive charge in the outermost band. A hole as well as an electron move to the surface where they produce ROS (superoxide anion) as well as hydrogen and hydroxyl radicals when water molecules are oxidized, which are used for the disinfection purpose through oxidizing the organic compounds in cell wall and cell membrane, changing the structure and function of protein and damaging DNA [78]. Multi resistant strains of bacteria, fungi, yeasts, and fungi can be inactivated by using titanium oxide irradiated with UV light, as discussed by Bogdan et al. [79]. It is a contradiction among several researchers in terms of photocatalytic inactivation of sheathed as well as non-sheathed viruses. Still now, only one article has been reported, which ensured the killing of SARS-CoV by using photocatalytic titanium apatite filter after six hours exposure with UV light [80].

The capacity of a virus to cause infection is lowered when spike protein is damaged on exposure to UV light coupled photocatalyst. Second-generation photocatalysts with other metal atoms have been developed by researchers to overcome the problem that low catalytic process of titanium oxide in sunlight as well as high combining ability of electron and hole in the valence band of titanium oxide. These new catalysts, such as S-doped and N-doped TiO_2 inactivate the infectious microbes under visible light and even interior lighting. These have not been used against viruses still now. Furthermore, more hydroxyl radicals are produced when silver nanoparticles are accumulated on the facets of titanium oxide nanoparticles; as a result, these inactivate bacteriophage MS2 efficiently [81]. To get water free from bacteriophage MS2, Ag-, and Cu-doped TiO_2 nanowires exhibited efficiency in dark as well as UV light.

The doped titanium oxide nanoparticles have increased activity to inactivate microbes in the presence of light because they have a narrow bandgap as compared to titanium, silver, and copper nanoparticles [82, 83]. Mixed nanoparticles of titanium oxide and silica have increased capacity to absorb bacteriophage MS2 due to high surface area of silica [84]. Pt-doped titanium oxide nanoparticles coated onto the surface of glass slide, because of high photocatalytic activity, have the potential to immobilize influenza A (H3N2) virus present in aerosols [85]. Byrnes et al. developed such photocatalytic agents that were active against bacteria and supposed the use of developed agents to be tested against SARS-CoV-2 [78]. Some of those materials are $BiVO_4$, $CuY_xFe^{2-}{}_xO_4$, $CuMn_2O_4$, $CuFeO_2$, $ZnMn_2O_4$, $CuCo_2O_4$, $BaCr_2O_4$, $LaFeO_8$, $NiCo_2O_4$, $La_{0.9}Sr_{0.1}CoO_3$, $LaCoO_3$, and $SrCr_2O_4$, but to use them against SARS-CoV-deactivation, their toxicity level must be investigated.

12.3.3 INACTIVATION BY NANOTECHNOLOGY-BASED SOLUTIONS

Particles of SARS-CoV-2 are larger as studied through cryo-electron microscopy, and these particles function as large particles when exposed to air and cause disease and these particles are near the larger end of nanoparticles having a range of size between 70–90 nm [86, 87]. These liquid droplets containing virus came from a person having infection during coughing, sneezing, suctioning, or during his normal breathing process. These particles or droplets come from respiratory tract along with bacterial and epithelial cells forming the lining of the tract. Size of droplets have a wide range. Larger size droplets are more harmful than those having smaller size and water is removed from them after exposure to air by evaporation process. It is due to evaporation the diameter and settling velocity of droplets is reduced but larger droplets evaporation rate is not much to decrease their settling but of smaller droplets there will be opposite case because in this condition solid residues come close to one another and held strongly due to respiratory secretions during water loss. Droplet nuclei is an important parameter of virus transmission [88, 89] such as a virion having 100 nm size and droplet nuclei having a diameter of one micrometer contains irregular packing of approximately 370 virions and if droplet nuclei diameter is increased having 10 micrometer diameter, it could have three lac 60,000 virions. Determination of size of droplet nuclei is through the constituent part with greater volume such as epithelial or bacterial cell. Ventilation systems and N95 masks contain medium for filtration have a great number of network of fibers through which air is passed. These filters have the ability to trap particles mainly by three arrangements. First one is impaction which helps to inhibit particles to diverge and causing it to strike with fiber. This process is used to dismiss particles having 500 nm diameter. The second mechanism is interception which is for the particles that will diverge with airstream flow lines, and the distance between airstream and particle center is smaller than its radius and is used for particles having 200 nm diameter. Third is diffusion and is very important for the removal of particles and removes particles having a diameter of less than 200 nm. The most penetrating particles are those having 300 nm diameter and are difficult to remove by the above three mechanisms [90].

Deposition of virus coated droplet nuclei on filter media depends on size larger size droplets will not go too deep, but smaller droplets will go in-depth to fibrous matrix. Facepiece masks use for filtration purposes, particle deposition can be changed through cyclical breathing process. Droplet nuclei have the ability to absorb moisture, so in humid air, they absorb water and swell, causing filter fibers to retain particles which results in their redistribution or breakdown.

In order to enhance the effectiveness and protection of air filters and masks, different strategies are followed for advancement of process for COVID-19. We can improve capturing of virus and retention, specifically those having a diameter of 300 nanometers, or by controlling the rearrangement of particles after humid air exhalation and immediate inactivity of microbes such as enveloped viruses and by increasing the performance of filtration of personal masks so that they can be reused. By combining the electrostatic and mechanical process of fabrics used in cloth masks, efficiency is increased more than 80% and 90% for particles having size greater and less than 300 nanometer [91].

Nanofibers are produced having size smaller than micrometer by using a process known as electrospinning. Masks containing thin layer of nanofibers have potential to trap even smallest droplets of viruses and bacteria and inhibit them to penetrate deep in mask. On surface of filter, layering of titanium oxide nanofibers by process of electro spinning have the ability to capture droplets of sub-micrometer size and their destruction is done by exposing them to sunlight or UV irradiation. Polyamide 11 nanofibers having thick film of micrometer are deposited on filter of polypropylene, titanium oxide nanoparticles are sprayed directly by electrospinning [92]. Uniform coating of titanium oxide nanoparticles was seen by electron microscopy without aggregation. These coated fibers showed excellent activity in terms of photocatalysis and bactericidal form and also in photo induced hydrophilicity.

12.4 NANOMEDICINE APPROACH FOR COVID THERAPEUTICS

Nanocarriers are involved in loading and delivering for a variety of 'active moieties' like nucleic acids, antivirals, and biologics. For SARS-COV-2, a suitable contrast of a therapeutic agent and nanocarrier is mandatory in formulation of nanomedicine. This approach can improve the therapeutic index by re-formulation of the accepted/trial drugs, mentioning their side effects and limitations.

As therapeutic developments against COVID-19 resemble with oncology so this approach can be nurtured by taking into consider the platform for therapeutics against cancer [93, 94]. Development of these therapeutics involve:

- Side effects related to drugs with proper knowledge of associated mechanism;
- A carefully examined strategy should be selected for the maximum impact of nanomedicine on the therapeutic Index.

In fact, a developmental platform for nanomedicine requires smart design of a nanocarrier for the delivery of drugs and strategies for the track developments enforcing more research [95, 96]. Knowledge and guidelines associated with drugs against virus and cancer can be helpful for a fruitful and fast research in development of COVID-19 treatment drugs.

12.4.1 NANOCARRIER SELECTION TO BYPASS CONVENTIONAL DRUGS

A suitable nanocarrier selection can eliminate many limitations in drug delivery, for example, toxic auristatin conjugates for hematological cancer treatment with the disadvantage of less drug pay-loads. This limitation was solved with the development of polymeric nanoparticles giving advantage of high drug (auristatin) payload for effective tumor repression [97]. Intolerable side effects of Aurora B kinase observed in a trial phase were avoided by combining it with polyethylene glycol/polylactide nanoparticles. Moreover, nucleic acid containing drugs also face limitations associated with intracellular delivery and unstable system of circulation [98–101]. Formulation of lipid nanoparticles loaded with nucleic acid drugs eliminated its conventional limitations with the aid of targeting the liver [102]. Similarly, silica mesoporous nanoparticles coated with lipid offered advantages of biocompatibility and more time for systematic circulation for the delivery of an antiviral drug, ML336. A high through output method, FIND was also reported, which screen these lipid nanoparticles for the *in vivo* delivery promoting nanocarriers as "immuno-oncology" therapeutics with the elimination of associated toxicity [103–105].

12.4.2 CHEMICALLY ENGINEERED DRUGS

A better generic approach involves some chemical modification in a drug molecule which enhance its compatibility with the specific class of nanocarriers, keeping the same physical/chemical properties [106, 107]. For example, hydrophobic doxorubicin drug was chemically altered to improve its compatibility with lipid bilayer nanoparticles which are specific for ionizable and amphiphilic drug candidates [108]. Pro-drug synthesis is also a useful approach for the enhanced association with the nanoparticles providing the advantage of controlled and targeted release, e.g., synthesis of antiretroviral candidates' prodrugs (against HIV) involves incorporation of fatty acid esters which were coated by poloxamer for a stable and efficient nanocrystal formation which was revealed through *in vivo* research in mice and rhesus [109–111]. Lipid bilayer nanocarriers loaded with cholesterol modified hydroxychloroquine (HCQ) drug provided benefits of lower toxicity, prolonged drug release, and reduced pulmonary fibrosis by inhibiting proliferation in the lungs of rats. It is useful for SAR-COV-2 suffering which also involves pulmonary fibrosis associated with viral loading [112]. An anticancer hydrophobic-hydrophilic drug conjugate (*Chlorambucil irinotecan*) synthesis by using hydrolysable ester linkage and then their self-assembly associated formation of nanoparticles provided enhanced drug retention, cellular uptake, and better accumulation of tumors [113, 114]. Similarly, pro-drug formation involving conjugation of cabazitaxel to fatty acids with polyethylene glycol-lipid results in nanoparticle formation during self-assembly and hence excellent anticancer activity with minimized toxicity [115].

12.4.3 NANOMEDICINE FOR COMBINATIONAL DRUG THERAPEUTICS

Another way of treating COVID-19 is the combination of drug therapeutics which provides benefits of less dosages of drug, variety of therapeutic targets and lower resistance development avoiding many side effects [116, 117]. Despite of carrying single drug, nanocarriers loaded with various drugs having different physical/chemical properties are promising candidates to achieve full potential of these combined therapeutics with controlled synergistic ratios, overlapped pharmacokinetics and reduced side effects after association [118]. Combination of hydrophilic/hydrophobic drugs and their loading in nanocarrier is useful to achieve their release in sequence, ratiometric loading followed by controlled release of the drugs; chemo-therapeutics/co-delivery of siRNA, co-delivery of RNAi-Plasmid DNA and micro-RNA [31].

Long lasting profiles of plasma drugs and their better level in lymph nodes are achieved by combining antiretroviral drugs, ritonavir, lopinavir (hydrophobic) and tenofovir (hydrophilic) using macaques *in-vivo* model [120]. FDA has also approved a treatment for acute leukemia associated to liposomal nanocarriers loaded with daunorubicin and cytarabine (anticancer drugs). Multi antiretroviral drugs loading in pegylated-magneto-liposomal nanocarriers showed excellent activity against HIV in primary cells of CNS with *in vivo/vitro* BBB trans-migration [121]. This multifunctional nano-platform can be advantageous against SARS-COV-2 which could spread in CNS. However, optimized nano-formulations remains a task which includes the analysis like:

- How these combined therapeutics interact;
- Their release profile, toxicity, and synergistic ratios [122, 123].

Screening of nanoparticles by high through output method can be useful to understand their interacting mechanism or synergism, but this method demands the mimicry of targeted tissues 3-D environment to analyze the drugs release profile [124]. Pre-clinical translational models for animals can be helpful, but differences between models of diseases in humans and animals remains an issue [125]. In short, scientist in nanomedicine can take advantage of all these opportunities in order to have a valid combination of therapeutics with the most suitable nanocarrier.

12.4.3.1 DELIVERY OF VACCINE

The knowledge gained on human immune system response with similarity of SARS-COV and MERS-COV to SARS-COV-2 can be helpful to develop a vaccine against COVID-19 [126, 127]. An approach in vaccine formation involves loading of nanoparticles with multiple antigenic moieties conjugated by physical or chemical methods has become an alternative to many conventional strategies [128–130]. Besides protecting antigen native structure, improved delivery and antigen presentation to the antigen-presenting cells (APCs), nanocarriers also offer several advantages:

- Since a variety of viruses including the SARS-COV-2 is nanosized thus, they can be specifically targeted by nanoparticles;

- Administration of these nanoparticles through oral, subcutaneous, intranasal, and intramuscular routes is advantageous to target the specific areas, e.g., lymph nodes eradicating barriers like tissues [131–133].

Researchers have also revealed an anti-protective role by cell processed as well as humoral immunity against SARS-COV-2 [134, 135]. Nanoparticles are developed in such a way to target B cells, T cells, macrophages, neutrophils, and monocytes (innate immune system). These nanoparticles with modified APCs can be helpful for various strategies to develop vaccine against COVID-19 [136, 137]. Several mechanisms and nanoparticles can also improve the immunity of T cells by increased antigen presentation to dendritic cells (DCs) [138].

The best advantage of nanocarrier based vaccine is nanoparticles either own the intrinsic property of adjuvants for the loaded antigens or helpful in the delivery of molecular adjuvants. Pre-clinical stages of WHO prepared vaccines for COVID-19 based on nanoparticles have been enlisted in Table 12.5.

12.5 NANOMEDICINE APPROACH FOR COVID VACCINE

The history of vaccine reveals its success in developing immunity against many infectious diseases, mainly through antibodies neutralization. For the COVID-19 vaccine formulation, the major issue is of selecting those approaches which can stimulate immunity against the virus with the involvement of both B cells and T cells. Another challenge is the fast development of strategies for the next-generation vaccines, which can also be addressed to a specific group of individuals with a compromise in the immune system [139]. All the proposed strategies based on vaccines against COVID-19 are important and may overlap when combined with nanocarrier [126, 140]. The nano-strategy for vaccine development demands a very suitable nanocarrier and enhanced focus on APCs which can complement each other to provide strong immune effects. Nanocarrier selection/design follows two strategies which are given below;

12.5.1 ANTIGEN DEPENDENT NANOCARRIER SELECTION

Antigen loading on the nanocarriers involve several factors like target location, bio-stability, physiochemical properties and required profile for the release of immunogens. Physio-sorption of antigen on nanoparticles depends on surface charges and hydrophobic interactions (non-covalent). The amphoteric nature of antigens makes them highly suitable for immobilization on nanocarriers, e.g., chitosan loaded on dextran-sulfate-polymeric nanoparticles, carbon nanotubes and inorganic nanoparticles (Gold NPs) [141–144]. In such cases antigen release is dependent on biological pH, temperature, and ionization. Nanocarriers loaded with encapsulated and matrix entrapped antigens are beneficial to avoid its biochemical deterioration. Poly(lactide-coglycolide)-PLGA nanoparticles are highly suitable for entrapping antigens with prolonged drug release [145]. Antigens suitable for such nanoparticles are *B. anthraces* spores, malaria antigens "tetanus toxoid," antigens of Listeria monocytogens and HBsAg (surface antigen of HBV) providing strong immune response at cellular and humoral level [146].

12.5.2 mRNA-BASED NANOCARRIERS

Lipid nanoparticles loaded with mRNA are under trial stage to provide a vaccine for COVID-19. Extracellular RNA can degrade the naked mRNA; thus a platform for safer delivery to the target is mandatory [147, 148]. Moreover, mRNA also embraces the ability of penetration in the lipid membrane and recognition of specific receptors of cells. Cellular machinery is then triggered by exogenous mRNA presence in cytosol for its complete translation into protein [149].

Lipid nanoparticles size range from 80 to 200 nm, which is similar to the size of infectious viruses [150]. These nanoparticles are synthesized by self-assembled cationic lipid and hold the ability for efficient delivery of mRNA into the cytoplasm. Selecting the intramuscular/intradermal routes are helpful for release kinetics of mRNA and translation into protein with both B and T cells response for immunity [151]. These lipid nanoparticles can be fabricated through some modifications like:

- Cationic lipid and cholesterol nanoparticles;
- Cationic lipids, cholesterol, and PEG-Lipid nanoparticles.

Cholesterol increases the stability of the system while PEG-Lipid can enhance the half-life of the formulation. Besides, lipid nanoparticles other nanocarriers for mRNA are protamine nanoliposomes, polyethylenimine nanoparticles, chitosan nanoparticles and PEG-lipid functionalized dendrimer nanoparticles with the size ranging from 100 to 600 nm [152–154].

12.5.3 DNA-BASED NANOCARRIERS

Naked DNA just like mRNA can also be degraded by nucleases leading to their incomplete delivery and immune response. Nanocarriers based on synthetic/natural polymers, inorganic particles, and cationic lipids are the most suitable for formulation of DNA containing vaccines. Polymeric nanoparticles with encapsulation of DNA can avoid its biological degradation resulting in controlled and targeted release of drug [155, 156]. For the specific antigen-antibody response PLGA nanotransporters are the extensively researched for the development of DNA based vaccines. They can improve the DNA loading and release with the prevention against degradation in biological system. These PLGA nanoparticles can be synthesized as:

- Cationic glycol-chitosan and PLGA;
- Polyethylenimine and PLGA [157, 158].

Nanocarriers with PEG conjugation induce shielding properties which can provide enhanced stability, protection against phagocytes, avoiding non-specific protein interactions and toxicity [159, 160]. Electroporation technology is the current development for the efficient delivery of mRNA and DNA to their targets after inducing pores in the cell membranes [145, 161, 162].

PLGA nanoparticles coated with DNA have been found to provide T as well as B cells immune reaction in pigs with this technology [163]. Research on vaccine formulation for COVID-19 using electroporation is ongoing with the clinical trials of intradermally administrated DNA plasmid encrypting the SARS-COV-2' S protein [164].

12.5.4 VACCINE ADJUVANTS NANOPARTICLES

Vaccine adjuvants nanoparticles-VANs are believed to provide immune response with safety and high efficiency. Vaccine adjuvants are crucial in COVID-19 pandemic situation to reduce the antigen dosage according to requirement, which lead to more unit production and hence availability to greater population [165]. Among many vaccine competitors for trial for COVID-19 five competitors are developed by combining antigen and adjuvant. Nanoparticles based NVX-CoV2373 vaccine for COVID-19 has been developed by combining a Matrix M adjuvant will soon be under clinical trials. Strategies for vaccine adjuvants nanoparticles can be helpful in improving designs of vaccine for COVID-19. Mechanism related to VANs is associated with alerting immune cells against the specific antigens to produce an immune response. VANs in such way enhance the efficacy of the immune system and are also termed as "Danger Signals" which can be characterized as PAMPs and DAMPs (damage associated molecular patterns) [166, 167]. PAMPs and DAMPs are derived from the same virus and pattern recognition receptors are there for recognizing them. Tolls like receptor is the example of pattern recognition receptors which can be exhibited through the immune cells to provide T cells and B cells advising through release of erythrogenic cytokines (Figure 12.6) [141, 168, 169]. Adjuvants regulate the signals for developing immune response against the coming antigen thus, improving the safety. VANs are designed in a manner which can act as nanocarriers for the delivery of molecular adjuvants or possess physiochemical property to provide pro/anti immunity route eliminating the limitations like fast clearance of bloodstream, poor targeting of immune cells and no antigen-adjuvant localization. Polymeric nanoparticles can encapsulate small molecules providing the advantage of targeted delivery (lymphoid organ-specific) and controlled exposure [170, 171]. The moderate dosage associated to combination of antigen, cyclic dinucleotide adjuvant and liposomal nanoparticles offers safe and efficient immune response.

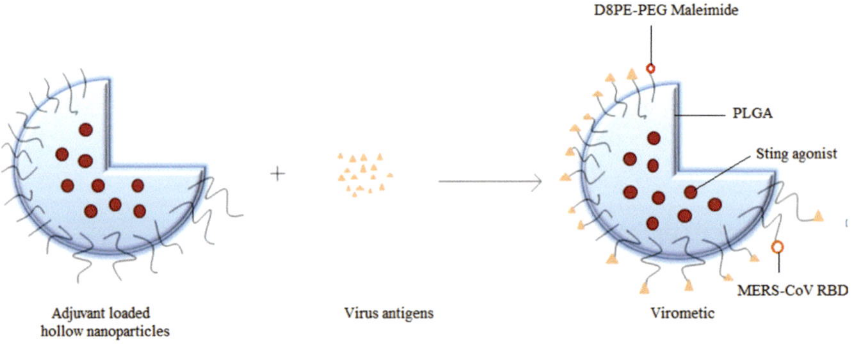

FIGURE 12.6 Synthesis of virion-nanoparticle adjuvants to stimulate humoral and CD4^{+} cell response.

Source: Adapted from: Ref. [31]; Open access source.

To achieve high dosage effects, lymph node targeting by vaccine adjuvants nanoparticles is the useful strategy while adjuvanticity is increased by targeting the DCs. *In vivo* research by using PLGA-calcium-phosphate nanoparticles combined with antigen and adjuvant combination revealed that improved antigen uptake, greater titers for antibody and APC activation enhanced the efficiency immunogenic response [172, 173]. Further studies showed T cells priming and efficient cross-presentation can be triggered by encapsulation of antigen-adjuvant resulting in co-localized compartments in the cells to activate the DCs [174, 175]. Another combination of PLGA nanoparticles with TLR4 and TLR7 molecular adjuvants synergistically activate the APCs to produce a long-lasting antigen response [176]. Codelivery of PLGA nanoparticles with immunoregulatory drugs (adjuvants) can induce antigen-specific peripheral response to tolerate the auto-reactive T cells thus, inhibiting the autoimmune response [177–182].

12.5.5 NANOPARTICLES WITH INTRINSIC ADJUVANTICITY

Nanoparticles have the potential of producing the intrinsic adjuvanticity sometimes, so they are also referred as VANs [183]. Hydrophobic nature, surface chemistry and many physiochemical characteristics of nanoparticles together are capable of producing the intrinsic adjuvant like mechanism [184–186]. For example, OH groups in poly(propylene sulfide) nanoparticles can activate the intrinsic adjuvanticity and enhances the immunity of the cells [185]. Co-loading of antigen with alumina nanoparticles can induce autophagy in DCs which promote the cross-dispensing of antigen to T cells leading to greater immunity at cellular and hormonal level [183]. Gold, PLG, and poly(γ-glutamic acid) nanoparticles have been found to increase adjuvanticity through DCs activation as well. Hydrophobic nature of gold nanoparticles also enhances the *in vivo*/*vitro* expression of inflammatory cytokines [187, 188]. In fact, vaccine adjuvants can enhance the antibody response and improves the overall efficacy of vaccines in elders, comprising a greater number of vulnerable groups with high mortality rate due to COVID-19 suffering [189, 190].

Aging is the key factor for weaker immune system due to immune senescence. It is related to decreased levels of interferon, T cells, immune-globulin M, neutrophils chemotaxis and cell division/proliferation rate [191]. Vaccine for influenza was developed through adjuvant technologies like complexes stimulating immune system, oil in water emulsion, microparticles, ionic liposomes and virosomes [192]. With the special focus on old population (greater than 70 years) an adjuvant "AS01" was developed which was based on liposomes for the units of herpes zoster vaccine [193, 194] In short, adjuvants addition significantly regulates the immune system of elders with lower risk of viral diseases like influenza and pneumonia during clinical trials providing another platform to develop the vaccine for COVID-19 [195].

12.6 CURRENT NANOTECHNOLOGY TO FIGHT COVID

It is necessary to avoid the spread of COVID among healthcare workers (HCWs) and the general public through PPE, face masks, or other material which confine the droplets of aerosol, stop their spread, and kill them. So, such materials can be formulated by using the nanomaterials that perform the same function with efficiency, as silver nanoparticles loaded onto the surface of filter kill bacteriophage MS2 [52].

12.6.1 GRAPHENES AND DICHALCOGENIDES

In biomedical applications such as diagnostics, therapeutics, safety/security, and environmental monitoring, grapheme, and dichalcogenides of transition metals have much importance. Pristine graphene is being used in biosensors, while its derivatives in detection and disinfection of microbes and enzyme assay [196, 197]. In the last decade, it was used for the first time to investigate the activity of enzymes, inhibition of viral helicase [198].

At that time, it was used for hepatitis C virus (HCV) as well as severe acute respiratory syndrome coronavirus (SARS-CoV), because of adherence of nucleotides of their nucleic acids of these viruses onto its surface containing hexagonal units. Further than its uses in therapeutics and diagnosis, when used on gloves, gowns, and masks, it holds viruses as well as bacteria which have diameter greater than 300 nm [199]. MoS_2 nanosheets belong to the 2D nanocarrier class and have good physiological stability, that is why these could be modified to perform the functions of therapeutic and disinfection molecules efficiently than nanographene as well as gold nanomaterials. TMDC absorbs light in the near-IR region that penetrates into the tissues leading towards chemo-photothermal treatment with less phototoxicity [200].

Mostly 2D materials have planar configuration in the form of sheet and various morphologies (nanoflowers) that is why they have large surface area onto which virus adhere. Nanoflower has thin radiating petals varying dimensions up to microns, for example, TMDCs-WSe_2, WS_2, $MoSe_2$, and MoS_2 are prepared directly at temperature up to 300°C in aqueous phase in atomically thin forms [201–204]. Here, it is advantageous that the crystal phase of 2D materials can be controlled. As TDMC has variable morphology, large surface area as well as edge reactivity, it has got more attention. At edges, it has high density due to dangling bonds, so nanoparticles and other nanomaterials can be used for its functionalization followed by its use in nanomedicine for detection and inactivation of microbes as well as hindrance in functions of the cells [205]. Due to its exceptional characteristics, as it is stable in air, available as a free-standing molecule and has the ability to anchor onto the substrate, it is being used for the inactivation of virus in aerosol, onto surfaces, face masks, etc.

12.6.2 MXenes

Another class of emerging material for the combat of COVID is MXenes which are 2D carbides and nitrides used to develop such surfaces which encapsulate and destroy the metabolic machinery of the viruses. Due to this reason, these can be used in the face masks and PPE.

These have hydrophilicity as well as zeta-potential in solutions ranging –30 and –80 mV. $Ti_3C_2T_x$ MXene adsorb strongly amino acids of viral spike peplomers followed by inactivation as well as killing of the virus [206]. It acts as a magnet for the proteins. It kills the microbes actively through light, when they come into contact with its surface [207–209]. These undergo plasmon resonance in the presence of visible light and IR source that is why these convert light into heat efficiently, as, $Ti_3C_2T_x$ gets plasmon resonance at 780 nm and after adherence of virus onto its surface; it is sterilized by red light, infrared lamp as well as solar light.

There are many biocompatible MXenes, such as $Ti_3C_2T_x$, $Ta_4C_3T_x$, Nb_2CT_x, etc. As these have properties of charge transfer and hydrophilicity, these kill the microbes [70, 210, 211]. Titanium carbide MXenes are the cheapest and have no harmful effects (ecological and toxicological) on the environment, these are used most commonly [212]. It is need of time to synthesize the single-layer MXene flakes of nanometer size on the required surfaces. Many other materials that can be used instead of MXenes are metal oxides and metal-organic frameworks due to their porous nature as well as antiviral properties.

Almost 50% of people suffering from COVID have kidney injury and need renal replacement therapy (RRT). When such patients do not get kidney transplanted in time, their survival rate lowers day by day [213, 214]; as, kidney removes toxic material from blood, supports fluid and electrolyte homeostasis and help in bone mineralization. In case of kidney failure, hemodialysis is preferred to remove the toxins from blood; in this process, two parallel membranes are used, one containing patient's blood and other semi-permeable membrane containing dialyzer that absorbs toxins and excess electrolytes from blood across their concentration gradients. In this way, the patient's blood is free from any harmful material, while diasylate is used for once.

Keeping in view the cost as well as problems of COVID patients, there should be such dialysis technology that is convenient and efficient for patients in all respective. MXenes used as novel sorbents can be reused, have small size as well as lightweight, for example, Ti_3C_2 MXene can be used for the removal of uremic toxin [215]. Researchers have assumed them as potential material to remold the renal replacement therapy [216].

12.7 SCOPE OF MISCELLANEOUS NANOTECHNOLOGY APPROACHES

Nanotechnology is not limited for the conventional methods of therapeutic and vaccine designs, but presents use of advanced bio-mimetic approaches as well as nanomaterials in preventing outbreak of COVID like diseases. Carbon quantum dots (CQDs) (Figure 12.7) having size <10 nm and surface potential ranging –7.9 to –39.2 mv, that were post-synthetic functionalized, were utilized for reducing the infectious effect of human coronavirus (HCoV-229E) by Szunerits and his co-workers [217]. These inhibited not only the spread of infection in Huh-7 cells but also inactivate the metabolic machinery of HCoV-229E. Carbon quantum dots functionalized with boronic acid inactivated these viruses with maximum efficiency of 5.2 ± 0.7 μg mL^{-1}. These boronic acid CQDs are used in the form of biomimetic nanodecoys such as liposomal articulations, renovated lipoproteins, and cell-membrane nanocomposites, which help in entrapping these viruses when their receptors of S-protein interact with cell membrane containing these nanodecoys [217].

Infection of Coxsackie A-21 virus can be hindered by using the liposomal surface engineered with antiviral antibodies [219]. Nanodecoys used in the cell membrane of mosquito entrap Zika virus and inactivate it [220]. Spike-protein (haemagglutinin, HA) of Influenza A virus contains multiple linking sites and can form bonds with other viral proteins; that is why, Hackenberger and his coworkers used it to inactivate the viruses [221]. Such interaction can be observed in case of viral trimeric HA viral ectoderm and surface glycan at the host cell containing the ending sialic acid residues (Sia) (solid symmetrical 3D folding resembling bacteriophage capsule). Symmetric icosahedral bacteriophages Qβ having 25 nm diameter contains K16 residues in its protein coat; these residues interact with sialic acid ligands to inactivate the virus.

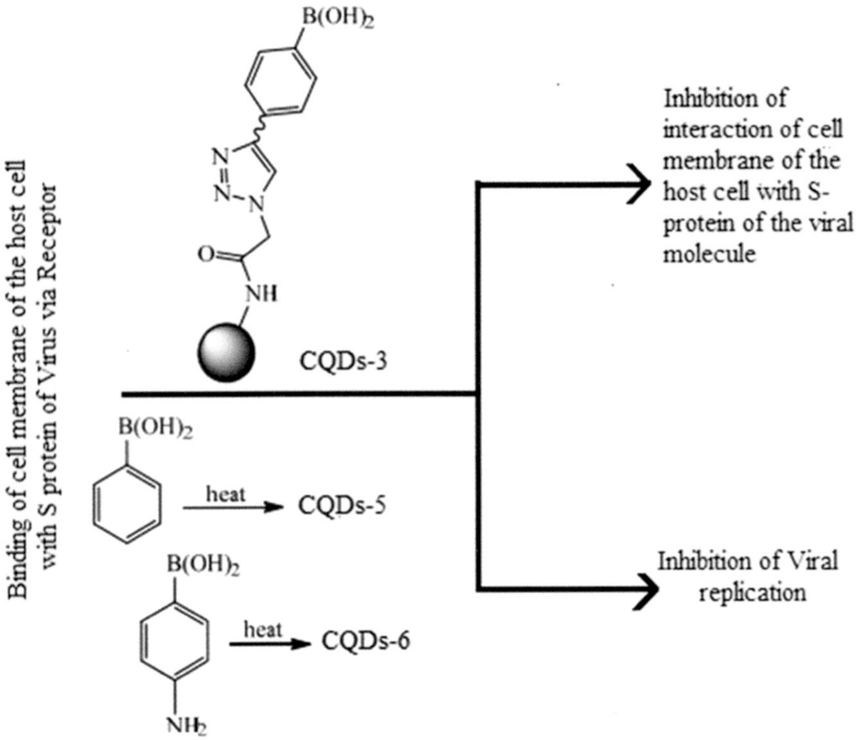

FIGURE 12.7 Synthesis of carbon dots through hydrothermal carbonization followed by their effect on attachment of virion.

Source: Adapted from: Ref. [218]; Open access source.

Covering of Qβ capsids with envelop of A/X31 virus and minimizing the interaction with host cell has been demonstrated by cryoelectron tomography in Figure 12.19. Inactivation of virus by nanoparticles present in phage capsid is being investigated by *in vitro*, *in vivo*, and *ex vivo* analysis.

12.8 CURRENT CHALLENGES AND FUTURE PROSPECTS

Nanotechnology is not only providing new approaches to treat the infectious diseases efficiently, improved mode of action of drugs but also novel nano-therapeutics and diagnostics. For example, nanoparticles, nanocarriers, and nano vaccines are being developed that are post synthetically functionalized with suitable functional groups. Such systems have a greater surface to diameter ratio, nano-size, and ability to modify their surface that can perform multiple functions, followed by their use in capturing the virus from entering into the cells and inactivating them.

Pharmaceuticals have to undergo many biological barriers while exhibiting antiviral from their management point [222–224]. To control the transmission of viral diseases, the size of therapeutics is important, so that they may reach inaccessible sites in the body, without causing quiescent infection as well as with constant duplication but at a very low rate [225]. This problem can be overcome by using such drug transporters that have nanoparticles, which get entered into all subcellular parts without causing any infections due to their ultra-small size, specific structural network, and characteristics. Hence, these are having been utilized to get through all these hindrances [226].

Nanomaterials such as dendrimers as well as silver nanoparticles have been proved excellent to treat viral diseases as they inactivate the viruses through different means. These are immunologically active because they: (i) enter into the sub-cellular parts of the cell membrane [227]; (ii) transfer drugs where they are required [227, 228]; (iii) large drug loading capacity [229]; and have biomimetic characteristics [230, 231]. Besides all these properties, these nanostructures also carry viral antigens across the cell membrane in a controlled way to inactivate the viruses without causing any infection through stimulating the sac-like DCs or B cells, antigen cross-exhibition, and activate a cellular/humoral immune response. On the whole, clinically, these are not only used to diagnose, control, detect, and treat the viral infections but also carry nanodrugs up to their required site. Delivery of nanodrugs can be upgraded by using such precursors that direct drug to the targeted site [232, 233]. Some such systems are available used; right now, formulation of nanovaccine is on the horizon due to platform of nanotechnology [234, 235].

As nano vaccines are safe in use, constructive, and cost-effective, so these should be stable at room temperature when encapsulated within the pore of nanoparticles, delivered to the required location, and administered once through compatible way. These efficiently process, recognize as well release antigens in a controlled manner after uptake by the mucosa/gut related lymphoid tissues and phagocytic cells followed by protection from proteolytic or enzymatic degradation at premature level. NP-based vaccines carry proteins as well as peptides to suitable tissues or cells to stimulate a satisfactory immune response [236, 237].

Still now, no vaccine has been developed for SARS-CoVs, RSV, and acquired immunodeficiency syndrome (HIV/AIDS). So, in case of COVID, the following alternative values should be considered:

- The metallic nanoparticles could be used for transmission and inactivation of COVID cells. As nanoparticles of silver prevent entrance of HIV-1 virus into the cell membrane of the host by interaction with cell receptors, in the same fashion, gold nanoparticles functionalized with biodegradable polymers inactivate HIV-1 and some subclasses of influenza virus (e.g., H1N1, H3N2, H5N1) [143, 238, 239].
- QDs, metal-grafted GO, nanocomposites, and nanophytotherapeutics can be used [240].
- Nanocarriers that are biodegradable (carbon nanotubes) should be considered for the transfer of antiviral drugs, for example, ribavirin, and Isoprinosine; these interact chemically with the surface of single-walled carbon nanotube and carry then to cell membranes [241].
- Such system should be explored that delivers drug efficiently, localize virus as well as target the specific tissue or organ. By using nanotechnological insights, nanotrap particles have been prepared against influenza virus, which can be further utilized against some other viruses [242].
- Use of nanomaterials that are biocompatible as well as have large drug-carrying capacity is encouraging to control the inflammation of COVID-19. Someone prepared nanoparticles by combining squalene, an autonomous lipid, and adenosine, an autonomous immuno-regulator followed by confinement with α-tocopherol, a natural antioxidant. When vascular endothelial barrier dysfunction is used on the location of inflammation, such systems carry therapeutics to the targeted position, in this way, the survival rate of patient increases. On delivery of adenosine and antioxidants simultaneously not only lowers the side effects but also enhances the potential of therapeutics, for example in hypercytokinemia by COVID-19 [119].
- To control the pandemic condition of COVID, it is critical to perform reliable test, as a novel biosensor based upon nanotechnology has been developed by Qui et al. [30, 219] for the identification of SARS-CoV-2.

12.9 CONCLUSION

The novel coronavirus is an infectious disease that has infected almost 2 million people, all over the world who are mainly suffering from heart, respiratory, and hemodynamic problems. To prevent its transmission, lockdown was imposed that affected the economy of the world. As there is no particular treatment against this infection, mostly precautionary measures or some symptomatic treatment is being used in clinics and hospitals, to avoid the entry of the virus into a host body. The use of some other treatments such as nucleoside analogs to reduce the synthesis of viral RNA, or directly change in the molecular assembly of the viral molecule is under clinical trials. In the conventional treatment against COVID, there are many challenges when the drug is administered intravenously, so nanotechnology is being used to develop the advanced treatment procedures and vaccine for COVID-19. As there is no certain antiviral agent against COVID, so already present therapeutics are being used to target the multifaceted molecular interactions. Still now, no vaccine has been developed that could fight it off. According to literature, some nano based vaccines and drugs have been used against other types of coronavirus to stimulate the immunity in patients, but in future, researchers should work on the direct use of nanomaterials as vaccine or vaccine adjuvants; for this purpose, a related animal model should be used. Meanwhile, however, the ability to overcome a crisis, novel solutions, smart management, and the utilization of advanced and modern technologies, discretely exploring the regime of emerging nanotechnology, could be very useful in lowering the present and future epidemics.

KEYWORDS

- **avian influenza virus**
- **carbon quantum dots**
- **central nervous system**
- **COVID-19**
- **nanomedicine**
- **nanotechnology**
- **nano-vaccine**

REFERENCES

1. Lukashev, A., & Zamyatnin, A., (2016). Viral vectors for gene therapy: Current state and clinical perspectives. *Biochemistry, 81*(7), 700–708. Moscow.
2. Escors, D., & Breckpot, K., (2010). Lentiviral vectors in gene therapy: Their current status and future potential. *Archivum Immunologiae et Therapiae Experimentalis, 58*(2), 107–119.
3. Walther, W., & Stein, U., (2000). Viral vectors for gene transfer. *Drugs, 60*(2), 249–271.

4. Kostarelos, K., (2020). *Nanoscale Nights of COVID-19*. Nature Publishing Group.
5. Yin, H., et al., (2014). Non-viral vectors for gene-based therapy. *Nature Reviews Genetics, 15*(8), 541–555.
6. Vincent, M., De Lázaro, I., & Kostarelos, K. (2017). Graphene materials as 2D non-viral gene transfer vector platforms. *Gene Therapy, 24*(3), 123–132.
7. Watkins, K., (2018). Emerging infectious diseases: A review. *Current Emergency and Hospital Medicine Reports, 6*(3), 86–93.
8. Cojocaru, F. D., et al., (2020). Nanomaterials designed for antiviral drug delivery transport across biological barriers. *Pharmaceutics, 12*(2), 171.
9. Gupta, A., et al., (2020). COVID-19: Emergence of infectious diseases, nanotechnology aspects, challenges, and future perspectives. *Chemistry Select, 5*(25), 7521.
10. Itani, R., Tobaiqy, M., & Al Faraj, A., (2020). Optimizing use of theranostic nanoparticles as a life-saving strategy for treating COVID-19 patients. *Theranostics, 10*(13), 5932.
11. Mainardes, R. M., & Diedrich, C., (2020). The potential role of nanomedicine on COVID-19 therapeutics. *Future Science*.
12. Vazquez-Munoz, R., & Lopez-Ribot, J. L., (2020). Nanotechnology as an alternative to reduce the spread of COVID-19. *Challenges, 11*(2), 15.
13. Fehr, A. R., & Perlman, S., (2015). Coronaviruses: An overview of their replication and pathogenesis. In: *Coronaviruses* (pp. 1–23). Springer.
14. Cornillez-Ty, C. T., et al., (2009). Severe acute respiratory syndrome coronavirus nonstructural protein 2 interacts with a host protein complex involved in mitochondrial biogenesis and intracellular signaling. *Journal of Virology, 83*(19), 10314–10318.
15. Lei, J., Kusov, Y., & Hilgenfeld, R., (2018). Nsp3 of coronaviruses: Structures and functions of a large multi-domain protein. *Antiviral Research, 149*, 58–74.
16. Beachboard, D. C., Anderson-Daniels, J. M., & Denison, M. R., (2015). Mutations across murine hepatitis virus nsp4 alter virus fitness and membrane modifications. *Journal of Virology, 89*(4), 2080–2089.
17. Zhu, X., et al., (2017). Porcine delta coronavirus nsp5 inhibits interferon-β production through the cleavage of NEMO. *Virology, 502*, 33–38.
18. Cottam, E. M., Whelband, M. C., & Wileman, T., (2014). Coronavirus NSP6 restricts autophagosome expansion. *Autophagy, 10*(8), 1426–1441.
19. Kirchdoerfer, R. N., & Ward, A. B., (2019). Structure of the SARS-CoV nsp12 polymerase bound to nsp7 and nsp8 co-factors. *Nature Communications, 10*(1), 1–9.
20. Imbert, I., et al., (2006). A second, non-canonical RNA-dependent RNA polymerase in SARS Coronavirus. *The EMBO Journal, 25*(20), 4933–4942.
21. Egloff, M. P., et al., (2004). The severe acute respiratory syndrome-coronavirus replicative protein nsp9 is a single-stranded RNA-binding subunit unique in the RNA virus world. *Proceedings of the National Academy of Sciences, 101*(11), 3792–3796.
22. Ma, Y., et al., (2015). Structural basis and functional analysis of the SARS coronavirus nsp14–nsp10 complex. *Proceedings of the National Academy of Sciences, 112*(30), 9436–9441.
23. Xu, X., et al., (2003). Molecular model of SARS coronavirus polymerase: Implications for biochemical functions and drug design. *Nucleic Acids Research, 31*(24), 7117–7130.
24. Hao, W., et al., (2017). Crystal structure of middle east respiratory syndrome coronavirus helicase. *PLoS Pathogens, 13*(6), e1006474.
25. Chen, Y., et al., (2009). Functional screen reveals SARS coronavirus nonstructural protein nsp14 as a novel cap N7 methyltransferase. *Proceedings of the National Academy of Sciences, 106*(9), 3484–3489.

26. Deng, X., et al., (2017). Coronavirus nonstructural protein 15 mediates evasion of dsRNA sensors and limits apoptosis in macrophages. *Proceedings of the National Academy of Sciences, 114*(21), E4251–E4260.
27. Shi, P., et al., (2019). PEDV nsp16 negatively regulates innate immunity to promote viral proliferation. *Virus Research, 265*, 57–66.
28. Weiss, C., et al., (2020). Toward nanotechnology-enabled approaches against the COVID-19 pandemic. *ACS Nano, 14*(6), 6383–6406.
29. Sivasankarapillai, V. S., et al., (2020). On facing the SARS-CoV-2 (COVID-19) with combination of nanomaterials and medicine: Possible strategies and first challenges. *Nanomaterials, 10*(5), 852.
30. Qiu, G., et al., (2020). *Dual-Functional Plasmonic Photothermal Biosensors for Highly Accurate Severe Acute Respiratory Syndrome Coronavirus 2 Detection, 14*(5), 5268–5277.
31. Nikaeen, G., Abbaszadeh, S., & Yousefinejad, S., (2020). Application of nanomaterials in treatment, anti-infection and detection of coronaviruses. *Nanomedicine, 15*(15), 1501–1512.
32. Kirchdoerfer, R. N., et al., (2016). Pre-fusion structure of a human coronavirus spike protein. *Nature, 531*(7592), 118–121.
33. Walls, A. C., et al., (2017). Tectonic conformational changes of a coronavirus spike glycoprotein promote membrane fusion. *Proceedings of the National Academy of Sciences, 114*(42), 11157–11162.
34. Freeling, J. P., et al., (2015). Anti-HIV drug-combination nanoparticles enhance plasma drug exposure duration as well as triple-drug combination levels in cells within lymph nodes and blood in primates. *AIDS Research and Human Retroviruses, 31*(1), 107–114.
35. Song, W., et al., (2018). Cryo-EM structure of the SARS coronavirus spike glycoprotein in complex with its host cell receptor ACE2. *PLoS Pathogens, 14*(8), e1007236.
36. Masters, P. S., (2006). The molecular biology of coronaviruses. *Advances in Virus Research, 66*, 193–292.
37. Ziebuhr, J., Snijder, E. J., & Gorbalenya, A. E., (2000). Virus-encoded proteinases and proteolytic processing in the *Nidovirales. Journal of General Virology, 81*(4), 853–879.
38. Cui, J., Li, F., & Shi, Z. L., (2019). Origin and evolution of pathogenic coronaviruses. *Nature Reviews Microbiology, 17*(3), 181–192.
39. Maier, H. J., et al., (2013). Infectious bronchitis virus generates spherules from zippered endoplasmic reticulum membranes. *MBio, 4*(5).
40. Fung, T. S., & Liu, D. X., (2019). Human coronavirus: Host-pathogen interaction. *Annual Review of Microbiology, 73*, 529–557.
41. Shereen, M. A., et al., (2020). COVID-19 infection: Origin, transmission, and characteristics of human coronaviruses. *Journal of Advanced Research.*
42. Kampf, G., et al., (2020). *Persistence of Coronaviruses on Inanimate Surfaces and Their Inactivation with Biocidal Agents, 104*(3), 246–251.
43. Sim, W., et al., (2018). *Antimicrobial Silver in Medicinal and Consumer Applications: A Patent Review of the Past Decade (2007–2017), 7*(4), 93.
44. Kaiser, J. P., Zuin, S., & Wick, P. J. S. O. T. T. E., (2013). *Is Nanotechnology Revolutionizing the Paint and Lacquer Industry? A Critical Opinion, 442*, 282–289.
45. Sohal, I. S., et al., (2018). *Ingested Engineered Nanomaterials: State of Science in Nanotoxicity Testing and Future Research Needs, 15*(1), 29.
46. Elechiguerra, J. L., et al., (2005). *Interaction of Silver Nanoparticles with HIV-1, 3*(1), 1–10.

47. Rogers, J. V., et al., (2008). *A Preliminary Assessment of Silver Nanoparticle Inhibition of Monkeypox Virus Plaque Formation, 3*(4), 129.
48. De Gusseme, B., et al., (2010). *Biogenic Silver for Disinfection of Water Contaminated with Viruses, 76*(4), 1082–1087.
49. Park, S., et al., (2018). *Disinfection of Waterborne Viruses Using Silver Nanoparticle-Decorated Silica Hybrid Composites in Water Environments, 625*, 477–485.
50. Zodrow, K., et al., (2009). *Polysulfone Ultrafiltration Membranes Impregnated with Silver Nanoparticles Show Improved Biofouling Resistance and Virus Removal, 43*(3), 715–723.
51. Du, T., et al., (2018). *Glutathione-Capped Ag2S Nanoclusters Inhibit Coronavirus Proliferation Through Blockage of Viral RNA Synthesis and Budding, 10*(5), 4369–4378.
52. Joe, Y. H., Park, D. H., & Hwang, J. J. J. O. H. M., (2016). *Evaluation of Ag nanoparticle coated air Filter Against Aerosolized Virus: Anti-Viral Efficiency with Dust Loading, 301,* 547–553.
53. Grass, G., et al., (2011). *Metallic Copper as an Antimicrobial Surface, 77*(5), 1541–1547.
54. Murray, J. P., Laband, S. J. J. A., & Microbiology, E., (1979). *Degradation of Poliovirus by Adsorption on Inorganic Surfaces, 37*(3), 480–486.
55. Warnes, S. L., Little, Z. R., & Keevil, C. W. J. M., (2015). *Human Coronavirus 229E Remains Infectious on Common Touch Surface Materials, 6*(6).
56. Van, D. N., et al., (2020). *Aerosol and surface stability of SARS-CoV-2 as compared with SARS-CoV-1, 382*(16), 1564–1567.
57. Han, J., et al., (2005). *Efficient and Quick Inactivation of SARS Coronavirus and Other Microbes Exposed to the Surfaces of Some Metal Catalysts, 18*(3), 176–180.
58. Líbalová, H., et al., (2018). *Toxicity of Surface-Modified Copper Oxide Nanoparticles in a Mouse Macrophage Cell Line: Interplay of Particles, Surface Coating and Particle Dissolution, 196*, 482–493.
59. Shi, M., et al., (2017). *The Roles of Surface Chemistry, Dissolution Rate, and Delivered Dose in the Cytotoxicity of Copper Nanoparticles, 9*(14), 4739–4750.
60. Borkow, G., et al., (2010). *A Novel Anti-Influenza Copper Oxide Containing Respiratory Face Mask, 5*(6), e11295.
61. Kim, H. E., et al., (2019). *Differential Microbicidal Effects of Bimetallic Iron-Copper nanoparticles on Escherichia coli and MS2 Coliphage, 53*(5), 2679–2687.
62. Sametband, M., et al., (2014). *Herpes Simplex Virus Type-1 Attachment Inhibition by Functionalized Graphene Oxide, 6*(2), 1228–1235.
63. Ziem, B., et al., (2017). *Size-dependent inhibition of herpesvirus cellular entry by polyvalent nanoarchitectures, 9*(11), 3774–3783.
64. Ziem, B., et al., (2016). *Highly Efficient Multivalent 2D Nanosystems for Inhibition of Orthopoxvirus Particles, 5*(22), 2922–2930.
65. Gholami, M. F., et al., (2017). *Functionalized Graphene as Extracellular Matrix Mimics: Toward Well-Defined 2D Nanomaterials for Multivalent Virus Interactions, 27*(15), 1606477.
66. Marks, R. M., et al., (2001). *Probing the Interaction of Dengue Virus Envelope Protein with Heparin: Assessment of Glycosaminoglycan-Derived Inhibitors, 44*(13), 2178–2187.
67. Bugatti, A., et al., (2007). *Heparin-Mimicking Sulfonic Acid Polymers as multitarget Inhibitors of Human Immunodeficiency Virus Type 1 Tat and gp120 Proteins, 51*(7), 2337–2345.
68. Ye, S., et al., (2015). *Antiviral Activity of Graphene Oxide: How Sharp Edged Structure and Charge Matter, 7*(38), 21571–21579.

69. Song, Z., et al., (2015). *Virus Capture and Destruction by Label-Free Graphene Oxide for Detection and Disinfection Applications, 11*(9, 10), 1171–1176.
70. Rasool, K., et al., (2016). *Antibacterial Activity of $Ti_3C_2T_x$ MXene,* 10(3), 3674–3684.
71. Jung, J. H., et al., (2010). *A Graphene Oxide Based Immuno-Biosensor for Pathogen Detection, 122*(33), 5844–5847.
72. Singh, R., Hong, S., & Jang, J. J. S. R., (2017). *Label-Free Detection of Influenza Viruses Using a Reduced Graphene Oxide-Based Electrochemical Immunosensor Integrated with a Microfluidic Platform, 7*, 42771.
73. Govorov, A. O., & Richardson, H. H. J. N. T., (2007). *Generating Heat with Metal Nanoparticles, 2*(1), 30–38.
74. Loeb, S., et al., (2018). *Solar Photothermal Disinfection Using Broadband-Light Absorbing Gold Nanoparticles and Carbon Black, 52*(1), 205–213.
75. Nazari, M., et al., (2017). *Plasmonic Enhancement of Selective Photonic Virus Inactivation, 7*(1), 1–10.
76. Maeda, K., & Domen, K. J. T. J. O. P. C. C., (2007). *New Non-Oxide Photocatalysts Designed for Overall Water Splitting Under Visible Light, 111*(22), 7851–7861.
77. Dunnill, C. W., & Parkin, P. J. D. T. I., (2011). *Nitrogen-Doped TiO_2 thin Films: Photocatalytic Applications for Healthcare Environments, 40*(8), 1635–1640.
78. Byrne, J. A., et al., (2015). *A Review of Heterogeneous Photocatalysis for Water and Surface Disinfection, 20*(4), 5574–5615.
79. Bogdan, J., Zarzyńska, J., & Pławińska-Czarnak, J. J. N. R. L., (2015). *Comparison of Infectious Agents Susceptibility to Photocatalytic Effects of Nanosized Titanium and Zinc Oxides: A Practical Approach, 10*(1), 1–15.
80. Han, W., et al., (2004). *The Inactivation Effect of Photocatalytic Titanium Apatite Filter on SARS Virus, 31*(11).
81. Liga, M. V., et al., (2011). *Virus Inactivation by Silver Doped Titanium Dioxide Nanoparticles for Drinking Water Treatment, 45*(2), 535–544.
82. Behnajady, M. A., & Eskandarloo, J. C. E. J. H., (2013). *Silver and Copper Co-Impregnated onto TiO_2-P25 Nanoparticles and Its Photocatalytic Activity, 228*, 1207–1213.
83. Rao, G., et al., (2016). *Enhanced Disinfection of Escherichia coli and Bacteriophage MS_2 in Water Using a Copper and Silver Loaded Titanium Dioxide Nanowire Membrane, 10*(4), 11.
84. Liga, M. V., et al., (2013). *Silica Decorated TiO_2 for Virus Inactivation in Drinking Water-Simple Synthesis Method and Mechanisms of Enhanced Inactivation Kinetics, 47*(12), 6463–6470.
85. Kozlova, E., et al., (2010). *Inactivation and Mineralization of Aerosol Deposited Model Pathogenic Microorganisms Over TiO_2 and Pt/TiO_2, 44*(13), 5121–5126.
86. Monteil, V., et al., (2020). *Inhibition of SARS-CoV-2 Infections in Engineered Human Tissues Using Clinical-Grade Soluble Human ACE2, 181*(4), 905–913.
87. Kim, J. M., et al., (2020). *Identification of Coronavirus Isolated from a Patient in Korea with COVID-19, 11*(1), 3.
88. Dutheil, F., Baker, J. S., & Navel, V. J. E. P., (2020). *COVID-19 as a Factor Influencing Air Pollution?, 263*, 114466.
89. Lu, J., et al., (2020). In: Wenzhe, S., Zhisheng, L., Deqian, Z., Chao, Y., Bin, X., & Zhicong, Y., (eds.), *COVID-19 Outbreak Associated with Air Conditioning in Restaurant* (Vol. 26, No.7, pp. 1628–1631). Guangzhou, China.
90. Hinds, W. C., (1999). *Aerosol Technology: Properties, Behavior, and Measurement of Airborne Particles*. John Wiley & Sons.

91. Konda, A., et al., (2020). *Aerosol Filtration Efficiency of Common Fabrics Used in Respiratory Cloth Masks, 14*(5), 6339–6347.
92. Lee, B. Y., et al., (2010). *Titanium Dioxide-Coated Nanofibers for Advanced Filters, 12*(7), 2511–2519.
93. Van, D. M. R., et al., (2019). *Smart Cancer Nanomedicine, 14*(11), 1007–1017.
94. Lammers, T. J. I. J. O. P., (2013). *Smart Drug Delivery Systems: Back to the Future vs. Clinical Reality, 454*(1), 527–529.
95. Pauletti, G. M., et al., (1997). *Improvement of Oral Peptide Bioavailability: Peptidomimetics and Prodrug Strategies, 27*(2, 3), 235–256.
96. Zhang, J., Kale, V., & Chen, M. J. T. A. J., (2015). *Gene-directed Enzyme Prodrug Therapy, 17*(1), 102–110.
97. Szebeni, J., et al., (2018). *Roadmap and Strategy for Overcoming Infusion Reactions to Nanomedicines, 13*(12), 1100–1108.
98. Qi, R., et al., (2017). *Nanoparticle Conjugates of a Highly Potent Toxin Enhance Safety and Circumvent Platinum Resistance in Ovarian Cancer, 8*(1), 1–12.
99. Ashton, S., et al., (2016). *Aurora Kinase Inhibitor Nanoparticles Target Tumors with Favorable Therapeutic Index in Vivo, 8*(325), 325ra17–325ra17.
100. Draz, M. S., et al., (2014). *Nanoparticle-Mediated Systemic Delivery of siRNA for Treatment of Cancers and Viral Infections, 4*(9), 872.
101. Davis, M. E., et al., (2010). *Evidence of RNAi in Humans from Systemically Administered siRNA Via Targeted Nanoparticles, 464*(7291), 1067–1070.
102. Ku, S. H., et al., (2016). *Chemical and Structural Modifications of RNAi Therapeutics, 104*, 16–28.
103. LaBauve, A. E., et al., (2018). *Lipid-Coated Mesoporous Silica Nanoparticles for the Delivery of the ML336 Antiviral to Inhibit Encephalitic Alphavirus Infection, 8*(1), 1–13.
104. Sago, C. D., et al., (2018). *High-Throughput in Vivo Screen of Functional mRNA Delivery Identifies Nanoparticles for Endothelial Cell Gene Editing, 115*(42), E9944–E9952.
105. Zhang, Y., et al., (2018). *Nanoparticle Anchoring Targets Immune Agonists to Tumors Enabling Anti-Cancer Immunity Without Systemic Toxicity, 9*(1), 1–15.
106. De Clercq, E., & Field, H. J. J. B. J. O. P., (2006). *Antiviral Prodrugs-the Development of Successful Prodrug Strategies for Antiviral Chemotherapy, 147*(1), 1–11.
107. Pertusat, F., et al., (2012). *Medicinal Chemistry of Nucleoside Phosphonate Prodrugs for Antiviral Therapy, 22*(5), 181–203.
108. Cern, A., et al., (2017). *New Drug Candidates for Liposomal Delivery Identified by Computer Modeling of Liposomes' Remote Loading and Leakage, 252*, 18–27.
109. Zhao, Y., et al., (2016). *Augmenting Drug-Carrier Compatibility Improves Tumor Nanotherapy Efficacy, 7*(1), 1–11.
110. Alotaibi, K. D., et al., (2018). *Phosphorus Speciation in a Prairie Soil Amended with MBM and DDG Ash: Sequential Chemical Extraction and Synchrotron-Based XANES Spectroscopy Investigations, 8*(1), 1–9.
111. Hobson, J. J., et al., (2019). *Semi-Solid Prodrug Nanoparticles for Long-Acting Delivery of Water-Soluble Antiretroviral Drugs within Combination HIV Therapies, 10*(1), 1–10.
112. Liu, L., et al., (2017). *Cholesterol-Modified Hydroxychloroquine-Loaded Nanocarriers in Bleomycin-Induced Pulmonary Fibrosis, 7*(1), 1–11.
113. Huang, P., et al., (2014). *Combination of Small Molecule Prodrug and Nanodrug Delivery: Amphiphilic Drug-Drug Conjugate for Cancer Therapy, 136*(33), 11748–11756.
114. Hu, Q., et al., (2015). *Complete Regression of Breast Tumor with a Single Dose of Docetaxel-Entrapped Core-Cross-Linked Polymeric Micelles, 53*, 370–378.

115. Wang, H., et al., (2017). *New Generation Nanomedicines Constructed from Self-Assembling Small-Molecule Prodrugs Alleviate Cancer Drug Toxicity, 77*(24), 6963–6974.
116. Shibata, A., et al., (2013). *Polymeric Nanoparticles Containing Combination Antiretroviral Drugs for HIV type 1 Treatment, 29*(5), 746–754.
117. Destache, C. J., et al., (2009). *Combination Antiretroviral Drugs in PLGA Nanoparticle for HIV-1, 9*(1), 1–8.
118. Zhong, H., et al., (2020). *Acid-Triggered Release of Native Gemcitabine Conjugated in Polyketal Nanoparticles for Enhanced Anticancer Therapy, 21*(2), 803–814.
119. Dormont, F., et al., (2020). *Squalene-Based Multidrug Nanoparticles for Improved Mitigation of Uncontrolled Inflammation in Rodents, 6*(23), eaaz5466.
120. Kraft, J. C., et al., (2018). *Mechanism-Based Pharmacokinetic (MBPK) Models Describe the Complex Plasma Kinetics of Three Antiretrovirals Delivered by a Long-Acting anti-HIV Drug Combination Nanoparticle Formulation, 275*, 229–241.
121. Jayant, R. D., et al., (2018). *Multifunctional Nanotherapeutics for the Treatment of Neuro AIDS in Drug Abusers, 8*(1), 1–12.
122. Ma, L., Kohli, M., & Smith, A. J. A. N., (2013). *Nanoparticles for Combination Drug Therapy, 7*(11), 9518–9525.
123. Chou, T. C., & Talalay, P. J. A. I. E. R., (1984). *Quantitative Analysis of Dose-Effect Relationships: The Combined Effects of Multiple Drugs or Enzyme Inhibitors, 22*, 27–55.
124. Zervantonakis, I. K., et al., (2012). *Three-Dimensional Microfluidic Model for Tumor Cell Intravasation and Endothelial Barrier Function, 109*(34), 13515–13520.
125. Kopetz, S., Lemos, R., & Powis, G. J. C. C. R., (2012). *The Promise of Patient-Derived Xenografts: The Best Laid Plans of Mice and Men, 18*(19), 5160–5162.
126. Lurie, N., et al., (2020). *Developing Covid-19 Vaccines at Pandemic Speed, 382*(21), 1969–1973.
127. Ahn, D. G., et al., (2020). *Current Status of Epidemiology, Diagnosis, Therapeutics, and Vaccines for Novel Coronavirus Disease 2019 (COVID-19), 30*(3), 313–324.
128. Park, Y. M., et al., (2013). *Nanoparticle-Based Vaccine Delivery for Cancer Immunotherapy, 13*(5), 177–183.
129. Lin, L. C. W., et al., (2018). *Advances and Opportunities in Nanoparticle-and Nanomaterial-Based Vaccines Against Bacterial Infections, 7*(13), 1701395.
130. Kanekiyo, M., et al., (2013). *Self-Assembling Influenza Nanoparticle Vaccines Elicit Broadly Neutralizing H1N1 Antibodies, 499*(7456), 102–106.
131. Slütter, B., et al., (2010). *Nasal Vaccination with N-trimethyl Chitosan and PLGA Based Nanoparticles: Nanoparticle Characteristics Determine Quality and Strength of the Antibody Response in Mice Against the Encapsulated Antigen, 28*(38), 6282–6291.
132. Li, A. V., et al., (2013). *Generation of Effector Memory T Cell-Based Mucosal and Systemic Immunity with Pulmonary Nanoparticle Vaccination, 5*(204), 204ra130–204ra130.
133. Ballester, M., et al., (2011). *Nanoparticle Conjugation and Pulmonary Delivery Enhance the Protective Efficacy of Ag85B and CpG Against Tuberculosis, 29*(40), 6959–6966.
134. Yang, Z. Y., et al., (2004). *A DNA Vaccine Induces SARS Coronavirus Neutralization and Protective Immunity in Mice, 428*(6982), 561–564.
135. Graham, R. L., et al., (2012). *A live, Impaired-Fidelity Coronavirus Vaccine Protects in an Aged, Immunocompromised Mouse Model of Lethal Disease, 18*(12), 1820.
136. Banchereau, J., & Steinman, R. M. J. N., (1998). *Dendritic Cells and the Control of Immunity, 392*(6673), 245–252.

137. Steinman, R. M., & Banchereau, J. J. N., (2007). *Taking Dendritic Cells into Medicine, 449*(7161), 419–426.
138. Joffre, O. P., et al., (2012). *Cross-Presentation by Dendritic Cells, 12*(8), 557–569.
139. Loutfy, M. R., et al., (2003). *Interferon Alfacon-1 Plus Corticosteroids in Severe Acute Respiratory Syndrome: A Preliminary Study, 290*(24), 3222–3228.
140. Amanat, F., & Krammer, F. J. I., (2020). SARS-CoV-2 vaccines: Status report. *Immunity, 52*(4), 58–589.
141. Irvine, D. J., et al., (2015). *Synthetic nanoparticles for Vaccines and Immunotherapy, 115*(19), 11109–11146.
142. Salazar-González, J. A., Gonzalez-Ortega, O., & Rosales-Mendoza, S. J. E. R. O. V., (2015). *Gold Nanoparticles and Vaccine Development, 14*(9), 1197–1211.
143. Zhao, L., et al., (2014). *Nanoparticle Vaccines, 32*(3), 327–337.
144. Pati, R., Shevtsov, M., & Sonawane, A. J. F. I. I., (2018). *Nanoparticle Vaccines Against Infectious Diseases, 9*, 2224.
145. Suk, J. S., et al., (2016). *PEGylation as a Strategy for Improving Nanoparticle-Based Drug and Gene Delivery, 99*, 28–51.
146. Hamdy, S., et al., (2011). *Targeting Dendritic Cells with Nano-Particulate PLGA Cancer Vaccine Formulations, 63*(10, 11), 943–955.
147. Lung, P., Yang, J., & Li, Q. J. N., (2020). *Nanoparticle Formulated Vaccines: Opportunities and Challenges, 12*(10), 5746–5763.
148. Geall, A. J., et al., (2012). *Nonviral Delivery of Self-Amplifying RNA Vaccines, 109*(36), 14604–14609.
149. Reichmuth, A. M., et al., (2016). *mRNA Vaccine Delivery Using Lipid Nanoparticles, 7*(5), 319–334.
150. Kranz, L. M., et al., (2016). *Systemic RNA Delivery to Dendritic Cells Exploits Antiviral Defense for Cancer Immunotherapy, 534*(7607), 396–401.
151. Kanasty, R., et al., (2013). *Delivery Materials for siRNA Therapeutics, 12*(11), 967–977.
152. Pardi, N., et al., (2015). *Expression Kinetics of Nucleoside-Modified mRNA Delivered in Lipid Nanoparticles to Mice by Various Routes, 217*, 345–351.
153. Brito, L. A., et al., (2014). *A Cationic Nanoemulsion for the Delivery of Next-Generation RNA Vaccines, 22*(12), 2118–2129.
154. Kaczmarek, J. C., et al., (2016). *Polymer-Lipid Nanoparticles for Systemic Delivery of mRNA to the Lungs, 128*(44), 14012–14016.
155. Pardi, N., et al., (2018). *mRNA Vaccines—a New Era in Vaccinology, 17*(4), 261.
156. Wang, G., et al., (2011). *Intranasal Delivery of Cationic PLGA Nano/Microparticles-Loaded FMDV DNA Vaccine Encoding IL-6 elicited Protective immunity Against FMDV Challenge, 6*(11), e27605.
157. Lim, M., et al., (2020). *Engineered Nanodelivery Systems to Improve DNA Vaccine Technologies, 12*(1), 30.
158. Zhao, K., et al., (2013). *Preparation and Efficacy of Newcastle Disease virus DNA Vaccine Encapsulated in PLGA Nanoparticles, 8*(12), e82648.
159. Long, Q., et al., (2017). Improving the cycle life of lead-acid batteries using three-dimensional reduced graphene oxide under the high-rate partial-state-of-charge condition. *Journal of Power Sources, 343*, 188–196.
160. Pack, D. W., et al., (2005). *Design and Development of Polymers for Gene Delivery, 4*(7), 581–593.

161. Steitz, J., et al., (2006). *Effective Induction of Anti-Melanoma Immunity Following Genetic Vaccination with Synthetic mRNA Coding for the Fusion Protein EGFP.TRP2, 55*(3), 246–253.
162. Chen, C., et al., (2018). Effect of glycine functionalization of 2D titanium carbide (MXene) on charge storage. *Journal of Materials Chemistry A, 6*(11), 4617–4622.
163. Hutnick, N. A., et al., (2012). *Intradermal DNA Vaccination Enhanced by Low-Current Electroporation Improves Antigen Expression and Induces Robust Cellular and Humoral Immune Responses, 23*(9), 943–950.
164. Smith, T. R., et al., (2017). *Development of an Intradermal DNA Vaccine Delivery Strategy to Achieve Single-Dose Immunity Against Respiratory Syncytial Virus, 35*(21), 2840–2847.
165. Gallucci, S., & Matzinger, P. J. C. O. I. I., (2001). *Danger Signals: SOS to the Immune System, 13*(1), 114–119.
166. Akira, S., Uematsu, S., & Takeuchi, O. J. C., (2006). *Pathogen Recognition and Innate Immunity, 124*(4), 783–801.
167. Iwasaki, A., & Medzhitov, R. J. N. I., (2004). *Toll-Like Receptor Control of the Adaptive Immune Responses, 5*(10), 987–995.
168. Platanias, L. C. J. N. R. I., (2005). *Mechanisms of Type-I-and Type-II-Interferon-Mediated Signaling, 5*(5), 375–386.
169. Tan, X., et al., (2018). *Detection of Microbial Infections Through Innate Immune Sensing of Nucleic Acids, 72*, 447–478.
170. Hanson, M. C., et al., (2015). *Nanoparticulate STING Agonists are Potent Lymph Node-Targeted Vaccine Adjuvants, 125*(6), 2532–2546.
171. Hamdy, S., et al., (2007). *Enhanced Antigen-Specific Primary CD4+ and CD8+ Responses by Codelivery of Ovalbumin and Toll-Like Receptor ligand Monophosphoryl lipid A in Poly (D, L-lactic-co-glycolic acid) Nanoparticles, 81*(3), 652–662.
172. Elamanchili, P., et al., (2007). *"Pathogen-Mimicking" Nanoparticles for Vaccine Delivery to Dendritic Cells, 30*(4), 378–395.
173. Sokolova, V., et al., (2010). *The Use of Calcium Phosphate Nanoparticles Encapsulating Toll-Like Receptor Ligands and the Antigen Hemagglutinin to Induce Dendritic Cell Maturation and T Cell Activation, 31*(21), 5627–5633.
174. Blander, J. M., & Medzhitov, R. J. S., (2004). *Regulation of Phagosome Maturation by Signals from Toll-Like Receptors, 304*(5673), 1014–1018.
175. Hoffmann, E., et al., (2012). *Autonomous Phagosomal Degradation and Antigen Presentation in Dendritic Cells, 109*(36), 14556–14561.
176. Kasturi, S. P., et al., (2011). *Programming the Magnitude and Persistence of Antibody Responses with Innate Immunity, 470*(7335), 543–547.
177. Maldonado, R. A., et al., (2015). *Polymeric Synthetic Nanoparticles for the Induction of Antigen-Specific Immunological Tolerance, 112*(2), E156–E165.
178. Look, M., et al., (2014). *The Nanomaterial-Dependent Modulation of Dendritic Cells and its Potential Influence on Therapeutic Immunosuppression in Lupus, 35*(3), 1089–1095.
179. Yeste, A., et al., (2012). *Nanoparticle-Mediated Codelivery of Myelin Antigen and a Tolerogenic Small Molecule Suppresses Experimental Autoimmune Encephalomyelitis, 109*(28), 11270–11275.
180. Turley, D. M., & Miller, S. D. J. T. J. O. I., (2007). *Peripheral Tolerance Induction Using Ethylene Carbodiimide-Fixed APCs Uses Both Direct and Indirect Mechanisms of Antigen Presentation for Prevention of Experimental Autoimmune Encephalomyelitis, 178*(4), 2212–2220.

181. Getts, D. R., et al., (2011). *Tolerance Induced by Apoptotic Antigen-Coupled Leukocytes is Induced by PD-L1+ and IL-10–Producing Splenic Macrophages and Maintained by T Regulatory Cells, 187*(5), 2405–2417.
182. Hunter, Z., et al., (2014). *A Biodegradable Nanoparticle Platform for the Induction of Antigen-Specific Immune Tolerance for Treatment of Autoimmune Disease, 8*(3), 2148–2160.
183. Li, H., et al., (2011). *Alpha-Alumina Nanoparticles Induce Efficient Autophagy-Dependent Cross-Presentation and Potent Antitumor Response, 6*(10), 645–650.
184. Hamad, I., et al., (2010). *Distinct Polymer Architecture Mediates Switching of Complement Activation Pathways at the Nanosphere-Serum Interface: Implications for Stealth Nanoparticle Engineering, 4*(11), 6629–6638.
185. Reddy, S. T., et al., (2007). *Exploiting Lymphatic Transport and Complement Activation in Nanoparticle Vaccines, 25*(10), 1159–1164.
186. Thomas, S. N., et al., (2011). *Engineering Complement Activation on Polypropylene Sulfide Vaccine Nanoparticles, 32*(8), 2194–2203.
187. Shima, F., et al., (2013). *Manipulating the Antigen-Specific Immune Response by the Hydrophobicity of Amphiphilic Poly (γ-glutamic acid) Nanoparticles, 34*(37), 9709–9716.
188. Moyano, D. F., et al., (2012). *Nanoparticle Hydrophobicity Dictates Immune Response, 134*(9), 3965–3967.
189. Liu, K., et al., (2020). Clinical features of COVID-19 in elderly patients: A comparison with young and middle-aged patients. *Journal of Infection, 80*(6), e14–e18.
190. Konnerth, H., et al., (2020). Metal-organic framework (MOF)-derived catalysts for fine chemical production. *Coordination Chemistry Reviews, 416*, 213319.
191. Franceschi, C., et al., (2000). *Inflamm-Aging: An Evolutionary Perspective on Immunosenescence, 908*(1), 244–254.
192. Fulop, T., et al., (2011). *Aging, Immunity, and Cancer, 11*(61), 537–550.
193. Weinberger, B. J. C. O. I. P., (2018). *Adjuvant Strategies to Improve Vaccination of the Elderly Population, 41*, 34–41.
194. Lal, H., et al., (2015). *Efficacy of an Adjuvanted Herpes Zoster Subunit Vaccine in Older Adults, 372*(22), 2087–2096.
195. Cunningham, A. L., et al., (2016). *Efficacy of the Herpes Zoster Subunit Vaccine in Adults 70 years of Age or Older, 375*(11), 1019–1032.
196. Stanford, M. G., et al., (2019). *Self-Sterilizing Laser-Induced Graphene Bacterial air Filter, 13*(10), 11912–11920.
197. Tu, Y., et al., (2013). *Destructive Extraction of Phospholipids from Escherichia Coli Membranes by Graphene Nanosheets, 8*(8), 594.
198. Nguyen, A. T., et al., (2015). *Crystal Networks in Silk Fibrous Materials: From Hierarchical Structure to Ultra Performance, 11*(9–10), 1039–1054.
199. Jang, H., et al., (2013). *Discovery of Hepatitis C virus NS3 Helicase Inhibitors by a Multiplexed, High-Throughput Helicase Activity Assay Based on Graphene Oxide, 52*(8), 2340–2344.
200. Gaurav, K., Mittal, G., & Karn, A., (2020). *A Short Review on the Development of Novel Face Masks During COVID-19 pandemic.*
201. Yin, W., et al., (2014). *High-Throughput Synthesis of Single-Layer MoS_2 Nanosheets as a Near-Infrared Photothermal-Triggered Drug Delivery for Effective Cancer Therapy, 8*(7), 6922–6933.
202. Sokolikova, M. S., et al., (2019). *Direct Solution-Phase Synthesis of 1T'WSe_2 Nanosheets, 10*(1), 1–8.

203. Mahler, B., et al., (2014). *Colloidal Synthesis of 1T-WS2 and 2H-WS2 Nanosheets: Applications for Photocatalytic Hydrogen Evolution, 136*(40), 14121–14127.
204. Sun, D., et al., (2015). *Formation and Interlayer Decoupling of Colloidal $MoSe_2$ Nanoflowers, 27*(8), 3167–3175.
205. Zhu, Q. L., & Xu, Q., (2014). Metal-organic framework composites. *Chemical Society Reviews, 43.*
206. Jing, X., et al., (2018). *Multifunctional Nanoflowers for Simultaneous Multimodal Imaging and High-Sensitivity Chemo-Photothermal Treatment, 29*(2), 559–570.
207. Chen, C., et al., (2018). *Effect of Glycine Functionalization of 2D Titanium Carbide (MXene) on Charge Storage, 6*(11), 4617–4622.
208. Nguyen, V. H., et al., (2020). *Novel Architecture Titanium Carbide ($Ti_3C_2T_x$) MXene Cocatalysts toward Photocatalytic Hydrogen Production: A Mini-Review, 10*(4), 602.
209. Wong, Z. M., et al., (2018). *Enhancing the Photocatalytic Performance of MXenes via Stoichiometry Engineering of Their Electronic and Optical Properties, 10*(46), 39879–39889.
210. Low, J., et al., (2018). *TiO_2/MXene Ti_3C_2 Composite with Excellent Photocatalytic CO_2 Reduction activity, 361*, 255–266.
211. Rasool, K., et al., (2017). *Efficient Antibacterial Membrane Based on Two-Dimensional Ti_3C_2Tx (MXene) Nanosheets, 7*(1), 1–11.
212. Pandey, R. P., et al., (2018). *Ultrahigh-Flux and Fouling-Resistant Membranes Based on Layered Silver/MXene ($Ti_3C_2T_x$) Nanosheets, 6*(8), 3522–3533.
213. Nasrallah, G. K., et al., (2018). *Ecotoxicological Assessment of Ti_3C_2Tx (MXene) using a Zebrafish Embryo Model, 5*(4), 1002–1011.
214. Naicker, S., et al., (2020). *The Novel Coronavirus 2019 Epidemic and Kidneys, 97*(5), 824–828.
215. Meng, F., et al., (2018). *MXene Sorbents for Removal of Urea from Dialysate: A Step Toward the Wearable Artificial Kidney, 12*(10), 10518–10528.
216. Hojs, N., Fissell, W. H., & Roy, S. J. C. J. O., (2020). *Ambulatory Hemodialysis-Technology Landscape and Potential for Patient-Centered Treatment, 15*(1), 152–159.
217. Rao, L., Tian, R., & Chen, X. J. A. N., (2020). *Cell-Membrane-Mimicking Nanodecoys Against Infectious Diseases, 14*(3), 2569–2574.
218. Innocenzi, P., & Stagi, L., (2020). Carbon-based antiviral nanomaterials: Graphene, C-dots, and fullerenes. A perspective. *Chemical Science, 11*(26), 6606–6622.
219. Magee, W. E., & Miller, O. V. J. N., (1972). *Liposomes Containing Antiviral Antibody Can Protect Cells from Virus Infection, 235*(5337), 339–341.
220. Rao, L., et al., (2018). *A Biomimetic Nanodecoy Traps Zika Virus to Prevent Viral Infection and Fetal Microcephaly Development, 19*(4), 2215–2222.
221. Lauster, D., et al., (2020). *Phage Capsid Nanoparticles with Defined Ligand Arrangement Block Influenza Virus Entry, 15*(5), 373–379.
222. Sanhai, W. R., et al., (2008). *Seven Challenges for Nanomedicine, 3*(5), 242–244.
223. Duncan, R., & Gaspar, R., (2011). *Nanomedicine (s) Under the Microscope, 8*(6), 2101–2141.
224. Ferrari, M., (2005). *Cancer Nanotechnology: Opportunities and Challenges, 5*(3), 161–171.
225. Cojocaru, F. D., et al., (2020). *Nanomaterials Designed for Antiviral Drug delivery transport Across Biological Barriers, 12*(2), 171.

226. De Oliveira, M. P., et al., (2005). *Tissue Distribution of Indinavir Administered as Solid Lipid Nanocapsule Formulation in mdr1a (+/+) and mdr1a (–/–) CF-1 Mice, 22*(11), 1898–1905.
227. Caron, J., et al., (2010). *Squalenoyl Nucleoside Monophosphate Nanoassemblies: New Prodrug Strategy for the Delivery of Nucleotide Analogues, 20*(9), 2761–2764.
228. Qasim, M., et al., (2014). *Nanotechnology for Diagnosis and Treatment of Infectious Diseases, 14*(10), 7374–7387.
229. Kumar, A., et al., (2012). *Gold Nanoparticles Functionalized with Therapeutic and Targeted Peptides for Cancer Treatment, 33*(4), 1180–1189.
230. McNeil, S. E., (2011). Unique benefits of nanotechnology to drug delivery and diagnostics. In: *Characterization of Nanoparticles Intended for Drug Delivery* (pp. 3–8). Springer.
231. Sanvicens, N., & Marco, M., (2008). *Multifunctional Nanoparticles-Properties and Prospects for Their Use in Human Medicine, 26*(8), 425–433.
232. Gagliardi, M. J. T. D., (2017). *Biomimetic and Bioinspired Nanoparticles for Targeted Drug Delivery, 8*(5), 289–299.
233. Petros, R. A., & DeSimone, J. M., (2010). *Strategies in the Design of Nanoparticles for Therapeutic Applications, 9*(8), 615–627.
234. Maurer, P., et al., (2005). *A Therapeutic Vaccine for Nicotine Dependence: Preclinical Efficacy, and Phase I Safety and Immunogenicity, 35*(7), 2031–2040.
235. Roldão, A., et al., (2010). *Virus-Like Particles in Vaccine Development, 9*(10), 1149–1176.
236. Greenwood, B., (2014). *The Contribution of Vaccination to Global Health: Past, Present and Future, 369*(1645), 20130433.
237. Nandedkar, T. D., (2009). *Nanovaccines: Recent Developments in Vaccination, 34*(6), 995–1003.
238. Sportelli, M. C., et al., (2020). *Can Nanotechnology and Materials Science Help the Fight Against SARS-CoV-2?, 10*(4), 802.
239. Kerry, R. G., et al., (2019). *Nano-Based Approach to Combat Emerging Viral (NIPAH virus) Infection, 18*, 196–220.
240. Shaligram, S., & Campbell, A., (2013). *Toxicity of Copper Salts is Dependent on Solubility Profile and Cell Type Tested, 27*(2), 844–851.
241. Zhu, S., et al., (2019). *Anti-Betanodavirus Activity of Isoprinosine and Improved Efficacy Using Carbon Nanotubes Based Drug Delivery System, 512*, 734377.
242. Singh, L., et al., (2017). *The Role of Nanotechnology in the Treatment of Viral Infections, 4*(4), 105–131.
243. Zhang, H.; Penninger, J.M.; Li, Y.; Zhong, N.; Slutsky, A.S. Angiotensin-converting enzyme 2 (ACE2) as a SARS-CoV-2 receptor: Molecular mechanisms and potential therapeutic target. *Intensive Care Med. 2020*, 46, 586–590.

CHAPTER 13

Recent Developments in Therapies and Strategies Against COVID-19

MISBAH HAMEED,[1] M. ZIA-UL-HAQ,[2] and MARIUS MOGA[3]

[1]*Institute of Pharmacy, Lahore College for Women University, Lahore, Pakistan, E-mail: misbahmajid1@gmail.com*

[2]*Office of Research, Innovation and Commercialization, Lahore College for Women University, Lahore–54000, Pakistan*

[3]*Faculty of Medicine, Transilvania University of Brasov, Brasov–500036, Romania*

ABSTRACT

COVID-19 is a new pandemic challenge experienced worldwide. Extensive research is going on through all parts of the world to combat the virus. The virus genome has been explored, but still, no vaccine is available against the virus. Thus, search is under process to find out the effective treatment against COVID-19 to reduce the complications due to the disease as well as to reduce the mortality rate. The treatment strategy against COVID-19 is based on the mechanism of action of purposed drugs, their potential therapeutic outcomes, their safety profiles specifically related to the study design of proposed clinical trials. All the repurposed drugs are being trialed on the basis of previous data available and especially those drugs which showed positive outcomes against MERS and SARS are explored for their effectiveness against COVID-19. The treatment is segregated into two major categories, primary, and Adjunctive therapies. In the following section, the drugs included in both categories are discussed in detail along with their potential use against COVID-19.

13.1 INTRODUCTION TO COVID-2 PANDEMIC

The causative agent of corona disease (COVID-2019) is beta coronavirus that was named novel coronavirus (2019-nCoV) by World Health Organization (WHO) but latter named severe acute respiratory syndrome-2 (SARS-CoV-2) by The International Committee of Taxonomy of Viruses as it causes the acute respiratory syndrome and the genome of new corona strain resembles Phylogenetically to severe acute respiratory syndrome coronavirus (SARS-CoV) that was the disease-causing agent of 2002. SARS-CoV-2 was declared a pandemic by WHO on 11th March 2020 [1].

Till now no specific treatment strategy has been developed. COVID-19 disease shows various clinical presentations varies largely from asymptomatic patients to critical respiratory failure in some patients. It is noted that 85% of the patients suffering from COVID-19 show pyrexia while only 45% are febrile on early stage of disease. Around 67.7% of patients have a cough among which 33.4% patients complained of sputum. Dyspnea, sore throat, and nasal congestion are reported in 18.6%, 13.9%, and 4.8% of patients thus are comparatively less common. Other indications include headache, muscle, and bone pains in 13.6%, 14.8% and 11.4% of the cases. Gastrointestinal (GI) symptoms like nausea, vomiting in 5% while diarrhea is observed in 3.7% of the cases (Table 13.1) [2].

Critical effects on the lung tissues can cause acute respiratory distress syndrome (ARDS) that can lead to septic shock, which is very critical, especially in patients above 60 years of age and the important cause of intensive care unit (ICU) stay and death from COVID-19. Old age, smoking, and other comorbid medical disorders further complicate the situation as such patients has high concentration of ACE2 receptors. A study conducted by indicated that leading medical conditions like hypertension, diabetes, and cardiovascular and cerebrovascular diseases complicate the patient's condition [3].

COVID-19 has resulted in unprecedented challenges to the healthcare systems worldwide in developed as well as underdeveloped countries. Till now, we have no clinically proven therapeutics for COVID-19Furthermore. Furthermore, a significant number of preclinical researches associated with treatment of allied viruses SARS and MERS was reported but as the outbreak associated with these viruses exist. Along with the development of an effective vaccine or therapeutic agents, healthcare professionals worldwide are exploring already available options to treat the COVID-19 patients and focusing on drug repositioning and repurposing of already existing treatments [4, 5]. These "repurposed" drugs are already having FDA approval in the USA but for other conditions. Some of these repurposed drugs like

TABLE 13.1 Coronavirus Worldwide Pandemics from Till February Year 2021

Disease	Incubation Duration	Cases Reported	Deaths Reported	Mortality	Treatment Used	Vaccination
SARS-CoV-1 (2003)	2–7 days	8,098	774	9.6%	Ribavarin, corticosteroids, immunosuppressive agents	Not available
MERS-CoV (MERS 2012)	5 days	2,574	885	34%	Antivirals, monoclonal antibodies	Not available
SARS-CoV-2 (COVID- 19)	2–14 days	136,996,364	2,951,832	2.1%	Antivirals, corticosteroids, monoclonal antibodies, azithromycin	Available

Remdesivir, Azithromycin, Ritonavir, Hydroxychloroquine (HCQ), and Ruxolitinib has entered in to clinical trials against COVID-19. Clinical current management of disease includes measures to control the spread of disease and to provide supportive care like oxygen maintenance and in critical cases, mechanical ventilator support (Table 13.2).

TABLE 13.2 Differences between Flu and COVID-19 Symptoms

Flu	COVID-19
Causative agent influenza viruses	Causative agent SARS-CoV-2
Serial interval of virus is 3 days thus spread faster	Serial interval of virus is 5–6 days take longer time to spread
Vaccine is available	vaccine is available
Mild symptoms	Symptoms vary from mild flu-like to acute respiratory distress syndrome
Children are commonly attacked by flu	Initial data reveals very rare cases in children however new variants are affecting children as well
Severe influenza infection occurs in children, pregnant women, elderly especially with chronic medical conditions	Infection can occur in all ages, but elderly and patients with other chronic medical conditions are at higher risk
Mortality is low	Mortality is high

Largely two strategies are being explored for the management of COVID-19. The first one is to target key enzymes of the virus, thus interfering with the replication of the virus and inhibiting its growth inside the host cell. For this purpose, antivirals already existing with effective action against some CoVs like SARS-CoV, MERS-CoV, HIV, and HCV are being repurposed to be tested against COVID-19 for their action. Search for the targets for binding of the drugs on the surface of the host cell may also be evaluated as a potential COVID-19 therapy for inhibiting viral entry.

The other approach is the use of immunoglobulins, interferons, monoclonal antibodies, and tyrosine kinase inhibitors for immunomodulation, particularly at an early stage of the disease, to boost immunity against the virus and in critical cases to prevent acute lung damage and organ impairment caused by uncontrolled immune response.

The incubation duration of the virus after exposure to the virus is 14 days. The severity of the symptoms varies in different patients as well as in different parts of the world. In 80% of the patients, few mild symptoms are observed. In 15% of the patients, the symptoms are severe, and hypoxia may develop and may involve lung in more than 50% of patients, especially in elderly patients. While in 5% of patient's respiratory failure or multiple organ damage may occur in late stages of the disease due to increased cytokine, this may lead to ICU admission resulting in increased tumor necrosis factor-alpha (TNF-α) and interleukin-2 (IL-2). The major cause leading to the death due to COVID-19 is uncontrolled pulmonary inflammation (Table 13.3).

TABLE 13.3 Drugs Repurposed for Treatment of COVID-19 Virus Their Mechanism of Action

Drug	Mechanism of Action
Remdesivir	Interacts and inhibits viral RdRp
Ribavirin	Prevents viral RNA-dependent RNA polymerase enzyme release
Lopinavir/ritonavir	Inhibits 3-chymotrypsin-like protease activity 3-chymotrypsin-like protease activity
Favipiravir	Prevents release of RNA-dependent RNA polymerase
Oseltamivir	Viral neuraminidase enzyme inhibitor
Umifenovir	Targets the S protein/ACE2 interface and stops the host cell fusion with viral envelope
Hydroxychloroquine and Chloroquine	Increase intracellular levels of zinc which in turn inhibits RNA-dependent RNA polymerase
Nitric oxide and epoprostenol	Improve oxygenation by reducing the mean pulmonary artery pressure in critical COVID-19 patients
Baricitinib	Inhibits Janus kinase 1 and 2 having a role in triggering effect on cytokine-induced phosphorylation of STAT
Ruxolitinib	Potent JAK1 and JAK2 inhibitor and inhibits clathrin-mediated endocytosis
Tocilizumab	Inhibits interleukin-6 receptor (IL-6R)
Camrelizumab	Targets programmed cell death 1 (PD-1) receptors
Meplazumab	An anti-CD147 antibody that inhibits entry of virus in the host cell
Eculizumab	Blocks the C5b production which stops complex C5b-9 and thus formation of membrane attack complex (MAC).
Bevacizumab	Prevents VEGF contact with endothelial receptors, KDR, and Flt-1
Corticosteroids	Inhibits pro-inflammatory genes that code for synthesis of cytokines, inflammatory enzymes, chemokines, and cell adhesion molecules
Renin angiotensin aldosterone system (RAAS) antagonists	Increases expression of ACE2 on lung cells
NSAID nonsteroidal anti-inflammatory drugs	Decreases the fever caused because of COVID-19

TABLE 13.3 *(Continued)*

Drug	Mechanism of Action
Convalescent plasma therapy	Transfer antibodies prepared in recovered COVID-19 patients
Azithromycin	Immunomodulatory action
Anticoagulants	Inhibit the attachment of virus to surface receptor (Spike) S1 via conformational changes.
Ascorbic acid	Enhances the maturation of T lymphocytes
Interferons	Increases the antiviral response of host
Anthelmintics	Potential to hinder viral replication and induce immunomodulation in host cells
Colchicine	Reduces IL-1 beta activation shows strong anti-inflammatory effects
Thiazolidinediones	Up regulate ACE2 receptor

13.2 POTENTIAL THERAPIES AND STRATEGIES AGAINST COVID-19

Overall therapeutic management can be divided into two groups:

- Primary therapies; and
- Adjunctive therapies.

13.2.1 PRIMARY THERAPIES

13.2.1.1 ANTIVIRAL AND ANTIRETROVIRALS

13.2.1.1.1 Nucleotide Analogs

Nucleoside analogs are a class of antiviral drugs that proves to be effective against different viruses such as hepatitis B, C, and HIV. Nucleoside analogs are further classified into three classes:

1. **Mutagenic Nucleosides:** This targets the viral dependence on RdRp that cause the replication of RNA from RNA template like ribavirin.
2. **Obligate Chain Terminators:** This targets additional DNA synthesis and incorporation as it lacks the reactive 3′-hydroxyl group needed for this process like azidothymidine (AZT).
3. **Delayed Chain Terminators:** This targets the process of transcription like Remdesivir.

13.2.1.1.2 Remdesivir

One of the clinical agents that were trialed in the current pandemic is Remdesivir (GS-5734). It was developed by Gilead Sciences. The drug was discovered to fight against RNA-based viruses, such as EBOV and the Coronaviridae viruses such as Middle East respiratory syndrome (MERS) and severe acute respiratory syndrome (SARS) [6].

Remdesivir possess a wide spectrum of activity, many researchers worldwide assessed its antiviral potential both *in vitro* and *in vivo* against SARS, MERS zoonotic coronaviruses (CoVs), circulating human CoVs HCoV-OC43 and HCoV-229E [7, 8] including its activity against CoVs including its prophylactic and therapeutic potential against MERS in an *in vivo* nonhuman primate model [9].

- ➢ **Mode of Action:** Remdesivir interferes the viral RNA-dependent RNA polymerase (RdRp), interacts with intact exon proofreading's ability and resulting in early cessation of viral RNA transcription. Remdesivir (developmental code GS-5734), is a prodrug that is metabolized to an alanine metabolite (GS-704277) in the cells, converted then into the monophosphate derivative and finally to active nucleoside triphosphate derivative (Figure 13.1) [6].

Remdesivir's broad-spectrum antiviral activity. It interferes with the viral RdRp and hinders chain termination in different RNA viruses, CoVs (MERS, SARS, contemporary human CoV) [7].

The outbreak of COVID-19 initiated the use of the Remdesivir on trials basis. In China, a randomized, placebo-controlled clinical trial (NCT04252664, since suspended) for Remdesivir was registered to estimate its potential use in patients suffering from mild to moderate COVID-19 infection [10]. Another trial (NCT04257656, since terminated) was registered in which Remdesivir administered to critical COVID-19 patients was having respiratory disease. In both trials, the dosage regimen was to administer 200 mg of the drug IV as a loading followed by 100 mg of the drug for consecutive 9 days. Both trials were planned to measure the outcomes till 28 days, and parameters monitored include fever, saturation level of oxygen and respiratory rate [10]. In the USA, as the cases of COVID-19 were at initial stages at the start of February, some of the hospitalized patients with critical conditions received Remdesivir with the same dosage for 4–10 days and showed improvement in respiratory symptoms [1]. Another study reported 53 hospitalized patients in USA, Europe, and Japan were given the drug in the same dosage. The mortality observed was 13.2% while clinical progress was witnessed in 62% of treated patients [12].

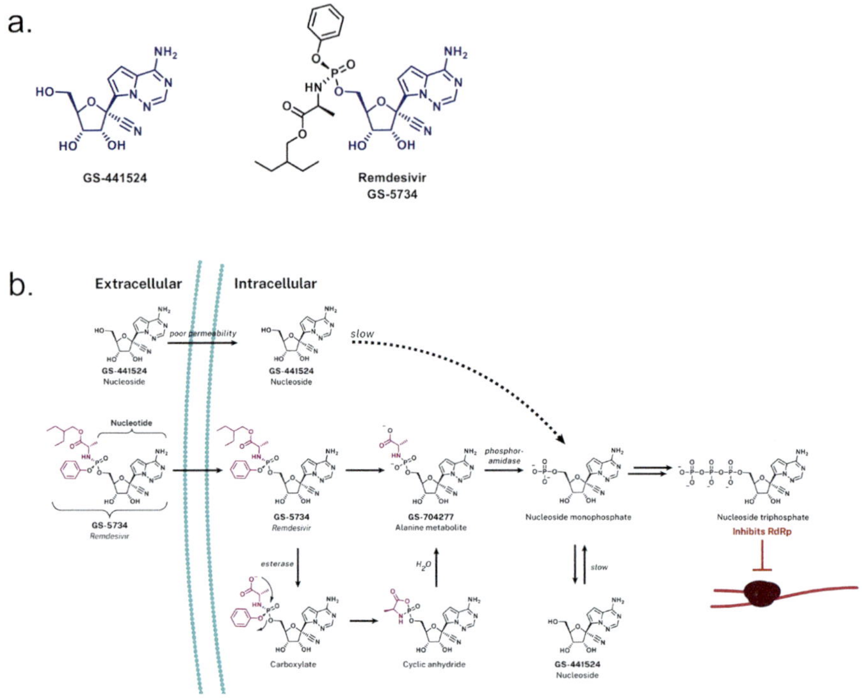

FIGURE 13.1 Remdesivir conversion into active metabolite in the cell.
Source: Adapted from: Ref. [6].

Approximately 70% of the patients receiving Remdesivir in the USA showed less dependency on oxygen, and many patients with critical symptoms and mechanically ventilated were extubated [12].

IV infusions of Remdesivir given at doses between 3 mg and 225 mg were tolerated well by the patients and showed no signs of kidney or liver toxicity. Remdesivir showed a half-life of approximately 35 hours and linear pharmacokinetics; however, after administration of multiple doses, elevation in levels of reversible aspartate aminotransferase (AST) and alanine transaminase (ALT) were observed. No adjustments of doses in hepatic or liver diseases are recommended at this stage however it is suggested not to start the dose if the glomerular filtration rate is low [13].

Overall adverse effects observed in COV ID-19 patients induce due to Remdesivir use include damage to hepatic function, transient GI symptoms, acute kidney injury (AKI), gastroparesis, or rectal bleeding, nausea, vomiting, skin rash and diarrhea [14]. Remdesivir has not shown any side effects on renal activity in patients with Ebola virus (EBOV) disease, but it should be noted that formulation contains sulfobutylether-β-cyclodextrin, which has good solubilizing activity and its use should be monitored in patients with renal impairment. Remdesivir shows rapid distribution, metabolism, and clearance thus clinically significant interactions are very rare. Co-administration of Remdesivir with carbamazepine, phenobarbitone, primidone, phenytoin, and rifampicin should be avoided as being enzyme inducers they can cause decrease in plasma concentrations of the Remdesivir. Remdesivir is not FDA approved, and for patient use, it is provided for compassionate use, enrollment in a clinical trial or expanded access [13].

An important consideration is that Remdesivir has patents until 2038. Although Gilead has focused on increasing the production of the drug to meet worldwide demand but concern is that many countries in the world would simply not be able to afford it.

13.2.1.1.3 Ribavirin

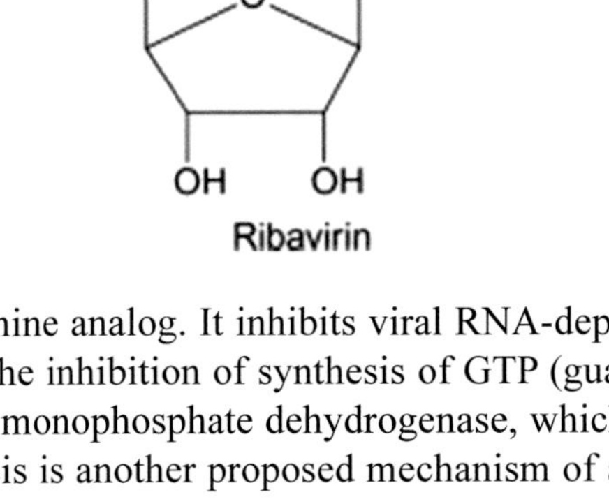

Ribavirin

Ribavirin is a guanine analog. It inhibits viral RNA-dependent RNA polymerase enzyme. The inhibition of synthesis of GTP (guanosine 5'-triphosphate) *via* inosine monophosphate dehydrogenase, which is needed for the viral RNA synthesis is another proposed mechanism of action of ribavirin.

Another mechanism proposed for ribavirin is that it increases the reaction of interferon-stimulated genes (ISG), thus increasing the sensitivity cell to exogenous interferon and also increasing the synthesis of endogenous interferon [15]. It is used against infections like hepatitis C virus (HCV) [16].

Pharmacokinetic studies of ribavirin showed that it is absorbed rapidly after oral administration with maximum concentration-time up to 1.5 hours, show rapid distribution but slow elimination. It shows absorption from proximal small bowel through concentrative N1 sodium-dependent nucleoside transporters. It shows extensive absorption but have about 50% absolute bioavailability because of first-pass effect. Have high apparent volume of distribution due to its distribution into nonplasma compartments, shows no plasma proteins binding [10].

Ribavirin inhibited COVID-19 virus reproduction at very small doses in the model using Caco-2 cells, and results are accordant with studies of ribavirin against other CoVs such as CoV-NL63, HCoV-43 and MERS-CoV-16, but not SARS-CoV-126. It is currently being investigated as a combination therapy with some other drugs against COVID-19. Ribavirin in combination with lopinavir/ritonavir showed some effectiveness against COVID-19 in patients and in tissue culture. Ribavarin when co-administered with lopinavir-ritonavir and a corticosteroid, it reduces the death rate in COVID-19 patients resulting from acute respiratory distress syndrome (ARDS). Some clinical trials using the combination of ribavirin with lopinavir-ritonavir and interferon-α (NCT04254874; ChiCTR2000029308) are underway [10]. Ribavirin has been proposed by National Health Commission (NHC) for the treatment of COVID-19 [17].

Ribavirin dosage strategy used in MERS trials was 2,000 mg loading dose followed by 1,200 mg 8 hourly for 4 days then 600 mg 8 hourly for 4–6 days and drug are given orally similarly in trials against SARS COV high doses of ribavirin up to 1.2 g to 2.4 g orally every 8 hours was required [18].

Ribavirin may expose the patients to severe side effects and may cause hematologic toxicity at high doses. As shown in SARS trials, a high dose of ribavirin causes hemolytic anemia in approximately 60% of patients. In MERS trials, it was observed that approximately 40% of patients on combination therapy of ribavirin with interferon required blood transfusions while 75% of the patients suffering from SARS presented elevated transaminase levels. Severe side effects like hematologic and liver toxicity were also observed when ribavirin was used in trials against SARS. It uses is contraindicated in pregnancy [19].

13.2.1.1.4 Lopinavir/Ritonavir

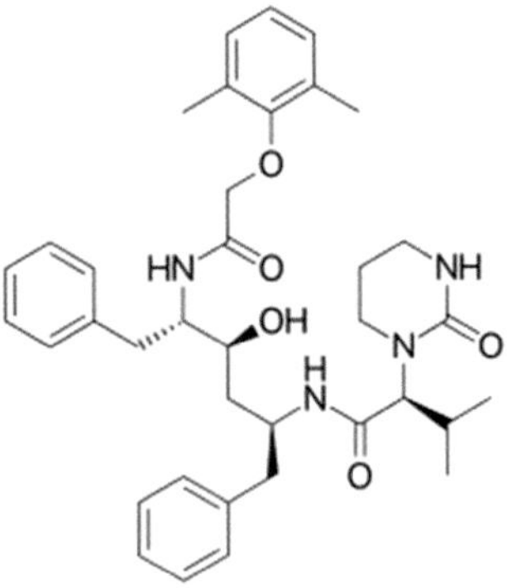

Lopinavir

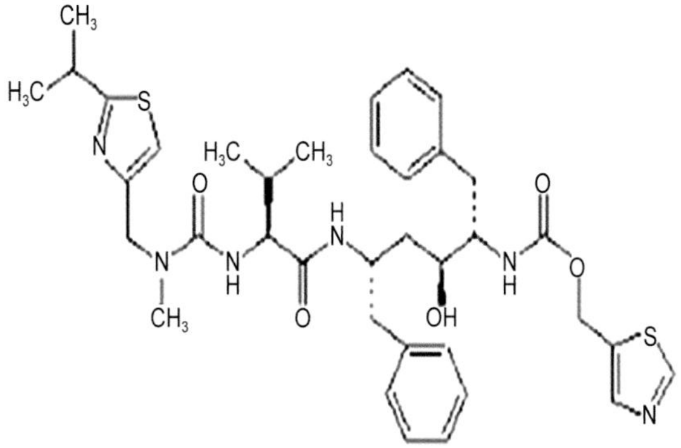

Ritonavir

Lopinavir is a protease inhibitor and is prepared from structurally similar ritonavir antiretroviral agents. Aspartic protease is essential for the cleavage of proteins from precursor polypeptide strand of virus, which is needed for structural and functional proteins. The inhibition of protease results in immature and non-effective virions [20]. Lopinavir is a selective inhibitor of the HIV type 1 (HIV-1), which is required for mature infective virus production. The drug blocks infectivity by blocking the maturation of HIV-1. Lopinavir is a highly potent. These two drugs are available as formulation because when co-administered, ritonavir at low doses improves the pharmacokinetic profile and the activity of lopinavir against HIV-1 protease [21].

Lopinavir/ritonavir is approved by FDA against HIV as an oral combination therapy. *In vitro* activity of the combination has also been proved against some CoVs by inhibiting 3-chymotrypsin-like protease activity [22]. Limited data is available on the efficacy of the Lopinavir/ritonavir when used in combination against SARS and MERS. It was also demonstrated in trials that its administration at early peak replication phase, i.e., within 7–10 days is beneficial while delayed initiation of the therapy has no effects [23]. Animal trials of combination of Lopinavir/ritonavirin against MERS-CoV was effective [20]. Based on previous results, it was selected for use against COVID-19. A study including 199 hospitalized patients with severe COVID-19 symptoms did not show significant clinical improvement or mortality when compared to conventional care [24]. However, it has been a part of a number of trials against COVID-19 including a two arms SOLIDARITY trial in which it was tested in combination with and without of the addition interferon-β and has been recommended as a possible therapy for against COVID-19 [25].

Side effects like GI abnormality, Pancreatitis, hepatotoxicity, and cardiac issues are also observed. Lopinavir is extensively metabolized by liver enzymes like CYP3A4 and CYP3A5, while the addition of ritonavir results in high concentrations of lopinavir by inhibiting the CYP3A4 enzyme. Lopinavir/ritonavir is mainly excreted by fecal route and less the 2% is by urinary excretion. Transference of lopinavir across the placenta is low; however, the addition of ritonavir increased the fetal exposure and may cause low birth weight, premature delivery, stillbirth, and small for gestational age infants [25].

13.2.1.1.5 Favipiravir

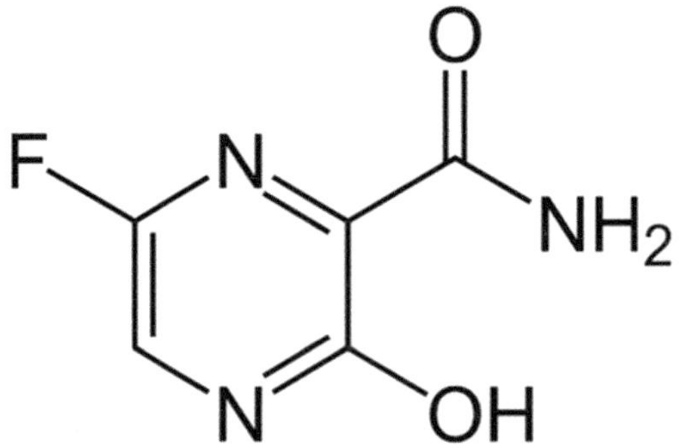

Favipiravir also known as T-705 was developed in Japan in 2002, is a pyrazine carboxamide derivative, a guanine analog, it competes with purine nucleosides and inhibits RNA-dependent RNA polymerase which is key enzyme of virus thus interfere with replication process. Favipiravir is a prodrug. It is ribosylated and phosphorylated inside the cell and is then converted into favipiravir ibofuranosyl-5′-triphosphate. It is a broad-spectrum antiviral and has been approved in some Asian countries like Japan for use against influenza viruses type A and B. It is also effective flavivirus, arenavirus, bunyavirus, and filoviruses. It has been proved effective against EBOV trials. In a study on patients suffering with EBOV, it was observed that patients receiving additional favipiravir along with WHO-recommended supportive therapy showed high survival rate [26].

Favipiravir has been used in a number of clinical trial for COVID-19. A trial including 80 patients was conducted in Shenzhen (ChiCTR2000029600) and resulted that patients receiving favipinavir demonstrated relatively shorter virus clearance time, but later this article was temporarily withdrawn.

The dosage favipinavir accepted in China is one day loading dose of 32,000 mg daily in two 1,600 mg doses followed by 1,200 mg for 2–14 days [27]. In another prospective and randomized study with 120 patients showing moderate to severe COVID-19 symptoms was compared with Arbidol. Differences in recovery rate was observed on day 7 in patients with moderate symptoms, while no significant change was observed in patients with severe symptoms [28].

Maximum plasma concentration of Flavipinavir occurs after 2 hours of administration with a half-life of 2–2.5 hours. It shows high (54%) plasma protein binding. It shows rapid clearance by the liver and kidneys. The drug is well-tolerated and may show mild adverse effect [26].

Transient thrombocytopenia and elevated liver enzyme levels was observed with elevated doses of favipiravir in animals having Lassa virus infection. Favipiravir use in an EBOV patient resulted in corrected QT (QTc) interval prolongation at high doses. The drug is teratogenic and should not be used in pregnancy.

13.2.1.1.6 *Oseltamivir*

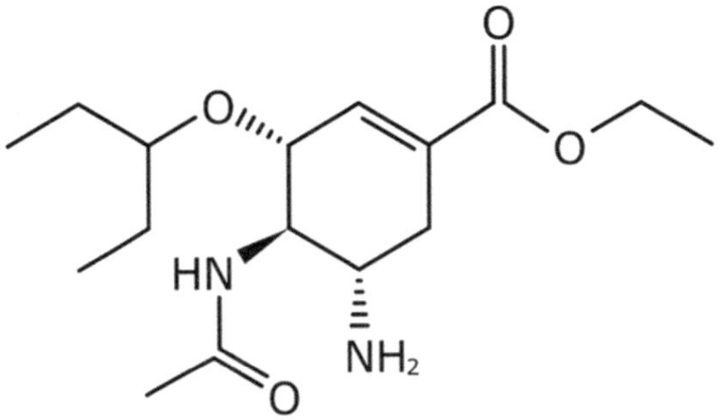

Oseltamivir is a viral neuraminidase enzyme blocker. The inhibition of the enzyme restricts the progeny influenza virus release from the infected cells and inhibits new viral cycles. Progeny virions bind to the cell surface glycoproteins through sialic acid. Neuraminidase removes this sialic acid resulting in the release of progeny virions. The neuraminidase inhibitors hinder the final stage of release of new virion [29].

Oseltamivir is used against viruses like influenza A type "A H1N1, A H2N2, type A H3N2, type A H5N1," and type B influenza viruses. It also has activity against influenza strain that caused the pandemic of 1918 Spanish flu [30]. Several clinical trials included oseltamivir but did not show any therapeutic intervention and once influenza has been excluded the role of oseltamivir has been decreased. It is also under trials for its effectiveness along with HCQ and Azithromycin. Few other clinical trials have been registered (NCT04261270 and ChiCTR2000029603) for the evaluation of the role of oseltamivir in combination and alone against COVID-19. A study conducted in Wuhan however do not demonstrate its positive outcome on COVID-19 patients [31]. The dose approved for COVID-19 is 75 mg for 5 days in combination with other drugs.

13.2.1.1.7 Umifenovir

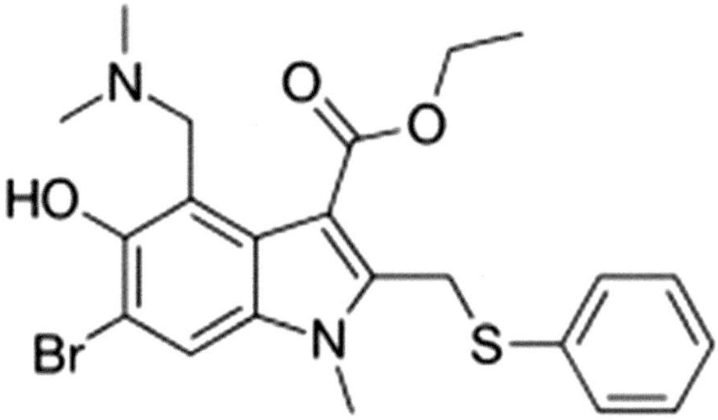

Umifenovi targets the S protein/ACE2 interaction thus stops the fusion of the host cell with membrane viral envelope. Thus, inhibits the entry of the virus into the host cell. Studies revealed that it also has some modulatory effect on the immune system of the host as it stimulates the humoral immune response, that cause the production of interferon and activates the phagocytic function of macrophages [32].

Umifenovir is effective against a number of different viruses that includes human influenza type A and B virus, hepatitis B virus (HBV), and avian coronavirus [33]. The drug is approved for clinical use against influenza type A and type B only in some countries like Russia and China. The drug is suggested to be used for COVID-19 based on its *in vitro* data available against SARS. The drug is being investigated along with pegylated interferon-β atomization (NCT04254874) in mild COVID-19 patients. Another nonrandomized study including 67 patients showed low mortality and high hospital discharge rates [34]. The dose of 200 mg PO every 8 hourly is given (NCT04260594) for COVID-19 treatment.

13.2.1.2 *HYDROXYCHLOROQUINE (HCQ) AND CHLOROQUINE*

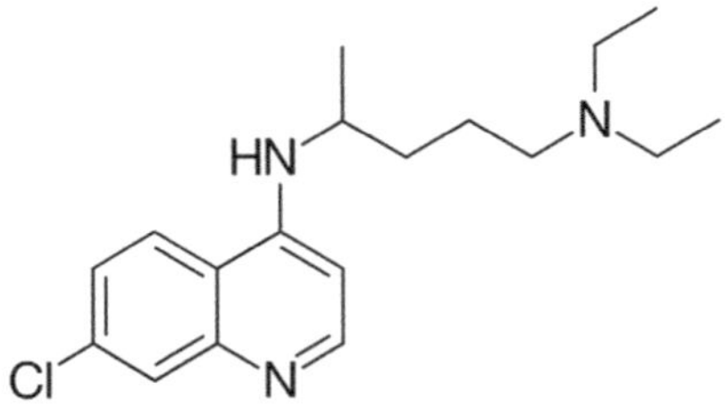

Chloroquine

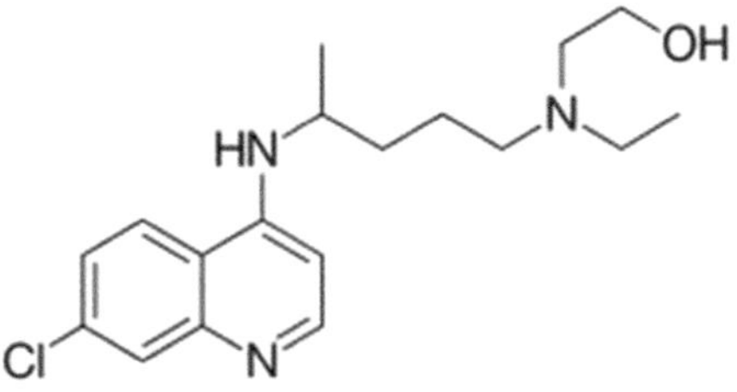

Hydroxychloroquine

Hydroxychloroquine (HCQ) and Chloroquine has long been used in malaria. HCQ is a derivative of "Chloroquine" with much less toxicity as compared to chloroquine. HCQ and Chloroquine are effective against rheumatoid arthritis, lupus erythematosus, and influenza A and B virus, HIV-1, and SARS COV-1. Based on previous data it has being trialed against COVID-19 treatment. HCQ and Chloroquine has multiple mechanism of action which supports its usage in the treatment of COVID-19.

Zinc inhibits RNA polymerase activity in retrovirus RNA and SARS-CoV. Chloroquine results in increased intracellular levels of zinc that inhibits RNA-dependent RNA polymerase that is required for RNA synthesis thus, inhibits the pathogenesis of positive-stranded RNA viruses. This is also observed that the presence of Zinc enhances the uptake of chloroquine by the cell, so the combination of two is being investigated [35]. Another mechanism reported is that ACE2 is one of the receptors that are used by SARS-COV virus for host cell entry, chloroquine restricts the terminal glycosylation of the ACE2 in *in-vitro* testing thus is suggested to be used as a prophylactic as well as treatment agent against COVID-19 [36]. One reason for the death among COVID-19 patients is cytokine storm which cause respiratory distress, and there is an evidence that HCQ and chloroquine has an effect to reduce cytokine storm.

A number of trials are underway to evaluate the efficacy of HCQ and chloroquine in COVID-19 and its emergency use has been allowed by FDA in COVID-19. A study presented that the use of chloroquine and hydroxyl chlorochine leads to improvement in clinical symptoms of the patients because of its anti-inflammatory properties [37]. Some encouraging results has been observed in China. In another study conducted in France in which 26 patients received HCQ 600 mg daily along with azithromycin and were compared with control. On 6th day all the patients receiving HCQ and Azithromycin together did not show virus. The same research group conducted a follow up study using a combination of both drugs on 80 patients. Results were encouraging as no virus was detected in 83% of patients on day 7, while in 93% of patients on 8th day [38].

The dose approved for COVID-19 patients was based on preliminary trials. In China, 500 mg of dose twice-daily was approved while in South Korea, 500 mg once daily was the approved dose of chloroquine in old and critically ill patients. Chloroquine and HCQ show serious side effects, especially in high doses. Common side effects include nausea, vomiting, diarrhea, hypokalemia, AV conduction defects, hypotension, circulatory collapse, and hemodynamic complications.

HCQ side effects are nausea, abdominal pain, rashes, and headaches. Bruising or infection are very rarely observed. Toxicity to the back of the eyes when HCQ has been used for over five years is noted, but it is also rare. Safe sun exposure is recommended due to a risk of skin damage.

HCQ is known to have integration if concurrently used with drugs, including increasing plasma digoxin levels, impairing antiepileptic drug activity, and enhancing the effects of hypoglycemic treatments and if given concurrently.

13.2.1.3 NITRIC OXIDE AND EPOPROSTENOL

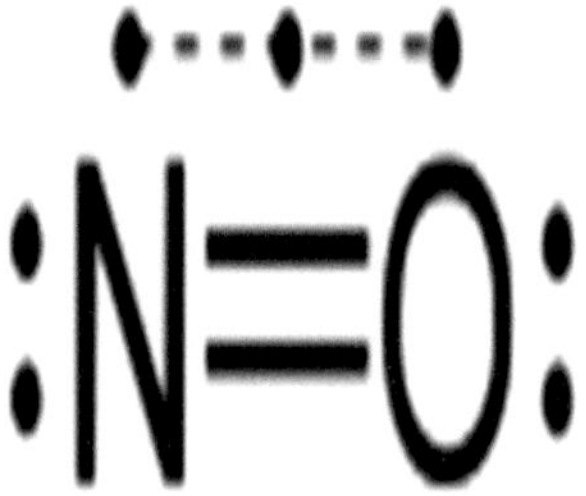

It has been suggested that inhaled pulmonary vasodilators can be essential therapy in patients on mechanical ventilation and showing ARDS and hypoxia. For this purpose, nitric oxide (iNO) and epoprostenol (iEPO) has been studied as inhaled pulmonary vasodilators in patients on ventilation. COVID-19 patients with serious ARDS when treated with iNO, showed improved oxygenation as iNO reduces the mean pulmonary artery pressure. Nitric oxide treatment can be pivotal in the world's fight against COVID-19 infection. It has also previously demonstrated certain *in vitro*

antiviral activity against SARS-CoV thus could have potential effectiveness against COVID-19 virus [26]. In one of the study iNO was administered for more than 3 days. On 1st day 30 ppm was given and was followed by 20 on 2nd day and 10 ppm on 3rd day. Some more clinical trials (NCT04305457, NCT04306393, NCT04312243) are underway to estimate the effectiveness of iNO in critical COVID-19 patients having pulmonary distress. FDA has permitted the usage of INO in critical COVID-19 patients. The Society of Critical Care Medicine suggested its usage in COVID-19 patients when patients are non-compliant to other strategies. Inhaled epoprostenol iEPO is a natural prostaglandin having vasodilator effect. Reported dose of iEPO is up to 50 ng/kg per minute [39].

13.2.2 ADJUNCTIVE THERAPIES

13.2.2.1 IMMUNOMODULATORY AGENTS

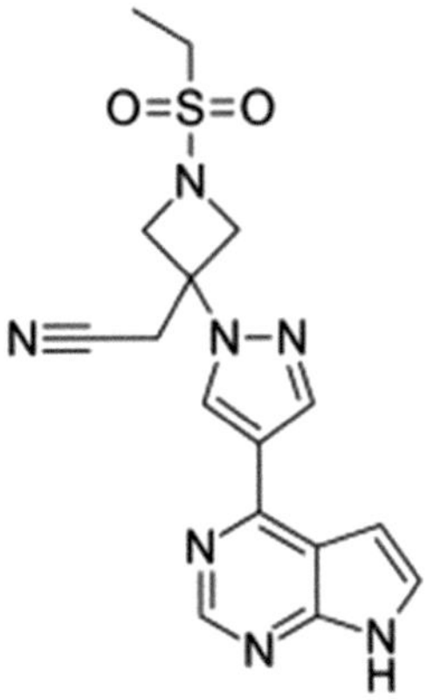

13.2.2.1.1 Baricitinib

Baricitinib inhibits Janus kinase 1 and 2. It has a role in triggering effect on cytokine-induced phosphorylation of STAT, which when transported to nuclear region, regulates gene transcription. Member of this family includes JAK1, JAK2, JAK3, and tyrosine kinase 2 (Tyk2) [40]. Studies reported that it activates different cytokines which stops the phosphorylation of STATs and causes temporary changes in neutrophil and lymphocyte numbers [10]. AP2-associated protein kinase 1 (AAK1) is an important manager of clathrin-mediated endocytosis and its disruption can restrict the passage of the virus into the host cells and further accumulation of virus intracellular. In a trial (NCT04321993) Baricitinib was suggested to be effective in COVID-19 patients showing acute respiratory disease as it will help reduce the entry of virus and also reduce the associated inflammation. It has also been used in combination with antivirals like ritonavir, Remdesivir, and lopinavir. The combination is suggested to be more effective as it will decrease viral infectivity by interfering with its entrance into the cells as well as reduce viral replication and will increase the host inflammatory response.

Baricitinib is considered a good agent to be used in combination with other drugs because of its pharmacokinetic properties that include low plasma protein binding and minimum interface with CYP enzymes (cytochromes P450). However, its usage is also associated with some serious side effects, especially the risk of infections from some opportunistic pathogens, particularly when used with immunosuppressing agents such as corticosteroids. In some patients using baricitinib, tuberculosis infection was observed. Thus, it is suggested that patients receiving Baricitinib should be verified for tuberculosis infection before and during therapy. In addition to this, pulmonary embolism and deep venous thrombosis has also been reported [41].

13.2.2.1.2 Ruxolitinib

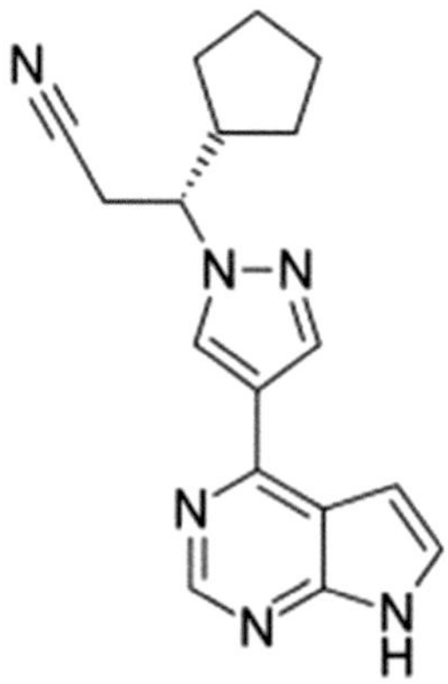

Ruxolitinib is also a potent JAK1 and JAK2 inhibitor administered orally. It was approved by FDA against myelofibrosis in November 2011. It shows its effect by inhibiting clathrin-mediated endocytosis but a pharmacokinetic study showed that the unbound plasma concentration of the drug required to produce this effect is much more than the tolerated therapeutic dose. Thus, it is unlikely to reduce the viral infectivity at therapeutic dose on the contrary, it may inhibit JAK resulting in reduced inflammatory response. A clinical trials for determining the efficacy of Ruxolitinib are underway [10].

13.2.2.1.3 Tocilizumab

Tocilizumab is a monoclonal whole antibody that has been designed to counter the interleukin-6 receptor (IL-6R), which is one of the cytokine linked with the development of some autoimmune diseases. Different cells like B-cells and T-cells, monocytes, fibroblasts, and lymphocytes produce IL-6. IL-6 is also associated with T-cell activation, initiation of protein synthesis in hepatic acute-phase and the instigation of immunoglobulin secretion. Tocilizumab is used in case serious cytokine release syndrome. FDA has permitted phase II clinical trials to evaluate the efficacy of tocilizumab in pneumonia associated with COVID-19 in hospitals. The practice of tocilizumab in patients having severe COVID-19 in China showed positive outcomes to control lung inflammation. Thus "seventh edition of the Chinese Clinical Guidance for COVID-19 Pneumonia Diagnosis and Treatment" included tocilizumab as an option to be used in critical COVID-19 patients showing prevalent lung lesions and higher IL-6 levels [42]. However, some serious side effects associated with the drug has also been observed, such as drug-induced liver injuries and acute liver failure. It can also result in concomitant opportunistic serious infections like Tuberculosis, specially when used in combination with immunosuppressants or corticosteroids.

13.2.2.1.4 Camrelizumab

Camrelizumab is a humanized whole monoclonal antibody. It is targeted to receptors involved programed cell death 1 (PD-1). These PD-1 receptors are located on T cells and works as negative regulators of T cell activity. Camrelizumab blocks the attachment of PD-10s to its ligand, PD-L1, and inhibits tumor cell escape from the immune system.

After exposure to certain antigen, PD-1 are rapidly expressed on T-cells, resulting in the interaction of T-cell receptor with burdened histocompatibility complex (MHC). Different pro-inflammatory mediators such as "IL-2, IL-6, IL-7, and IL-15" in help out in regulation of PD-10s of T-cells. This interaction results in signals that tolerate T-cells to their specific antigenic sites, thus neutralize their effector functions. Studies on animal models showed that blocking PD-1 or PD-L1 results in reduced T cell death, it also regulates cytokine production, and reduces organ failure and death in rate in sepsis [43]. Camrelizumab is being investigated to be used in different types of malignancies such as hepatocellular carcinoma and Hodgkin lymphoma. It is also being investigated for its effectiveness COVID-19 patients, especially those presenting with serious lymphocytopenia-associated pneumonia. Camrelizumab is currently under trials (NCT04268537) to assess its effectiveness in COVID-19 [44].

Camrelizumab is usually considered to have a good safety profile. A most serious side effect is reactive capillary hemangioma which is self-limiting and not life-threatening.

13.2.2.1.5 Meplazumab

Meplazumab is an anti-CD147 antibody. CD147 has the ability to bind to spike protein (SP) and facilities the viral entry in the host cell. A recent study revealed that COVID-19 virus can invade the human host cell by using this CD147-spike protein (SP) route. Meplazumab has the ability to inhibit the binding of CD147 to SP, thus prevent the entry into the host cell. Meplazumab has been used in various trials in COVID-19 patients and trials has resulted in speedy recovery of COVID-19 patients suffering from pneumonia [45].

13.2.2.1.6 Eculizumab

Eculizumab is a "humanized monoclonal IgG antibody." It has the ability to bind with the C5 complement protein and prevents its conversion into C5a and C5b; thus, by blocking the formation of C5b, it inhibits terminal C5b-9 complex or membrane attack complex (MAC) formation [46].

As complement system has been recognized as a vital host facilitator for MERS-CoV and SARS-CoV-induced diseases and activation of this complement system could control pro-inflammatory reaction against infection. Eculizumab is under trials to find its effectiveness in COVID-19 patients with severe ARDS (NCT04288713).

13.2.2.1.7 Bevacizumab

Bevacizumab is a recombinant, humanized monoclonal antibody. It neutralizes vascular endothelial growth factor (VEGF) and averts its contact with endothelial receptors, KDR, and Flt-1 [47]. The vascular permeability damage in critical COVID-19 patients is estimated to reduce pulmonary edema. This is evident that critical COVID-19 patients have significant pulmonary mucus and inflammatory exudation more than the SARS infective patients. Bevacizumab has been suggested as a promising agent and is being tested in the treatment for serious COVID-19 patients in clinical trials [48].

It has been long used as an antitumor drug. However, it may produce reversible myocardial toxicity or other associated dysfunction. Its use may result in hypertension; thus, blood pressure should be monitored during and after treatment with bevacizumab.

13.2.2.2 CORTICOSTEROIDS

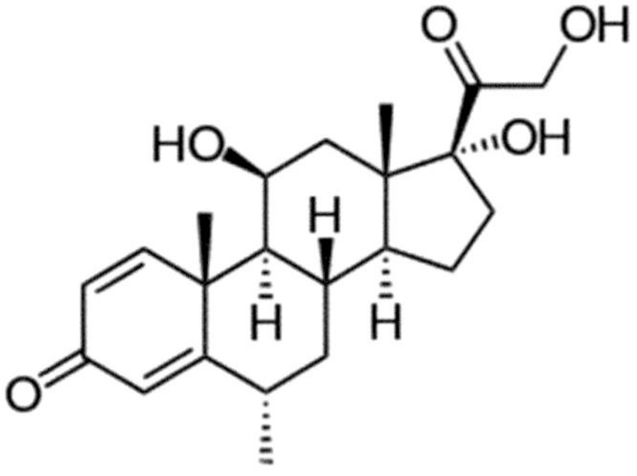

Methylprednisolone

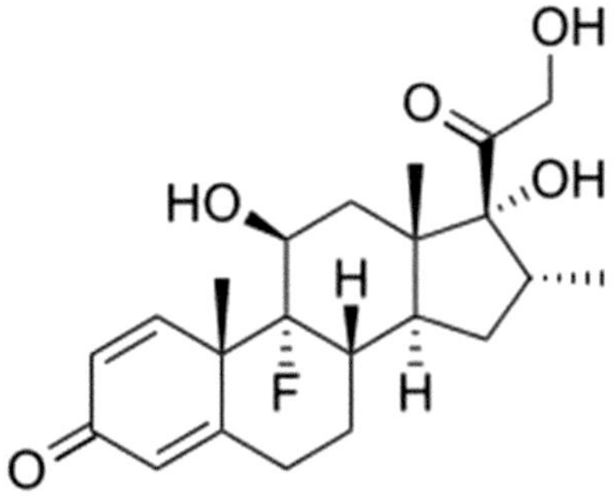

Dexamethasone

Corticosteroids inhibits many inflammatory factors. Corticosteroids stop pro-inflammatory genes that code cytokines, chemokines, inflammatory enzymes, cell adhesion molecules and receptors to address the inflammatory process and produce homeostasis. Corticosteroids like methylprednisolone and dexamethasone are strong anti-inflammatory and anti-fibrotic agents, inhibit cytokine response and hasten the process to overcome pulmonary and systemic inflammation in case of pneumonia. Corticosteroids can inhibit some inflammatory genes and previously used in various viral diseases. Corticosteroids such as methylprednisolone can improve deregulated immune response that is caused by sepsis that increase the blood pressure. Previously the clinical outcomes of corticosteroids in SARS and MERS patients were not encouraging but still number of clinical trials are underway to evaluate its activity in COVID-19. Recently a study group in England releases preliminary results of randomized, controlled clinical trials, and results proved that dexamethasone can reduce the mortality by one third when used in low doses in critical COVID-19 patients [49]. In another study conducted in 201 patients treated with prednisolone showed that it may be effective to decrease the death rate in patients having ARDS associated with COVID-19 [50]. Methylprednisolone reduced fever and hypoxia and shortened the duration of disease in another study conducted in 42 patients [51].

Similarly, Dexamethasone has showed some efficacy on ARDS by minimizing ventilator duration and mortality rate in COVID-19 patients even without severe ARDS. It was demonstrated in trials that use of corticosteroids in the first week was linked with reduced viral clearance.

The doses of methylprednisolone used in different trials for COVID-19 patients is 1–2 mg/kg daily IV for 5–7 days. Chinese Thoracic Society recommends that the dose of methylprednisolone should be ≤ 0.5 to 1 mg/kg daily [52].

Corticosteroids show different anti-inflammatory potential with different kinetic profiles. For intensive and rapid effect, intravenous treatment may be required. Oral and intravenous dexamethasone is being evaluated in the RECOVERY trial. Should be used with caution in pregnancy as dexamethasone cross the placental barrier, thus, prednisolone or hydrocortisone are recommended in pregnant patients as they are converted into inactive forms by the placenta.

13.2.2.3 RENIN ANGIOTENSIN ALDOSTERONE SYSTEM (RAAS) ANTAGONISTS

Coronavirus enters human cells by binding its viral spike protein to the membrane-bound form of the monocarboxypeptidase angiotensin-converting enzyme 2 (ACE2). ACE2 is important in regulating the renin-angiotensin-aldosterone system (RAAS), as it metabolizes angiotensin II to produce angiotensin-(1–7). Animal studies have shown that angiotensin-converting-enzyme (ACE) inhibitors and angiotensin-receptor blockers (ARBs) can control ACE2 expression, thus can increase the availability of target molecules for COVID-19 virus [53].

As ACE2 is located in the lower respiratory tract, it is one of the major targets of the SARS-CoV-2 infection. It has also been observed that diseases like diabetes, hypertension, and coronary artery disease for which RAAS inhibitors are prescribed are often observed in patients suffering from COVID-19 patients.

In experimental mouse models, it was observed that exposure to SARS-CoV-1 spike protein resulted in acute lung injury, which is limited by RAAS blockade [54].

In another small study, elevated plasma angiotensin II levels were observed in patients with COVID-19. Restoration of ACE2 by giving recombinant ACE2 resulted to reverse lung-injury process in preclinical models of some viral infections [55]. Some trials are underway to assess the efficacy and safety RAAS modulators, recombinant human ACE2 and the ARB losartan in COVID-19 patients.

A recombinant human ACE2 is proved to be safe effective in acute respiratory distress syndrome. Patients when treated with rhACE2 showed a rapid decrease in elevated angiotensin-II levels and IL-6 plasma concentration.

Reduced expression of cellular membrane ACE2 may hinder the entry of SARS-CoV-2 into the cells, but it may cause activation of AT1R leading to lung tissue injury, higher ACE2 expression on the lung cell surface, will result in the higher chances of viral entry and reduce chance of lung injury because of reduced AT1R activation. Thus ACEi/ARB or rhACE2 may be effective against COVID-19 infection but more investigation is needed. It should also be considered that sudden withdrawal of RAAS inhibitors should be avoided in patients with heart failure or myocardial infarction.

13.2.2.4 NONSTEROIDAL ANTI-INFLAMMATORY DRUGS (NSAIDS)

13.2.2.4.1 Ibuprofen

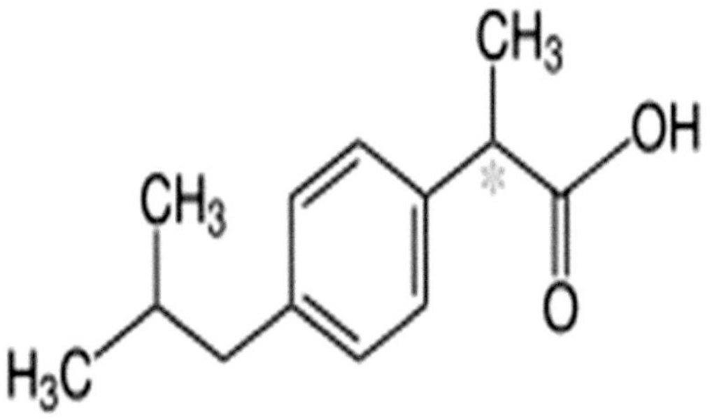

Ibuprofen

Fever is common in COVID-19 infection for which antipyretics like Ibuprofen and acetaminophen are taken commonly by patients in order to reduce the discomfort associated with fever. Most recently, the safety related to the use of Ibuprofen in COVID-19 patients has been questioned as some cases have reported the worsening of the symptoms in these patients. It has also been demonstrated that Ibuprofen has better fever reduction efficacy as compared to acetaminophen. Fever has an efficacy in reducing and limiting the viral illness; thus, it can be hypothesized that the reduction in fever by using Ibuprofen may worsen the symptoms of COVID-19 by reducing the natural defense mechanism of the body against the virus. Another important mechanism is that it is easier to unloaded oxygen from hemoglobin and supply it to tissues when the temperature is higher than normal body temperature. Based on initial reports from Italy, WHO cautions against ibuprofen usage in COVID-19 patients; however latter on WHO as well as the European Medicines Agency (EMA) recommended that use of nonsteroidal anti-inflammatory drugs (NSAIDs) should not be stopped when clinically indicated [56].

NSAIDs inhibit the enzyme cyclooxygenase (COX), which convert arachidonic acid to prostaglandin H_2 (PGH_2), then some other enzymes convert PGH_2 to several other prostaglandins and to thromboxane A_2. Ibuprofen is a nonselective COX inhibitor, and it inhibits both isoforms of COX, that is COX-1 and COX-2 [57].

A part from antipyretic Ibuprofen is also being trialed in Argentina as a possible treatment for COVID-19 by using its hypertonic solution via inhalation. The clinical trials started in June, 2020.

13.2.2.4.2 Indometacin

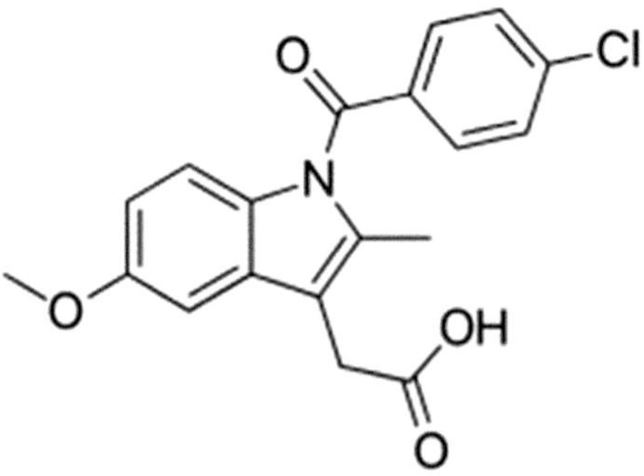

Indometacin is also one of the important NSAIDS which is usually recommended for the treatment of fever, pain, swelling, and inflammation and commonly prescribed in gout and arthritis. It inhibits the production of prostaglandins and also inhibits COX enzyme which is involved in the production of prostaglandins.

A study to evaluate the use of NSAID in SARS-CoV also looked at indomethacin. The results of the study suggested that indomethacin showed good *in vitro* antiviral activity against canine coronavirus, inhibiting virus replication and provide protection to the host cell from damage induced by virus, this antiviral activity was also noticed *in vivo* and also against human SARS-CoV at a dose of 1 mg/kg [58].

13.2.2.5 Convalescent Blood Products

In convalescent plasma (CP) therapy, blood from people recovered from an infectious illness is used to transfer antibodies prepared to the patients suffering from it, to help them recover. The use of CP to protection or treatment of infectious diseases is almost 100 years old. It has been used prophylactically as well as a treatment strategy in previous outbreak like Spanish flu and diseases like polio, rabies, measles, Ebola, and hepatitis B. Results of case studies conducted during the MERS and SARS coronavirus outbreaks also supported the fact that CP can be used in COVID-19 and is safe to be used and can cause faster viral clearance, especially in early disease course.

Patients recovered from COVID-19 develop antibodies against Coronavirus following 2–3 weeks of infection. These antibodies are detectable through various quantitative assays like ELISA. These antibodies are found to be protective in action, suggesting that this therapy could be of use in humans as well. A number of studies has been reported and suggested the use of CP in critically ill COVID-19 patients. It is to be noted that most of the studies conducted were observational and non-randomized, additional treatment interventions were also used, such as steroids, antivirals, and other medicines. Although there is incomplete and limited data available to date from various trials conducted worldwide, including China, Netherlands, and Iraq, US FDA announced emergency use authorization (EUA) of CP in hospitalized patients of COVID-19 on 23rd of August 2020 [59].

All the trials conducted using CP suggest preferably high antibody titer should be given at early stages of infection before the development of serious and life-threatening inflammatory conditions.

Over 72,000 people have been given CP in the US, of which initial safety data for 5,000 patients has been published which suggested that CP is a relatively safe intervention. Severe adverse events incidence was found to be less than 1%. General risks observed in plasma transfusion are allergic reactions, transfusion-associated circulatory and acute lung injury, and aggravation of immune-mediated tissue damage by antibody-dependent enhancement (ADE). However, these effects have not been observed with CP.

13.2.2.6 Azithromycin

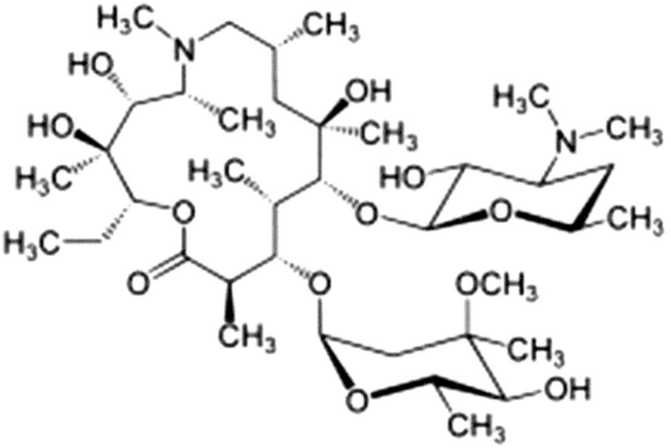

Azithromycin is an antibiotic used against various bacterial infections. It belongs to the macrolide group of antibiotics. Azithromycin prevents bacterial growth by inhibiting the synthesis of protein. It binds to the 50S ribosomal subunit of the bacterial cell and inhibits the process of translation of mRNA. It is used in chest infections such as nose and throat infections, pneumonia, skin infection, and sexually transmitted infections. It has been suggested to be used in COVID-19 infection. It has been proven that Azithroymcin has good activity against Ebola and Zika viruses. Previously, has been part of adjunctive therapy to provide some immunomodulatory and anti-inflammatory results along with bacterial coverage of some respiratory tract infections like influenza. Currently, azithromycin has been tested in a number of trials along with HCQ as a treatment strategy in COVID-19 patients.

Pfizer has announced some encouraging results of the use of Azithromycin with HCQ for the trials conducted in France. Trials were conducted in 20 patients out of which 6 were given azithromycin and HCQ at a time as a combination therapy which showed highest virologic cure rate. Around 100% clearance of viral population in nasopharyngeal swabs was reported in these 6 patients when compared with controls and those who received single therapy [60]. However, another study reported that full and rapid viral clearance is unexpected and also reported significant comorbidities. The dose used in these trials is an initial dose of 500 mg followed by a daily dose of 250 for days 2–5, cotreated with 600 mg of HCQ for 10 days [61].

13.2.2.7 ANTICOAGULANTS

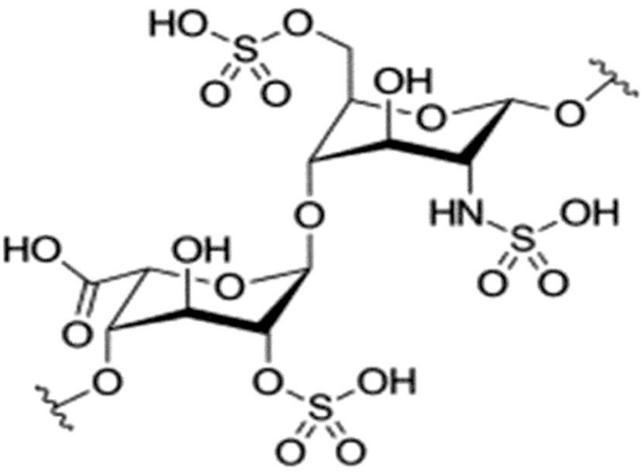

Heparin

It has been observed that disseminated intravascular coagulation and high d-dimer levels are one of the predictors that worsen the outcomes in COVID-19 patients as hypercoagulable state can result in micro and macro thrombosis. It has been reported that the use of anticoagulants may reduce the rate of mortality in COVID-19 patients.

Heparin is one of the anticoagulants suggested for the treatment. It has good anti-inflammatory properties. It can inhibit viral attachment to surface receptor (Spike) S1 via conformational changes [62]. Anticoagulants can be administered in patients were rapidly progressing respiratory deterioration are observed. It may possibly involve some additional mechanism apart from prevention of thrombosis when used in COVID-19 patients [63].

13.2.2.8 ASCORBIC ACID

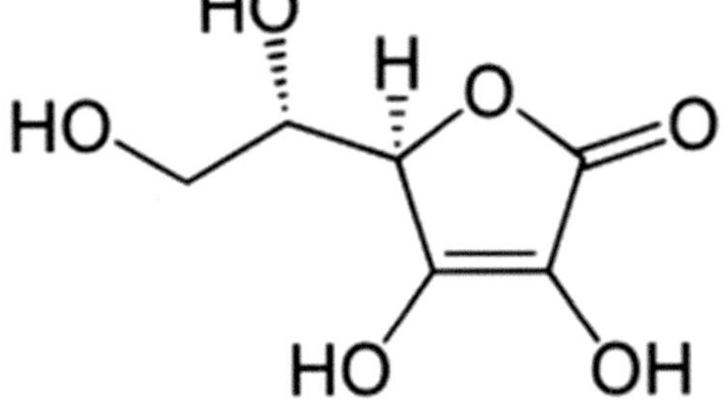

Ascorbic acid is one of the essential nutrients that plays many significant roles. Vitamin C in the form of *ascorbate* is very important as it performs various physiological functions. It serves as an enzyme substrate, a cofactor, and an electron donor. It performs various functions which include the synthesis of carnitine, collagen, neurotransmitters, and catabolism of tyrosine and the metabolism of microsome. It has the ability to neutralize free radicals, function as a potent antioxidant and assist to reverse cellular damage [64]. Ascorbic acid can be effective antiviral as well especially against influenza viruses. It is suggested that vitamin C enhances the maturation of T lymphocytes which are required against viral infections. It also inhibits free radicals' production and cytokines remodulation needed for systemic inflammatory syndrome.

A number of trials are underway to understand the role of vitamin C in COVID-19. A trials in China are evaluating the effectiveness of Vitamin C in high doses in COVID-19 patients. The suggested dose is 1,500 mg as supportive therapy, while high doses by IV route has also been evaluated. The dose between 2–10 g/day is given by IV route which resulted in high oxygen index and eventually recovery of all patients [26].

13.2.2.9 INTERFERONS

Interferons are the signaling proteins that are released in the body in response to the viral infections. IFN-I is a cytokine that is released after viral infection. It is immediately recognized as IFNAR receptors are present on the plasma membrane of most cells. Where it induces signal transducer and activator of transcription 1 (STAT1) phosphorylation. STAT1 in return activate ISG, which interfere with viral replication, spreading, and activating the adaptive immune response. ISGs has several pattern recognition receptors (PRRs) for recognition of infectious agents. The ISGs has role in decreasing membrane fluidity, reducing the membrane fusion and the escape of the virus. ISGs also can prevent viral cycle at several steps because of some antiviral proteins [65].

Interferon treatment presented inadequate activity against SARS-CoV and MERS-CoV. IFNβ1 controls CD73 levels in the pulmonary endothelium resulting in subsequent adenosine secretion. Adenosine has a strong anti-inflammatory effect that provide the endothelial barrier. Interferon treatment could thus reduce vascular escape in ARDS but is not sufficient for patients showing ARDS [66].

It is assumed that in severe lung injury associated COVID-19, IFN-I-mediated reaction aggravates, resulting in high tissue damage. IFN-1 is especially helpful if when given at the early infection stage. Administration of an anti-interferon agent may prove to be of some help when given at a late stage.

Interferons like IFNα is used in combination with antivirals like ribavirin. [National Health Commission of the People's Republic of China. (2020). *Diagnosis and Treatment Protocol for COVID-19 Patients* (tentative 8th edition). Updated on 8 September 2020. English translation available at http://regional.chinadaily.com.cn/pdf/DiagnosisandTreatmentProtocolforCOVID-19Patients (Tentative 8th edition).pdf. Accessed 13 November 2020)].

Clinical trials are underway in different countries to assess the activity of interferons against COVID-19. In one of the registered trials, IFNα2b is used in along with lopinavir/ritonavir. While in another reported trials IFNß1b is administered subcutaneously along with lopinavir/ritonavir and ribavirin.

13.2.2.10 ANTHELMINTIC DRUG

13.2.2.10.1 Ivermectin

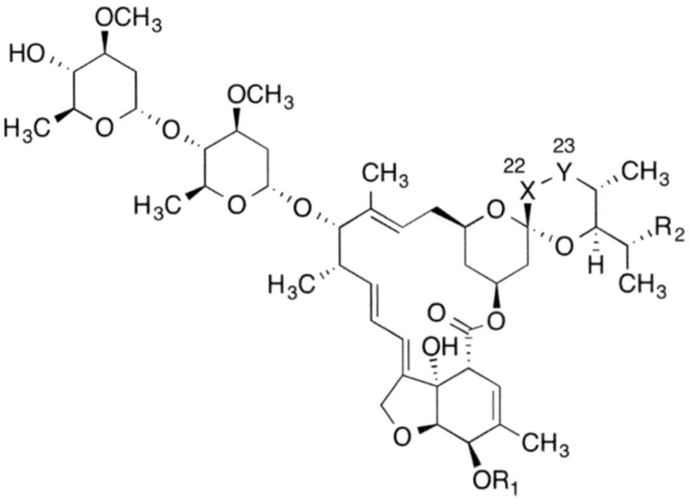

Ivermectin is one of the anti-anthelmintic drugs that has been used in the treatment of various infections in mammals. Ivermectin is a broad-spectrum highly lipid-soluble drug and has different effects on parasites such as nematodes, arthropods, mycobacteria, and flavivirus. A part from its good antiparasitic and antiviral activity, it can induce immunomodulatory effects in the host cells. It also inhibits the proliferation of cancer cells; it also has a role in regulating glucose and cholesterol. Ivermectin increase the influx of Cl-ions in invertebrates cell membrane by activating specific ivermectin-sensitive ion channels. The resulting hyperpolarization causes muscle paralysis of anthelmintics. It has been discovered that ivermectin inhibits the interaction between integrate molecules of human immunodeficiency virus (HIV)-1 with its nuclear transport receptor importin α/β. Another study showed that it has the potential to hinder viral replication of some viruses, such as dengue virus, flavivirus, yellow fever virus, and influenza [67].

Effectiveness of Ivermectin against COVID-19 virus *in vitro* cell culture has been reported. It inhibits nuclear import of viral proteins. However, these inhibition effect against COVID-19 virus has not been observed *in vivo*. FDA issued a statement on April 10, 2020, concerning self-medication of ivermectin against COVID-19 with reference to recently published *in vitro* study of ivermectin and has cleared the fact that this type of studies are usually only the early stages of drug development.

13.2.2.10.2 Niclosamide

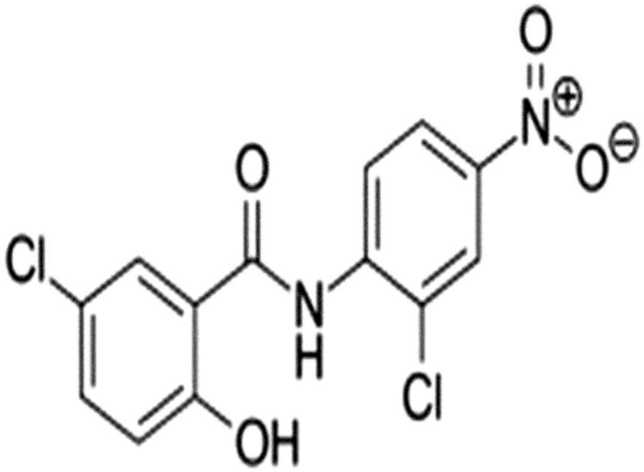

Niclosamide is also an anthelmintic drug and is commonly used to treat tape-worm infestations. It is FDA approved as an anthelmintic for over 50 years now for the past five years it has seen increasing interest in its anticancer use. Niclosamide works by inhibiting glucose uptake, process of oxidative phosphorylation, and anaerobic metabolism in the tapeworms.

It is SARS-CoV virus replication inhibitor. Studies showed its effective-ness in Vero E6 cells and Vero B4 cells against coronavirus and MERS-CoV replication [68].

13.2.2.10.3 Colchicine

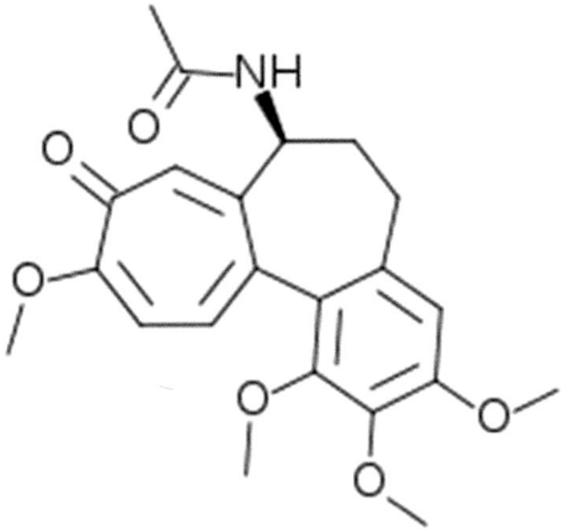

Colchicine is an anti-inflammatory drug that is commonly used in gout. It acts by hindering the inflammatory complex in neutrophils and monocytes and finally activation of IL-1beta. Colchicine also has inhibitory effects on macrophages. It has been used in COVID-19 patients who present with myopathies and the results and has shown reduction in inflammation associated with the cardiac myocytes [69]. There are a number of ongoing studies investigating colchicine for cytokine storm.

13.2.2.10.4 Teicoplanin

Teicoplanin is an antibiotic that is used as a prophylactic agent and in the treatment of some serious Gram-positive bacterial infections, such as methicillin-resistant *Staphylococcus aureus* and *Enterococcus faecalis*. It is a semisynthetic glycopeptide in nature. It is produced from the fermentation of *Actinoplanes teichomyceticus*. It has a spectrum of activity similar to that of vancomycin. It acts by inhibiting bacterial cell wall synthesis.

Teicoplanin has been shown to effectively prevent the entry of Ebola, SARS, and MERS envelope pseudotyped viruses into the cytoplasm. At low micromolar range (IC50, 330 nM), it has an inhibitory action on transcription- and replication-competent virus-like particles. Studies also revealed that teicoplanin also inhibits cathepsin L and cathepsin B the activities of the host cell's which results in splitting of viral glycoprotein and causing the exposure of the receptor-binding structures of its core genome and its consequent release into the cytoplasm of the host cells. It is suggested that teicoplanin can has a potential role as a novel inhibitor specifically against cathepsin L-dependent viruses [70, 71].

13.2.2.11 THIAZOLIDINEDIONES

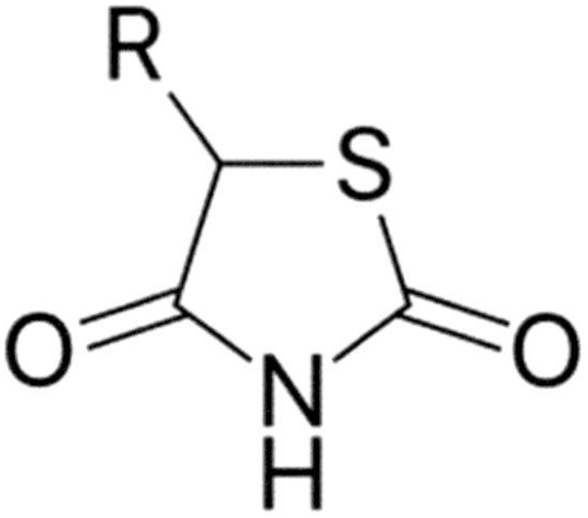

The thiazolidinediones are known as glitazones after ciglitazone, the prototypical drug of this class. These are heterocyclic compounds with a five-membered C_3NS ring. The group was introduced in the late 1990s and is used in the treatment of diabetes mellitus type 2. Thiazolidinedione has shown efficiency against pulmonary disease induced by respiratory syncytial virus (RSV) or H1N1 influenza infection; however, their role in COVID-19 treatment is still not explored [72]. Thiazolidinediones upregulate ACE2 receptor, which is a binding target for COVID-19 virus in host cells. More studies and clinical trials are needed to establish any efficacy of this group against COVID-19 disease.

13.2.2.11.1 Nitazoxanide

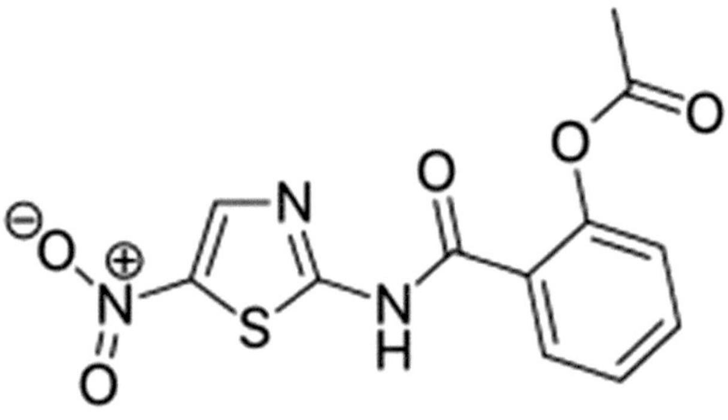

Nitazoxanide is a broad-spectrum antiviral and antiparasitic agent. It is used for the treatment of different helminthic, protozoal, and viral infections. Nitazoxanide is the prototype agent of the thiazolides, which is a group having synthetic nitrothiazolyl-salicylamide derivatives with antiviral and antiparasitic activity. Tizoxanide, an active metabolite of nitazoxanide also antiparasitic drug of the thiazolide class. Clinical trials of nitazoxanide against influenza has been done and shown inhibitory effect on a broad range of influenza virus subtypes. The drug is also effective against influenza viruses which develop some resistance to neuraminidase inhibitors like oseltamivir Nitazoxanide is also being investigated as a potential treatment for chronic hepatitis B, chronic hepatitis C, norovirus gastroenteritis and rotavirus.

Nitazoxanide and its metabolite tizoxanide have shown inhibitory effects against MERS-CoV in LLC-MK2 cell lines. It has inhibition effects against other coronavirus strains. Nitazoxanide has shown inhibitory effects on pro-inflammatory cytokines in peripheral blood mononuclear cells (PBMCs), but its effectiveness against COVID-19 virus still needed to be explored [11].

13.3 CONCLUSION

COVID-19 pandemic is the greatest global public health emergency of time. Till now, no single treatment strategy is available for COVID-19. Extensive trials and studies are underway around the globe to evaluate effective management strategies for the treatment of COVID-19. However, the search for optimal agents to treat or prevent the infection still remains ill-defined, and results or evidence for appropriate therapy remains inconclusive and keep on changes. While certain studies are encouraging and potential benefits of therapy outweighs the relatively low or minor risks of adverse effects.

It should be noted that progression of disease can occur rapidly even in stable patients and also viral load is highest in the early stage of the disease. The timing of initiation of therapy is also needed to be well defined. It is also noted that no single treatment is effective against the disease, so multiple drug combinations with appropriate doses and keeping in view the possible side effects and condition of the patient should be selected. Patients with pulmonary complications and who are hospitalized are at high risk. Clinical trials carried out worldwide suggested that pneumonia caused by COVID-19 can be treated with different antiviral therapies, specially beginning with those pre-existing drugs that has no serious side effects. However, it should be noted that many of the results of therapeutic effects are circumstantial, and controlled clinical trials must be carried out to evaluate the actual efficacy of these drugs. It is also suggested that commencement early drug treatment against COVID-19 may prevent severe symptoms, specifically serious like damage of lung making a difference in saving the lives of patients all over the world.

KEYWORDS

- **immune modulator**
- **interleukin-2**
- **RNA-dependent RNA polymerase**
- **severe acute respiratory syndrome**
- **tumor necrosis factor-alpha**
- **World Health Organization**

REFERENCES

1. Lu, R., et al., (2020). Genomic characterization and epidemiology of 2019 novel coronavirus: Implications for virus origins and receptor binding. *Lancet, 395*(10224), 565–574.
2. Guan, W. J., et al., (2020). Clinical characteristics of coronavirus disease 2019 in China. *N. Engl. J. Med., 382*(18), 1708–1720.
3. Kakodkar, P., Kaka, N., & Baig, M. N., (2020). A comprehensive literature review on the clinical presentation, and management of the pandemic Coronavirus disease 2019 (COVID-19). *Cureus, 12*(4), e7560.
4. Zia-Ul-Haq, M., et al., (2021). *Alternative Medicine Interventions for COVID-19* (Vol. XII, p. 284). Springer, Cham: Springer Nature Switzerland AG.
5. Zia-Ul-Haq, M., Dewanjee, S., & Riaz, M., (2021). *Carotenoids: Structure and Function in the Human Body* (Vol. XVI, p. 859). Springer Nature Switzerland AG: Springer International Publishing.
6. Eastman, R. T., et al., (2020). Remdesivir: A review of its discovery and development leading to emergency use authorization for treatment of COVID-19. *ACS Cent. Sci., 6*(5), 672–683.
7. Brown, A. J., et al., (2019). Broad-spectrum antiviral Remdesivir inhibits human endemic and zoonotic deltacoronaviruses with a highly divergent RNA dependent RNA polymerase. *Antiviral Res., 169*, 104541.
8. Varga, A., Lionne, C., & Roy, B., (2016). Intracellular metabolism of nucleoside/nucleotide analogues: A bottleneck to reach active drugs on HIV Reverse Transcriptase. *Curr. Drug Metab., 17*(3), 237–252.

9. de Wit, E., et al., (2020). Prophylactic and therapeutic Remdesivir (GS-5734) treatment in the rhesus macaque model of MERS-CoV infection. *Proc. Natl. Acad. Sci. U S A, 117*(12), 6771–6776.
10. Saber-Ayad, M., Saleh, M. A., & Abu-Gharbieh, E., (2020). The rationale for potential pharmacotherapy of COVID-19. *Pharmaceuticals, 13*(5). Basel.
11. Cao, J., Forrest, J. C., & Zhang, X., (2015). A screen of the NIH Clinical Collection small molecule library identifies potential anti-coronavirus drugs. *Antiviral Res., 114*, 1–10.
12. Grein, J., et al., (2020). Compassionate use of Remdesivir for patients with severe Covid-19. *N. Engl. J. Med., 382*(24), 2327–2336.
13. Sanders, J. M., et al., (2020). Pharmacologic treatments for Coronavirus disease 2019 (COVID-19): A review. JAMA.
14. Wang, W., et al., (2020). Detection of SARS-CoV-2 in different types of clinical specimens. *JAMA, 323*(18), 1843–1844.
15. Loustaud-Ratti, V., et al., (2016). Ribavirin: Past, present and future. *World J. Hepatol., 8*(2), 123–130.
16. Glue, P., (1999). The clinical pharmacology of ribavirin. *Semin. Liver Dis., 19*(Suppl 1), 17–24.
17. Sun, Y., et al., (2020). Diagnosis and treatment of emergency surgeries in otorhinolaryngology, head and neck surgery during the covid-19 outbreak: A single-center experience. *World J. Otorhinolaryngol Head Neck Surg.*
18. Stockman, L. J., Bellamy, R., & Garner, P., (2006). SARS: Systematic review of treatment effects. *PLoS Med., 3*(9), e343.
19. Arabi, Y. M., et al., (2020). Ribavirin and interferon therapy for critically ill patients with middle east respiratory syndrome: A multicenter observational study. *Clin. Infect. Dis., 70*(9), 1837–1844.
20. Chu, C. M., et al., (2004). Role of lopinavir/ritonavir in the treatment of SARS: initial virological and clinical findings. *Thorax, 59*(3), 252–256.
21. Yao, T. T., et al., (2020). A systematic review of lopinavir therapy for SARS coronavirus and MERS coronavirus-A possible reference for coronavirus disease-19 treatment option. *J. Med. Virol., 92*(6), 556–563.
22. Cao, B., et al., (2020). A trial of lopinavir-ritonavir in adults hospitalized with severe Covid-19. *N. Engl. J. Med., 382*(19), 1787–1799.
23. Muralidharan, N., et al., (2020). Computational studies of drug repurposing and synergism of lopinavir, oseltamivir and ritonavir binding with SARS-CoV-2 protease against COVID-19. *J. Biomol. Struct. Dyn.*, 1–6.
24. Oldfield, V., & Plosker, G. L., (2006). Lopinavir/ritonavir: A review of its use in the management of HIV infection. *Drugs, 66*(9), 1275–1299.
25. Chandwani, A., & Shuter, J., (2008). Lopinavir/ritonavir in the treatment of HIV-1 infection: A review. *Ther. Clin. Risk Manag., 4*(5), 1023–1033.
26. Wu, R., et al., (2020). An update on current therapeutic drugs treating COVID-19. *Curr. Pharmacol. Rep.*, 1–15.
27. Du, Y. X., & Chen, X. P., (2020). Favipiravir: Pharmacokinetics and concerns about clinical trials for 2019-nCoV infection. *Clin. Pharmacol. Ther., 108*(2), 242–247.
28. Cai, Q., et al., (2020). *Experimental Treatment with Favipiravir for COVID-19: An Open-Label Control Study.* Engineering (Beijing).
29. Moscona, A., (2005). Neuraminidase inhibitors for influenza. *N. Engl. J. Med., 353*(13), 1363–1373.

30. Tumpey, T. M., et al., (2002). Existing antivirals are effective against influenza viruses with genes from the 1918 pandemic virus. *Proc. Natl. Acad. Sci. U S A, 99*(21), 13849–13854.
31. Wang, D., et al., (2020). Clinical characteristics of 138 hospitalized patients with 2019 novel coronavirus-infected pneumonia in Wuhan, China. *JAMA, 323*(11), 1061–1069.
32. Boriskin, Y. S., et al., (2008). Arbidol: A broad-spectrum antiviral compound that blocks viral fusion. *Current Medicinal Chemistry, 15*(10), 997–1005.
33. Glushkov, R. G., et al., (1999). *[Mechanisms of arbidole's immunomodulating action]. Vestn Ross. Akad. Med. Nauk, 3*, 36–40.
34. Wang, Z., et al., (2020). Clinical features of 69 cases with Coronavirus disease 2019 In WUHAN, China. *Clin. Infect. Dis., 71*(15), 769–777.
35. Xue, J., et al., (2014). Chloroquine is a zinc ionophore. *PLoS One, 9*(10), e109180.
36. Vincent, M. J., et al., (2005). Chloroquine is a potent inhibitor of SARS coronavirus infection and spread. *Virol. J., 2*, 69.
37. Tang, W., et al., (2020). Hydroxychloroquine in patients with mainly mild to moderate coronavirus disease 2019: Open-label, randomized controlled trial. *BMJ, 369*, m1849.
38. Gautret, P., et al., (2020). Clinical and microbiological effect of a combination of hydroxychloroquine and azithromycin in 80 COVID-19 patients with at least a six-day follow up: A pilot observational study. *Travel Med. Infect. Dis., 34*, 101663.
39. Alessandri, F., Pugliese, F., & Ranieri, V. M., (2018). The role of rescue therapies in the treatment of severe ARDS. *Respir Care, 63*(1), 92–101.
40. Iwata, S., & Tanaka, Y., (2016). Progress in understanding the safety and efficacy of Janus kinase inhibitors for treatment of rheumatoid arthritis. *Expert Rev. Clin. Immunol., 12*(10), 1047–1057.
41. Chen, Y. C., et al., (2020). Safety of baricitinib in East Asian patients with moderate-to-severe active rheumatoid arthritis: An integrated analysis from clinical trials. *Int. J. Rheum Dis., 23*(1), 65–73.
42. Fu, B., Xu, X., & Wei, H., (2020). Why tocilizumab could be an effective treatment for severe COVID-19*? J. Transl. Med., 18*(1), 164.
43. Fang, W., et al., (2018). Camrelizumab (SHR-1210) alone or in combination with gemcitabine plus cisplatin for nasopharyngeal carcinoma: Results from two single-arm, phase 1 trials. *Lancet Oncol., 19*(10), 1338–1350.
44. Markham, A., & Keam, S. J., (2019). Camrelizumab: First Global Approval. *Drugs, 79* (12), 1355–1361.
45. Varghese, P. M., et al., (2020). Host-pathogen interaction in COVID-19: Pathogenesis, potential therapeutics and vaccination strategies. *Immunobiology*.
46. Ricklin, D., et al., (2010). Complement: A key system for immune surveillance and homeostasis. *Nat. Immunol., 11*(9), 785–797.
47. Totzeck, M., Mincu, R. I., & Rassaf, T., (2017). Cardiovascular adverse events in patients with cancer treated with bevacizumab: A meta-analysis of more than 20 000 patients. *J. Am. Heart. Assoc., 6*(8).
48. Cascella, M., et al., (2020). *Features, Evaluation, and Treatment of Coronavirus (COVID-19).* In StatPearls. 2020 © StatPearls Publishing LLC.: Treasure Island, FL.
49. Ledford, H., (2020). Coronavirus breakthrough: Dexamethasone is the first drug shown to save lives. *Nature, 582*(7813), 469.
50. Wu, C., et al., (2020). Risk factors associated with acute respiratory distress syndrome and death in patients with Coronavirus disease 2019 pneumonia in Wuhan, China. *JAMA Intern. Med., 180*(7), 1–11.

51. Wang, Y., et al., (2020). *Early, Low-Dose and Short-Term Application of Corticosteroid Treatment in Patients with Severe COVID-19 Pneumonia: Single-Center Experience from Wuhan, China.* medRxiv. 2020.03.06.20032342.
52. Shang, L., et al., (2020). On the use of corticosteroids for 2019-nCoV pneumonia. *Lancet, 395*(10225), 683–684.
53. Jarcho, J. A., et al., (2020). Inhibitors of the renin-angiotensin-aldosterone system and COVID-19. *The New England Journal of Medicine, 382*(25), 2462–2464.
54. Kuba, K., et al., (2005). A crucial role of angiotensin-converting enzyme 2 (ACE2) in SARS coronavirus-induced lung injury. *Nat. Med., 11*(8), 875–879.
55. Gu, H., et al., (2016). Angiotensin-converting enzyme 2 inhibits lung injury induced by respiratory syncytial virus. *Sci. Rep., 6*, 19840.
56. Sodhi, M., & Etminan, M., (2020). Safety of Ibuprofen in patients with COVID-19: Causal or Confounded? *Chest, 158*(1), 55–56.
57. Rao, P., & Knaus, E. E., (2008). Evolution of nonsteroidal anti-inflammatory drugs (NSAIDs): Cyclooxygenase (COX) inhibition and beyond. *J. Pharm. Pharm. Sci., 11*(2), 81s–110s.
58. Amici, C., et al., (2006). Indomethacin has a potent antiviral activity against SARS coronavirus. *Antivir. Ther., 11*(8), 1021–1030.
59. Bloch, E. M., et al., (2020). Deployment of convalescent plasma for the prevention and treatment of COVID-19. *J. Clin. Invest., 130*(6), 2757–2765.
60. Gautret, P., et al., (2020). Hydroxychloroquine and azithromycin as a treatment of COVID-19: Results of an open-label non-randomized clinical trial. *Int. J. Antimicrob. Agents, 56*(1), 105949.
61. Molina, J. M., et al., (2020). No evidence of rapid antiviral clearance or clinical benefit with the combination of hydroxychloroquine and azithromycin in patients with severe COVID-19 infection. *Med. Mal. Infect., 50*(4), 384.
62. Mycroft-West, C., et al., (2020). *The 2019 Coronavirus (SARS-CoV-2) Surface Protein (Spike) S1 Receptor Binding Domain Undergoes Conformational Change Upon Heparin Binding.* bioRxiv, 2020.02.29.971093.
63. SHI, C., et al., (2020). *The Potential of Low Molecular Weight Heparin to Mitigate Cytokine Storm in Severe COVID-19 Patients: A Retrospective Clinical Study.* medRxiv. 2020.03.28.20046144.
64. Gropper, S. A. S., Smith, J. L., & Groff, J. L., (2009). *Advanced Nutrition and Human Metabolism*. Australia; United States: Wadsworth/Cengage Learning.
65. Schneider, W. M., Chevillotte, M. D., & Rice, C. M., (2014). Interferon-stimulated genes: A complex web of host defenses. *Annual Review of Immunology, 32*, 513–545.
66. Ranieri, V. M., et al., (2020). Effect of intravenous interferon β-1a on death and days free from mechanical ventilation among patients with moderate to severe acute respiratory distress syndrome: A randomized clinical trial. *JAMA, 323*(8), 725–733.
67. Laing, R., Gillan, V., & Devaney, E., (2017). Ivermectin-old drug, new tricks? *Trends in Parasitology, 33*(6), 463–472.
68. Gassen, N. C., et al., (2019). SKP2 attenuates autophagy through beclin1-ubiquitination and its inhibition reduces MERS-Coronavirus infection. *Nature Communications, 10*(1), 1–16.
69. Deftereos, S., et al., (2013). Colchicine and the heart: Pushing the envelope. *J. Am. Coll. Cardiol., 62*(20), 1817–1825.

70. Wang, Y., et al., (2016). Teicoplanin inhibits Ebola pseudovirus infection in cell culture. *Antiviral Res., 125*, 1–7.
71. Baron, S. A., et al., (2020). Teicoplanin: An alternative drug for the treatment of coronavirus COVID-19. *Int. J. Antimicrob. Agents, 105944*(10.1016).
72. Arnold, R., Neumann, M., & König, W., (2007). Peroxisome proliferator-activated receptor-γ agonists inhibit respiratory syncytial virus-induced expression of intercellular adhesion molecule-1 in human lung epithelial cells. *Immunology, 121*(1), 71–81.

CHAPTER 14

An Overview of COVID-19 Treatment

SAFFORA RIAZ,[1] FARKHANDA MANZOOR,[1] DOU DEQIANG,[2] and NAJMUR RAHMAN[3]

[1]*Department of Zoology, Lahore College for Women University, Lahore, Pakistan, E-mail: riazsaffora@gmail.com (S. Riaz)*

[2]*College of Pharmacy, Liaoning University of Traditional Chinese Medicine, Dalian Campus, China*

[3]*Department of Pharmacy, Shaheed Benazir Bhutto University, Sheringal, Pakistan*

ABSTRACT

Novel Coronavirus identified in Wuhan, China, spread the global pandemic. COVID-19 has become the leading cause of death internationally due to reasons of a significant public health crisis. The fast extension of the COVID-19 pandemic has made the advancement of a SARS-CoV-2 antibody worldwide for human well-being and financial need. Pharmacologic specialists endorsed the effectiveness of repurposing drugs or novel and improved treatments by created tested antibodies for COVID-19. It might be helpful to a reduction in the rate of mortality all through the general population. The conceivable part of plant-determined standard antiviral mixtures for improving plant-based medications against COVID has been suggested. Lipid-epitomized mRNA nucleoside-adjusted immunization encoded the SARS-CoV-2 RBD was created. A solitary vaccination of mRNA-RBD evoked both potent killing counter-acting agent and cell reactions and gave a near-complete assurance against wild SARS-CoV-2 disease in the lungs of hACE2. A single portion of mRNA-RBD gave long-term insurance against the SARS-CoV-2 test. However, the different reactions after vaccination and human re-infection by SARS-CoV-2 have raised many questions about a potential SARS-CoV-2 vaccination.

14.1 INTRODUCTION

SARS-CoV-2 coronavirus 2 is an enveloped RNA virus that causes the severe respiratory syndrome. In the past few years, mortality due to COVID-19 was 125 million and 50 million infections due to clinical disease [1]. COVID-19 common symptoms are cough, myalgia, chills, headache, and fever that appear in a patient after an average of six days of infection. It was proven that major organs directly affected by the coronavirus were the lungs, where pulmonary infiltrates' consolidations evolved within 7–10 days. The mortality rate was approximately 9.6%, and the initial onset of SARS-CoV patients become dependent on ventilator support until most patients had recovered [2–4]. Coronavirus infection epidemic arose in Arabian Peninsula in the year 2012 with a 35% mortality rate. The spread of infection occurs due to the shedding of viral particles during SARS-CoV-2 infection [5]. COVID-19 patients worldwide present the same pattern of the symptoms, but patients with no symptoms appear but infected were 20% [6, 7]. Severe atypical pneumonia is the common feature among MERS-CoV sand SARS-CoV. However, acute kidney injury (AKI) and gastrointestinal (GI) symptoms were prominent differences among MERS and COVID-19. The investigators attributed that supportive care is the only treatment of the coronavirus. Both viruses bind to different receptors as MERS binds to the human, and SARS binds to the angiotensin-converting enzyme receptor [8].

14.2 SARS-COV-2-INDUCED PNEUMONIA MECHANISMS

Pneumonia induced by microorganism is a complex mechanism, a clinical and preclinical exploration of the infection clarify numerous viewpoints. In the host, viral infection-induced the immunological response. When a response is initiated at times of infection cytokine storm cause the coagulation and affects the tissues. Microvascular aspiratory apoplexy and microvascular lung vessels obstructive-thrombo-provocative disorder-related lung injury may occur in COVID-19 [9].

In many cells and tissues, leukocytes delivered the IL-6 on an enormous number of cells and tissues. While interleukin 6 is sometimes unable to compete with the microorganisms' levels that cause sickness, tumor putrefaction factor α, interleukins family proteins interferon-gamma, get affected.

The separation of B lymphocytes advances the development and hindrance of certain classes of the cells. Intense stage proteins were created that were useful in thermoregulation of the focal sensory system and bone support. Albeit IL-6 assumed favorable to incendiary part and it can likewise have calming impacts. IL-6 would be useful during cardiovascular illnesses, infections, immune system issues, and a few kinds of malignancy. Cytokine discharge disorder (CRS) occurred in the severe pathogenesis represented by fever and various organ dysfunctions, and IL-6 is the primary marker. The interleukins-1β may prevent fibrosis in the lungs because SARS-CoV-2 binds to Toll-Like Receptor of IL-1β that activates after virus contact [10].

14.2.1 SEVERITY OF ILLNESS

On account of gentle Illness, patients suffered from manifestations of a respiratory tract after viral disease contact, nasal blockage, including mild fever, hack (dry), sore throat, discomfort, migraine, muscle agony, or anxiety. The common symptoms are lack of taste and smell, looseness of the bowels, and dyspnea. Other respiratory manifestations include moderate pneumonia and severe pneumonia related to fever, serious dyspnea, respiratory problem, tachypnea, and hypoxia. Nevertheless, the fever might be mild or even missing that should be interpreted cautiously.

14.2.2 ACUTE RESPIRATORY DISTRESS SYNDROME

Lungs of corona patients affected by hypoxia and clinical determination are suffered from acute respiratory distress syndrome. Acute respiratory distress syndrome generally presents a respiratory distress picture. The CT examination, chest imaging used incorporates chest radiograph, or two-sided opacities showing by lung ultrasound disclosed the lung breakdown. A ventilator could manage pneumonic edema. Acute respiratory inception of the edema is demonstrated after heart failure and different causes like liquid over-burden. Echocardiography can be helpful for monitoring and ruling out this cause (Figure 14.1) [11].

14.3 CATEGORIES OF COVID-19 PATIENTS

In case of SARS-CoV-2, there are three different categories of patients, which are described in subsections.

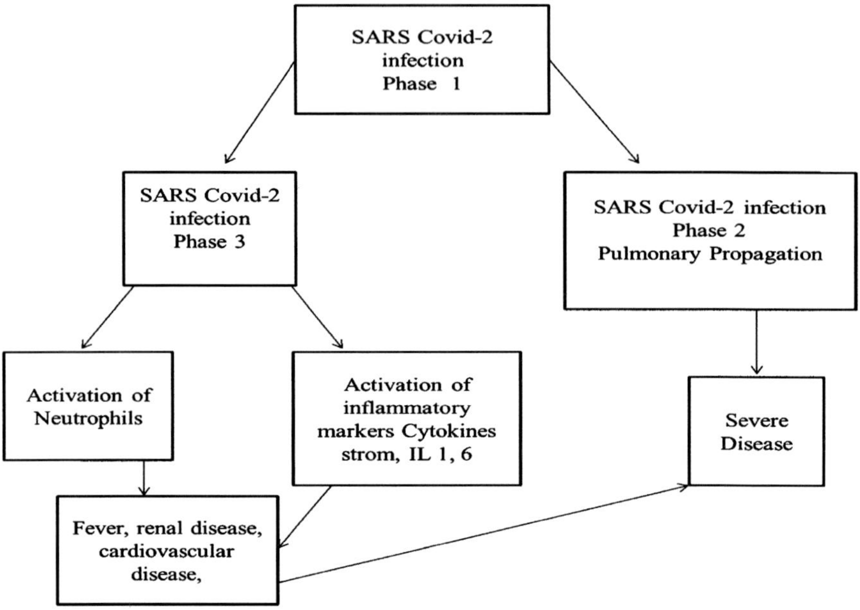

FIGURE 14.1 Flow chart showing pneumonia induced by SARS-CoV-2 virus.

14.3.1 IN CASE OF CATEGORY 1

Patients have COVID-19 infections with clear HRCT without lung involvement and no respiratory distress, not dependent on oxygen with no desaturation on exertion.

14.3.2 CATEGORY 2 PATIENTS

COVID-19 infection, raised IL-6 and involvement of lungs on HRCT, not dependent on oxygen with no desaturation on exertion.

14.3.3 CATEGORY 3 PATIENTS

COVID-19 infection, oxygen dependence, desaturation on exertion, raised IL-6, and involvement of lungs on HRCT.

14.4 TREATMENT

The early spread of COVID-19 pandemic for tending to respiratory disability was the oxygen treatment because there is no antibody and definitive antiviral treatment suggested for COVID-19 to date. Non-obtrusive (NIV) and intrusive mechanical ventilation (IMV) might be important hard-headed to oxygen treatment in instances of a respiratory disorder. Acute Respiratory Distress Syndrome (ARDS) is one of the COVID complications that harm the lungs. It provokes the clinicians to investigate the condition for managing respiratory disappointment [12–16]. In critical patients, acetaminophen via nasal cannula as oxygen supportive therapy for fever control should be given. In SpO 2 above 97 or 94, the patient suffered from mild to moderate disease; in SpO2 $\leq$ 90, the patient has a high degree of infection and depends on the mechanical ventilator to maintain the level of O_2 in the body. If the white blood cell count is high, antibiotics should be given because sometimes bacterial and viral pneumonia show the same symptoms. Currently, no specific anti-COVID treatment is recommended. Third-generation antibiotics such as cephalosporins may be used in case of mixed infection [17].

Various categories of drugs and treatment regimens have been used or recommended according to the clinical conditions, as given in Figure 14.2. Each of them will be described below in detail.

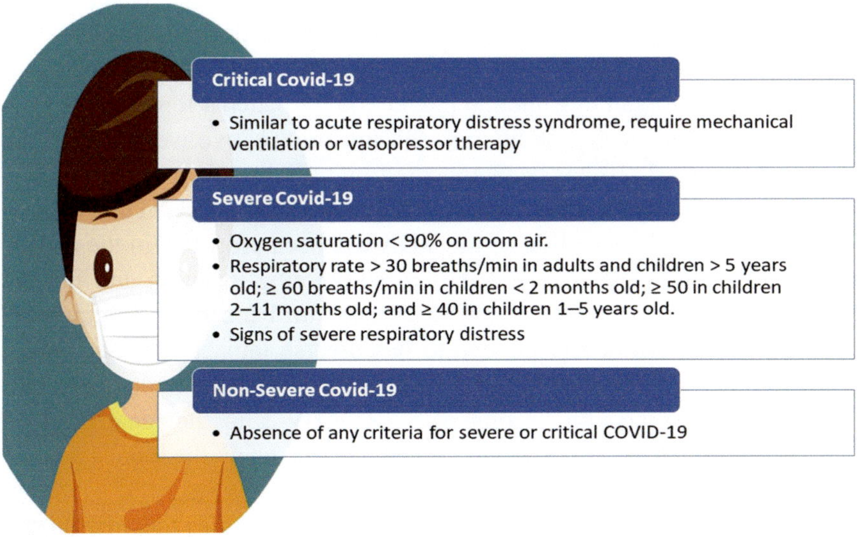

FIGURE 14.2 COVID-19 patients sub-groups based on clinical indicators.

14.4.1 VITAMINS

Fundamentally COVID-19 sick patients were treated with intravenous (IV) vitamin C high dosages with the expectation of recovery of patients. Nonetheless, it is not important for the standard convention because no proof for its viability for COVID-19 diseases was accounted for. At the same time, standard doses of vitamin C are by and large unknown, so its high dosages may result in nausea, cramps, and an expanded danger of the kidney.

Vitamin D against COVID-19 has ensured many beneficial effects. Individuals with low Vitamin D levels might be more helpless to cope with the infection of respiratory tract contaminations. Individuals who took Vitamin D supplements are less inclined to create intense respiratory infection when compared with those individuals who have a low degree of Vitamin D. Vitamin D may secure against COVID-19 by boosting our body's regular protection framework. Vitamin D might be defensive against infectivity and seriousness from COVID-19 through both genomic and non-genomic pathways by interceded resistant and non-insusceptible activity on a few issues. Antimicrobial peptide, cathelicidin produce by the respiratory epithelial cells and upgrades the intrinsic insusceptible framework created by the Vitamin D. Antimicrobial peptide acts against microbes and growths as well as straightforwardly have antiviral activity against respiratory infections [18, 19]. Vitamin D has immunomodulatory impacts on the versatile insusceptible framework that appeared to downregulate the activity of TH1 and TH17 and enhanced the separation of Treg. These stimuli cause a decline in the creation of pro-inflammatory cytokines, interleukins, and tumor necrosis factors. Therefore, multi-organ dysfunction in COVID-19 patients forecasted by the reducing cytokine storm condition with high provocative weight [20, 21]. Up-regulation of IL-10 has been appeared by utilizing vitamin D, which is considered the likely treatment for COVID-19 [22]. Likewise, in the lungs of COVID-19 patients, actuation of the VDR has been proposed in the aspiratory stellate cells may assume a part in smothering irritation and fibrotic changes. Vitamin D has been appeared to control the renin-angiotensin-aldosterone framework and believe to has diverse impacts among tissues. ACE2 articulation seemed to hinder Oral alfa-calcidiol (1α-hydroxyvitamin D), the principle receptor section of SARS-CoV-2, in the renal rounded cells. Therefore, vitamin D applies a defensive impact on the kidney against COVID by diminishing viral passage into cells [23].

During SARS-CoV-2 disease ACE2 in the lungs is downregulated causes an increase of angiotensin II, which is considered to be the reason for heart injury, myocarditis, and acute respiratory distress syndrome [24]. ACE2 articulation expands by using vitamin D after concealment of renin [25]. These impacts might decrease cardiovascular injury, particularly in COVID-19 patients, the increase of angiotensin II and subsequently diminish the danger of ARDS. This system is thought to help alleviate the bradykinin storm, which has been appeared to underlie the numerous organ brokenness in COVID-19 [26].

Pleiotropic impacts of Vitamin D against endothelial can cause the relieved vascular spillage, blood vessel, and venous apoplexy in COVID-19 patients. It has appeared in the essential dermal human microvascular endothelial cell model that Vitamin D3, 25(OH)D3 and 1,25(OH)2D3 settled vascular endothelial layers utilizing a non-genomic pathway [27, 28]. Despite numerous systems recommending possible advantages of Vitamin D for COVID-19, 1,25(OH)2D. It is as yet not clear whether this biologic activity could boost the creation of killing antibodies and be adverse in the setting of reaction to COVID-19 contamination or COVID-19 immunization. Further examinations are needed to explore this part of Vitamin D activities.

14.4.2 CORTICOSTEROIDS

Corticosteroids are recommended in case of pneumonia caused by a viral infection or to treat a respiratory issue. The side effects of corticosteroids in treating COVID-19 disease cause overflowing lung irritation, promoting respiratory failure, intense respiratory distress condition, and demise.

Early experience and review investigation reported that potential mortality due to COVID-19 decreases by utilizing corticosteroids [29–31].

14.4.2.1 DEXAMETHASONE

Various corticosteroids, Dexamethasone, Prednisone, methylprednisolone, are great beneficial drugs. They are cheap, readily available, and effective. The COVID-19 treatment rules propose dexamethasone to people hospitalized in acute conditions [32–35]. In COVID-19 cases, dexamethasone was recommended to be more advantageous. Before recommending the dexamethasone COVID, 19 patients' symptoms were assessed [36–37]. Dexamethasone has been accessible worldwide and a most fundamental medication reported by the guidelines of the health agencies and the world. It is suggested for the COVID-19 patients hospitalized without a ventilator's help or may require oxygen. In the COVID-19 patients in the principal seven-day stretch of ailment, sickness might be overwhelmed by dynamic viral replication playing an optional immune pathological role. At that stage, dexamethasone has a more notable mortality advantage [38–40].

14.4.3 IMMUNOMODULATORY OR ANTIVIRAL DRUGS

For treatment of COVID-19 infection among patients, drugs that were used for flu were also suggested. As immunomodulatory drugs, chloroquine and hydroxychloroquine (HCQ) were proposed. The use of HCQ reduced viral load was significantly associated with the viral disappearance shown in a non-randomized trial of macrolides azithromycin. In particular, these drugs inhibit the mobilization and activation of neutrophils, stimulate the alveolar macrophages phagocytosis, induce the downregulation of cell surface adhesion molecules, production of pro-inflammatory cytokines [41–45]. Chloroquine can act in prolongation of viral infection. Thought to be used as HCQ with azithromycin can work in prolongation and heart arrhythmias [46].

14.4.3.1 REMDESIVIR

Remdesivir may be recommended for hospitalized COVID-19 patients because of its clinical benefit recovery and improvement in patients. A simple prodrug remdesivir has substantial clinical advantages, expected fruitful fundamental outcomes dependent on its delivered beneficial results [47]. General mortality is the main endpoint result of any preliminary clinical trials; advanced remdesivir caused do not show a satisfactory reduction in mortality [48]. Regardless of all analysis and alerts, the FDA has endorsed remdesivir to be utilized for COVID-19. Therefore, remdesivir advised against COVID-19 with mild infection [49, 50].

14.4.3.2 OSELTAMIVIR

Tamiflu (oseltamivir) against SARS-CoV is an antiviral drug utilized for flu (influenza). Docking with key proteins showed the similarity in binding like neuraminidase. No clinical information proposes that oseltamivir is viable in treating SARS-CoV even it is used as an antiviral drug has the attention. Due to the huge viability of Tamiflu (oseltamivir) become an intriguing issue with the scourge of COVID illness 2019. Oseltamivir is thought to be useful in the treatment of COVID because it has an antiviral impact. The revealed investigation of the antiviral effect of oseltamivir against SARS-CoV-2 could positively affect the treatment of COVID-19 [51].

14.4.3.3 FAVIPIRAVIR AND OTHER ANTIVIRAL MEDICATIONS

Avigan (favipiravir) is affirmed in Japan and China against influenza is an antiviral medicine that has shown preventive impact on SARS-CoV-2 contaminated human cells. Flu infection may be just the trouble, so favipiravir is safe in case of flu infection. For reappearing flu infections, favipiravir was affirmed in China and Japan in 2014. Favipiravir used to treat flu infection by joining RNA of the virus and stimulated the mutagenesis by acting as a mutagen. No legislative approval about Favipiravir use against coronavirus is reported [52–55].

14.4.3.4 COLCHICINE

A repurposable medication Colcrys utilized for the treatment of gout. Colchicine can bring down the number of cases of COVID-19 hospitalized patients when it passes through preliminary clinical trials. If cytokine storm initiated in the case of COVID-19 infection, Tocilizumab (Actemra) could work in a very useful way comparatively with colchicine [56].

14.4.3.5 TOCILIZUMAB

Tocilizumab is an FDA-approved drug that acts on to monoclonal neutralizer IL-6 receptor, as it is a monoclonal antibody that is administered to patients suffering from infection other than COVID-19. Tocilizumab has been shown to improve clinical outcomes in genuine cases of COVID-19 pneumonia by immense lower mortality. However, the use of Tocilizumab produced conflicting results for the treatment of COVID patients. Patients with COVID-19 suggested positive outcomes when treated with Tocilizumab. Guidelines of The Infectious Disease Society of America and NIH guidelines recommend Tocilizumab for the hospitalized COVID-19 patients having respiratory decompensation. Use of Tocilizumab recommended after the clinical trials are performed randomly and report the reduction in mortality rate [57–60].

14.4.3.6 NAFAMOSTAT

Nafamostat has been used to treat disseminated intravascular coagulation as a proteinase inhibitor by acting as antithrombin and antiplasmin. It is also used in the treatment of pancreatitis. Nafamostat hinders viral limit by acting on the receptors of a subordinate host cell of corona infected patients. In lung tissues, multinucleated goliath cell shape changed by the viral burden and fewer antibodies level. A hemostat was proposed anyway, but it fails to obtain any basic positive outcomes. It is a viral envelope film mix inhibitor suggested treating COVID [61].

14.4.4 ANTI-PARASITIC DRUGS

Treatment with the anti-parasitic drugs could help lessen the viral burden and accelerate recovery in patients with gentle to-direct COVID-19. Anti-parasitic drugs are utilized to treat tropical infections such as scabies, onchocerciasis, and helminthiases. Likewise, it is assessed for its capability to diminish the pace of intestinal sickness transmission executing by mosquitoes in humans [62].

14.4.4.1 IVERMECTIN

Ivermectin is an oral prescription used to treat infections accomplished by parasites. Specialists and campaigners promote the ivermectin use as a solution for COVID-19 solution all over the world. Ordinarily, ivermectin is used to treat ecto and endoparasites, i.e., head lice in people. Now the medication has been allowed to treat COVID-19 patients. The use of ivermectin is yet under trial according to the guidelines of the World Health Organization (WHO). Evidence about the role of ivermectin on the reduction of viral have very low certainty. Ivermectin is recommended for two reasons; first of all, our cells are protected due to their antiviral reactions. Second, restrict the entry of infectious agents into cells by limiting the binding of spike protein on the cell membrane receptors [63].

14.4.5 SEROTHERAPY

Antibodies taken from the blood of recovered individuals address a remedial option at present. The natural defense mechanism of the COVID-19 positive patients produced antibodies that protect their body from re-infection of the virus. From the blood serum of the infected patient, antibodies can be extracted and used to treat the patient by developing passive immunity. The progress in results and its danger to profit proportion have few potential well-being concerns, and there are many functional difficulties with this methodology [64].

14.4.6 INTERFERON THERAPY

During the spread of the corona, interferons were utilized to treat patients. Interferon β can suppress the infection was proposed as an appropriate treatment method [68]. Viral protein replication in SARS-CoV can be fundamentally reduced by the interferon (IFN-I). It is realized that interferon safeguards against COVID to get away innate insusceptibility right off in the disease course. Therefore, interferons have become an appealing strategy for the treatment of COVID-19. The consequences of interferon therapy are significant due to versatile humoral and cell reactions in COVID patients [65].

14.4.7 NEW DRUGS RECOMMENDATION FOR COVID

Viral RNA fragments could be used to create novel drugs that affect the virus's machinery by targeting the centered mRNA of the virus [66]. Drugs targeting different viral proteins and enzymes that play a vital role in protein replication are protease, helicase, and RNA polymerase; spike glycoprotein could be used for drug development. New drugs are novel that target the COVID-19 at the molecular level by arresting the mechanism of mRNA. It was a valuation point that viral replication can be diminished up to 90% using siRNA-based RNAi technology [67].

14.4.8 TREATMENT BY TRANSFUSION OF PLASMA

COVID-19 patients recovered patients plasma have antibodies against corona is recommended and used as plasma therapy. A broad number of clinical fundamentals are in progress to choose the prosperity and practicality of the treatment, and starter results were promising. When people recover from corona patients, blood contains antibodies that the immune system made to fight the COVID. Antibodies are found in the plasma of blood. Plasma taken from recovered patients has been used in history to treat infectious diseases. It is comprehensively acknowledged to be secured. Earlier exploration had found that patients with (or at risk for) outrageous COVID-19 who got mending plasma inside three days of assurance were more disinclined to pass on than patients who got recovering plasma later in their infection. To give plasma, an individual should fulfill a couple of guidelines. They probably patients recovered from corona infection had no virus in their plasma after serology test but a high quantity of antibodies in their plasma. Blood characterization of plasma donor and patient ought to have a similarity. At whatever point plasma is given, it is assessed for other overpowering ailments, similar to HIV. Plasma taken from one donor is adequate plasma to treat one to three patients. Transfusion of plasma should not provide the prolonged safe system nor make the supporter more defenseless against getting re-infection with the disease [68].

14.4.9 TREATMENT WITH IMMUNOGLOBULINS AND ANTIBODIES

Monoclonal antibodies unequivocal are similarly being endeavored against SARS-CoV-2. The human monoclonal antibody has different binding sites. Some antibodies bind to confining receptor region, other human monoclonal antibodies that attach to the spike glycoprotein. Based on their binding sites, various types of vaccines have been explored. The development of hyper immunoglobulins formation is still under working to treat corona infected patients. It would be more remarkable and successfully applicable than plasma therapy. It contains recuperating serum, immunoglobulin G (IgG) of humans, and its efficacy can be increased by developing recombinant polyclonal antibodies [69, 70].

14.4.10 MESENCHYMAL STEM CELL THERAPY

The mesenchymal stem cell can be used in treatment. Moreover, thought to be utilized as they can apply to fix the damaged lung tissues has no apoptotic alleviating effect and remove the alveolar fluid by propelling [71]. In different countries such as China and Sweden applicability of therapy by stem cells is under trial. It can decrease the hyperactivity of CD4+ T and CD8+ T cells and suppress the IL-10. After stem cell therapy, lungs become impenetrable to SARS-CoV-2 and have a high relieving effect [72, 73].

14.4.11 ANTICOAGULANT

Coagulation markers such as D-dimer, prothrombin detected in the COVID-19 patients' blood undergo coagulation. Venous thromboembolism and anticoagulant treatment are common in COVID-19 patients. Patients were prescribed to get thromboprophylaxis. Enoxaparin is a blood thinner medicine that is used to treat the circulatory issue as anticoagulation. Heparin is also preferred for anticoagulation as a prophylactic dose for all patients with COVID [74].

14.5 DIFFERENT THERAPIES

Respiratory assistance of the lungs is compulsory when the disease achieves a complex clinical picture. The efficacy of different therapies in combating COVID-19 is still under trial to evaluate their safety for patients. It provides more options for the treatment of coronavirus disease. Complement-targeting therapeutics were used to treat autoimmune diseases are now being suggested in COVID-19 treatment. In cases with mild to moderate disease, supportive therapies with bed rest, high intake of water, and sufficient calories are recommended that provide them relief from chest congestion. A mechanical ventilator supports patients in a severe case of disease. In more critical patients, extracorporeal membrane oxygenation could be performed to maintain the oxygen saturation in the blood of the patient [75].

14.6 THE VACCINE FIRST HUMAN TRIAL

In the meantime, the logical examination is developing to build up a SARS-CoV-2 antibody. More than 100 competitor vaccines are being developed worldwide; out of them, only 8 or 10 are in clinical examination. In this 'antibody gaming,' Chinese scientists have all the earmarks of being ahead, having finished a stage I examination. A few investigations are continuous, particularly in the US, and the UK. The after-effects of immunization I clinical trials take place in Wuhan (China). After clinical trials, glycoproteins spiked antibody communicating to adenovirus type 5 get the reactogenicity and immunogenicity and then distributed in the world [76].

14.6.1 VACCINE TRIALS AND IMMUNIZATION

The improvement of a counter-acting agent is in progress. Vaccination is undertrials from the last 12 to 18 months evaluated for more broad use. Fundamentally four counter-acting agents are used effectively for COVID-19 to affect safe response. Vaccine effect firstly as crippled or inactivated contamination; secondly inhibit the copying or non-replicating viral vectors, to inoculate viral proteins inside the body; third nucleic-destructive based vaccinations, make copies of viral protein using host machinery; fourth, using protein-based antibodies to inject viral protein piece or disease like particle inside the body [77]. Around 90 vaccinations are going through powerful new development and some of them have adequately positive results [75].

Vaccine prepared in the UK is a glycoprotein in nature and can be helpful to neutralize the adenovirus. Its use can be safe and develop the humoral response. Another excellent vaccination primers consolidate immunizer is RNA vaccination. It is a novel sort of immunizer where an RNA of a viral antigenic protein is implanted into individuals to create a safe response. The immune response of the synthesized RNA vaccine was disseminated after the innate viral progressions [79]. The use of mRNA inoculation development gives a specific advantage of fast headway over various antibodies due to its valuable natural ability to speedily change over into protein inside the cell (Table 14.1) [80].

14.6.2 VACCINE DELIVERY SYSTEM

SARS-COV-2 vaccines development race moved with unprecedented speed, and authorization for the use of the vaccine on an emergency basis get approval worldwide. Now, attention should be taken to the verification, allocation, and distribution of vaccines. Improvement in the delivery of vaccines has also taken place. The microneedle patches containing specific ligands embedded in liposomes taken up by the Langerhans cells in the skin show the safe response [82]. Various decisions that can be researched in the vaccination of vaccines suggest that it should be subjected to mucosal to acquaint antigens with mucosa-related lymphoid tissues. At present open

TABLE 14.1 Currently Recommended Vaccines and Their Effectiveness [81]

SL. No.	Name of Vaccine	Status	Recommendation for Age Group	Dosage	Efficacy of Vaccine
1.	Pfizer-BioNTech	Used in US	Anyone 16 and older.	Two shots, 21 days apart	95% efficacy
2.	Moderna	Used in US	Adults 18 and older.	Two shots, 28 days apart	94.1% effective
3.	Johnson & Johnson	Used in US	Adults 18 and older.	Single shot	72% overall efficacy
4.	Oxford-AstraZeneca	Approved for other countries. Not used in US	Adults 18 and older	Two doses, four to 12 weeks apart	76% effective
5.	Novavax	Still completing clinical trials	Adult's age 18–84	2 doses, three weeks apart	86.3% efficacy
6.	Sputnik V-AstraZeneca	Authorized in Algeria, Bolivia, Serbia, the Palestinian territories, and Mexico	$\geq$ 18 years of age	2 doses	91.4% effective
7.	Sinovac/Sinopharm vaccines	Authorization for use in Asian countries	Above 60 years	2 doses	79.34% effective

through oral course consolidate rotavirus, typhoid, cholera, and poliovirus have inoculated. Fast dissolving tablets that can be put into the mouth may be a viable alternative for vaccination that reduced swallowing difficulties in children and old subjects. The mixture uses dried vaccination covered onto spots without needle powder implantation like ballistic powder imbuement or intradermal powder. This method could even pass on the inoculation clearly into the cytoplasm of the cells [83].

14.6.3 COVID-19 VACCINES CHALLENGES

The world is in urgent need of powerful antibodies against the coronavirus disease 2019 (COVID-19). Right now, there are 78 immunization applicants, progressing 201 preliminaries and expanding. Among which 12 immunizations are affirmed, moving the use of these antibodies continuously in various parts of the world. In Nepal, the COVID-19 immunization program was started on January 27th, 2021. The public authority of India gave a gift of 10 million antibody doses for the Nepalese populace to forestall COVID-19. The public administration of Nepal chose to begin mass immunization, beginning by inoculating well-being and security laborers. There is a requirement for long-haul checking of unfavorable medication responses, and a genuine requirement for observing by pharmacovigilance focuses inside a country. Randomized controlled clinical preliminaries are needed to affirm immunization adequacy in the world. Pharmacogenomics study confirms the dissimilarities in genomic grouping related to the reaction of immunization. Randomized controlled clinical preliminaries are required to prove immunization adequacy in the world. Coronavirus strains are different in different countries of the world. While the course of immunization, careful measures should be taken [84–87].

14.6.4 HESITANCY OF PEOPLE TOWARD THE VACCINE

By November 2020, more than 10 million individuals had been infected. More than a quarter-million passed on of COVID-19 in the US after developing the vaccines misperception about the improvement in the level of antibodies COVID-19 immunization circulated in the public media [88–91].

People of the US and other countries show their hesitancy towards the vaccination, notwithstanding the difficulties related to costs, access, effectiveness, and coordination of immunization. Immunization reluctance is not a novel wonder in the US reluctancy and hesitancy of people towards the vaccines is always cause of reappearance of the diseases in the history as the measles and polio. Now the people show reluctant behavior for immunization in the era of the COVID-19 pandemic. Essentially, there are populace subgroups throughout the planet with high antibody aversion revealed before the pandemic. While there is a significant expectation for the COVID-19 immunization, little is thought about antibody reluctance specifically for COVID-19. Distinguishing explicit populaces and their qualities concerning antibody reluctance will help fill in as critical parts of a fruitful inoculation technique when a COVID-19 immunization is free for everyone [92].

COVID-19 immunization that assures the security and efficacy of the vaccine on antibody development can guarantee the reliability of the people on the vaccines. Racial and ethnic minorities had higher antibody aversion in bunch correlations. This could be clarified dependent on an assortment of components that existed before the COVID-19 pandemic. Previously antibody reluctance was too less accessibility of the medical experts, less authentic biomedical and medical services, lower support of minorities in clinical preliminaries, and cost-related concerns. Socially skilled techniques for general well-being and exploration have shown a guarantee in improving well-being results and commitment to COVID-19 immunizations. People living in country regions, those with lower family salaries, and lower levels of instruction were bound to be reluctant about getting inoculated with a COVID-19 antibody. Up until now, there have been conversations on antibody prioritization. It is recommended that at priority vaccination be given to medical practitioners exposed to the virus while dealing with the COVID-19 patients. People also show hesitancy due to the high cost of the vaccine. So, policymakers assure the commitment for access to vaccination and free immunizations for everyone. The hesitancy of people for vaccines can be reduced by convincing the people by addressing the following points:

- Vaccination against COVID-19 is everyone's personal choice. So, if people get vaccinated, then people can get protect themselves from getting infected and sick.
- Due to vaccination immune system boost up, and when people get exposed to the virus, their body would be ready to fight against the virus.
- Older and vulnerable group of people who suffered from chronic and various medical complications such as diabetes and heart disease can be safer when get vaccinated. In this way, they can help the community by getting vaccinated.

- If people will show positive behavior for vaccination, lives will get normal after eradicating the coronavirus pandemic.
- must keep in mind side effects of the vaccine are very rare. It may not harm the people. If symptoms usually appear, they are temporary.

Hesitancy for vaccines affects people of all different ethnicities. A vaccine cannot reduce the pandemic unless communities are not agreed to get vaccinated. After scientific approval, policymakers should create and underwrite emotionally supportive networks that introduce the advancement of COVID-19 immunization programs. A few impediments may have affected the consequences [93–96].

14.6.5 ATTITUDES OF PEOPLE TOWARDS VACCINATION

Globally vaccines can reduce the burden of coronavirus infection due to their effective interventions. People of developing countries and even developed countries show a negative attitude towards vaccines—people's unwillingness to vaccination pressing problem in reducing the risk of corona infection. Among the people of the Jordon, the public has less acceptability for COVID-19 vaccine. People of Bangladesh who get infected with the vaccine provided by India now have no reliability on a vaccine. In a global survey, about 48% of the world, the population is still confused and unassured to vaccination beneficial effects. China's population comparatively relies on the beneficial effects of the vaccines, and they get vaccinated in context to protect themselves from the virus [97]. Possibly more hazardous because people of lower financial positions are bound to be uncertain or reluctant to be immunized. Satisfaction and convincing the local community by media and other campaigns about vaccination can build up individuals' trust. People should advocate the current realities of the beneficial effects of vaccines to reduce their reluctance [98]. A case study showed that social media also plays an essential role in developing trust in antibody development, diminishing immunization reluctance [99, 100].

14.6.6 PSYCHOLOGICAL CONSIDERATION OF VACCINATION

Indeed, even the best immunizations do not work for everybody. Like the measles antibody, a few immunizations are exceptionally effective, decreasing contamination rates by about 98%. Viability or how much the antibody lessens disease rates in “this present reality”—outside of the exceptionally controlled clinical-preliminary setting—is frequently lower than the underlying adequacy rate. Besides, these announced adequacy rates depend on a generally short subsequent period, and it is obscure how the immunization will perform over the long run. Even though immunization viability relies vigorously upon antibody-related variables attributes, cognitive, and social behavior can significantly influence the resistant framework of antibody reaction. Every Immune System has a different response to a vaccine. All immunizations challenge the invulnerable framework. Level of antibodies increases after immunization—because of the quick and vague intrinsic invulnerable reaction [101]. The first response of the body to antigen remains for a couple of days. The immunization response varies from individuals to individuals. One primary factor that balances this reaction is whether the immunization beneficiary has recently experienced the antigen the protein outside of microbe either through disease or vaccination. The body responds to a quicker and fiercer immunizer safe reaction than an essential resistant response [102]. However, there are less significant views about stress, depression, and Other psychological factors that influence the level of antibody production. Immunization is not just useful for members and straightforwardly appropriate to clinical settings yet, in addition, an accommodating worldview to evaluate the resistant framework's capacity to react to microbes—even the same antibody given the difference. A few investigations reported that depression changes various aspects of the antibody reactions [103]. People having zoster infections were treated with varicella-zoster. Depressed people have a low response because the number of produced antibodies was less than healthy people. Other mental elements that anticipated a more inadequate response to immunization include high-quality negative influence, low characteristic positive influence, high neuroticism, and low confidence. US citizens during the pandemic developed the psychological issue represented by the nervousness named chronophobia. Due to which their immunity gets affected due to mental weakness factors like neuroticism.

Incidentally, the dread of COVID-19 itself may decrease an antibody's capacity to present invulnerability against the infection. The pervasiveness of mental manifestations and clinical determinations has expanded during the overall pandemic. There is a direct relationship with immunization reactions or synergistically cooperating with pressure to anticipate antibody response [104]. COVID-19 pandemic itself has irritated many danger factors for immunization reactions, like pressure and inactivity. Earlier exploration recommends that mental interventions can improve antibody responsiveness. Consequently, right now is an ideal opportunity to recognize those factors, consul the people so the danger of resistant reaction can be eliminated [105].

14.6.7 COVID-19 VACCINE PROMOTION PROGRAM AND BEHAVIORALLY STRATEGIES

COVID-19 vaccination started from the start of 2021 at twist speed yield a protected and viable antibody. However, this critical milestone is just the initial step. The US public has initially participated in the vaccination trials. The Center to any effective procedure is to reconstruct trust in the care of immunization trials and the honesty of the endorsement interaction. At the start of immunization programs, different celebrities have been vaccinated as a volunteer [106]. Those who are vaccinated need to be warned about transient adverse effects of the vaccines to stay away from harmful exposure from ill-equipped people. The current vaccination does not completely protect the individuals. Awareness about the effectiveness of the vaccine can be made by the advertisement, by developing campaigns in educational institutes, at the workplace. People should show the evidence of vaccination when entered in stores or other public places, in-cafe eating, event congregations, centers, bars, and other public spots with a danger of transmission. Airlines are considering making vaccination a condition for worldwide air travel [107]. These methodologies could give a solid motivating force to get immunized. The level of the agreeableness of these methodologies will rely upon the public's insights about COVID-19 [108].

14.7 NATURAL ANTIVIRAL PLANT EXTRACTS USE FOR COVID-19

Plants contain many useful extracts that were used in combination to treat various diseases in the past. Few plants have antiviral components that may be used for the treatment of COVID-19. The relationship between the positive effects of therapeutic plants and the presence of certain metabolites can be liable for specific effects under trials. It was recommended that terpenoids, alkaloids, stilbenes, and flavonoids are the major regular powerful combination for the progression of antiviral plant-based drugs. Mass testing of different therapeutics plant extracts with antiviral properties could be associated with the antiviral combinations. After their development, they may be used to treat COVID-19 [109].

During the pandemic, various ethnobotanists and traditional healers suggested natural herbs to develop a beneficial viral inactivation system. Another strategy is to develop an antiviral insusceptible response by routine eating of specified plants or plant extracts as nutrition. Medicinal Plants can induce improvements by the high antiviral potential to restrict the risk of SARS-CoV2 and relative infections. Various plant combinations can be used to treat viral infection based on a traditional system of medicines that need a scientific rationale.

Thymus vulgaris, *Curcuma longa*, *Rosmarinus officinalis*, *Ocimum basilicum*, *Melissa officinalis*, and *Mentha piperita* depict naturally powerful combinations to treat viral infection. Onions (*Allium cepa*), apples (*Malus domestica*), green tea (*Camellia sinensis*) and buckwheat (*Fagopyrum esculentum*) are highly effective against COVID because they have proteases in them [110]. Iranian specialists recommended Gillan's plants that have alkaloids and are helpful in eradicating the viral infection. Consistently using *Echium amoenum* tea, a mix of *Stachys schtschegleevi* and *Origanum vulgare* are encouraged to hinder infection [111].

Flavonoid scutellarein from the base of *Scutellaria baicalensis* naturally having antiviral compounds has been used to treat SARS-CoV-2. Its antiviral Flavonoids control infection by their ATPase activity. The triterpenes of *Camellia japonica* were reported for massive antiviral action against the COVID [112].

The bisbenzylisoquinoline alkaloids, e.g., tetrandrine, fangchinoline, and cepharanthine isolated from *Stephania tetrandra* have been reported for anti-SARS-CoV effects. The restricted alkaloid lycorine from *Lycoris radiata* generally showed unique obstruction of SARS-CoV [113].

14.8 NANOMEDICINE FOR COVID-19

Nanotechnologists are working to explore suitable ways and means of nanotechnology to enhance the efficacy, safety, and delivery of drugs. Association with nanotechnology is nanobodies that are little sections of the immune response [114]. The job of nanotechnology in antiviral exploration and its fruitful possibilities for COVID-19 are more effective than expected due to the following variables:

- Nanomaterials and SARS-CoV-2 can straightforwardly contact and battle with one another because of comparability in size;
- At present FDA-affirmed nanomaterials are close to the size of SARS-CoV-2 (60–140 nm can diminish the symptoms of current antiviral medications;

- Various medications can be conveyed by using Nanomaterials works with controlled/directed medication discharge by improving the strength of mRNA antibodies. SARS-CoV-2 and future dangers presented by other irresistible infections can be constrained by including nanotechnology [115].

Flu immunizations, aspiratory surfactant (PS)-biomimetic liposomes were intended for heterosubtypic invulnerability potentiation directed by cytotoxic T lymphocytes that express the CD8+ protein [116]. Nanotechnology advances immune response articulation other than this antibody in creating adjuvants for immunizations. In any case, understanding the contamination replication cycle is key to a sensible antiviral procedure. Notwithstanding the way that we may eventually come to understand viral life cycles in an unforeseen manner. Despite the above nanomaterials, mercaptobenzoic acid-modified gold nanomaterials were also used for HIV (human immunodeficiency virus) through the multivalent confining technique. New types of globular glycofullerenes were used against counterfeit Ebola contamination sickness. Nanomaterials for the delivery of antiviral drugs and antibodies are used. Due to similarities between SARS-CoV-2 and different diseases, nanomaterials can deliver antiviral drugs with better potency. FDA-approved nanomaterials, including liposomes, PLGA nanoparticles, etc., can be used to encapsulate antiviral medicines, transportation of various drugs, and cotransport drugs for better treatment results. Nanomaterials can be helpful to redesign drugs for SARS-CoV-2 by using virus protein modified with antibodies ensuring good results [117]. Medicine mixes can be furthermore attempted and co-passed on by nanomaterials. Possibly nanomaterials will in a little used to co-pass on angiogenesis factors (or various meds to help mollify hypoxia) and antiviral prescriptions to create better outcomes [118].

14.9 OZONE THERAPY FOR COVID-19

Gamma interferon induction, cytokines, and interferons, and cytokines modulation is an immunological response in response to ozone therapy. More realistic standard treatment regimens of ozone therapy against SARS are a monotherapy as documented. In clinical practice, due to evidence of antiviral activity of ozone, the therapeutic applicability of ozone therapy in COVID-19 is increasing [119].

Ozone is triatomic oxygen pharmacologically produced by ultraviolet (UV) radiation and lightning and powerful oxidant in nature. SARS-CoV-2 is rich in cysteine ozone intact by forming disulfide bridges in high quantities in the virus oxidase cysteine residues by ozone.

In the first phase, inhibition of Cellular penetration, viral receptors inactivation, ozone's action by oxidation is used for the specific creation of the bond structure of the cell membrane. Replication of endogenous COVID-19 is blocked by the transductor on which ozone acts directly, and receptors' activity can regulate it. Ozone shows its anti-inflammatory activity through the; therefore, it could protect from acute coronary syndromes and ischemia-reperfusion damage in the lungs of patients affected by COVID-19. Humoral and cellular immune systems stimulated by the ozone through induction in cytokines linked genes the activation of pathways related to the transcriptional factors nuclear factor of activated T-cells. Ozone therapy is not useful in crucial and critical conditions, but ozone therapy has shown its efficacy at the early stage of viral infection [78, 120–122].

14.10 CONCLUSION

COVID-19 pandemic forced us to promote existing research knowledge and disseminate updated knowledge about COVID-19 diagnosis and therapeutics options among society. Healthcare workers (HCWs) must be remaining updated with up-to-date knowledge. More testing facilities must be provided by the government, enabling early diagnosis and delivering supportive treatments. Researchers have found present moment remedial methodologies and long-haul immunization arrangements to lessen the spread of COVID-19 infection and mortality rate. Anticipation and treatment of COVID-19 by locally existing plant species recorded. Despite huge advancement and good after-effects of created antibody numerous hindrances remain. Despite the development of vaccine challenges encompassing large-scale manufacturing and transportation to millions or billions of doses to other countries of the world. Since some immunization types, like mRNAs, vaccines are very sensitive and degraded at room temperatures. An additional challenge is that the new, more infectious variants of the coronavirus developed, threatening the vaccine rollout strategy. There is a need for long-term monitoring of adverse drug reactions (ADR). Randomized clinical trials are required to monitor the efficacy of a vaccine.

KEYWORDS

- **antiviral compounds**
- **cytokine discharge disorder**
- **gastrointestinal**
- **immunization**
- **medicinal herbs**
- **SARS-CoV-2**
- **vaccine**

REFERENCES

1. Lu, R., Zhao, X., Li, J., Niu, P., Yang, B., Wu, H., et al., (2011). Genomic characterization and epidemiology of 2019 novel coronavirus: Implications for virus origins and receptor binding. *Lancet, 395*, 565–574.
2. Lee, N., Hui, D., Wu, A., Chan, P., Cameron, P., Joynt, G. M., et al., (2003). A major outbreak of severe acute respiratory syndrome in Hong Kong. *New England Journal of Medicine, 348*, 1986–1994.
3. Fani, M., Teimoori, A., & Ghafari, S., (2020). Comparison of the COVID-2019 (SARS-CoV-2) pathogenesis with SARS-CoV and MERS-CoV infections. *Future Virology, 15*, 317–323.
4. Zumla, A., Hui, D. S., & Perlman, S., (2015). Middle east respiratory syndrome. *Lancet, 386*, 995–1007.
5. Lee, S., Kim, T., Lee, E., Lee, C., Kim, H., Rhee, H., et al., (2020). Clinical course and molecular viral shedding among asymptomatic and symptomatic patients with SARS-CoV-2 infection in a community treatment center in the Republic of Korea. *JAMA Internal Medicine, 180*, 1447–1452.
6. Huang, C., Wang, Y., Li, X., Ren, L., Zhao, J., Hu, Y., et al., (2020). Clinical features of patients infected with 2019 novel coronavirus in Wuhan, China. *Lancet, 395*, 497–506.
7. Chen, G., Wu, D., Guo, W., Cao, Y., Huang, D., Wang, H., et al., (2020). Clinical and immunological features of severe and moderate coronavirus disease 2019. *The Journal of Clinical Investigation, 130*, 2620–2629.
8. Rabaan, A. A., Al-Ahmed, S. H., Haque, S., et al., (2020). SARS-CoV-2, SARS-CoV, and MERS-COV: A comparative overview. *Le Infezioni in Medicine, 28*, 174–184.
9. Ciceri, F., Beretta, L., Scandroglio, A. M., Colombo, S., Landoni, G., Ruggeri, A., et al., (2020). Microvascular COVID-19 lung vessels obstructive thromboinflammatory syndrome (MicroCLOTS): An atypical acute respiratory distress syndrome working hypothesis. *Critical Care and Resuscitation, 22*, 95–97.
10. Conti, P., Ronconi, G., Caraffa, A., Gallenga, C. E., Ross, R., Frydas, I., & Kritas, S. K., (2020). Induction of pro-inflammatory cytokines (IL-1 and IL-6) and lung inflammation

by Coronavirus-19 (COVI-19 or SARS-CoV-2): Anti-inflammatory strategies. *Journal of Biological Regulators and Homeostatic Agents, 34*, 327–331.
11. Ronco, C., Reis, T., & Husain-Syed, F., (2020). Management of acute kidney injury in patients with COVID-19. *The Lancet Respiratory Medicine, 8*, 738–742.
12. Zhou, F., Yu, T., Du, R., Fan, G., Liu, Y., Liu, Z., et al., (2020). Clinical course and risk factors for mortality of adult inpatients with COVID-19 in Wuhan, China: A retrospective cohort study. *Lancet, 395*, 1054–1062.
13. Gattinoni, L., Coppola, S., Cressoni, M., Busana, M., Rossi, S., & Chiumello, D., (2020). COVID-19 does not lead to a "typical" acute respiratory distress syndrome. *American Journal of Respiratory and Critical Care Medicine, 201*, 1299–1300.
14. Wu, C. N., Xia, L. Z., Li, K. H., Ma, W. H., Yu, D. N., Qu, B., et al., (2020). High-flow nasal-oxygenation-assisted fibreoptic tracheal intubation in critically ill patients with COVID-19 pneumonia: A prospective randomized controlled trial. *British Journal of Anaesthesia, 125*, 166–168.
15. Sousa, F. H., Casanova, V., Findlay, F., Stevens, C., Svoboda, P., Pohl, J., et al., (2017). Cathelicidins display conserved direct antiviral activity towards rhinovirus. *Peptides, 95*, 76–83.
16. Quraishi, S. A., De Pascale, G., Needleman, J. S., Nakazawa, H., Kaneki, M., Bajwa, E. K., et al., (2015). Effect of cholecalciferol supplementation on vitamin d status and cathelicidin levels in sepsis: A randomized, placebo-controlled trial. *Critical Care Medicine, 43*, 1928–1937.
17. World Health Organization (WHO), (2020). Clinical management of severe acute respiratory infection (SARI) when COVID-19 disease is suspected. Interim guidance. *Pediatr. Med. Rodz., 16*(1), 9–26.
18. Jiang, J. S., Chou, H. C., & Chen, C. M., (2020). Cathelicidin attenuates hyperoxia-induced lung injury by inhibiting oxidative stress in newborn rats. *Free Radical Biology and Medicine, 150*, 23–29.
19. Lu, L., Zhang, H., Dauphars, D. J., & He, Y. W., (2021). A potential role of interleukin 10 in COVID-19 pathogenesis. *Trends in Immunology, 42*, 3–5.
20. McElvaney, O. J., Hobbs, B. D., Qiao, D., McElvaney, O. F., Moll, M., McEvoy, N. L., et al., (2020). A linear prognostic score based on the ratio of interleukin-6 to interleukin-10 predicts outcomes in COVID486 19. *EBioMedicine, 61*, 103026.
21. Heine, G., Niesner, U., Chang, H. D., Steinmeyer, A., Zugel, U., Zuberbier, T., et al., (2008). 1,25- dihydroxyvitamin D3 promotes IL-10 production in human B cells. *European Journal of Immunology, 38*, 2210–2218.
22. Ashtari, F., Toghianifar, N., Zarkesh-Esfahani, S. H., & Mansourian, M., (2015). Short-term effect of high-dose vitamin D on the level of interleukin 10 in patients with multiple sclerosis: A randomized, double492 blind, placebo-controlled clinical trial. *Neuroimmunomodulation, 22*, 400–404.
23. McLaughlin, L., Clarke, L., Khalilidehkordi, E., Butzkueven, H., Taylor, B., & Broadley, S. A., (2018). Vitamin D for the treatment of multiple sclerosis: A meta-analysis. *Journal of Neurology, 265*, 2893–2905.
24. Evans, R. M., & Lippman, S. M., (2020). Shining light on the COVID-19 pandemic: A vitamin D receptor checkpoint in defense of unregulated wound healing. *Cell Metabolism, 32*, 704–709.
25. Ali, R. M., Al-Shorbagy, M. Y., Helmy, M. W., & El-Abhar, H. S., (2018). Role of Wnt4/β-catenin, Ang II/TGFβ, ACE2, NF-κB, and IL-18 in attenuating renal ischemia/

reperfusion-induced injury in rats treated with Vit D and pioglitazone. *European Journal of Pharmacology, 831*, 68–76.
26. Wu, J., Deng, W., Li, S., & Yang, X., (2021). Advances in research on ACE2 as a receptor for 2019-nCoV. *Cellular and Molecular Life Sciences, 78*, 531–44.
27. Hanff, T. C., Harhay, M. O., Brown, T. S., Cohen, J. B., & Mohareb, A. M., (2020). Is there an association between COVID-19 mortality and the renin-angiotensin system? A call for epidemiologic investigations. *Clinical Infectious Diseases, 71*, 870–874.
28. Ledford, H., (2020). Coronavirus breakthrough: Dexamethasone is the first drug shown to save lives. *Nature, 582*, 469.
29. Wu, C., Chen, X., Cai, Y., Zhou, X., Xu, S., Huang, H., et al., (2020). Risk factors associated with acute respiratory distress syndrome and death in patients with coronavirus disease 2019 pneumonia in Wuhan, China. *JAMA Internal Medicine, 180*, 934–943.
30. Ruan, S. Y., Lin, H. H., Huang, C. T., Kuo, P. H., Wu, H. D., & Yu, C. J., (2014). Exploring the heterogeneity of effects of corticosteroids on acute respiratory distress syndrome: A systematic review and meta-analysis. *Critical Care, 18*, 1–9.
31. Bosco, J. L., Silliman, R. A., Thwin, S. S., Geiger, A. M., Buist, D. S., Prout, M. N., et al., (2010). A most stubborn bias: No adjustment method fully resolves confounding by indication in observational studies. *Journal of Clinical Epidemiology 63*, 64–74.
32. Zhou, F., Yu, T., Du, R., Fan, G., Liu, Y., Liu, Z., et al., (2020). Clinical course and risk factors for mortality of adult inpatients with COVID-19 in Wuhan, China: A retrospective cohort study. *The Lancet, 395*, 1054–1062.
33. Collins, R., Bowman, L., Landray, M., & Peto, R., (2020). La magia de la aleatorización versus el mito de la evidencia a partir de la práctica clínica (The magic of randomization versus the myth of real-world evidence). *New England Journal of Medicine, 382*, 674–678.
34. Arabi, Y. M., Mandourah, Y., Al-Hameed, F., Sindi, A. A., Almekhlafi, G. A., Hussein, M. A., et al., (2018). Corticosteroid therapy for critically ill patients with Middle East respiratory syndrome. *American Journal of Respiratory and Critical Care Medicine, 197*, 757–767.
35. Waterer, G. W., & Rello, J., (2021). Steroids and COVID-19: We need a precision approach, not one size fits all. *Infectious Diseases and Therapy,* 9, 701–705.
36. Lanthier, L., Mayette, M., Huard, G., Plourde, M. E., & Cauchon, M., (2020). In patients hospitalized for COVID-19, does dexamethasone reduce 28-days mortality compared to standard treatment? *La Revue Medicine Interne, 41*, 790–791.
37. Russell, C. D., Millar, J. E., & Baillie, J. K., (2020). Clinical evidence does not support corticosteroid treatment for 2019-nCoV lung injury. *The Lancet, 395*, 473–475.
38. Ni, Y. N., Chen, G., Sun, J., Liang, B. M., & Liang, Z. A., (2019). The effect of corticosteroids on mortality of patients with influenza pneumonia: A systematic review and meta-analysis. *Critical Care, 23*, 1–9.
39. Monedero, P., Gea, A., Castro, P., Candela-Toha, A. M., Hernandez-Sanz, M. L., Arruti, E., et al., (2021). Early corticosteroids are associated with lower mortality in critically ill patients with COVID-19: A cohort study. *Critical Care, 25*, 1–3.
40. Ahmed, M. H., & Hassan, A., (2020). Dexamethasone for the treatment of coronavirus disease (COVID-19): A review. *SN Comprehensive Clinical Medicine, 2*, 2637–2646.
41. Gordon, C. J., Tchesnokov, E. P., Feng, J. Y., Porter, D. P., & Gotte, M., (2020). The antiviral compound remdesivir potently inhibits RNA-dependent RNA polymerase from middle east respiratory syndrome coronavirus. *Journal of Biological Chemistry, 295*, 4773–4779.

42. De Wit, E., Feldmann, F., Cronin, J., Jordan, R., Okumura, A., Thomas, T., et al., (2020). Prophylactic and therapeutic remdesivir (GS-5734) treatment in the rhesus macaque model of MERS-CoV infection. *Proceedings of the National Academy Sciences, 117*, 6771–6776.
43. Williamson, B. N., Feldmann, F., Schwarz, B., Meade-White, K., Porter, D. P., Schulz, J., et al., (2020). Clinical benefit of remdesivir in rhesus macaques infected with SARS-CoV-2. *Nature, 585*, 273–276.
44. Chen, N., Zhou, M., Dong, X., Qu, J., Gong, F., Han, Y., et al., (2020). Epidemiological and clinical characteristics of 99 cases of 2019 novel coronavirus pneumonia in Wuhan, China: A descriptive study. *Lancet, 395*, 507–513.
45. Wang, Z., Yang, B., Li, Q., Wen, L., & Zhang, R., (2020). Clinical features of 69 cases with coronavirus disease 2019 in Wuhan, China. *Clinical Infectious Diseases, 71*, 769–777.
46. Zarogoulidis, P., Papanas, N., Kioumis, I., Chatzaki, E., Maltezos, E., & Zarogoulidis, K., (2012). Macrolides: From in vitro anti-inflammatory and immunomodulatory properties to clinical practice in respiratory diseases. *European Journal of Clinical Pharmacology, 68*, 479–503.
47. Kollias, A., Kyriakoulis, K. G., Dimakakos, E., Poulakou, G., Stergiou, G. S., & Syrigos, K., (2020). Thromboembolic risk and anticoagulant therapy in COVID-19 patients: Emerging evidence and call for action. *British Journal of Haematology, 189*, 846, 847.
48. Lamb, Y. N., (2020). Remdesivir: First approval. *Drugs, 80*, 1355–1363.
49. Spinner, C. D., Gottlieb, R. L., Criner, G. J., López, J. R., Cattelan, A. M., Viladomiu, A. S., et al., (2020). Effect of remdesivir vs standard care on clinical status at 11 days in patients with moderate COVID-19: A randomized clinical trial. *JAMA, 324*, 1048–1057.
50. Jiang, Y., Chen, D., Cai, D., Yi, Y., & Jiang, S., (2021). Effectiveness of remdesivir for the treatment of hospitalized COVID-19 persons: A network meta-analysis. *Journal of Medical Virology, 93*, 1171–1174.
51. Hayden, F. G., Treanor, J. J., Fritz, R. S., Lobo, M., Betts, R. F., Miller, M., Kinnersley, N., et al., (1999). Use of the oral neuraminidase inhibitor oseltamivir in experimental human influenza: Randomized controlled trials for prevention and treatment. *JAMA, 282*, 1240–1246.
52. Zhang, X. W., & Yap, Y. L., (2004). The 3D structure analysis of SARS-CoV S1 protein reveals a link to influenza virus neuraminidase and implications for drug and antibody discovery. *Journal of Molecular Structure Theochem., 68*, 137–141.
53. Goldhill, D. H., Langat, P., Xie, H., Galiano, M., Miah, S., Kellam, P., et al., (2019). Determining the mutation bias of favipiravir in influenza virus using next-generation sequencing. *Journal of Virology, 93*.e01217–01218.
54. Shiraki, K., & Daikoku, T., (2020). Favipiravir, an anti-influenza drug against life-threatening RNA virus infections. *Pharmacology and Therapeutics, 209*, 107512.
55. Ison, M. G., & Scheetz, M. H., (2021). Understanding the pharmacokinetics of favipiravir: Implications for treatment of influenza and COVID19. *EBioMedicine, 63*, 103204.
56. Pilkington, V., Pepperrell, T., & Hill, A., (2020). A review of the safety of favipiravi-a potential treatment in the COVID-19 pandemic? *Journal of Virus Eradication, 6*, 45–51.
57. Khambholja, K., & Asudani, D., (2020). Potential repurposing of favipiravir in COVID-19 outbreak based on current evidence. *Travel Medicine and Infectious Disease, 35*, 101710.
58. Joshi, S., Parkar, J., Ansari, A., Vora, A., Talwar, D., Tiwaskar, M., et al., (2021). Role of favipiravir in the treatment of COVID-19. *International Journal of Infectious Disease, 102*, 501–508.

59. Prieto-Pena, D., & Dasgupta, B., (2021). Biologic agents and small-molecule inhibitors in systemic autoimmune conditions: An update. *Polish Archives of Internal Medicine, 131*, 171–181.
60. Singh, T. U., Parida, S., Lingaraju, M. C., Kesavan, M., Kumar, D., & Singh, R. K., (2020). Drug repurposing approach to fight COVID-19. *Pharmacological Reports, 72*, 1479–1508.
61. Kewan, T., Covut, F., Al-Jaghbeer, M. J., Rose, L., Gopalakrishna, K. V., & Akbik, B., (2020). Tocilizumab for treatment of patients with severe COVID-19: A retrospective cohort study. *EClinicalMedicine, 24*, 100418.
62. Rojas-Marte, G., Khalid, M., Mukhtar, O., Hashmi, A. T., Waheed, M. A., Ehrlich, S., et al., (2020). Outcomes in patients with severe COVID-19 disease treated with tocilizumab: A case-controlled study. *QJM: An International Journal of Medicine, 113*, 546–550.
63. Toniati, P., Piva, S., Cattalini, M., Garrafa, E., Regola, F., Castelli, F., et al., (2020). Tocilizumab for the treatment of severe COVID-19 pneumonia with hyperinflammatory syndrome and acute respiratory failure: a single-center study of 100 patients in Brescia, Italy. *Autoimmunity Reviews, 19,* 102568.
64. Caly, L., Druce, J. D., Catton, M. G., Jans, D. A., & Wagstaff, K. M., (2020). The FDA-approved drug ivermectin inhibits the replication of SARS-CoV-2 in vitro. *Antiviral Research, 178*, 104787.
65. Hensley, L. E., Fritz, E. A., Jahrling, P. B., Karp, C., Huggins, J. W., & Geisbert, T. W., (2004). Interferon-β 1a and SARS coronavirus replication. *Emerging Infectious Diseases, 10*, 317–319.
66. Lokugamage, K. G., Hage, A., Schindewolf, C., Rajsbaum, R., & Menachery, V. D., (2020). *SARS-CoV-2 is Sensitive to Type I Interferon Pretreatment* (Vol. 21, pp. 1–9). BioRxiv.
67. Ton, A. T., Gentile, F., Hsing, M., Ban, F., & Cherkasov, A., (2020). Rapid identification of potential inhibitors of SARS-CoV-2 main protease by deep docking of 1.3 billion compounds. *Molecular informatics, 39*, 2000028.
68. Jin, Z., Du, X., Xu, Y., et al., (2020). Structure of Mpro from COVID19 virus and discovery of its inhibitors. *Nature, 582*, 289–293.
69. Li, G., De Clercq, E., (2020). Therapeutic options for the 2019 novel coronavirus (2019-nCoV). *Nature Reviews Drug Discovery, 19*, 149–150.
70. Lloyd, E. C., Gandhi, T. N., & Petty, L. A., (2021). Monoclonal Antibodies for COVID-19. *JAMA, 325*, 1015.
71. Cao, X., (2020). COVID-19: Immunopathology and its implications for therapy. *Nature Reviews Immunology, 20*, 269, 270.
72. Ankrum, J., (2020). Can cell therapies halt cytokine storm in severe COVID-19 patients. *Science Translational Medicine, 12,* 540–550.
73. Leng, Z., Zhu, R., Hou, W., et al., (2020). Transplantation of ACE2- Mesenchymal stem cells improves the outcome of patients with covid-19 pneumonia. *Aging and Disease, 11*, 216–228.
74. Buonaguro, F. M., Puzanov, I., & Ascierto, P. A., (2020). Anti-IL6R role in treatment of COVID-19-related ARDS. *J. Transl. Med., 14*(1), 165.
75. Zhu, F. C., Li, Y. H., Guan, X. H., Hou, L. H., Wang, W. J., Li, J., et al., (2020). Safety tolerability and immunogenicity of a recombinant adenovirus type-5 vectored COVID-19 vaccine. A dose-escalation open-label non-randomized first-in-human trial. *Lancet, 13*, 1845–1854.

76. Klein, A., (2020). Drug trials underway new scientist 245:3270-85 E Callaway e race for coronavirus vaccines. *A Graphical Guide Nature, 7805*, 576–577.
77. Dhama, K., Sharun, K., Tiwari, R., et al., (2020). COVID-19 an emerging coronavirus infection advances and prospects in designing and developing vaccines immunotherapeutics and therapeutics. *Human Vaccines & Immunotherapeutics, 6*, 1232–1238.
78. Zia-Ul-Haq, M., Dewanjee, S., & Riaz, M. 2021). *Carotenoids: Structure and Function in the Human Body* (Vol. XVI, p. 859). Springer Nature Switzerland AG: Springer International Publishing.
79. Leanh, T., Andreadakis, Z., Kumar, A., et al., (2020). COVID19 vaccine development landscape. *Nature Reviews Drug Discovery,* 5, 305–306.
80. Lurie, N., Saville, M., Hatchett, R., & Halton, J., (2020). Developing covid-19 vaccines at pandemic speed. *New England Journal of Medicine, 21*, 1969–1973.
81. https://www.yalemedicine.org/news/covid-19-vaccine-comparison (accessed on 6 August 2021).
82. Dhama, K., Patel, S. K., Pathak, M., Yatoo, M. I., Tiwari, R., Malik, Y. S., et al., (2020). An update on SARS-CoV-2/COVID-19 with particular reference to its clinical pathology pathogenesis immunopathology and mitigation strategies. *Trav. Med. Infect. Dis., 37*, 101–755.
83. Biasio, L. R., Bonaccorsi, G., Lorini, C., & Pecorelli, S., (2020). Assessing COVID-19 vaccine literacy a preliminary online survey. *Hum. Vaccines Immunother.*, 1–9.
84. Cutler, D. M., & Summers, L. H., (2020). The COVID-19 pandemic and the $16 trillion virus. *JAMA, 324*(15), 1495–1496.
85. Ball, P., (2020). Anti-vaccine movement could undermine efforts to end coronavirus pandemic researchers warn. *Nature, 581*, 251.
86. Dror, A. A., Eisenbach, N., Taiber, S., Morozov, N. G., Mizrachi, M., Zigron, A., et al., (2020). Vaccine hesitancy. The next challenge in the fight against COVID-19. *European Journal of Epidemiology, 35*(8), 775–779.
87. Badur, S., Ota, M., Öztürk, S., Adegbola, R., & Dutta, A., (2020). Vaccine confidence is the key to restoring trust. *Human Vaccines & Immunotherapeutics, 5*, 1007–1017.
88. McAteer, J., Yildirim, I., & Chahroudi, A., (2020). The vaccines act: Deciphering vaccine hesitancy in the time of COVID 19. *Clinical Infectious Diseases, 71*(15), 703–705.
89. Harrison, E. A., & Wu, J. W., (2020). Vaccine confidence in the time of COVID-19. *European Journal of Epidemiology, 4*, 325–330.
90. Price, J. H., Dake, J. A., Murnan, J., Dimmig, J., & Akpanudo, S., (2005). Power analysis in survey research importance and use for health educators. *American Journal of Health Education, 4*, 202–209.
91. Webb, F. J., Khubchandani, J., Striley, C. W., & Cottler, L. B., (2019). Black-white differences in willingness to participate and perceptions about health research results from the population based health street study. *Journal of Immigrant and Minority Health, 21*(2), 299–305.
92. Randolph, H. E., & Barreiro, L. B., (2020). *Herd immunity Understanding COVID-19 Immunity 52*(5), 737–741.
93. Altmann, D. M., Douek, D. C., & Boyton, R. J., (2020). What policymakers need to know about COVID-19 protective immunity. *The Lancet, 395*(10236), 1527–1529.
94. Neumann-Bohme, S., Varghese, N. E., Sabat, I., Barros, P. P., Brouwer, W., Van, E. J., et al., (2020). Once we have it will we use it. A European survey on willingness to be vaccinated against COVID-19. *Eur. J. Health Econ., 21*(7), 977–982.

95. Peretti-Watel, P., Seror, V., Cortaredona, S., Launay, O., Raude, J., Verger, P., et al., (2020). A future vaccination campaign against COVID-19 at risk of vaccine hesitancy and politicization. *The Lancet Infect. Dis., 20*(7), 769–770.
96. Habersaat, K. B., Betsch, C., Danchin, M., Sunstein, C. R., Bohm, R., Falk, A., et al., (2020). Ten considerations for effectively managing the COVID-19 transition. *Nat. Hum. Behav., 4*(7), 677–87.
97. Cacciapaglia, G., Cot, C., & Sannino, F., (2020). Second wave COVID-19 pandemics in Europe a temporal playbook. *Sci. Rep., 10*(1), 15514.
98. Martin, L. R., & Petrie, K. J., (2017). Understanding the dimensions of anti-vaccination attitudes the vaccination attitudes examination (VAX) scale. *Ann. Behav. Med., 51*(5), 652–660.
99. Lee, S. A., (2020). Coronavirus Anxiety Scale A brief mental health screener for COVID-19 related anxiety. *Death Stud., 44*(7), 393–401.
100. Butler, M. J., & Barrientos, R. M., (2020). The impact of nutrition on COVID-19 susceptibility and long-term consequences. *Brain Behavior and Immunity, 87*, 53–54.
101. Choon, L. W. G., Narang, V., Lu, Y., Camous, X., Nyunt, M. S. Z., et al., (2019). Hallmarks of improved immunological responses in the vaccination of more physically active elderly females. *Exercise Immunology Review, 25*, 20–33.
102. Christ, A., Lauterbach, M., & Latz, E., (2019). Western diet and the immune system an inflammatory connection. *Immunity, 51*(5), 794–811.
103. Cohen, S., (2021). Psychosocial vulnerabilities to upper respiratory infectious illness implications for susceptibility to coronavirus disease 2019 (COVID-19). *Perspectives on Psychological Science, 16*(1), 161–174.
104. Fitzpatrick, K. M., Harris, C., & Drawve, G., (2020). Living in the midst of fear depressive symptomatology among US adults during the COVID-19 pandemic. *Depression and Anxiety, 37*(10), 957–964.
105. Hao, F., Tan, W., Jiang, L., Zhang, L., Zhao, X., Zou, Y., et al., (2020). Do psychiatric patients experience more psychiatric symptoms during COVID-19 pandemic and lockdown. A case-control study with service and research implications for immunopsychiatry. *Brain Behavior and Immunity, 87*, 100–106.
106. Harris, V., Ali, A., Fuentes, S., Korpela, K., Kazi, M., Tate, J., Parashar, U., et al., (2018). Rotavirus vaccine response correlates with the infant gut microbiota composition in Pakistan. *Gut Microbes, 9*(2), 93–101.
107. Luchetti, M., Lee, J. H., Aschwanden, D., Sesker, A., Strickhouser, J. E., Terracciano, A., & Sutin, A. R., (2020). The trajectory of loneliness in response to COVID-19. *American Psychologist, 75*(7), 897–908.
108. Lynn, D. J., & Pulendran, B., (2018). The potential of the microbiota to influence vaccine responses. *Journal of Leukocyte Biology, 103*(2), 225–231.
109. Balachandar, V., Mahalaxmi, I., Kaavya, J., Vivekanandhan, G., Ajithkumar, S., Arul, N., Singaravelu, G., et al., (2020). COVID-19 Emerging protective measures. *Eur. Rev. Med. Pharmacol. Sci., 24*, 3422–3425.
110. Dong, Y., Dai, T., Wei, Y., Zhang, L., Zheng, M., & Zhou, F., (2020). A systematic review of SARS-CoV-2 vaccine candidates. *Sig. Transduct. Target Ther., 5*, 237.
111. Mahmood, N., Nasir, S. B., & Hefferon, K., (2020). *Plant-Based Drugs and Vaccines for COVID- Vaccines, 9*, 15.
112. Naja, F., & Hamadeh, R., (2020). Nutrition amid the COVID-19 pandemic. A multi-level framework for action. *Eur. J. Clin. Nutr., 74*, 1117–1121.

113. Panyod, S., Ho, C. T., & Sheen, L. Y., (2020). Dietary therapy and herbal medicine for COVID-19 prevention. A review and perspective *Tradit. J. Complement. Med., 10*, 420–427.
114. Zhang, D. H., Wu, K. L., Zhang, X., & Deng, S. Q., (2020). Peng B In silico screening of Chinese herbal medicines with the potential to directly inhibit 2019 novel coronavirus. *Integr. J. Med., 18*, 152–158.
115. Sampangi-Ramaiah, M. H., Vishwakarma, R., & Shaanker, R. U., (2020). Molecular docking analysis of selected natural products from plants for inhibition of SARS-CoV-2 main protease. *Curr. Sci., 118*, 1087–1092.
116. Monajjemi, M., Mollaamin, F., & Shojaei, S., (2020). An overview on Coronaviruses family from past to Covid-19. Introduce some inhibitors as antiviruses from Gillan's plants. *Biointerface Res. Appl. Chem., 10,* 5575–5585.
117. Yang, Y., Islam, S., Wang, J., Li, Y., & Chen, X., (2020). Traditional Chinese medicine in the treatment of patients infected with 2019-new coronavirus (SARS-CoV-2): A review and perspective. *Int. J. Biol. Sci., 16*, 1708–1717.
118. Bocci, V., Zanardi, I., & Travagli, V., (2011). Oxygen/ozone as a medical gas mixture. A critical evaluation of the various methods clarifies positive and negative aspects. *Med. Gas. Res., 28*(1), 6.
119. Rowen, R. J., (2019). Ozone and oxidation therapies as a solution to the emerging crisis in infectious disease management: A review of current knowledge and experience. *Med. Gas. Res., 4*, 232–237.
120. Rowen, R. J., & Robins, H., (2020). A plausible penny costing effective treatment for coronavirus- ozone therapy. *J. Infect. Dis. Epidemiol., 6*, 113.
121. Walls, A. C., Park, Y. J., Tortorici, M. A., Wall, A., McGuire, A. T., & Veesler, D., (2020). Structure-function and antigenicity of the SARS-CoV-2 Spike Glycoprotein. *Cell, 181*, 281–292.
122. Zia-Ul-Haq, M., et al., (2021). *Alternative Medicine Interventions for COVID-19* (Vol. XII, p. 284). Springer, Cham: Springer Nature Switzerland AG.

Index

D

I

O

P

Q